Internal Medicine Training Notes and Survival Guide

Kehua Zhou

Internal Medicine Training Notes and Survival Guide

An Insider's Roadmap for the Journey from Resident to Attending Physician

Springer

Kehua Zhou
Appleton, WI, USA

ISBN 978-1-0716-4038-8 ISBN 978-1-0716-4039-5 (eBook)
https://doi.org/10.1007/978-1-0716-4039-5

This Springer imprint is published by the registered company Springer Science+Business Media, LLC, part of Springer Nature.
The registered company address is: 1 New York Plaza, New York, NY 10004, U.S.A.

This book is dedicated to my patients who are the heart and soul of my medical practice and the driving force behind my dedication to healing and compassion. The courage, resilience, and trust of my patients inspire me to strive for excellence every day. In the strength, stories, and trust of my patients, I find motivation, purpose, and the privilege of serving as their physician.

Preface

As an internal medicine physician, I have independently practiced hospital medicine at multiple hospitals in Wisconsin, USA, for 4 plus years. Before that, I was an internal medicine resident physician. After I graduated from medical school in 2010, my journey to medicine changed a couple of times before my application to internal medicine training.

Before and during my internal medicine residency training, I often sought a single source or book that is easily accessible, convenient, and succinct to satisfy my cravings for knowledge and to fulfill the requirements of my internal medicine residency training. Yet, I was unable to find such a source that met my expectations. Besides clinical skills learned and honed in actual clinical practices, I remember my days and nights reading UpToDate and Medscape websites, scouring through *Pocket Medicine: The Massachusetts General Hospital Handbook of Internal Medicine*, discussing journal articles and guidelines in Journal Clubs, reading and learning from simulating patient cases through the Medical Knowledge Self-Assessment Program® (MKSAP) and the UWorld®, asking questions and seeking answers, and learning experiences from my senior residents and attendings.

During my 3 years (June 2017 through June 2020) of internal medicine residency training, I took daily notes based on the aforementioned sources and experiences. By the time I graduated from my internal medicine residency training in June 2020, I had compiled four notebooks of handwritten internal medicine training notes. For the past 4 plus years while practicing as a hospitalist physician at multiple hospitals in Wisconsin, I typed the notes into a single Word file and revised and updated the notes based on the available guidelines and medical knowledge to the best of my ability. Additionally, I also added summaries, clinical pearls, takeaway messages, and references to the available notes.

The notes were based on my personal learning and practicing experiences. Although I did revise all of the notes/excerpts to ensure the knowledge and information was up-to-date while avoiding plagiarism, experienced clinicians can still trace much of the information from their original aforementioned sources. Like science and technology, medical knowledge of the notes stands on the shoulders of giants.

Like all internal medicine physicians, I value and remain thankful for my learning experiences and appreciate the knowledge and skills that the patients and my attending physicians of various specialties have taught me. The notes not only prepared me to be a competent internal medicine physician but also helped me prepare and pass the American Board of Internal Medicine board exam. Even during my clinical practice at this moment, I still go back to these notes for guidance, especially when taking care of patients with unusual presentations.

Structure of the Book

This book comprises over 200,000 words, with the majority of the notes presented as one to a few sentences, rendering the information succinct, easy to understand, and digest. The notes also provide simple, yet important key information in patient care including but not limited to the workup and management of various clinical scenarios. This book is divided into daily notes (in the format of a diary with the original dates *but with updated knowledge and information*) during residency training (57%), notes for outpatient medicine and clinical subspecialties (25%), and notes as a hospitalist (18%).

The daily notes were based on knowledge and experiences I learned from actual clinical cases (workup, medication regimen, patient education, and sometimes patient and family interactions). The notes for outpatient medicine and clinical subspecialties were based on specific topics/subspecialties and were heavily clinically oriented with a focus on patient care. The addition of notes as a hospitalist was based on my job duties as a hospitalist, which requires knowledge and understanding of acute neurological and neurosurgical issues, various types of cancers, and some common yet complicated or uncommon clinical scenarios of infectious diseases.

Hospitalist physicians nowadays often work as universal admitters for the majority of adult patients in the hospital. My current duties as a hospitalist include taking care of patients with acute neurological condition(s). The notes of the neurology ward were originally based on the Emergency Neurological Life Support® (ENLS®) course. Meanwhile, many of my patients have a history of cancer or are on active cancer treatments. I thus also reorganized my notes that were taken while I was a resident rotating in the oncology clinics and at a National Cancer Institute-designated cancer center. As a hospitalist physician, I see the complexity yet acuity of infectious diseases daily. While taking care of patients with life-threatening infections, I admire my infectious disease colleagues' work and am always thrilled to have guidance from them. Yet from time to time, I'm often the one solely tasked with the heavy duty of initial workups and treatments and even the final plan for my patients with severe infections. As a result, I compiled the notes for common inpatient infectious disease consultations.

Intended Use

On top of providing understanding and pathophysiology for some important yet difficult-to-grasp topics in internal medicine training, the notes also provide many clinical pearls and curbside recommendations. Yet, the notes do not provide much of the fundamental anatomy, physiology, or pharmacological basic knowledge and only encompass a negligible fraction of pediatrics. Nonetheless, this book provides a comprehensive framework for the learning and practicing of internal medicine after graduation from medical school, during and after residency training. Possible audiences for this book include resident physicians, practicing physicians, physician assistants, and nurse practitioners in the field of internal medicine.

After years of practice, I learned that nothing can be guaranteed in the medical field. A patient's condition may change instantaneously with or without our awareness. While this book may shed light on the clinical practices of internal medicine, many of the times, in both the acute care and outpatient settings, this book does not intend to provide many of the basic foundations for the clinical practice in internal medicine. The notes were based on actual patients I encountered during my residency training and practices, often without detailing the specific backgrounds or any other patient information. Thus, the workup and management of symptoms and disorders in this book may necessitate fine and careful tailoring for their use in actual clinical practices.

This book was based on the training and practices of a general internal medicine physician in the USA. The notes were updated based on the most up-to-date medical knowledge to the best of my ability. Nonetheless, the intent of the author of this book was not to guide any clinic practices but rather provide a framework for trainees' learning and physicians' and associated health care providers' review of knowledge and may also help with the preparation of board examinations in internal medicine. Readers of this book who are not familiar with the topic are recommended to seek additional knowledge and training before applying the information or knowledge in this book to actual patient care.

As an internal medicine physician, I have participated in many if not all aspects of the patient's care on which the notes were originally based. However, I recognize and admit the limitations in the clinical training and practices as a general internal medicine physician. This is especially true in some specialty situations, rather than following management examples of this book, consulting specialists and experts are more appropriate and should be strongly encouraged and advocated, especially in life-saving situations. Patient care is not a solo show; it involves interactions among people, and effective communication with patients (and patients' family members), specialists, and healthcare providers is of the utmost importance to good patient care.

Lastly, this book is not meant to guide patient management but rather to serve as a tool for internal medicine clinicians to study and better understand patient care and interventions. It may also be used by clinicians to refresh his or her knowledge.

Appleton, WI, USA Kehua Zhou

Disclaimer

The information provided in this book is intended for educational purposes only and should not be construed as medical advice or a substitute for professional medical care. While every effort has been made to ensure the accuracy and reliability of the information presented, the author and publisher make no representations or warranties, express or implied, regarding the completeness, suitability, or applicability of the content for any particular purpose.

Medical knowledge and practices are constantly evolving, and recommendations may change over time. For any knowledge and information with questions, readers of the book are advised to refer to specific updated guidelines and standards of care protocols and seek recommendations from experts in the specific field regarding specific topics or patient conditions.

The author and publisher disclaim any liability for any loss, injury, or damage incurred as a consequence, directly or indirectly, of the use and application of the information contained in this book. Reliance on any information provided herein is solely at the reader's own risk.

Furthermore, reference to specific products, procedures, or services does not imply endorsement or recommendation by the author or publisher. Readers are encouraged to conduct their own research and exercise judgment in evaluating the appropriateness of any recommendations or treatments mentioned in this book.

By using this book, readers agree to indemnify and hold harmless the author and publisher from any claims, damages, or losses arising from their use of the information herein.

Contents

Part I
Diary Notes During Residency Training

Chapter 1
The Journey Begins with the ICU and Cardiology Rotation

July 2nd, 2017 Through July 31st, 2017

After graduating from medical school outside the United States, I studied physical therapy for 3 years and then practiced physical therapy and wound care for 4 years. I was fortunate to enter the internal medicine training program at Buffalo 7 years after my medical school graduation.

My journey to medicine at that time felt like painting on a piece of blank canvas. It started with my intern month at the intensive care unit (ICU) and cardiology floor. While taking care of ICU patients under the chair physician of the critical care medicine unit occupied the majority of our time, the ICU team of residents was also responsible for taking care of the cardiology floor patients with a cardiologist. Thus, the notes of this chapter were essentially a mixture of critical care medicine and cardiovascular medicine.

Although the first month of residency still involved a small portion of scut work, the learning to practice medicine did start from information gathering (reviewing medical records, taking a thorough history of present illness, performing a pertinent yet detailed physical examination, presenting labs and imaging results, and explaining current ongoing treatments). The goals of the first month, retrospectively, really focused on thorough history taking and physical examination for patient interaction; whereas ordering workups and management for patients were largely left to senior residents and my attending physicians. The whole process nonetheless was very daunting for a foreign medical graduate who had been off clinical practice of medicine for 7 years.

I appreciated the patience and efforts of my senior resident and attending physicians in teaching me while caring for sick patients. Additionally, I did have my co-intern together with medical students on the team. Both my co-intern and I were foreign medical graduates while the medical students were from the local medical school for that month; undoubtedly the medical students often outperformed me and my co-residents. I still remember my co-intern and I went to the ICU at 3–4 a.m. to see patients and stayed late and long hours to complete daily progress notes and

K. Zhou, *Internal Medicine Training Notes and Survival Guide*,
https://doi.org/10.1007/978-1-0716-4039-5_1

History and Physical notes. Yet, my senior resident kept on telling me the notes were in no way important as compared to good patient care which in fact is partially but not necessarily true when I think of it nowadays.

My daily notes did start from the beginning of my residency training. In this Chapter, topics covered include code status, fluid resuscitation, sepsis and septic shock, case presentation in daily rounding, preoperative cardiac evaluation, stress ulcer prophylaxis, hypertensive urgency/emergency management, congestive heart failure, acute myocardial infarction, stroke, diabetic ketoacidosis, hyperosmolar hyperglycemic state, and respiratory failure together with some knowledge of mechanical ventilation. At the end of the first rotation, the canvas remains a collection of a few small colored dots despite my revision and updates up to the last moment of submission of the book for publication.

7/2/2017

1. **Code status**: full code vs. Do Not Resuscitate (DNR)/Do Not Intubate (DNI) vs. partial code (DNR only and ok for intubation or DNI only and ok for resuscitation).
2. **Clinical Institute Withdrawal Assessment (CIWA)** protocol is used for alcoholic patients; lorazepam is preferred over diazepam for liver failure. May order scheduled Ativan or Librium for 1–2 days if the patient is in active withdrawal.
3. While acute kidney failure (AKI) often is caused by dehydration or hypovolemia and should be treated with intravenous fluid, other causes of AKI are not uncommon in actual practices. **Fractional Excretion of Sodium (FENa)** % = 100 × (Scr × Una) / (Sna × Ucr): FENa < 1% indicates prerenal while >4% indicates post-renal kidney injury (FENa 1%–4% indicates intrinsic kidney injury); UNa (urine random sodium excretion rate) <20 mmol/L indicates prerenal while >40 mmol/L indicates either intrinsic or postrenal kidney injury.
4. **Gabapentin and vancomycin** together with many other medications require renal dose adjustment in renal failure.
5. **Haloperidol** 2–5 mg im/iv or Zyprexa 5 mg iv can be used for irritability in hospitalized patients.
6. In septic and hemorrhagic shock, **morning cortisol check** may be necessary to rule out adrenal insufficiency.
7. **Albumin + Lasix** can be used for **anasarca** associated with poor nutritional status (low serum albumin).
8. Typical workup and management of **gastrointestinal (GI) bleeding**: fecal occult blood testing, hematocrit and hemoglobin lab check q6h, packed red blood cell (PRBC) transfusion (1 unit raises hemoglobin by 1 g/dL), proton pump inhibitor pantoprazole 40 mg iv bid after 80 mg iv bolus. Additional testing may include anemia panel (serum folate, B12, iron, ferritin, total iron binding capacity, and reticulocytes), hemolysis workup (haptoglobin, LDH, direct Coombs test, and peripheral blood smear), and disseminated intravascular coagulation (DIC) panel (platelet count, PT, aPTT, fibrinogen).

9. Urinary tract infections due to **extended-spectrum beta-lactamase (ESBL)** positive bacteria require treatment with carbapenems (most often sensitive) or fluoroquinolones (sometimes resistant).
10. **Ventilator weaning requirements**: mentation alert with spontaneous breathing, medical conditions leading to intubation like lung disease being treated, and Rapid Shallow Breathing Index (RSBI, also known as Yang Tobin Index) = f/Vt (f is respiratory frequency, Vt is tidal volume in liters). An RSBI < 105 indicates likely successful extubation.
11. **Typical ventilator settings**: typical tidal volume 6 mL/kg, 100% FiO_2, PEEP at 5 cmH_2O, RR 14–16. If low SO_2, can increase FiO_2 and/or PEEP. If high CO_2 retention, we can increase RR and/or tidal volume.
12. **Stroke etiologies and workup**: (1) Etiologies: atrial fibrillation (Afib), patent foramen ovale (PFO), carotid plaque, hypercholesterolemia, hypercoagulability. (2) Workup: Holter/telemetry to assess for arrhythmia; echocardiogram to assess for thrombus and vegetation, with bubble study to assess for PFO, atrial septal aneurysm if suspected embolic stroke; carotid ultrasound/Doppler or CT angiogram of the neck for carotid artery stenosis, lipid panel, HA1c. Additional workup includes TSH, homocysteine, and hypercoagulability workup (thrombophilia workup if suspicion of hypercoagulability). May order procalcitonin, erythrocyte sedimentation rate (ESR), C reactive protein (CRP), and blood culture if infection is suspected (atypical stroke presentation, immunosuppressant use, combined ischemic and hemorrhagic strokes).
13. Cardene = nicardipine; **hypertensive crisis** (hypertensive emergency + hypertensive urgency) = sBP > 180 or dBP > 120. Hypertensive emergency has target organ damage while hypertensive urgency does not. Treatment of hypertensive crisis: decrease mean arterial pressure (MAP) by 25% in minutes to 14 h with IV medications like Cardene drip, as-needed hydralazine IV or as-needed labetalol IV; or oral captopril 12.5–100 mg tid, clonidine 0.2 mg tid.
14. To-do list in **daily rounding**: I/O, flow sheet for night events, all medications (including IV drips), vital signs, labs and imaging studies (including ultrasounds and echocardiogram if any), vent settings, and physical exams.
15. Additionally, **overnight and the-day-before events** for **daily rounding**: CIWA protocol (dosing of meds, vital range, flow sheet from nurses); vent settings (FiO_2, RR, PEEP, tidal volume); meds and drips and pressors; vital signs (including Tmax) and trends, and overnight events.
16. Colistin = polymyxin E, Keppra = levetiracetam (inhibits presynaptic calcium channels), VATS = video-assisted thoracoscopic surgery, TIPS = transjugular intrahepatic portosystemic shunt.
17. **Tuberculosis (TB)** isolation discontinuation requires **negative sputum acid-fast test daily × 3 days**.
18. **Rheumatoid arthritis (RA)** can also have tenosynovitis. In RA, physical examination usually reveals boggy tender joints. **Workup for RA** includes serology for rheumatoid factor (RF), cyclic citrullinated peptide (CCP) antibodies (more specific), ESR, CRP, antinuclear antibodies (ANA), and uric acid.

19. **Diagnosis of RA** requires: inflammatory arthritis involving three or more joints (3 points); positive rheumatoid factor (RF) and/or anti-citrullinated peptide (2–3 points); elevated levels of CRP and/or ESR (1 point); similar diseases including particularly psoriatic arthritis, acute viral polyarthritis, SLE, gout and pseudogout have been ruled out; duration over 6 weeks (1 point). The diagnosis of RA requires 6/10 points, morning stiffness >30 min, and duration of symptoms >6 weeks. Treatment: NSAIDs and glucocorticoids + disease-modifying antirheumatic drugs (DMARDs) which take 3–6 months for efficacy. **DMARDs** include **conventional synthetic DMARDs** (including methotrexate, sulfasalazine, leflunomide, and hydroxychloroquine), **targeted synthetic DMARDs** (JAK inhibitors: tofacitinib and baricitinib), and **biologic DMARDs** (e.g., etanercept, infliximab, adalimumab, rituximab, abatacept, and golimumab).
20. **Methotrexate (MTX)**: stop 3 months before pregnancy; typical dosage is 7.5–25 mg (optimal dose is 25 mg) once a week, no alcohol before and after methotrexate, watch for liver function tests (LFTs), CBC, CMP. Test for Hep B and C first before prescribing methotrexate. When prescribing methotrexate, will also need to prescribe folate 1000 mg qd; use leucovorin if stomatitis.
21. Methotrexate may require up to **6 months to take effect** and thus must be observed for 6 months. If no improvement with methotrexate, add a TNF alpha inhibitor or IL-6 inhibitor Actemra (tocilizumab), or add a combination of sulfasalazine and hydroxychloroquine.
22. **Treatment algorithm for RA**: Use **methotrexate with or without low dose prednisone** (maximum 3 months for steroid) as initial treatment; if failure, **combine MTX with hydroxychloroquine (Plaquenil) and sulfasalazine** or use of biologic DMARD (with or without MTX) or JAK inhibitors (with or without MTX) ⇒ switch to other TNF inhibitors.
23. The use of **TNF inhibitors** increases the risk of lymphoma and tuberculosis (TB). TNF inhibitor is contraindicated in demyelinated disease and requires screening for TB before prescribing.
24. **High CCP** levels indicate a worse prognosis, will need a TNF inhibitor after 3–6 months' treatment of methotrexate.

7/2/2017

1. Make sure room numbers are right; check the code status of patients.
2. Update events of the day for ICU patients.
3. Spiking temperature in ICU patients: need **BUS (blood, urine, sputum) cultures**.
4. **Elevated blood pressure** etiologies and solutions: identify and treat the cause while giving symptomatic labetalol or hydralazine. Common causes include pain, anxiety, and dyspnea, rarely thyroid and adrenal gland dysfunctions.
5. **Hepatic encephalopathy** treatment: lactulose +/− rifampin 550 mg bid, may also correct zinc deficiency (evidence is limited for zinc correction or supplementation).
6. **Metabolic acidosis**: if high anion gap, will need to check for osmolar gap and rule out toxicant ingestion. If **non-anion gap metabolic acidosis**, check urine

electrolytes Na+, K+, CL+. Urine anion gap = K+Na−Cl; useful to identify causes of non-anion gap metabolic acidosis; it is a reverse representation of renal NH_4 secretion. If negative, it means sufficient NH_4 secretion (Type II RTA), and positive means insufficient secretion of NH_4 (Type I RTA).

7. **Steven Johnson Syndrome** treatment: triamcinolone, Benadryl, hydroxyzine im q4h, prednisolone. Timely transfer to the burn unit with a focus on supportive care remains standard.
8. **Dyspnea and tachycardia** with concerns for pneumonia: if chest X-ray (CXR) is negative or no change but still concerned with pneumonia, do CT for post-obstructive pneumonia (especially in lung cancer patients). **Procalcitonin (use cut point of 0.3–0.5)** is usually very sensitive and specific for pneumonia diagnosis.
9. **Ventricular tachycardia (VTach)**, patient stable, could be SVT + LBBB. A brief run of tele Vtach in a stable patient, do 12 lead EKG, SVT with RVR ⇒ consider giving adenosine or metoprolol.
10. Treatment for confirmed **stable Vtach**: 150 mg iv amiodarone over 10 min, or sotalol after cardiology consultation. If unstable, follow advanced cardiac life support (ACLS) protocols.
11. **Non-sustained VTach**: greater than or equal to 3 beats of VTach ≥100 bpm, but less than 30 s. Treatment is goal- or etiology-directed medical optimization.
12. **Sustained VTach**: ≥30 s or hemodynamic instability. Additional treatment besides amiodarone bolus followed by drip includes intravenous **lidocaine** (preferred in acute myocardial ischemia or infarction) or intravenous **procainamide** after cardiologist consultation.
13. **Uncomplicated urinary tract infection (UTI)** treatment: Bactrim, fosfomycin, nitrofurantoin, ampicillin, or Cipro as outpatient.
14. Presurgery: **succinylcholine** during intubation can increase plasma K+, thus no K+ supplementation before surgery.
15. Never document a physical exam you did not do. BRBPR = bright red blood per rectum.
16. **Propofol** sedation increases serum triglyceride. **Diabetic diet**: regular diet with 1800–2000 calorie per day restriction for carbohydrates (130–220 g of carbs per day).
17. **Abnormal troponin and CKMB,** if suspicion is high for coronary artery disease while low suspicion for acute coronary syndrome, may order echo and stress test; if unsure about acute coronary syndrome, consult a cardiologist before ordering stress test.
18. **Pleural effusion** sometimes can be from congestive heart failure (usually bilateral or right-sided), and can benefit from Lasix/diuretics.
19. PVC → bigeminy, reentrant etiology, electrical alternans. PAC vs. PVC (compensatory pause).
20. **Case presentation**: CC (chief complaint), DDx (differential diagnoses), HPI (history of present illness), ED (emergency department) course, PMH (past medical history). Medications, FH (family history), SH (social history), VS (vital signs), PE (physical examination), and assessment and plan.

7/3/2017

1. **Admission medication reconciliation** (it may be performed by a pharmacy technician or registered nurse): medication list, confirm with the patient, dosing, and last dispense date/or last dosage time. Reach out to PCP for the medication list, call the nursing home/facility to get medication records (pharmacy, patient, and PCP), and/or show me the pills if necessary. Write down the medication names and quantity if no medical record is available.
2. **Health care proxy** (power of attorney for health) may have the information about the patient's health condition and medication list; may call the 24-h pharmacy number to get the medication list, vitamins, and inhalers.
3. **Code status**: what do you want to be done with your life? All treatments on board? If your heart stops beating, do you want chest compressions? If multiple co-morbidities and likely poor prognosis, will need to mention possible outcomes of cardiopulmonary resuscitation (chances for survival to discharge if **cardiac arrest: in-hospital = around 25%; out-of-hospital = 10%–12%**). Medical Orders for Life-Sustaining Treatment (MOLST) Form in the New York State.
4. Medical orders for life-sustaining treatment, witness, and code status are part of History & Physical.
5. **Lactic acidosis**: Type A—impaired oxygenation; Type B—insufficient metabolism or excessive production. D-lactic acidosis: short bowel allows undigested carbohydrates to reach the colon. Serum lactic acid does not detect D-lactic acidosis.
6. **Osmolar gap** >10 mOSM/kg = consider possible toxin ingestion (diabetic ketoacidosis can also have a high osmolar gap due to beta-hydroxybutyrate to acetone conversion by way of acetoacetate).
7. **Discharge summary**: major procedures, tests, and test results, may call the primary care doctor at admission and discharge, anything that you want to mention about this patient. This always serves as the final legal document for a patient's hospitalization. Discharge documentation distribution. Discharge summary can be done 1/2 day ahead (STAT for rehab or SNF), otherwise done in 24 h.
8. **Signout**: critical information transferring, why admitted, pertinent meds, night events, and action plans.
9. Daily **SOAP** (subjective, objective, assessment and plan) note: symptoms and change in conditions, do SOAP notes.
10. Hospitalized: avoid sleeping pills as they increase risks for fractures. Anxious and sleep difficulties, try to avoid benzos, go to see the patient if symptoms change, and check QT intervals. May use **Seroquel** short term in dementia patients and/or **trazodone** in otherwise relatively healthy or young patients for insomnia or agitation or anxiety. Add an addendum for important information if notes are completed in the morning.
11. **Penicillin allergy** in a patient with kidney failure, if G- infection, may use aztreonam which has no coverage against G+ or anaerobes, but is synergistic with aminoglycosides. The majority of patients with documented penicillin allergy can tolerate cephalosporins.

7/4/2017

1. **Oral levothyroxine to iv**: The American Association of Clinical Endocrinologists/ American Thyroid Association guidelines recommend an intravenous dose of 50%–70% of the patient's oral dose.
2. **K replacement**, hypokalemia: keep serum mag above 2, serum potassium above 4. No more than 10 mg/h for peripheral IV or no more than 20 mg/h for central line.

7/5/2017

1. **Cardiolite stress test** (Cardiolite/technetium), walk 5-–10 min, rest day 1, exercise day 2 in obese patients (BMI ≥ 30).
2. **Lexiscan**, also known as regadenoson, a pharmacological stressor for cardiac stress test.
3. Stop metoprolol and other beta blockers if **cocaine use**.
4. **Rapid shallow breathing index (RSBI)** = RR/Vt in liters, <100 is a good parameter for ventilator weaning.
5. **Heparin anticoagulation**: 0.3–0.5 anti-Xa Units/mL for acute myocardial infarction (AMI) for 48 h or until revascularization with percutaneous coronary intervention, angina and stroke; 0.5–0.7 anti-Xa Units/mL for PE, DVT and mechanic valve. Anti-Xa of 0.35 Units/mL corresponds to aPTT 66 s
6. **Percutaneous coronary intervention (PCI)**: drug-eluting stents require at least 6 m, preferably 1 year, of dual antiplatelet therapy (DAPT), then drop P2Y12 inhibitor like Plavix and keep aspirin. Metal stents require at least 30-day DAPT, then drop P2Y12 inhibitor like Plavix and keep aspirin.
7. The minimum recommended duration of dual antiplatelet therapy after stent placement is **1 month for bare-metal stents, 3 months for the sirolimus (Rapamune)-eluting stent** (Cypher), and 6 months for other drug-eluting stents.

7/6/2017

1. **Potassium replacement dosage** for serum potassium replenishment from 2 to 2.5, requires 100 mEq KCl tablet dosage; 2.5–3, requires 75 mEq KCl tablet dosage; 3–4, requires 100 mEq KCl tablet dosage. ESRD hypokalemia should be cautious and use a low scale for K supplementation.
2. **Hyperkalemia**: EKG showing peak T wave; stabilize with calcium gluconate; temporize with D50 25 g iv followed by regular insulin 5–10 u iv, HCO3, beta-agonist albuterol inhaler; eliminate with dialysis, Lasix, Lokelma (10 mg tid for 6 doses, if chronic hyperkalemia, do 10 mg daily), or Kayexalate 15 –30 g once.
3. Refractory hyperkalemia, acidosis, extreme electrolyte disturbances, intoxication, oliguria, and uremia should be treated with **dialysis**.
4. **Stress test contraindications**: acute coronary syndrome in 48 h, high-risk unstable angina, acute pulmonary embolism, severe symptoms of aortic stenosis, uncontrolled heart failure, arrhythmia, myopericarditis, and acute aortic dissection.

5. **No BiPAP** in acute pulmonary embolism, respiratory arrest, vomiting, pneumothorax, facial or nasopharyngeal trauma, esophageal or laryngeal surgery.
6. Standard Bruce protocol, modified Bruce protocol, submax/symptom-limited; hold nitrates, beta blocker, calcium channel blocker, ranolazine before and during stress test.
7. Lexiscan (regadenoson), Persantine (dipyridamole) stress test, dobutamine stress test: used for patients **unable to exercise**, recent myocardial infarction; may continue (but no initiation of) beta blocker in these patients.
8. Cardiolite (Sestamibi) stress test [also known as single photon emission computed tomography (SPECT) stress testing], PET (rubidium), Echo, and cardiac MRI are used in **uninterpretable baseline ECG**, such as paced rhythm, LBBB, resting T wave depression >1 mm, digoxin use, left ventricular hyperplasia (LVH). After intermediate EKG, **pharmacologic tests or tests for localization of ischemia** should be performed if concerns for heart disease.

7/8/2017

1. **Cocaine intoxication and hypertension** should be treated with diazepam and/or lorazepam (benzodiazepines), aspirin if chest pain ⇒ addition of nitroglycerin or nitroprusside (alternative: phentolamine (α_1 blockader) 5–10 mg iv q5–15 min). May use labetalol/carvedilol (alpha and non-selective beta-blockers) in combination with vasodilator (nitroglycerin and nitroprusside) at the same time.
2. **Chest pain in cocaine abusers**: obtain ECG, administer benzodiazepines, aspirin 325 mg oral (assuming aortic dissection not suspected), nitroglycerin 0.4 mg sublingual with or without continuous infusion, phentolamine (hold if sBP <100). If QRS widening on EKG (suggesting profound toxicity), administer sodium bicarbonate 1–2 mEq/kg IV push. Phentolamine: 1 –2.5 mg iv q 5–15 min.
3. **Hypertensive emergencies:** if symptoms are mainly neurologic and/or acute kidney injury, start nicardipine/clevidipine/labetalol; if is due to scleroderma, start captopril; if during pregnancy, use hydralazine, labetalol, oral nifedipine; if it is mainly cardiac- AMI (use nitroglycerin, esmolol, or metoprolol), CHF (use nitroglycerin, furosemide, or nitroprusside if no cardiac ischemia).
4. Nitroprusside can cause **coronary steal syndrome** (blood flow from a narrowed coronary artery was directed to other coronary vessels causing chest pain; it is also the mechanism of the pharmacological stress test). **Subclavian steal syndrome** = occlusion or stenosis of the subclavian artery proximal to the vertebral artery origin which may cause arterial insufficiency in the brain (ie, vertebrobasilar insufficiency) or upper extremity numbness and pain. **Coronary-subclavian steal** = coronary circulatory ischemia after coronary artery bypass surgery (CABG) using the internal mammary artery (IMA), worsening with **ipsilateral arm exercises** or movements (this happens when there is a proximal left subclavian artery stenosis causing retrograde flow from the LIMA to the distal left subclavian artery).
5. **Acute aortic dissection**: emergent surgery, pain control with IV opioids and esmolol to lower HR below 60 bpm while targeting sBP 100–120 mmHg or lowest tolerated pressure without compromising perfusion. If systolic blood pres-

sure remains elevated after heart rate is consistently <60 bpm, may use nitroprusside 0.25–0.5 μg/kg/min; titrate as needed by 0.5 μg/kg/min every 5 min.

7/9/2017

1. **Heart failure treatment**: congestion and perfusion- (a) warm and dry, continue outpatient treatment; (b) warm and wet, treat with diuretics; (c) cold and dry, use inotropes; cold and wet, use diuretics and inotropes and/or vasodilators.
2. **Acute myocardial infarction** treatment BMONASH: beta-blocker (avoid in acute decompensated congestive heart failure, but initiate before discharge), morphine, oxygen, nitrates, aspirin, statin, and heparin drip.
3. **Acute congestive heart failure** treatment LMNOP: Lasix (or bumetanide), morphine, nitrate, oxygen +/− noninvasive ventilation. Add ACEi or ARB if no hypotension; change to hydralazine and isosorbide dinitrate if renal dysfunction, especially in African Americans. Additional goal-directed treatments include angiotensin receptor-neprilysin inhibitor (ARNi), mineralocorticoid receptor antagonist (MRA), and sodium-glucose cotransporter 2 inhibitor (SGLT2i). Beta blockers should be added when appropriate in reduced ejection fraction heart failure before discharge.
4. **Advanced congestive heart failure**: IV **vasodilators** (nitroglycerin, nitroprusside-cyanide/thiocyanate toxicity, nesiritide); **inotropes** dobutamine <5 μg/kg/min; dopamine increases GFR and natriuresis but can cause vasoconstriction when >10 μg/kg/min; milrinone dosage decrease by 50% in renal failure; intra-aortic balloon pump (IABP); ventricular assistive device (LAVD and RVAD); transplantation.

7/19/2017

1. **Congestive heart failure (CHF) hypertension**: hydralazine and isosorbide dinitrate if renal dysfunction, especially in African Americans; metoprolol succinate, bisoprolol, or carvedilol (only these three beta blockers can decrease mortality in CHF); ACEi or ARB; spironolactone, eplerenone, loop diuretics better than hydrochlorothiazide.
2. **Stress ulcer prophylaxis indications:** mechanical ventilation >48 h; coagulopathy (platelet <50,000, INR > 1.5, or PTT > 2 times control); Hx of gastrointestinal ulceration or bleeding within last year; traumatic brain injury, traumatic spinal cord injury, or burn; ≥2 of the following: sepsis, ICU stay >1-week, occult gastrointestinal bleeding for 6 or more days, ≥250 mg/day hydrocortisone or 62.5 mg/day prednisone use.
3. **Anticoagulants**: direct thrombin (IIa) inhibitors, antithrombin (fluid phase thrombin inhibitors), Factor Xa inhibitor (direct vs indirect).
4. **Direct thrombin (IIa) inhibitors**: parental direct thrombin (IIa) inhibitors—bivalirudin, argatroban, desirudin; the only oral direct thrombin (IIa) is dabigatran (usual dosing is 150 mg bid, will need 5–10-day parenteral anticoagulation before initiation for treatment of venous thromboembolism)

5. **Direct Factor Xa inhibitors**: rivaroxaban (Xarelto 15 mg bid for 21 days then 20 mg daily for VTEs), apixaban (Eliquis 10 mg bid for 7 days then 5 mg bid for VTEs), edoxaban (Lixiana), betrixaban (Bevyxxa).
6. Novel oral anticoagulants (NOACs) except **apixaban** are not used in severe renal insufficiency.
7. **NOACs** are not used in valvular atrial fibrillation (defined as mechanical heart valve and rheumatic mitral stenosis that is severe or clinically significant or mitral valve area $\leq$1.5 cm^2), BMI > 40 kg/m^2 or body weight > 120 kg or pregnancy. Of note, NOAC may be used in obese patients with BMI > 40 kg/m^2 or weight > 120 kg per the updated International Society on Thrombosis and Hemostasis Scientific and Standardization Committee guidance.
8. **Benzodiazepines**: long acting—diazepam, clonazepam, flurazepam; intermediate acting—lorazepam, temazepam, oxazepam, alprazolam; short-acting—triazolam, midazolam. Appropriate for liver failure and seniors: lorazepam, oxazepam, and temazepam.

7/21/2017

1. **Revised cardiac risk index**: (a) high-risk surgical procedures: intraperitoneal, suprainguinal vascular, intrathoracic; (b) history of ischemic heart disease, i.e., myocardial infarction, chest pain, positive stress test, nitrate uses; (c) history of congestive heart failure, i.e., pulmonary edema, rales, S3, CXR showing pulmonary vascular redistribution; (d) cerebrovascular accident, transient ischemic attacks (TIAs); (e) preoperative treatment with insulin; (f) preoperative serum creatinine >2 mg/dL. If increased risks for major perioperative cardiac events, check whether any active cardiopulmonary symptoms (if yes, delay surgery and start treatments for symptoms) and check functional status (goal $\geq$4 METs), such as whether patient can climb up a flight of stairs or walking at ground level at 4 mph (if yes, patient is optimized and can proceed with surgery understanding the increased risks), if no, check cardiac stress test or coronary angiography and consult cardiologist.
2. **Hyponatremia** in hyperglycemia correction: corrected Na = measured Na + [2.4 × (measured serum glucose − 100)/100]
3. Commonly used **ventilation mode**: **Pressure-regulated volume control (PRVC)**—ventilator attempts to achieve a set tidal volume at the lowest possible airway pressure. Setting: tidal volume 6 mL/Kg, respiratory rate (12–20, usually around or slightly above patient's spontaneous respiratory rate), PEEP (5–8 cmH_2O), FiO_2.
4. **Synchronized intermittent mandatory ventilation (SIMV)**: the ventilator will deliver a mandatory (set) number of breaths with a set volume while at the same time allowing spontaneous breaths.
5. **pPEAK** = peak inspiratory pressure. High pPEAK causes: (a) tube kicking or obstruction (suction is needed); (b) acute loss of lung compliance (pneumothorax, chest X-ray is needed; auto-peep, pressure release is needed); (c) main stem intubation (endotracheal tube shift, do auscultation). Methods for solutions: disconnect the ventilator, suction, and bag ventilating the patient.

6. **Plateau pressure** represents alveolar pressure, ≤30–35 mmH_2O is normal. Normally pPEAK − plateau pressure ≤5 cmH_2O. High peak inspiratory pressure can cause barotrauma. **Inspiratory hold** = plateau pressure measure; **expiratory hold** = auto positive end-expiratory pressure (PEEP) measure. PEEP is the pressure from the ventilator to keep the alveoli open.
7. **Diabetic ketoacidosis (DKA)** diagnosis or definition: plasma glucose ≥ 250 or even normal, pH < 7.3, HCO_3 < 15, and moderate ketonemia or ketonuria.
8. **Hyperosmolar hyperglycemic state** diagnosis or definition: plasma glucose >600, elevated serum osmolality (>320 mOsm/kg), and impaired mental status.
9. **Typical insulin dosage requirement per day** (recommend slowly and gradually increase to this dosage): outpatient 0.2 u/kg; floor patient, healthy and thin 0.3 u/kg; sick average weight patient 0.4 u/kg; overweight and insulin resistant patient 0.5 u/kg; history of insulin resistance in morbid obese patients 0.6 u/kg. **Goal serum glucose in diabetes as outpatient** premeal target: <90–130 mg/dL and postmeal (2 h after a meal) target: <180 mg/dL as outpatient. **In-hospital goal** premeal: 140–180 mg/dL for critically ill patients and 100–140 mg/dL for non-critically ill patients (random glucose goal less than 180 mg/dL).
10. Commonly used **insulin types**: rapid-acting insulin- Lispro (Humalog), Aspart (Novolog), Glulisine (Apidra); short-acting insulin- regular (Novolin), Velosulin (used in insulin pump); long-acting- glargine (Lantus), detemir (Levemir), degludec (Tresiba).
11. **Correction factor for carbohydrates** = 1800/total daily dose of insulin. **Carbohydrate coverage of a meal** = total grams of carbohydrates/correction factor. This may be used as nutritional coverage for each meal.
12. High blood sugar correctional insulin dose = (actual glucose − target glucose)/correction factor
13. **Calculated serum osmolality** = 2 × Na + glucose/18 + BUN/2.8. Additional osmoles: protein, ion, urea, glucose, and toxicant ingestions of ethanol, methanol, ethylene glycol, isopropyl alcohol, or aspirin (salicylates).

7/22/2017 Treatment of Diabetic Ketoacidosis (DKA) or Hyperosmolar Hyperglycemic State (HHS)

1. **Fluid resuscitation**: (a) Normal Saline (NS) bolus at 1 L/h for 1 L; (b) half NS or NS at 250 mL/h or 500 mL/h for 1–2 L; (c) when glucose drops below 200 or 250 mg/dL in DKA or 300 mg/dL in HHS, change intravenous fluid to D5 + NS at 150–250 mL/h; insulin at 0.1 u/kg subcutaneous q2h.
2. **The DKA or HHS protocol**: finger stick glucose q1h, BMP q4h, with insulin dosing: bolus insulin 0.1 u/kg iv followed by 0.1 u/kg/h continuous, if glucose not falling 50%–70% per hour, double the dose. Alternative dosing: subcutaneous insulin 0.3 u/kg bolus, followed by 0.2 u/kg subcutaneous at 1 h later and 0.2 u/kg subcutaneous every 2 h. Short-acting insulin takes 15–30 min to work and has a duration of action of 4–6 h.
3. **Potassium supplementation in DKA**: if K < 3.3, give 20–40 mEq K/h; if K is 3.5–5.3, give 20–30 mEq K in each liter IV fluid. If K > 5.3 mEq/L, do not give K but check serum K every 2 h.

4. **Bicarb drip indications**: if serum pH <6.9, dilute $NaHCO_3$ (100 mmol) in 400 mL H_2O with 20 mEq KCL (add KCL in fluid only if concerns for hypokalemia) IV over 2 h, repeat lab every 2 h. Bicarb drip is also used in serum bicarb level <10 mEq.

7/23/2017 Fluid Resuscitation

1. **Obligatory water intake**: ingested water 500 mL, water in food 800 mL, water from oxidation 300 mL daily.
2. **Obligatory water output**: urine 500 mL, skin 500 mL, respiratory tract 400 mL, and stool 200 mL daily.
3. At least 1–2 L of NS are given ASAP to restore tissue perfusion in **hypovolemic shock**. A typical recommended dosage of fluid hydration of **30 mL/kg** fluid bolus is recommended in sepsis.
4. **IV fluid maintenance in NPO patients**: 2 L per day with D5 + 0.45%NS + 20 mEqKCL at 80 mL/h in a medium sized patient.
5. **Nasogastric tube feeding indications:** NPO status patients after 1–2 days in the severely malnourished, 3–5 days in the moderately malnourished, and within 7 days in the normally or overnourished. **Gastrostomy (PEG) or jejunostomy (PEJ) feeding indications**: expected tube feeding for more than 4–6 weeks or nasogastric tube feeding for ≥14 days.
6. **Chronic hypernatremia** (>48 h): D5 at 1.35 mL/kg/h × BW in kilos (**goal correction <8–10 mEq/L in 24 h**), remeasure serum sodium every 4–6 h.
7. **Acute hypernatremia** (<48 h): D5 at 3–6 mL/kg/h × BW in kilos until Na < 145 then D5 at 1 mL/kg/h, monitor glucose and Na q2h (Na 1–2 mEq/h, normalize in 24 h). If glucose is high, slow infusion rate or change to 2.5% glucose (this protocol is less commonly used in clinical practices as we usually do not know the duration of hypernatremia and because of the concerns of the adverse consequence of cerebral edema from rapid correction).
8. **Total body water** (TBW) = 0.5 in men or 0.6 in women × body weight in kilos. **Water deficit** = current TBW × ([serum Na/140] − 1).
9. **Acute/chronic hypernatremia**: hourly D5W infusion rate in mL/h based on water deficit in mL divided by 24 h or goal duration of sodium correction
10. **Hypotensive septic shock**: NS 0.9% 2-L bolus over 60 min; will need additional 500 cc bolus and even maintenance fluid thereafter if sBP < 90, lactate > 4 and increasing, HR > 110 bpm, or decreased urinary output < 30 mL/h or start of pressor support. Example of maintenance fluid of 70-year-old sepsis patient with fever and diverticulitis with a blood pressure of 145/85: basal needs 70 (body weight in kilos) + 40 = 110 mL/h; for additional loss in fever, can add 10–15 mL/h.
11. Example: 75-year-old male hospitalized with community-acquired pneumonia, temperature 39.5 °C, HR 80, BP 105/72, Weight 85 kg, Na 165, K 4.0. Order IV option 1: 0.45%NS at 140 (85 + 40 + 15) mL/h. Order IV option 2: D5W at 150 mL/h for 50 h (water deficit 0.5 × 85 × ([165–140]/140)) = 7.58 L; expected correction time 72 h, thus in reality should be 7580/72 = 105 mL/h.

12. **Fluid 4-2-1 rule** for iv fluid (normal saline) maintenance: 4 mL/kg/h for the first 10 kg, 2 mL/kg/h for second 10 kg, and 1 mL/kg/h thereafter.
13. In septic shock, **fluid resuscitation** should be 30 mL/kg/h for 2 L in the first 3 h.

7/25/2017

1. **Ventilator weaning trial** should happen after PEEP < 8 cmH_2O.
2. For **congestive heart failure** (either symptomatic or asymptomatic), ACEi or ARB use when LVEF ≤ 40%, spironolactone/eplerenone use when LVEF < 35%, SGLT2i when symptomatic LVEF > 40% and elevated natriuretic peptides or LVEF ≤ 40%; ARNi in LVEF < 40% but also recommended in patients with preserved ejection fraction; beta blocker if no hypotension and no acute symptoms. **ARNi** administration: (1) patient should be able to tolerate ARB or ACEi; (2) should wait at least 36 h after the last dose of ACEi (not ARB) when switching.
3. **Community-acquired pneumonia** is treated inpatient with iv ceftriaxone, azithromycin, and steroids (debatable, but I commonly use steroids especially if wheezing during exam or smoking history).
4. **CPAP vs BiPAP**: if hypercapnic, use BiPAP, usually 12/6, maximal 18/6 if obese.
5. **Delirium or anxiety**, avoid mentation-altering medications, but if absolutely needed, use trazodone, Seroquel, Ativan, or Haldol (Haloperidol). Some neurologists prefer Ativan to Haldol because of the shorter half-life of Haldol.
6. Non-ST elevated myocardial infarction (**NSTEMI**) or ST elevated myocardial infarction (STEMI) heparin protocol: 60 u/kg bolus followed by 13 u/kg/h (low standard protocol). **STEMI** will need consultation with a cardiologist STAT and follow STEMI protocol for cardiac catheterization.
7. Deep vein thrombosis (**DVT**) or pulmonary embolism (**PE**) heparin protocol: 80 u/kg bolus followed by 18 u/kg/h (high standard protocol)
8. **Heparin anti-Xa monitoring**: 0.3–0.5 for low standard in age > 75, high bleeding risks, acute myocardial infarction (AMI), unstable angina patients; 0.5–0.7 for high stand for DVT, PE, and mechanical valve replacement history patients.

7/26/2017

1. 40% FiO_2 **BiPAP** 16/8: if tolerated well and saturation improves, the patient can then be taken off BiPAP and placed on high flow or even nasal cannula. May get venous or arterial blood gas to confirm improvements before BiPAP removal.
2. **Nasal cannula oxygen**: low flow 1–15 lpm; standard face mask 5–10 lpm; partial rebreather mask and non-rebreather mask: >10 lpm. **High flow** 30–60 lpm (40%–100% FiO_2) ➔ BiPAP ➔ intubation.
3. **Pulmonary embolism**, may need echo if concerns for heart strain and tPA or thrombectomy. For **high mortality risk patients**, need to contact an interventional radiologist or interventional cardiologist for possible thrombolytics or mechanical thrombectomy.

4. Maalox (aluminum/magnesium/simethicone) provides quick relief for heartburn, gas, and bloating.
5. **GI cocktail** = Maalox 30 mL (aluminum hydroxide (Equiv. to dried gel, USP) 200 mg – Magnesium hydroxide 200 mg – Simethicone 20 mg) + Lidocaine viscous 15 mL + anticholinergic (antispasmodic) for dyspepsia
6. Simethicone is an oral anti-foaming agent for bloating, discomfort, or pain by gas
7. Pulmicort = budesonide, MiraLAX = polyethylene glycol, Colace = docusate, Singulair = montelukast, Fosamax = alendronic acid, Depakote/Depakene = valproic acid.
8. **Respiratory failure**: Type 1 hypoxic respiratory failure = $PaO_2 < 60$ mmHg with a normal or low $PaCO_2$; Type 2 hypercapnic respiratory failure = $PaCO_2 \geq 45$ mmHg.
9. **Bridging heparin with Eliquis**: stop heparin 1 h before starting Eliquis or stop heparin and start Eliquis simultaneously
10. **Metformin renal dosing**: when eGFR 30–45, may continue previous metformin but do not start; when eGFR < 30, metformin is contraindicated; eGFR > 45 no adjustment necessary.
11. **Xarelto dosing DVT**: 15 mg bid for 21 days followed by 20 mg daily after. In patients with chronic kidney disease, Xarelto will need renal adjustment dosing.

7/27/2017

1. When concerned for tachycardia, may trial **levalbuterol** (Xopenex) 1.25 mg q8h instead of Duonebs (ipratropium bromide/salbutamol). For intractable nausea and vomiting, may use **trimethobenzamide** or **dronabinol** if concerns for prolonged QTc.
2. Liver disease with significant edema and third spacing, may need to use albumin. No K supplement in end-stage renal disease (ESRD). Caution K supplement in acute kidney injury.
3. **Sepsis** is diagnosed if the suspected source of infection together with SIRS (Systemic Inflammatory Response Syndrome) criteria ≥ 2: T > 38 or < 36, heart rate > 90 bpm, RR > 20 or PaCO2 < 34 mmHg, WBC > 12,000/mm^3 or < 4000/mm^3 or > 10% immature bands. Sepsis is also diagnosed if suspected infection with an acute increase of ≥2 SOFA points (RR ≥ 22, altered mentation, and sBP ≤ 100 mmHg). **Septic shock** defines the use of a pressor(s) in sepsis to maintain MAP ≥65 mmHg and lactate >2 mmol/L despite adequate fluid resuscitation (30 mL/kg).
4. **Septic shock treatment (first line is norepinephrine) Neo-Synephrine dosing**: 0.9%NS + phenylephrine (Neo-Synephrine) 160 μg IV; 0.9%NS + phenylephrine (Neo-Synephrine) 32 μg IV. Higher concentrations require a central line.
5. **Pain inpatient treatment**: hydromorphone 0.5 mg iv q3h, morphine 0.2 mg iv q4h, or ketorolac 15 mg iv q6h. If alcoholic or diabetic, may add gabapentin 100 mg tid.
6. Ketorolac for moderate pain 4–6; Tylenol/ibuprofen/naproxen for mild pain 1–3; hydromorphone for severe pain 7–10. Oxycodone, hydrocodone, lidocaine patch, and capsaicin patch can also be used for pain management.

7. **Muscle relaxers**: methocarbamol (Robaxin), cyclobenzaprine (Flexeril), carisoprodol (Soma), gabapentin, metaxalone (Skelaxin).
8. **Constipation treatment**: docusate senna, polyethylene glycol, magnesium hydroxide 2400 mg q24h po, bisacodyl suppository 10 mg rectal daily, bisacodyl (Dulcolax) 5 mg po daily.

7/30/2017

1. For hemodialysis patients, digoxin starts at 0.25 μg iv now, 0.125 μg 6 h later, and then 0.125 μg every other day. The dosage is renally adjusted.
2. **Fentanyl drip for sedation** in ICU: fentanyl citrate 25 mg q2h iv prn for sedation.
3. **Vasopressors mechanism**: activation of alpha 1, beta 1, beta 2, or dopamine receptors (vasodilation vs vasoconstriction); calcium sensitizers (increase myocardial contractility, phosphodiesterase inhibitor ➔ increases inotropy and vasodilation).
4. **Norepinephrine** (Levophed): 0.4 mg/kg/min acts on both alpha 1 and beta 1 receptors; it is the preferred pressor for septic shock.
5. **Phenylephrine** (Neo-Synephrine) is a pure alpha-adrenergic agonist that can increase mean arterial pressure (MAP) via increased systemic vascular resistance; it may be used as an alternative to norepinephrine when norepinephrine causes arrhythmia. **Phenylephrine** is also the pressor in left ventricular outflow tract obstructions (**LVOTOs**) from hypertrophic cardiomyopathy and the most commonly used pressor to improve cerebral blood flow in **ischemic stroke**.
6. **Epinephrine** (beta1, beta2, and alpha1 agonist) increases cardiac output while increasing systemic vascular resistance and has variable effects on mean arterial pressure (MAP) at high doses. Epinephrine is alpha 1 predominant, mostly used in **anaphylaxis**; is a second line pressor after Levophed for septic shock and a second line pressor after Levophed and/or vasopressin for hypotension after cardiac surgery including coronary artery bypass grafting.
7. **Vasopressin also known as anti-diuretic hormone (ADH)** activates V1a receptors leading to vasoconstriction, activates V2 and V1b as well as oxytocin receptors promoting anti-diuresis and exerting procoagulant activity. It is used as adjunctive therapy as epinephrine to norepinephrine for septic shock and as a first line alternative for hypotension related to cardiac surgery.
8. **Ephedrine** works on alpha and beta receptors; it is only used in post-anesthesia-induced hypotension.
9. **Dopamine**, an alternative to Levophed in bradycardia and has a low risk for arrhythmia: 1–2 mg/kg/min as a vasodilator; 5–10 mg/kg/min stimulates beta 1 and increases cardiac output; >10 mg/kg/min stimulates alpha 1 and causes an increase in systemic vascular resistance.
10. **Dobutamine**: not a vasopressor but a vasodilator; it is contraindicated in idiopathic hypertrophic subaortic stenosis.
11. **Phenylephrine** can cause reflex bradycardia; **dopamine** can lead to diuresis, worsening hypovolemia; **epinephrine** causes mucosal ischemia; **dobutamine** causes hypotension.

12. **Transbronchial biopsy** is the method of diagnosis for sarcoidosis and bronchiolitis obliterans organizing pneumonia (BOOP, AKA cryptogenic organizing pneumonia) and hilar mass.
13. **Antiseizure meds**: levetiracetam (Keppra), phenytoin (Dilantin), diazepam (Valium), midazolam (Versed), pentobarbital.
14. **Syndrome of inappropriate antidiuretic hormone (SIADH)**: usually urine osmolality higher than serum osmolality; treatment includes urea 15 g daily [Ure-Na 15 g BID (to continue daily as outpatient)] and salt tablets 1 g daily to 2 g tid as appropriate. Drugs that cause SIADH: thiazide, vincristine, carbamazepine, tricyclic antidepressants (TCAs), selective serotonin reuptake inhibitors (SSRIs), clofibrates, oxytocin, morphine, nicotine.
15. **The HIV incubation period** is 6 months to 1 year.

7/31/2017 Lung Auscultation

1. **Vesicular breath sounds**, I:E = 3:1 over most lung surfaces
2. **Bronchial breath sounds**, I:E = 1:1 with a distinct pause
3. **Bronchovesicular breath sounds**, I:E = 1:1 normal over chest or post chest between the scapula.
4. **Ronchi (low-pitched wheezes)**: snoring, gurgling, or rattle-like, usually clears after cough
5. **Coarse crackles** are discontinuous, brief, popping sounds. Compared to fine crackles, they are louder and lower in pitch and last longer; also known as bubbling sounds.
6. **Early inspiratory crackles** = rales (severe airway obstruction); late inspiratory crackles = rales (restrictive defect).
7. **Wheeze**: continuous with musical quality- (**1**) High pitched squeaking, (**2**) Low-pitched snoring/moaning. Wheezes indicate narrowing of airways. Monophonic (throughout the respiratory cycle) vs polyphonic (COPD and severe asthma)
8. **Stridor** is caused by upper airway narrowing or obstruction, heard through a stethoscope; may be seen in 20% of extubated patients. In children, stridor becomes louder in supine, as seen in pertussis, croup, epiglottitis, and aspiration.

Takeaway Messages

1. Emphasis as a first-month intern is on information gathering and understanding of patients' diagnoses and treatments.
2. Case presentation and documentation is the major responsibility of interns.
3. Key to practicing medicine as an intern is to learn to stabilize patients quickly and to seek help in a timely fashion from senior residents and, if necessary, attending physicians.
4. Understand the treatment principles of congestive heart failure.
5. Levophed is the go-to pressor for septic shock, extreme bradycardia; phenylephrine is for left ventricular outflow tract obstructions (LVOTOs) or ischemic stroke; epinephrine is used in cardiac arrest (iv) and anaphylaxis (im); vasopressin is alternative to Levophed in septic shock and hypotension related to cardiac surgery.

Further Readings and References

1. Sterns, R.H., and E.J. Hoorn. *Overview of the treatment of hyponatremia in adults*, ed. M. Emmett. Waltham: UpToDate. Accessed October 31, 2023.
2. Santanilla, Jairo I. 2011. Chapter 3: The crashing ventilated patient. In *Emergency department resuscitation of the critically ill*. Dallas: American College of Emergency Physicians.
3. Pham, T., L.J. Brochard, and A.S. Slutsky. 2017. Mechanical ventilation: State of the art. *Mayo Clinic Proceedings* 92 (9): 1382–1400.
4. Wiethorn, E.E., C.M. Bell, and B.S. Wiggins. 2021. Effectiveness and safety of direct oral anticoagulants in patients with nonvalvular atrial fibrillation and weighing ≥ 120 kilograms versus 60-120 kilograms. *American Journal of Cardiovascular Drugs* 21: 545–551.
5. Rosovsky, R.P., E. Kline-Rogers, L. Lake, et al. 2023. Direct oral anticoagulants in obese patients with venous thromboembolism: Results of an Expert Consensus Panel. *The American Journal of Medicine* 136 (6): 523–533.
6. Heidenreich, P.A., B. Bozkurt, D. Aguilar, et al. 2022. 2022 AHA/ACC/HFSA guideline for the management of heart failure: A report of the American College of Cardiology/American Heart Association Joint Committee on clinical practice guidelines. *Journal of the American College of Cardiology* 79 (17): e263–e421.

Chapter 2
The General Internal Medicine Floor Rotation

August 1st, 2017 Through September 24th, 2017
Right after the ICU rotation, I spent 2 months on the general medicine floors at two different local teaching hospitals. The typical day of life began with rounding on patients, gathering patient data, and later presenting patient data and discussing the plan of care with my senior resident and attending physicians. With the education and guidance from senior residents and attending physicians, this again was a progressive learning process based on actual patient encounters and interactions. Usually around noon time, there were university-wide lectures covering major topics in general internal medicine, and in the evenings I kept on rewriting the notes from a piece of paper to the notebook.

Patients on the general medicine floor were usually admitted because of a wide range of acute conditions with multiple baseline co-morbidities. Among these diseases, topics covered in this chapter include acute and chronic kidney disease, acute coronary syndrome, pneumococcal vaccination, community-acquired pneumonia, COPD exacerbation, stroke, mechanical and prosthetic valves, hyponatremia, contaminated (blood, urine, and sputum) culture, liver failure, alcoholic cirrhosis, urinary tract and bloodstream infections, gastrointestinal bleeding, GERD, dysphagia and metabolic alkalosis. Although medicine has progressed rapidly in the past two decades, treatments for many diseases or conditions remain unsatisfactory or, on rare occasions, even nonexistent. As one step further, this chapter further touches on the topic of goals of care discussions.

Besides medical knowledge learned and skills honed during the two general medicine floor months, I also appreciated and benefited greatly from the correction of my progress notes by one of my attending physicians. She taught me the important principles of progress note writing to which I still cling. For medical documentation, copying and pasting are not tolerated in any academic or community hospital, yet efficient medical documentation remains of great significance no matter where you practice medicine in this country and regardless whether or not you are tasked with multiple other assignments on top of active patient care. Meanwhile, thorough

K. Zhou, *Internal Medicine Training Notes and Survival Guide*,
https://doi.org/10.1007/978-1-0716-4039-5_2

documentation of patient care can be equally important after stabilizing a patient's unstable or deteriorating conditions. My attending taught me to write succinct yet thorough progress notes without any redundancy. While many of my physician colleagues may argue against this tenet, I fully support the idea that the daily progress note should focus on diagnosis, plan of care, and documentation of patient interactions while de-emphasizing the reiteration of data that were already in the medical record system. This belief nonetheless has helped me to stay efficient in medical charting while maintaining accuracy.

8/1/2017

1. **Lacosamide** (Vimpat) has a bioavailability of 100%.
2. **Voiding trial**: remove Foley, if no self-voiding after 6 h, straight cath × 2–3 after measuring postvoid volume through bladder scan using ultrasound, reinsert Foley, and voiding trial failed.
3. **Atrial fibrillation** medications: amiodarone (not commonly used unless running out of options) IV 150 mg over 10 min; 0.5–1 mg/min maintenance dose (800 mg qd in divided doses × 1 week, then 600 mg qd in divided doses × 1 week, then 400 mg qd × 4–6 weeks, then 200 mg daily). Atenolol 25–100 mg daily. Carvedilol 3.125–25 mg bid. Diltiazem oral 120–480 mg daily, IV 0.25 mg/kg over 2 min; second bolus can be given if HR > 100, followed by a drip 5–15 mg/h. Esmolol IV 500 mg/kg over 1 min ⇒ 50–200/mg/kg/min. Metoprolol IV 2.5–5 mg over 2 min, no maintenance dosing; oral 25–100 mg bid, may use succinate 25–200 mg daily. Verapamil iv 0.075–0.15 mg/kg over 2 min, second bolus can be given in 15–30 min if needed; patient starts with nonsustained release verapamil dose 120–480 mg → may switch to extended-release.
4. **Angioedema**: if due to ACE inhibitor, threatening airway, treatment: give icatibant, if not available, give FFP, C1 esterase inhibitor Berinert. In reality (actual clinical practices), if anaphylaxis, give IV famotidine, Benadryl, and Solumedrol. If unstable, given epinephrine 0.3 or 0.5 mg intramuscular in the anterolateral aspect of the middle third of the thigh.
5. **Globulin gap**, also known as paraprotein gap or gamma gap, is the difference between the total protein and albumin. >4 g/dL is considered elevated, as seen in acute HIV, plasma cell dyscrasias, and generalized inflammation.
6. Monoclonal band on serum protein electrophoresis (SPEP) = **plasma cell dyscrasia**.
7. **CHA2DS2-VASc**: congestive heart failure, hypertension, age (75 years old), diabetes, stroke or TIA, vascular (PAD, MI, aortic plaque), age (65 years old), sex. If atrial fibrillation or flutter and CHA2DS2-VASc ≥2, the patient will need full anticoagulation unless contraindications.

8/2/2017

1. **Anemia workup**: occult blood, reticulocyte, transferrin, ferritin, iron, and total iron binding capacity, vitamin b12, folate, erythropoietin, hepatitis profile, hemoglobin, electrophoresis, kappa and lambda light chains, protein electropho-

resis, serum immunofixation, and immunoglobulin A, G, M and LDH, haptoglobin, Coombs testing, bone marrow biopsy.

2. **Post-pulmonary embolism workup**: (A) If positive familial history, age < 50, on oral contraceptives, or hormonal replacement therapy, send thrombophilia panel 2 weeks after completion of treatments, or 2 weeks after discontinuing warfarin, or 2 days after stopping direct oral anticoagulants and heparin, as thrombus, heparin, and warfarin can change results; (B) malignancy workup (routine cancer screening).
3. **Thrombophilia panel** includes lupus antibody with reflex, protein C and S, antithrombin III, prothrombin, cardiolipin ab, factor V Leiden, anticardiolipin ab, beta-2-glycoprotein I antibody, and homocysteine.
4. Of note, in patients with homozygous factor V Leiden, prothrombin gene mutations, or deficiencies of protein S, C, or antithrombin, lifelong anticoagulation is not necessary even in unprovoked venous thromboembolism. **Lifelong anticoagulation however may be appropriate in patients with recurrent, unprovoked and/or life threatening VTEs**.
5. **Flomax** (tamsulosin) takes 48 h to work, 0.4 mg oral daily; if not effective in 2–4 weeks, can increase to 0.8 mg daily.
6. **Foley catheter** should be changed every 4 weeks.
7. **Complicated UTI** should be treated with 7–14 days' antibiotics. **Gram-negative bacteremia**: continue antibiotics for 7–14 days. **Gram-positive bacteremia** usually requires long-term intravenous antibiotics.
8. **QTc normal value**: <440 ms in male and <460 ms in female.

8/5/2017

1. **COPD exacerbation** diagnosis requires acute changes in one or more of the following: increase in cough frequency and severity, increase in sputum production volume and/or change in sputum character, and worsening dyspnea.
2. **Management of COPD exacerbation**: provide supplemental oxygen to target SO_2 of 88%–92%, PO_2 of 60–70 mmHg; NPPV (like BiPAP, setting initially can be 8–12 cmH_2O inspiratory pressure, 3–5 cm H_2O expiratory pressure); albuterol 2.5 mg inhaler, ipratropium nebulizer, methylprednisolone 60–125 mg iv once with lower dosages thereafter, antibiotics.
3. **Severities of lung function impairment**: in patients with FEV1/FVC < 0.7, GOLD1 (FEV1 > 80%), GOLD2 (FEV1: 50%–80%), GOLD3 (FEV1: 30%–50%), GOLD4 (FEV1: <30%) predicted.
4. **Bacterial pathogens in COPD exacerbation** (probability high to low): H. influenzae > Moraxella catarrhalis > S. pneumoniae > Pseudomonas.
5. **Supplementary oxygen therapy**: Nasal cannula oxygen 0–6 lpm (FiO_2 = 21%–40%); venturi masks deliver FiO_2 up to 60% (2–12 lpm); simple masks (FiO_2 = 55%, 6–10 lpm); nonbreathing masks (FiO_2 = around 90% FiO_2). The inability to correct hypoxemia with relatively low FiO_2 should prompt consideration of pulmonary embolism, acute respiratory distress syndrome (ARDS), pulmonary edema, severe pneumonia, and others.

6. **Antibiotics** for COPD exacerbation: Levaquin 750 mg daily, ceftriaxone (with azithromycin), cefotaxime (with azithromycin), or moxifloxacin.
7. **Hypothalamic-pituitary-adrenal (HPA) axis** suppression happens in the following conditions: (1) Glucocorticoid ≥20 mg for greater than 3 weeks; (2) Evening/bedtime dose of greater than 5 mg prednisone for more than a few weeks; (3) Cushingoid appearance. In hospitalized patients with HPA suppression, stress dose steroids with hydrocortisone is usually necessary.
8. **Uncomplicated COPD** with no risk factors (<65 yo, FEV1 > 50%, <2 exacerbations/year, no cardiac disease), can be treated with azithromycin/clarithromycin, cephalosporins, TMP-SMX or doxycycline. **Complicated COPD** (1 or more risk factors) should be treated with levofloxacin, moxifloxacin, or Augmentin with azithromycin.
9. **Pneumococcal conjugate vaccine (PCV15 or PCV20)** for all adults 65 years or older as well as adults 19 through 64 years old who have certain chronic medical conditions or other risk factors. Per the CDC, "If PCV15 is used, a dose of PPSV23 should be given one year later. The minimum interval is 8 weeks after PCV 15 for PPSV 23 and can be considered in an immunocompromising condition (immunocompromised- alcoholism, chronic heart disease, not hypertension, chronic liver or kidney or lung disease, cigarette smoking, diabetes), cochlear implant, or cerebrospinal fluid leak. If PCV20 is used, no PPSV23 is necessary." "If PPSV 23 or PCV 13 administration history, give 1 dose of PCV20 at least 1 year after PCV13; give 1 dose of PCV15 or PCV20 at least 1 year after the most recent PPSV23."
10. **Causes of high troponin**: acute myocardial infarction, Takotsubo cardiomyopathy, heterophile antibodies, chronic kidney disease
11. **CT with contrast** is used for detecting inflammation, mass, acute changes and looking at arteries.
12. **Atrial fibrillation**: heart rate less than 110 with exertion/rest (if less stringent) is considered as rate controlled, around 80–90 s at rest is ideal.
13. **Adult constipation (urgent treatment)**: severe constipation treatment: suppositories (glycerin and bisacodyl); dis-impaction (manual fragmentation → enema with mineral oil) → if unsuccessful, order a water-soluble contrast enema (gastrografin or Hypaque) to rule out proximal impactions → water enema over sodium phosphate enema (fleet enema) or balanced electrolyte solution with polyethylene glycol.

8/8/2017

1. **Framingham risk score** for CVD risks in 10 years: age > 65 years old for males, >54 years old for females, diabetes, LDL + HDL, blood pressure.
2. **Primary prevention of stroke**: healthy diet, moderate alcohol consumption, non-smoking, physically active, no abdominal adiposity.
3. **Secondary prevention of stroke**: monotherapy with ACEi, ARB, or CCB or diuretics for blood pressure control or combination therapy (ACEi + CCB). Plus, aspirin or a P2Y12 inhibitor or dual antiplatelet therapy with aspirin and a P2Y12 inhibitor.

4. **Blood pressure goal** before thrombolytic therapy (Tenecteplase (TNK) is more commonly used than t-PA now) or mechanical thrombectomy in stroke: ≤185/110. After thrombolytic therapy or mechanical thrombectomy, blood pressure should be stabilized ≤180/105 for at least 24 h after thrombolytic treatment. Decrease blood pressure 15% during the first 24 h after stroke onset, and restart antihypertensive medications 24 h later.
5. **Secondary prevention of non-cardioembolic stroke or TIA of atherothrombotic, lacunar, or cryptogenic type**: aspirin (50–100 mg), clopidogrel 75 mg, or combination of aspirin-extended-release dipyridamole. In reality, it depends on which one patient is already on, and can be modified based on the original medication. Of note, **cilostazol** is an acceptable monotherapy for secondary stroke prevention in Asians.
6. For **carotid endarterectomy**, recommends aspirin (ASA) (81–325 mg daily) before surgery and continues indefinitely.
7. **Dual antiplatelet therapy (DAPT, aspirin, and clopidogrel) indications**: recent acute myocardial infarction, other carotid artery stenosis after stent placement; recently symptomatic intracranial large artery disease for 90 days followed by one antiplatelet therapy. For carotid artery stenting, DAPT should start before and continue for 30 days after carotid artery stenting, followed by single antiplatelet therapy.
8. Platelet **P2Y12 receptor blockers**: clopidogrel, ticlopidine, ticagrelor, prasugrel, and cangrelor. P2Y12 blockers block the binding of adenosine diphosphate to P2Y12.
9. **Acute ST elevated myocardial infarction (STEMI)**: aspirin 162–325 mg to all patients as soon as possible, then once the reperfusion strategy (percutaneous coronary intervention, fibrinolysis, or none) establishes, give P2Y12 blocker (use clopidogrel if fibrinolysis; use ticagrelor if no perfusion plans; use ticagrelor or prasugrel if percutaneous coronary intervention). **Door to needle** for thrombolysis in STEMI is ≤30 min; **door to balloon** for percutaneous coronary intervention is ≤90 min.
10. In patients treated with aspirin and a P2Y12 receptor blocker, if high risk for gastrointestinal bleeding, should start **gastrointestinal prophylaxis** with a proton pump inhibitor.
11. Patients with drug-eluting stents or bare metal stents without increased risk of bleeding or planned noncardiac surgery within 1 year, should continue DAPT for a minimum of 6–12 months. If tolerable, an **additional 18 months**.
12. For stable patients with a high risk of bleeding, a minimum of 4 weeks of uninterrupted DAPT for bare metal stents (BMA), and 1–3 months for drug eluting stents (DES) for patients with acute coronary syndrome. It is reasonable to extend these durations to 3 months for BMS and 6 months for DES.
13. Clopidogrel, prasugrel, and ticagrelor should be stopped 5, 7, and 3–5 days respectively **before surgery**.
14. Drug elimination in chronic kidney disease: azithromycin 5%–12% renally excreted; moxifloxacin 15%–21% renally excreted; pioglitazone 15%–30% renally excreted; ciprofloxacin 30%–57% renally excreted; amoxicillin

50%–70% renally excreted; digoxin 57%–80% renally excreted. Renal adjustment for dosing is necessary for >25%–30% of renally excreted medications.

15. **Phosphate nephropathy**: calcium-phosphate deposits in tubules and interstitium lead to acute kidney injury (in days to months). **Risk factors**: GFR < 60, >60 years of age, female, hypertension, diabetes, congestive heart failure, volume depletion, active colitis, and medications that may predispose to acute kidney injuries (renin-angiotensin-aldosterone system blockers, diuretics, lithium, and NSAIDs). Avoid the use of fleet enema if eGFR <30 ml/min.

8/9/2017

1. **Seizure precautions**: padding around the bed, mats around the bed.
2. **Clobazam** binds $GABA_A$ receptors to exert its anticonvulsant and anxiolytic effects. Taper clobazam, can add as needed diazepam, can also add gabapentin (also used in EtOH withdrawal).
3. **Hypernatremia**: check BMP Na q4h; treatment: D5W or 1/2NS or enteral water administration (free water flush via NG tube at 400 cc q6h)
4. **Chronic benzodiazepine use** can lead to a pharmacological syndrome including drowsiness, ataxia, fatigue, weakness, dizziness, vertigo, syncope, reversible dementia, depression, impaired intellect, psychomotor and sexual dysfunction, agitation, auditory and visual hallucinations, paranoid ideation, mania, delirium, depersonalization, sleepwalking, aggressivity, orthostatic hypotension, and insomnia.
5. List of **anti-epileptic drugs (AEDs)**: acetazolamide, carbamazepine, clobazam, clonazepam, eslicarbazepine acetate, ethosuximide, gabapentin, lacosamide, lamotrigine, levetiracetam, nitrazepam, oxcarbazepine, piracetam, phenobarbital, phenytoin, pregabalin, primidone, rufinamide, sodium valproate, topiramate, vigabatrin, zonisamide.
6. **Red urine**: urinalysis showing urine RBC <8 hpf → check CPK for possible myoglobinuria from rhabdomyolysis.
7. **Neurocheck** used in stroke, transient ischemic attack (TIA), and syncope.
8. **Possible renal cell carcinoma**: sometimes may not need biopsy, rather go directly for nephrectomy.
9. Drugs require caution in patients with chronic kidney disease (CKD): RAAS antagonist- avoid in renal artery stenosis, discontinue or reduce dosage if SCr increases >30% or K > 5.5; dose adjustment in CKD: ampicillin, cephalosporins, quinolones, trimethoprim, aminoglycosides.
10. **Hydrochlorothiazide** 12.5 mg (25 mg only increases diuresis effects) daily reaches maximal effects of blood pressure control; calcium channel blockers can be added on top of hydrochlorothiazide.

8/9/2017 extra

1. **HIV and infections:** CD4 < 400, oral candida; Strep Pneumonia in CD4 > 200. CD4 < 200, cryptosporidium, JC virus, PCP. CD4 < 100, histoplasma, C albicans (esophagus), toxoplasma. CD4 < 50, mycobacterium avium-intracellulare

(MAC), CMV, Cryptococcus. **PCP prophylaxis**: Bactrim (also helps with toxoplasma) or aerosolized pentamidine.

2. **Highly active anti-retroviral therapy (HAART)** standard of care for HIV: two nucleoside/nucleotide reverse transcriptase inhibitors (NRTIs) + a non-nucleoside reverse transcriptase inhibitor (NNRTI), a protease inhibitor (with ritonavir boosting), or an integrase inhibitor.
3. **HIV treatment**: emtricitabine (NRTI) + tenofovir alafenamide (NRTI) + dolutegravir (integrase inhibitor), or Biktarvy = emtricitabine (NRTI) + tenofovir alafenamide (NRTI) + bictegravir (integrase inhibitor). HIV post-exposure treatments: dolutegravir + tenofovir disoproxil fumarate + emtricitabine, or raltegravir + tenofovir disoproxil fumarate + emtricitabine.
4. Guaifenesin (with or without codeine) and benzonatate for cough.
5. First episode of unprovoked **pulmonary embolism** treatment: anticoagulation for 3–6 months (consider: serial D-dimer testing at 2–3 weeks and then again at 1–2 months after discontinuation of anticoagulation) or lifelong.
6. **Classic orthostatic hypotension** = drop in sBP ≥ 20 mmHg or dBP ≥ 10 mmHg within 3 min of standing or head-up-tilt. **Delayed orthostatic hypotension** = drop in sBP ≥ 20 mmHg or dBP ≥ 10 mmHg beyond 3 min of standing or head-up-tilt. **Postural autonomic tachycardia** = a heart rate of ≥120 beats/min or an increase of ≥30 beats/min upon transferring from supine to standing. **Autonomic impairment** = decrease in blood pressure without a corresponding increase in heart rate (<10 bpm).
7. **Orthostatic hypotension treatment**: midodrine 2.5 mg bid or fludrocortisone 0.1–0.2 mg daily, can be titrated up and used together if necessary. Droxidopa is used in orthostatic hypotension caused by autonomic dysfunction.
8. **Alcohol withdrawals** (time from last drink): 6–36 h for minor withdrawal, 6–48 h for seizures, 12–48 h for hallucinations, 48–96 h for delirium tremens.
9. Criteria for **community-acquired pneumonia-related** clinical stability: T ≤ 37 C; HR ≤ 100 bpm; RR < 24; sBP ≥ 90 mmHg; $SaO_2 \geq 90\%$ or $PO_2 \geq 60$ on room air; maintaining oral intake; normal mentation.
10. **Community-acquired pneumonia** requires 5 or more days of antibiotics. If afebrile for 48–72 h, and has no more than 1 sign of clinical instability, we can transition to oral antibiotics.
11. **Community-acquired pneumonia treatment**: prednisone 40 mg daily for 5 days, antibiotics 5–7 days (including azithromycin 500 mg daily for 3 days or 500 mg once on the first day followed by 250 mg daily for another 4 days). If fluoroquinolone is used, there is no need to use azithromycin.
12. Amlodipine takes 3 days to work and 6 weeks to peak; lisinopril 5 mg = captopril 25 mg; lisinopril works in 1 h. The initial dosage of lisinopril is 2.5–5 mg daily; the initial dosage of captopril is 6.5 mg tid and may go up to 50 mg tid.
13. **NIHSS**: level of consciousness; ask age and month; blink eye and squeeze hands; best gaze; visual fields; facial palsy; motor arm and leg drift; limb ataxia; sensation; best language/aphasia; dysarthria (slurred, unintelligible); extinction and inattention (formerly known as neglect).

14. **Discharge criteria**: able to eat, able to urinate, and has been having bowel movements, vitally stable, no acute medical issues, able to take care of patient self and activities of daily living (ADLs) with/without assistance depending on placement. **Discharge locations**: home, home therapy, skilled nursing facility, outpatient therapy, inpatient rehabilitation, hospice at home, or hospice at a facility.
15. **Pancreatic enzyme replacement**: Creon at 500 u/kg/meal. Stool elastase is used to diagnose chronic pancreatitis (moderate pancreatic insufficiency: 100–200 μg elastase/g fecal material; severe pancreatic insufficiency: <100 μg elastase/g fecal material). In pancreatitis, serum trypsin, lipase, and amylase are increased. Only **lipase** is specific for pancreatitis; amylase is also increased in parotitis.
16. **Roflumilast** 250 μg once daily for 4 weeks, followed by 500 μg once daily. It is a selective long-acting inhibitor of PDE-4 to treat inflammation in COPD and prevent exacerbation in severe COPD. **Roflumilast cream 3%** is approved for mild, moderate, and severe plaque psoriasis.
17. **Diarrhea** workup: fecal leukocyte, stool culture, stool ova and parasite, stool clostridium difficile toxin, and gastrointestinal panel PCR. If it remains uncontrolled, consider colonoscopy with biopsy and rule out microscopic colitis.

8/10/2017

1. **Aortic stenosis** symptoms: chest pain (exertional angina), syncope or presyncope, and shortness of breath.
2. **Aortic stenosis**: parvus (small pulse) and tardus (delayed pulse), symptoms appear when the valve orifice decreases to ≤1 cm^2 (normal >3 cm^2). **Severe aortic stenosis** if any of the following: aortic valve area ≤1 cm^2 (or AVA indexed to body surface area (BSA) <0.6 cm/m^2), peak aortic velocity ≥ 4 m/s, the pressure gradient ≥ 40 mmHg.
3. **Indications for aortic valve replacement**: severe high gradient aortic stenosis (≥40 mmHg) by history or on exercise testing; asymptomatic severe aortic stenosis with left ventricular ejection fraction <50%; patients with severe aortic stenosis when undergoing other cardiac surgeries.
4. **Cardiac catheterization indications**: NSTEMI (type I primary cardiac), STEMI, unstable angina. Type II NSTEMI is from noncardiac insult and may have selective cardiac catheterization after hospitalization.
5. **Percutaneous cardiac intervention (PCI)** = cardiac angiography + angioplasty + stent placement.
6. **Chest pain**, worse with exertion, better with rest/nitroglycerin. All three met = typical (cardiac) chest pain; met 2/3 = atypical chest pain; met 1/3 = noncardiac chest pain.
7. **Unstable angina/NSTEMI** treatment: anti-ischemic and other treatments (nitrates, O_2, ACEi/ARB/CCB, morphine, and beta-blocker), antiplatelet therapy, anticoagulation therapy with heparin drip or enoxaparin (may add nitroglycerin drip if uncontrolled angina or hypertension) for 48 h or till cardiac catheterization (could be longer if need for coronary artery bypass grafting) or percutaneous cardiac intervention (PCI).

8. **Percutaneous cardiac intervention (PCI)**: selective angiography (stress test once stabilizes) and conservative strategy if TIMI score ≤ 2; routine angiography and invasive strategy if TIMI score ≥ 3.
9. **The thrombolysis in myocardial infarction (TIMI) score**: age ≥ 65, ≥3 CAD risk factors, known CAD (stenosis ≥50%), aspirin use in past 7 days, severe angina (≥2 episodes in 24 h), EKG ST changes ≥0.5 cm, and positive cardiac markers.
10. **STEMI treatment**: needs emergent cardiac catheterization (door-to-needle time for thrombolysis <30 min or preferably door-to-balloon time <90 min); anticoagulation with heparin, enoxaparin, bivalirudin, or fondaparinux; immediate adjunct therapy including beta-blocker (avoid if HR < 60 bpm or > 110 bpm, acute moderate to severe heart failure, secondary or third-degree AV block), nitrate, morphine, oxygen, ACEi/ARB, and intensive statin/insulin.
11. **Indications for coronary artery bypass grafting (CABG) therapy**: triple vessel disease (e.g., RCA, LAD, LCx), two-vessel disease + diabetes, or single vessel disease with left main artery (LAD or LCx). **Multivessel coronary artery disease (MVD)** = greater than 70% stenosis in at least two major coronary arteries with a diameter of ≥2.5 mm or in one coronary artery in addition to greater than 50% stenosis of the left main trunk.
12. Amlodipine causes edema in 20% of heart failure patients.
13. Loperamide for diarrhea. Prochlorperazine is used for nausea and vomiting as well as anxiety and schizophrenia.
14. **Provoked** venous thromboembolism should be treated with 3 months' anticoagulation. **Provoking factors** include trauma, injury, oral contraceptives, pregnancy, and hospitalization. **Unprovoked and recurrent and cancer-associated venous thromboembolism** may require anticoagulation for the rest of life. Common novel anticoagulants: apixaban 10 mg bid for 7 days followed by 5 mg bid; rivaroxaban 15 mg bid for 21 days followed by 20 mg daily; dabigatran 150 mg bid requires at least 5 days of initial therapy with a parenteral anticoagulant.
15. **Unfractionated heparin** is preferred in eGFR ≤30, extensive clot burden, hemodynamical instability, anticipated need for discontinuation or invasive procedure including PCI, obesity, or poor subcutaneous absorption.

8/11/2017

1. **Axis**: check leads I and aVF (QRS should be upward normally). **RBBB**: RSR' in V1–V3, S wave in V5 and V6. **LBBB**: dominant S wave in V1, broad monophasic R wave in lateral leads (I, aVL, V5, and V6). **LPFB**: RAD, tall R (qR) wave in II, III, aVF. **LAFB**: LAD, deep S (rS) wave in II, III, and aVF.
2. **Treatment of chronic kidney disease (CKD)** grades 3–5 not yet on dialysis: Step 1 goal is to **treat hyperphosphatemia** to reduce serum phosphorus concentrations to ≤5.5 mg/dL (or closer to normal levels); hyperphosphatemia is usually common when eGFR ≤ 25–40 mL/min/1.73 m^2; treatment should focus on restricting dietary phosphate intake. Step 2: after **2–4 months** of unsatisfactory control of serum phosphate, need to prescribe phosphate binders. Calcium-

containing phosphate binders—calcium acetate/carbonate; non-calcium phosphate binders—aluminum salt, **sevelamer**, **lanthanum**. Additionally, will need to treat hypocalcemia and hyperparathyroidism with **ergocalciferol (Vit D2) or cholecalciferol (Vit D3)**. Step 3: If elevated PTH despite optimal ergocalciferol and phosphate binder **over 6 months**, give low-dose vitamin D derivatives (**calcitriol, alfacalcidol, or doxercalciferol**). Step 4: in moderate to severe hyperparathyroidism, use **cinacalcet** (cautious side effects: increased serum phosphate and decreased serum calcium). Maintain the serum bicarbonate concentration above 22 mEq/L (with **oral bicarbonate** if necessary). The target PTHi level in CKD 5 is **130–600 pg/mL**.

3. **Preprocedural evaluation for CABG**: CBC, PT/PTT/INR, clotting time, BMP, LFT, CXR. Beta-blockers, calcium channel blockers, and nitrates should be continued until surgery. Administration of temazepam immediately before CABG; IV small dose of midazolam before the arterial line; aspirin should be continued up to the time of surgery. Clopidogrel should be held 5 days and prasugrel should be held 7 days before surgery.
4. **Stress testing**: 48 h before stress testing, we should (NOT mandatory and varies for guidelines) stop beta-blockers, calcium channel blockers, and nitrates, but continue diuretics, ARBs, and ACEis. 12 h before vasodilator stress testing, caffeine (methylxanthines) should be stopped, if consumed, delay the test for at least 12 h after performing the resting imaging (2-day rest stress protocol). L-arginine can be continued during stress testing to give the effectiveness of medical therapy; however, if there is no prior history of CAD, L-arginine should be held before the stress test. No need to withhold amiodarone or statins. No need to withhold digoxin, estrogen, or diuretics, but order additional stress testing with concurrent myocardial imaging.
5. **Venous blood gas (VBG) versus arterial blood gas (ABG)**: the central venous pH is 0.03–0.05 (the same as HCO_3) pH units lower, PCO_2 4–5 mmHg higher than ABG. The peripheral venous pH is 0.02–0.04 pH units lower (HCO_3 1–2 mEq higher) and PCO2 3–8 mmHg higher than ABG.
6. **Anion gap** = Na-Cl-HCO_3; normal 12 +/− 4. **Delta corrected AG** = AG + 2.5 (4 − albumin). **Delta ratio (delta delta)** = [AG − 12]/[24-HCO_3]. HAGMA 0.8–2; NAGMA <0.4; mixed 0.4–0.8. Mixed HAGMA + metabolic alkalosis >2. NS 0.9% infusion can cause NAGMA; Ringer's lactate infusion can cause metabolic alkalosis.
7. Surgery will usually revoke DNR/DNI → recheck before surgery and after surgery. **Ferric gluconate** 125 mg in NS 0.9% 100 mL at a rate of 2 mL/min for severe iron deficiency.

8/13/2017

1. **Ranolazine** is used for uncontrolled angina despite medical therapies.
2. Six groups of advanced life support medical treatments for **acute myocardial infarction**: dual antiplatelet therapy, statin, ACEi, beta blocker, and nitrates.
3. **ACHS** = finger stick glucose before each meal and at bedtime.

4. **Drugs frequently causing Parkinsonism (extrapyramidal symptoms)**: antipsychotics (atypical and typical except clozapine and quetiapine), dopamine depleters (reserpine, tetrabenazine), anti-emetics (metoclopramide, levosulpiride). **Drugs infrequently cause Parkinsonism**: clozapine, quetiapine, lithium, SSRI, valproic acid, and phenytoin.
5. **Pneumonitis**: difficulty breathing and nonproductive cough; usually has a procalcitonin of less than 0.3.
6. **Pneumonia** = pneumonitis + consolidation and exudation due to infection, usually procalcitonin >0.3.
7. **Alzheimer's dementia**: In end-of-life dementia, get a palliative care consultation. While the process begins at diagnosis, hospice care begins after treatment is stopped and when it's clear that the person is not going to survive the illness.
8. **Two questions to establish a baseline**: what is your dad like before admission? What is his quality of life?
9. **Late-stage Alzheimer's disease**: loss of the ability to respond to their environment, to carry out conversations, and eventually to control movements.
10. **Dysphagia diet**: Pureed diet, dental soft, mechanical soft diet, transitional diet, or general diet for solid food; nectar thick, honey thick, or thin liquids for liquids.
11. **Adrenal insufficiency treatment**: hydrocortisone 50 mg iv q6h after hydrocortisone 100 mg iv once in hypotension.
12. **Hospice care discussions**: no transfer back to hospital, stop blood draws, no iv antibiotics or fluids, no hemodialysis, no feeding tube, continue meds (oral antibiotics if needed for comfort) to provide comfort.
13. **Pneumococcal vaccinations**: (A) 19–64 yo with intermediate risk of pneumococcal disease (smoker, CHF, chronic heart/lung disease, diabetes, alcoholic, and chronic liver disease), give 1 dose PCV15 (followed by a dose of PPSV23 given at least 1 year after the PCV15 dose) or 1 dose PCV20 or PCV21 alone. (B) ≥19 yo with high-risk factors (asplenia, immunocompromised, CSF leak, cochlear implant, and advanced kidney disease), give PCV 15 first, and at least 8 weeks later, give PPSV23. (C) >65 yo, if healthy with no intermediate or high-risk factor, give PCV15 followed by PPSV23 or PCV20 or PCV21 alone.
14. Definitions of **acute kidney injury**: increase in serum creatinine by 0.3 mg/dL within 48 h, or increase in creatinine to 1.5 × baseline which is known or presumed to have occurred within prior 7 days; or urine output <0.5 mL/kg/h for 6 h.

8/14/2017

1. **A-a gradient** = $[713 \times FiO_2 - (PCO_2/0.8)] - PaO_2$. Normally $2.5 + 0.21 \times$ age in years.
2. Normal A-a gradient was seen in high altitude and hypoventilation. Increased A-a gradient was seen in V/Q mismatch, diffusion limitation (fibrosis), and R-L shunt.
3. Surgery, if patients are on Plavix, ideally should be held 5 days before surgery; can check P2Y12 to confirm.

4. Daily weight at 6 a.m., strict Is and Os (important for congestive heart failure patients), vitals q4–8 h, and activity order are important orders for admission.
5. **Orbital cellulitis treatment**: initial treatment with vancomycin plus ceftriaxone and metronidazole (alternative vancomycin + Unasyn or Zosyn) with ophthalmologist or ENT consultation. With defervesce and symptom improvement, can switch to oral clindamycin 300 mg tid + Augmentin 875 mg q12h for 7 days.
6. **Goals of care discussions**: I hear that. Is it Okay if we talk about where we can go from here? I can't even imagine what it's like for you to live with an illness that keeps getting worse. You have been living with this disease for a long time. And, I think we are in a different place now. I wish we had a more effective treatment. I admire your spirit and everything you have done to fight this illness. I was hopeful too. Would it be all right if we talked about where we go from here?
7. **ESRD-HD treatment**: (A) doxercalciferol; (B) sevelamer; (C) Darbepoetin; (D) calcitonin (nasal spray)/cinacalcet; (E) sodium ferric gluconate 62.5 mg/5 mL every 2 weeks.
8. **Dementia with behavioral disturbance**: quetiapine 50 mg bid, citalopram 20 mg qd, trazodone 75 mg qhs.
9. **Ventricular tachycardia**: amiodarone drip → synchronized cardiovert.
10. Prevention of **ventricular fibrillation**: amiodarone 800–1600 mg in 1–2 doses for 1–3 weeks, followed by 400–600 mg daily for 1 month, followed by 200–400 mg once daily.
11. **Pulseless ventricular tachycardia** or ventricular fibrillation: seek specialist help; advanced life support 2 min/5 cycles × 2 (defibrillation/shocks between cycles), then amiodarone IV push 300 mg bolus, if not effective, give 150 mg additional, un-dilutional is preferred, maximal dose 2.2 g. Once the return of circulation, start amiodarone drip at 1 mg/min for 6 h, followed by 0.5 mg/h for 18 h then oral.
12. **Stable VTach**: seek specialist help; IV 150 mg amiodarone push over 10 min, then 1 mg/h for 6 h followed by 0.5 mg/h for at least 18 h with a total duration of infusion of 24 h and then transition to oral.
13. **Breakthrough stable VT**: seek specialist help; 150 mg amiodarone supplemental dose in 100 mL D5W or NS over 10 min.
14. **Clopidogrel** loading dose 300 mg or 600 mg, followed by 75 mg daily for up to 12 months in non-ST elevated myocardial infarction (NSTEMI) or unstable angina (UA).
15. **Plavix response assay**: platelet function P2Y12 reaction units: responsive (<194) vs. unresponsive (>194).

8/16/2017

1. **Community-acquired pneumonia** common symptoms: fever, chills, cough, purulent sputum, pleuritic chest pain, dyspnea plus imaging findings of lung infiltrates.
2. **Most common bacteria of community-acquired pneumonia**: Streptococcus, H. influenza, Moraxella.

3. **Wheezing**: bronchiolar/bronchial. Seen in pleural fluid, cardiac (heart failure), lung cancer, asthma, and pneumonia.
4. **Causes of metabolic alkalosis** with compensation: loop diuretics and hydrochlorothiazide, vomiting, antiacid use, hyperaldosteronism.
5. **Respiratory compensation for metabolic acidosis**: $PCO_2 = 1.5(HCO_3) + 8 +/- 2$
6. Patients on diuretics, for acute kidney injury, check urea rather than urine creatinine and Na (fractional excretion of urea).
7. **Contraction alkalosis** refers to the increase in blood pH that occurs as a result of fluid losses (volume contraction). The change in pH is especially pronounced with acidic fluid losses caused by vomiting. Rennin increase leads to angiotensin II increase and aldosterone increase → hypokalemia and metabolic alkalosis.
8. **Hypoxia** = consider massive pulmonary embolism; **cephalization** on imaging studies of the lungs = consider fluid overload.
9. Loop diuretics not working → add **metolazone** which is synergistic with loop diuretics.
10. **Afib** goal INR 2–3. **Mechanical aortic valve replacement** without additional risk factors goal INR 2–3; if additional risk factors like atrial fibrillation, hypercoagulable state, LV dysfunction (LVEF <35%), prior thromboembolism, goal INR is 2.5–3.5. **Mechanical mitral valve** replacement goal INR 2.5–3.5. **On-x valve** requires aspirin 81 mg daily plus INR targets 2.5 for the first 3 months and 1.5–2.0 thereafter but 2.5 if additional risk factors. If an indication for dual antiplatelet therapy, discontinue aspirin while keeping clopidogrel, usually within the first week to 1 month following PCI while patient on full anticoagulation with warfarin or NOAC.
11. **Bioprosthetic aortic valve replacement** (transcatheter aortic valve implantation) should be followed by aspirin and clopidogrel initiation for 3–6 months right after replacement. **Bioprosthetic surgical aortic valve replacement and bioprosthetic mitral valve replacement** should be followed by warfarin anticoagulation for 3–6 months. For mechanical On-X AVR and no thromboembolic risk factors, goal INR (1.5–2.0) may be reasonable starting ≥3 months after surgery, with aspirin 75–100 mg daily. "Mechanical bileaflet aortic valve without other risk factors does not require bridging, while those with thromboembolic risk factors, older-generation mechanical AVRs, or mechanical mitral valve replacements, all require bridging anticoagulation therapy".
12. Anticoagulation with a VKA to achieve an INR of 2.5 is reasonable for at least 3 months and as long as 6 months after surgical **bioprosthetic MVR or AVR** in patients at low risk of bleeding. Alternative: Patients receive intravenous heparin during valve implantation followed by chronic antiplatelet therapy after implantation: three (Evolut R/PRO) to **six (SAPIEN) months of dual antiplatelet** (aspirin 75 or 100 mg daily plus clopidogrel 300 mg loading dose followed by 75 mg daily) therapy followed by aspirin-only therapy.
13. If **bioprosthetic valve replacement, for patients on anticoagulants for atrial fibrillation** (AF): add clopidogrel to the anticoagulant drug (warfarin or a novel agent) for 3 months, and after that, continue with anticoagulant alone.

14. NOAC is a reasonable alternative to VKA in patients with AFib and native aortic valve disease, tricuspid valve disease, or mitral regurgitation (MR) and a CHA_2DS_2VASc score ≥2, as well as AFib 3 months' status post bioprosthetic MVR or AVR.
15. Clinical presentation of **hepatorenal syndrome**: a progressive rise in serum creatinine; often normal urine sediment; no or minimal proteinuria (<500 mg/day); very low Na excretion (<10 mg/dL); oliguria.
16. **Type I hepatorenal syndrome**: more serious type—twofold increase in creatinine to ≥2.5 mg/dL over ≤2 weeks. **Type II hepatorenal syndrome**: resistant to diuretics. Treatment of hepatorenal syndrome includes midodrine, albumin, and octreotide.
17. ≥8 ribs on chest X-ray = consider hyperinflated lung = consider COPD
18. **Pulmonary nodules**: (A) ≥8 mm serial CT scans at 3, 6, 9 to 12 months, 18–24 months ⇒ PET → biopsy. (B) for nodules ≤6 mm, routine follow-up CT is not required, but if suspicious morphology or upper lobe location or high risk, will need to repeat CT at 12 months. (C) pure ground glass nodules ≥6 mm ⇒ continued surveillance by serial CT scan in 6–12 months. If <6 mm, repeat CT is not needed. Then every 2 years for a total of 5 years. Resection if Solitary pulmonary nodule at least 15–20 mm. (D) a part-solid (subsolid) nodule with a part-solid component likely to be malignant: if ≥6 mm, CT at 3–6 months, then at 5 years.

8/17/2017 Hyponatremia

1. Classification I: true volume depletion (gastrointestinal losses, thiazide use, and heat); decreased tissue perfusion [congestive heart failure (CHF) or cirrhosis]; syndrome of inappropriate antidiuretic hormone (SIADH).
2. Classification II: hypovolemia (gastrointestinal losses, renal losses); normovolemia (SIADH, primary polydipsia, low salt); hypervolemia (CHF or cirrhosis).
3. Causes of hyponatremia in HIV: symptomatic infection, volume depletion, SIADH, and adrenal insufficiency.
4. **Causes of hyponatremia**: (A) effective arterial blood volume depletion (CHF and cirrhosis), true volume depletion, diuretic-induced hyponatremia, CHF and cirrhosis. (B) SIADH. (C) endocrine disorders (hypothyroidism, adrenal insufficiency [hypovolemia induced by ADH increase, secondary euvolemic hyponatremia as seen in ectopic Atrial Natriuretic Peptide (ANP) in malignancy, exercise, MDMA ecstasy]). (D) hyponatremia with a high or normal serum osmolarity (glucose, mannitol, diabetic ketoacidosis, pseudohyponatremia as seen in increased serum lipids and proteins).
5. **Urine sodium > 40** ≥ consider hypovolemic hyponatremia from renal loss → review history and medications, measure morning cortisol and ACTH stimulation test (low cortisol and positive ACTH stimulation tests- glucocorticoid and mineralocorticoid deficiency, diuretics, head injury/cranial injury → suspected cerebral salt wasting).

6. If morning cortisol and ACTH stimulation test normal → TSH increase? If yes = consider hypothyroidism; if no = consider SIADH.
7. Measure serum and urine osmolarity → urine Na → morning cortisol and ACTH stimulation test → TSH test. **Urine osmolarity is usually greater than serum osmolarity** in SIADH.
8. Mild to moderate symptoms of hyponatremia include headache, nausea, vomiting, fatigue, gait disturbance, and confusion. In chronic hyponatremia (>48 h), these symptoms are not associated with impending herniation. However, in more acute hyponatremia, these can evolve into seizures, respiratory arrest, and herniation.
9. **Goal of emergency therapy**: The goal of non-emergent therapy is to increase serum sodium by 4–6 mEq/L over several hours, but should be <8 mEq/L over 24 h. Can monitor urine osmolarity, K, Na.
10. Over correction risks: **osmotic demyelination** (central pontine myelinolysis).
11. If overcorrection, give desmopressin 1 μg once with or without D5W bolus 250–500 cc. **Risks of osmotic demyelination** include Na ≤ 105, hypokalemia, alcoholism, malnutrition, and liver disease.
12. **Emergency therapy for hyponatremia**: normal saline (NS) 3% 100 mL over 10–15 min to raise serum Na by 2–3 mEq/L. Non-emergent asymptomatic acute/subacute can give 50 mL NS 3% over 10 min or 100 mL NS3% at a slower rate. In chronic severe hyponatremia with mild to moderate symptoms, can give 50 mL NS 3% bolus or NS 3% at 15–30 mL/h. Consider using desmopressin 1–2 μg iv or subcu q8h for 24–48 h to prevent the risks for overcorrection.
13. SIADH can be treated with oral salt tablets (1 g daily to 2 g tid): 1 g oral salt = 35 mL NS 3%. **KCL increases serum sodium.**
14. **CHF with hyponatremia** treatment: restricting fluid intake; ARB/ACEi/loop diuretics; tolvaptan (not in liver disease, no more than 30-day duration).

8/18/2017

1. Weigh patient: initiate weight-based heparin dosing at 15 u/kg/h with bolus dosing at 65 u/kg for Non-ST elevated myocardial infarction (NSTEMI).
2. **Heyde's syndrome** = triad of aortic stenosis (AS), gastrointestinal bleeding, and acquired von Willebrand syndrome (AVWS); bleeding usually is from angiodysplasia in patients with aortic stenosis.
3. Do not fall off the original diagnostic hypothesis.
4. **Central venous pressure** in cm = height of observed jugular venous distention + 5 cm (perpendicular to ground)
5. **Bactrim penetrates** the bladder wall better.
6. **NSTEMI**: may or may not have chest pain or ST-T wave abnormality, but chest pain if any is usually relieved with nitro, and almost always has elevated troponin.
7. **Congestive heart failure (CHF) diuresis** until HCO_3/Creatinine goes up slightly. Metoprolol's mortality benefit for diastolic CHF is unsure.

8. **Absolute reticulocyte** count is the number of reticulocytes during the time the reticulocyte spends in blood circulation before maturation. The range of the reticulocyte percentage is **0.5%–2.5%** in adults.
9. Corrected reticulocyte percentage = reticulocyte percentage × (HCT/45). Reticulocyte index also known as **reticulocyte production index** (RPI) = (HCT/45) × reticulocyte percentage/maturation time (RPI > 3 = normal BM; RPI < 2 = inadequate BM). **Reticulocyte maturation time** is 1 (day) for RBC maturation when hgb level is 45%–36%, 1.5 (days) for RBC maturation when hgb level is 16%–25%, and 2.5 (days) for RBC maturation when hgb level is ≤15%.
10. Serum osmolarity < urine osmolarity is consistent with SIADH.
11. **Cullen's sign and Grey Turner's sign** = consider retroperitoneal bleeding.

8/20/2017

1. **Pleural effusion analysis**: cytology, triglyceride, adenosine deaminase (useful for the diagnosis of tuberculous pleurisy), LDH, protein (serum and pleural fluid), pH, glucose, cell count and differential, culture, and sensitivity.
2. **Bloody pleural fluid**: pleural fluid Hgb <1% is nonsignificant; hgb 1%–20% usually indicates cancer, pulmonary embolism, trauma, or pneumonia; >50% indicates hemothorax.
3. **Cloudy or turbid pleural fluid**: check triglyceride, high triglyceride indicates chylothorax.
4. **Putrid odor indicates an abundance of mast cells** = consider possible anaerobic infections.
5. **Light's criteria**: pleural fluid protein/total serum protein ratio > 0.5 and pleural fluid LDH/serum LDH > 0.6 or 2/3 upper limit for serum LDH. Additional serum albumin—pleural albumin <1.2. If all met, it is exudate.
6. **Differential cell count** in pleural fluid analyses: neutrophil predominant—pulmonary embolism, pneumonitis, pneumonia, and empyema. Lymphocyte predominant—TB pleurisy, cancer. Eosinophilia predominant—pneumothorax, hemothorax, asbestosis, Churg-Strauss. Mononucleosis—chronic inflammation.
7. Glucose low in pleural fluid analyses—infection (pneumonia), malignancy, TB, hemothorax, Churg-Strauss.
8. Pleural fluid pH < 7.2 with pneumonia, need to drain the fluid; **pH < 7.2 with malignancy = possible life expectancy of 30 days**. **Asbestosis has bloody pleural** fluid with high lymphocytes and high ESR.
9. **Mesothelioma symptoms**: chest pain, dyspnea, cough, hoarseness, night sweats, or dysphagia. Chest X-ray shows unilateral pleural wall thickening and pleural effusion.
10. Initial **evaluation of mesothelioma** includes CT of the chest with contrast, thoracentesis, and closed pleural biopsy. If not sufficient tissue was acquired to make a diagnosis → video-assisted thoracic surgery (VATS) or open thoracostomy. Prognosis: overall survival of 9–17 months after diagnosis. Biomarkers: soluble mesothelin-related peptide, fibulin-3, and osteopontin.

11. **Histology of mesothelioma**: epitheloid (60%)—tubulopapillary, acinar (glandular), adenomatoid and solid epithelioid. Sarcomatoid—malignant spindle cells, mimicking leiomyosarcomas and synovial sarcoma. Biphasic or mixed.
12. **Hypercalcemia of malignancy**: PTHrP release, ectopic PTH, osteolytic metastases with local release of cytokines including osteoclast activating factors, tumor production of 1,25-dihydroxyvitamin D (calcitriol).
13. **PTHrP**: squamous cell carcinoma, breast cancer cells in bone (increases receptor activation of nuclear factor kappa B ligand (Rank L) in bone)—RANK→osteoclast activation.
14. Osteoclast activating factor as seen in multiple myeloma.
15. **1,25-dihydroxyvitamin D** elevation: all cases of hypercalcemia in Hodgkin lymphoma and 1/3 in non-Hodgkin lymphoma.
16. **Ectopic PTH secretions** in ovarian, small cell, and squamous cell lung carcinoma, primitive neuroectodermal tumor, thyroid papillary carcinoma, metastatic rhabdomyosarcoma, and pancreatic malignancy.

8/21/2017

1. **Hypercalcemia work-up**: serum PTH, PTHrP, vitamin D metabolites (25 hydroxyvitamin D and 1,25-dihydroxyvitamin D), serum electrophoresis and serum free light chains.
2. **Symptoms of hypercalcemia**: painful bones, renal stones, abdominal groans, and psychiatric moans.
3. Calcium correction in hypoalbuminemia: calcium = serum calcium + 0.8 (normal albumin of 4 – serum albumin).
4. Patients with **severe serum calcium** > 14 or symptomatic hypercalcemia require NS 0.9% at 200–300 cc/h → 100–150 cc/h. Additionally, give immediate calcitonin 4 iu/kg, repeat in several hours if necessary, or zoledronic acid 4 mg iv over 15 min (or pamidronate).
5. If refractory hypercalcemia or severe renal impairment, may use **denosumab**.
6. Glucocorticoids are effective in the treatment of hypercalcemia in lymphoma, sarcoid, and other granulomatous diseases.
7. 15% calcium bonds to organic and inorganic anions, 40% bonds to albumin, 45% active ionized (free) calcium.
8. Zoledronic acid can cause fever; PO_4 insufficiency should be supplemented with K Phos Neutral/KPO_4.
9. Heparin and Lovenox can increase potassium, and so does beta blocker. Albuterol causes hypokalemia, so does sodium bicarbonate.
10. **Atrial fibrillation** treatments: beta blocker, diltiazem, amiodarone, or cardioversion with 120–200 J biphasic or 200 J monophasic shock.
11. **Supraventricular tachycardia**: vasovagal maneuver, adenosine 6 mg iv push followed by 12 mg iv push if not effective; or cardioversion with 50–100 J monophasic cardioversion.
12. Ventricular tachycardia or ventricular fibrillation: cardioversion ASAP if shockable rhythm with 120–200 J biphasic or 360 J monophasic cardioversion. Give epinephrine 1 mg IV/IO with repeat every 3–5 min if PEA. Consider amioda-

rone 300 mg once then additional 150 mg once (follow advanced cardiovascular life support protocols).

13. **For Bradycardia**, if symptomatic and unstable, give **atropine** 0.5 mg iv once, may repeat to a total dose of 3 mg. If not working, start **dopamine** drip at 5 μg/kg/min or epinephrine 2–10 mg/min. Or 1 mg **epinephrine** is mixed with 500 ml of NS or D5W at 2–10 μg/min and titrated to the patient's response. Cardiologist consult stat for **transcutaneous pacer** before permanent pacemaker.
14. **Combined with anticholinergic medications oxybutynin**, suprapubic catheterization markedly reduces bladder infection and kidney damage when the catheter is regularly irrigated and changed.
15. **Colovesical fistulas** are mostly a complication of diverticulitis, cancer, or Crohn's disease. Surgery to repair is usually recommended and patients require Foley catheter for 7–10 days after surgery.
16. **Enterococcus** infection is treated with penicillin or vancomycin iv.

8/24/2017

1. **Adrenal crisis**: diagnostic—serum cortisol and serum chemistry should be drawn and samples should be held for later measurement of ACTH, renin, and aldosterone if diagnosis of adrenal insufficiency is likely. Treatment is hydrocortisone 100 mg iv once followed by 50 mg iv q6h.
2. **ACTH measurement**: at least 24 h after the last dose of a short-acting glucocorticoid (i.e., hydrocortisone) and even longer after long-acting glucocorticoids like dexamethasone. If a long-acting glucocorticoid, replace it with hydrocortisone first then after several days, measure ACTH.
3. **Gastric antral vascular ectasia (GAVE)** is an uncommon but often severe cause of upper gastrointestinal bleeding, responsible for 4% of nonvariceal upper GI bleeding. It is diagnosed via endoscopy ("watermelon" stomach). Histology of GAVE: vascular ectasia of mucosal capillaries, focal thrombosis, spindle cell proliferation, and fibrohyalinosis. **Potential treatments**: antrectomy, estrogen, octreotide, methylprednisolone, or cyclophosphamide with some evidence.
4. **Pulmonary embolism severity index (PESI)** is used to assess mortality related to pulmonary embolism.
5. **Thrombolysis for pulmonary embolism** is used when persistent hypotension, shock, or drop in systolic blood pressure ≥40 mmHg from baseline. **It should also be considered when a patient has a high mortality risk**.
6. Respiratory therapy consultation for incentive spirometry. Acapella is used for mucous clearance.
7. **Metamucil** = meta orange psyllium fiber supplement which can be used in both diarrhea and constipation.
8. **Risks with proton pump inhibitors**: C diff colitis, pneumonia, low magnesium and muscle spasms, heart palpitations, interstitial nephritis, and fracture of hip, wrist, and spine.

9. **Vitamin D deficiency treatment**: ergocalciferol 50,000 iu every week for 8 weeks, followed by cholecalciferol 1000 iu daily indefinitely.
10. **Neuropathy diagnosis**: check b12, methylmalonic acid, Vit D, EMG, and TSH.
11. **Tiotropium** increases urinary retention. **Loperamide** is used for diarrhea.
12. **Calcium polycarbophil** is a stool stabilizer for constipation, diarrhea, and abdominal discomfort.
13. **Combivent Respimat** = ipratropium bromide and albuterol
14. Prolonged QTc in patients with pacemakers requires **QTc correction**: decrease QTc in paced rhythm by 48.3 ms at a heart rate of 66 and by 81.3 ms at a faster rate: 527 − 81.3 ms = 447 ms at HR 88 for corrected QTc.
15. **Liraglutide (Victoza)**: is an incretin (metabolize hormone) memetic, glucagon-like peptide-1 (GLP-1) agonist that stimulates insulin secretion, decreases prandial glucagon secretion, delays gastric emptying, causes GI discomforts, pancreatitis, and possible thyroid cancer, but less hypoglycemic episodes.
16. **GLP-1 agonists** including bid exenatide, daily liraglutide and semaglutide, and weekly albiglutide and dulaglutide in combination with base insulin are good for diabetes control.

8/25/2017

1. **COPD severity** based on FEV1: mild ≥80%, moderate 50%–80%, severe 30%–50%, very severe <30%.
2. **Hypertension** in adults can be treated with calcium channel blocker, then beta blocker. Hypertension in alcohol withdrawal can be treated with clonidine or metoprolol in the short term.
3. **Prazosin** is used for PTSD, nightmares, and urinary retention.
4. **Subclinical hypothyroidism**: normal free T4 in the presence of elevated TSH, treat only if TSH ≥ 10, especially if thyroid peroxidase antibody positive.
5. NSAIDs can increase cardiovascular disease risk. Usually, albumin is 60% of total protein.
6. QTc correction is necessary for pacer, RBBB, and LBBB.
7. Dysphagia II diet (ground food thick liquid); dysphagia I diet (pureed food with nectar thick liquids).
8. **PET** uses fluoro-deoxy-glucose to assess metabolisms of the human body.
9. **Smoking cessation treatment**: nicotine patch 21 g daily for 4 weeks, followed by 14 g daily for 4 weeks and 7 g daily for 4 weeks.
10. **Sepsis vs septic shock**: whether we can maintain blood pressure after 30 ml/kg intravenous fluid in the first 2–3 h. If not, it is likely septic shock. Severe sepsis is defined as sepsis with organ dysfunction, hypoperfusion, or hypotension.
11. In contrast to CPAP, auto-titrating positive airway pressure (APAP) devices deliver varying pressure based on the patient's needs. These varying pressures increase breathing synchrony.
12. Uncontrolled obstructive sleep apnea increases risks for **stroke and cardiac events**.
13. 1 beer = 154 calories. CPAP pressure typically 4–20 cm H_2O.
14. Ipratropium is short-acting and tiotropium is long-acting.

15. Acute kidney injury due to cardiorenal vs prerenal is dependent on volume status.
16. Mometasone is a corticosteroid inhalant. **Oral inhalation is used for asthma while nasal inhalation is for allergic rhinitis.**
17. **Urticaria treatment**: antihistamines (cetirizine or loratadine) and H2 blockers (ranitidine, famotidine, or cimetidine), a brief course of prednisone, and topical triamcinolone.
18. Typically, PVCs may go away with a stress test.

8/27/2017

1. Doxycycline and azithromycin can also decrease inflammation. Benzonatate is an antitussive, 100–200 mg tid prn for cough; guaifenesin is another antitussive.
2. **May-Thurner syndrome**: iliac vein compression syndrome → lower extremity vein compression causing dysfunction, swelling, pain or blood clots (DVTs) in the iliofemoral vein, accounts for 2%–3% lower extremity DVTs, typically in patients with 20–40 s of age. May-Thurner syndrome nowadays also known as **nonthrombotic iliac vein lesions** and can involve both the right and left iliac veins as well as other named venous segments. Symptoms include pain in a dependent position. Treatment includes **concomitant angioplasty and stenting** of the affected segment (followed by antiplatelet therapy and compression stockings) if not deep vein thrombosis, concomitant thrombolysis, and anticoagulation if DVT.
3. Pulmonary embolism may have an EKG showing S1Q3T3. Screening in patients with no other obvious reason for **hypercoagulability**: antithrombin, Protein C and S, Factor V Leiden, prothrombin G20210A, cardiolipin, lupus antibody, and homocysteine.
4. **Pulmonary embolism additional workups** include echo, troponin, lower extremity venous Doppler, and BNP.
5. Retinal detachment: more in anticoagulation, but not statistically significant.
6. Lidocaine patch and capsaicin patch, q12h for pain and can increase to q8h.
7. With the use of Lasix or diuretics, kidney function improves ≥ it possibly indicates the cause of kidney failure is **cardiorenal syndrome**.
8. Rate control **≤ 110 bpm** with activities and **< 85 bpm** at rest is ideal for AFib. **Heavy drinking takes 7 days** to develop dependence and possible withdrawal if stop drinking suddenly.
9. **Bone marrow suppression from alcohol** causes thrombocytopenia or even pancytopenia.
10. Diltiazem and verapamil can cause vasodilation and decrease blood pressure, but verapamil has less vasodilation and better heart rate control.
11. Dabigatran (Pradaxa) requires at least 5–10 days of initial therapy with a parenteral anticoagulant, then 150 mg oral bid. It has a reversible agent **idarucizumab**.
12. Blood culture typically is ordered with 2 sets. **Contaminated blood culture samples**: G+ bacilli from epithelium, usually only one of the bottles positive. **Blood culture contaminants**: coagulase-negative Staphylococcus, aerobic and

anaerobic diphtheroid, Propionibacterium species, bacillus, and viridians group streptococci. If one or more additional blood cultures were obtained within 48 h and all were negative, the isolate may be considered a contaminant.

13. **Sputum culture sample contamination criteria**: too many squamous cells and epithelial cells.
14. **Urine culture contaminants**: bacteria normally considered to be skin, vaginal, and rectal contamination, such as staph spp., not aureus in mixed culture, lactobacillus spp., diphtheroid (Corynebacterium spp), anaerobic gram negative bacilli (rods), viridian group streptococci, non-hemolytic strep, not enterococcus.
15. **Daptomycin should not be used in pneumonia** as it inhibits surfactants. Daptomycin also causes hepatotoxicity and creatinine kinase elevation (rhabdomyolysis).
16. **Allergic bronchitis treatment**: loratadine 10 mg daily, ranitidine 150 mg bid, Mometasone furoate 220 mg oral inhalation 2 puff bid with mouth rinse after.

8/29/2017

1. **Hypercapnic respiratory failure**: $PaCO_2 > 45$, acute (pH < 7.4), chronic (pH normal). Noninvasive ventilation (like BiPAP) is used in pH < 7.3, RR > 25, and increased work of breathing.
2. **Hypoxemic hypercapnic respiratory failure** refers to SO_2 < 90%–92% or PaO_2 < 60–70 mmHg together with CO_2 retention.
3. The development of acute hypercapnia with significant acidemia (pH < 7.2) and/or marked decrease in the level of consciousness may require **STAT intubation and mechanical ventilation**.
4. Non-invasive ventilation refers to positive pressure ventilation delivered through a noninvasive interface like a nasal mask, face mask, or helmet.
5. Unfractionated heparin is cleared through hepatic and renal mechanisms, whereas low molecular weight heparin is dependent on renal clearance.
6. **Metabolic encephalopathy (toxic metabolic encephalopathy)** is a broad category that describes abnormalities of water, electrolytes, vitamins, and other chemicals that adversely affect brain function.
7. Confusion is a state; **delirium** = confusion + superimposed hyperactivity of the nervous system. Acute toxic metabolic encephalopathy encompasses delirium and the acute confusional state in the absence of primary brain diseases.
8. **Asthma step-up treatment**: step 1 all need a short-acting beta agonist (SABA); step 2 add low-dose inhaled corticosteroid (ICS); step 3 low dose ICS + LABA OR low dose ICS + LAMA OR moderate dose ICS OR low dose ICS + leukotriene receptor antagonist (LTRA); step 4 increase ICS dose (with LABA), may add LAMA/LTRA; step 5 oral steroids.
9. **COPD control**: step 1 SABA prn; step 2 standing inhaled bronchodilator (LAMA is preferred over LABA); step 3 (ICS plus LABA) or LAMA; step 4 ICS + (LAMA and/or LABA), can add phosphodiesterase-4 (PDE-4) inhibitor roflumilast to prevent exacerbation.

10. COPD treatment: SABA [albuterol, levalbuterol (Xopenex) → **LAMA** (tiotropium, aclidinium, glycopyrrolate)] or/and LABA (Salmeterol, indacaterol, olodaterol, vinlanterol) → add ICS.
11. **COPD exacerbation diagnosis** requires worsening cough, dyspnea, or/and sputum. If only 1 out of 3 symptoms, it is mild, can increase bronchodilator. If at least 2 out of 3 symptoms, it is moderate or severe (complicated if at least 1 risk factor; uncomplicated if no risk factors), can add antibiotics. If C reactive protein >20–40 mg/L, antibiotics probably necessary.
12. Non-risk factors: age < 65, FEV1 > 50%, <2 exacerbations a year, no cardiac disease.
13. Antibiotics for **uncomplicated** COPD exacerbations, use macrolide or cephalosporins or doxycycline or TMP-SMX. For **complicated** COPD exacerbations, use fluoroquinolones, and Augmentin (if risk for pseudomonas, use Levaquin and culture sputum).
14. **Pseudomonas risks**: advanced COPD, previous isolation of pseudomonas from sputum, concomitant bronchiectasis, frequent administration of antibiotics, frequent hospitalizations, systemic steroid use.
15. Advair = fluticasone propionate and salmeterol.
16. ICS: flunisolide, fluticasone, budesonide, mometasone, ciclesonide, beclomethasone.

8/30/2017

1. **Osteomyelitis**: diagnosis with MRI, bone scan if MRI not possible; X-ray shows osteomyelitis → MRI (may not be necessary) and surgery (podiatrist or general surgeon, sometimes needs vascular surgery service to improve blood circulation as well).
2. **End-stage renal disease (ESRD)** causes angiodysplasia and gastrointestinal bleeding.
3. **Extended Spectrum Beta-Lactamase (ESBL) positive bacterium** is typically treated with meropenem or ertapenem. Piperacillin and tazobactam is only 57.9% sensitive and can be 98% sensitive if pep/tazo is combined with Amikacin; it is 29.6% sensitive with Cipro.
4. **Sepsis diagnosis requires two or more of the following of the SIRS criteria**: T > 38 or < 36; HR > 90, RR > 20 or $PaCO_2$ < 32; WBC > 12 or <4 or >10% immature bands; with a possible source of infection.
5. Alternatively, sepsis can also be made if meeting two or more of the following qSOFA criteria: RR ≥ 22, AMS, sBP ≤ 100 mmHg.
6. The frequently increased levels of serum **prolactin** levels were observed immediately after generalized and complex partial seizures.
7. **Septic shock**: sepsis and vasopressor therapy are needed to maintain MAP ≥65 and treat lactate >2 mmol/L despite adequate fluid resuscitation (30 mL/kg).
8. Conditions associated with **angiodysplasia** account for 20% upper GI bleed and 30% lower GI bleed, seen in: ESRD, von Willebrand disease, aortic stenosis, left ventricular assist device.

9. **Differentials mnemonic** for diagnosis workups: VITAMIN C- vascular, infectious, traumatic, autoimmune, metabolic, idiopathic/iatrogenic, neoplastic, and congenital.
10. **Spontaneous bacterial peritonitis (SBP)** refers to an ascitic fluid infection without an evident intra-abdominal surgically treatable source in cirrhosis and ascites. Typical symptoms may include fever, abdominal pain, or altered mentation.
11. The diagnosis of SBP is established by a positive ascitic fluid culture or polymorphonuclear neutrophils (PMNs) > 250 cells/mL in ascitic fluid. **Treatment of SBP**: empiric antibiotic treatment, give IV albumin 1.5 g/kg at diagnosis and 1 g/kg on day 3, discontinue beta blockers. Can use cefotaxime 2 g q8h or ceftriaxone 2 g daily for 5 days.
12. **Ceftriaxone for SBP prophylaxis** in hospitalized cirrhosis patients: GI bleed and cirrhosis; one or more episodes of SBP; ascitic fluid protein < 1.5 and creatinine > 1.2 or BUN > 25 or serum Na < 130 or Child-Pugh score ≥ 9.

8/31/2017

1. **Cellulitis treatment**: screen for DVT and treat with cefazolin (the majority of infection is caused by Streptococcus) or vancomycin if concerns of MRSA.
2. **Alcoholic cirrhosis treatment**: spironolactone to furosemide ratio 100–40; low salt diet, non-selective beta blocker (like nadolol 20 mg daily and hold if heart rate < 60 bpm, not appropriate in acute decompensated liver failure).
3. **Paracentesis indications**: anyone with ascites with signs and symptoms of infection like fever, hypotension, peripheral leukocytosis, encephalopathy, or acidosis. Any patient with first-time ascites also should get paracentesis.
4. **Paracentesis fluid analysis**: amylase, protein, albumin, cell count, LDH, culture, glucose.
5. **Hepatic encephalopathy** can have asterixis; fetor hepaticus = breath smells musty.
6. **Reye syndrome**: aspirin metabolites decrease beta-oxidation by reversible inhibition of mitochondrial enzymes. Reye syndrome typically happens after parents use aspirin to treat viral syndromes in children. It causes swelling in the liver and brain and thus death.
7. **Mallory bodies** (damaged intermediate filaments): intracytoplasmic eosinophilic inclusions in alcoholic hepatitis, but can also be seen in nonalcoholic steatohepatitis (NASH), cholestatic liver diseases, and primary biliary cirrhosis (PBC).
8. **Gamma-glutamyl transferase (GGT)** is not increased in bone disease but liver diseases; skeletal muscle injury or disease typically has AST ≫ ALT.
9. **Chronic hepatitis B**: consider liver biopsy if ALT 1–2 × upper limit normal (ULN) or immune tolerated phase if age > 40. Treat if moderate to severe inflammation or fibrosis on biopsy. Treatment: entecavir/tenofovir if lamivudine-resistant, PEG-IFN (pegylated interferon).

10. **HCV is treated with RNA polymerase inhibitor (RNAPi)** (sofosbuvir), ribonucleic analog to stop RNA replication (ribavirin), and sofosbuvir/velpatasvir (band name Epclusa).
11. Lab monitoring for patients on **HCV treatment**: CBC, INR, LFTs, GFR, HCV viral load, and TSH (if interferon is used) prior to starting treatment. Protease inhibitors are contraindicated if decompensated liver disease (ascites and encephalopathy) or CTP score ≥ 7. Discontinue if jaundice, nausea, vomiting, weakness, 10 × increase in ALT, or significant increase in bilirubin, or INR after 4 weeks.
12. **Autoimmune hepatitis**, Type 1: anti-smooth muscle antibody positive; Type 2 anti-liver/kidney microsome 1 (anti-lkm1) positive. **Treatment if ALT × 10 upper limit normal** (ULN), or ALT × 5 ULN and IgG × 2 ULN or bridging or multiacinar necrosis. **Treatment**: prednisone monotherapy; prednisone and azathioprine (can be used in cirrhosis); or budesonide if not cirrhotic + azathioprine.
13. **Alcoholic hepatitis** uses Maddrey's discriminant function (MDF). Consider treatment with steroids if the MDF score ≥32, and/or the MELD score > 20. Treatment includes **methylprednisolone** 32 mg/day or prednisolone 40 mg/day for 4 weeks with a 4–6-week taper. This is **contraindicated if active GI bleed, pancreatitis, untreated HBV, or uncontrolled infections**.
14. **Acetaminophen injury** (>10 g, recommended maximum daily dose <4 g) depletes glutathione stores; CYP2E1 (a member of the cytochrome P450 mixed-function oxidase system in the liver) can be induced by fasting, alcohol, and certain anti-convulsants and anti-TB treatments. **CYP2E1 inducers** cause liver injury with acetaminophen dosage even as low as 2 g/day. **Treatment of acetaminophen toxicity**: charcoal if within 4 h of ingestion; oral N-acetylcysteine 140 mg/kg loading dose → 70 mg/kg q4h × 17 additional doses. If IV (not preferred), give 150 mg/kg × 1 h → 50 mg/kg for 4 h → 100 mg/kg × 16 h.
15. **Fondaparinux 2.5 mg subcutaneously** is used in HIT, pork allergies, and religious reasons. DVT ppx dosage is 2.5 mg subcu daily.

9/3/2017

1. **Shock liver (ischemic hepatitis)** usually has AST and ALT greater than 1000 and significant elevation of LDH and total bilirubin.
2. The presence of hematuria is common in UTI (acute cystitis) but not in urethritis or vaginitis. Celiac disease antibodies: antigliadin peptide, **antitransglutaminase**, antiendomysial antibodies.
3. **Steroid taper indications**: glucocorticoid use ≥20 mg/day of prednisone for ≥3 weeks; evening/bedtime dose ≥5 mg of prednisone for more than a few weeks; or cushingoid appearance.
4. Two conditions requiring **immediate cessation of glucocorticoids** or a significant rapid reduction rather than tapering: steroid-induced psychosis nonresponsive to antipsychotic medications, and herpes-induced corneal ulceration.
5. **NAFL** (Non-alcoholic fatty liver) = steatosis and no inflammation. **NASH** = steatosis + inflammation +/− fibrosis on biopsy. Treatment: weight loss ≥10%,

exercise, diabetes control (liraglutide or pioglitazone may be beneficial), statins, vitamin E decreases steatosis but not fibrosis.

6. **Acute liver failure** = acute insult to liver + coagulopathy + encephalopathy. Fulminant hepatic failure (FHF) = encephalopathy within 2 weeks of the first manifestation of liver disease.
7. **Workup for acute liver failure**: PT/INR, PTT, ammonia, BUN/Cr, pH, lactate, acetaminophen level, ceruloplasmin, serum/urine copper, pregnancy test.
8. **Decompensated cirrhosis** = jaundice, variceal bleeding, encephalopathy, and/or ascites.
9. **Cirrhosis treatment**: decrease Na intake to 1–2 g/day, diuretics (spironolactone/furosemide = 100/40), avoid NSAIDs. If large volume paracentesis (>5-L ascitic fluid removal), will need to give 6–8 g albumin/L fluid, avoid large volume paracentesis if spontaneous bacterial peritonitis to minimize acute kidney injury.
10. **Hepatic hydrothorax** secondary to diaphragmatic defect often on the right side, less common on the left side; avoid chest tube, because it may develop spontaneous empyema.
11. **Spontaneous bacterial peritonitis (SBP)** treatment: third generation cephalosporins or Augmentin for 5 days; iv albumin 1.5 g/kg at diagnosis and 1 g/kg on day 3. If not responding, repeat paracentesis in 48 h.
12. **Indefinite prophylaxis of spontaneous bacterial peritonitis indications**: history of SBP; ascitic total protein < 1.5 plus Na < 130, creatinine > 1.2, BUN ≥ 25, or (CPS ≥ 9 and total bilirubin ≥ 3). Usually use Cipro 500 mg daily or Bactrim Double strength daily.
13. **Child-Pugh score for cirrhosis mortality**: bilirubin, albumin, INR, ascites, encephalopathy.
14. **Portosystemic encephalopathy** treatment: lactulose with a goal of 2–4 stools per day, with or without rifaximin 550 mg bid. Prevention of upper gastrointestinal bleeding: nadolol, propranolol (use carvedilol if nonresponsive)
15. **Ursodeoxycholic acid (UDCA) also known as ursodiol** is used for the treatment of primary sclerosing cholangitis (PSC) and primary biliary cholangitis (PBC), cholesterol gallstones.
16. **Pruritus in primary biliary cholangitis** treatment: cholestyramine (give 2–4 h after UDCA); if refractory symptoms, use naltrexone, or rifampin.
17. **Endoscopic retrograde cholangiopancreatography (ERCP)** is used in choledocholithiasis, primary sclerosing cholangitis, gallstone pancreatitis, and cholangitis. If ERCP is not successful, do percutaneous transhepatic cholangiogram.
18. A **hepatobiliary iminodiacetic acid (HIDA)** scan (hepatobiliary scan) is the most sensitive test to diagnose acute cholecystitis.

9/4/2017

1. Cellulitis, check for deep vein thrombosis as a differential. Selective beta-blockers (metoprolol, atenolol, and bisoprolol) are ok to use in COPD.

2. Use **Levaquin** with caution in old patients, because of its risks for tendonitis and tendon rupture especially in seniors >60 years old and with the concurrent use of prednisone.
3. Obstructive sleep apnea: check respiratory oxygen saturation overnight with result reports.
4. **Propafenone** is the last resort for SVT/VTs. Side effects of propafenone include herpes, hypersensitivity, agranulocytosis, and CNS disturbance.
5. Ventolin = albuterol sulfate. Singulair = montelukast sodium
6. **Lisinopril** at 2.5–5 mg is used for the heart, at 10–40 mg is for hypertension.
7. **Propranolol**: for hypertension, use 40 mg bid; for migraine, use 80 mg/day every 6 or 8 h; for thyrotoxicosis, use 10–40 mg every 6–8 h, which can go up to 60–80 mg every 6 h.
8. **Angiogram (contrast dye) kidney toxicity prevention**: NAC 600 mg bid and bicarb 1 h before and after showed no additional benefits while the normal saline infusion is effective in preventing contrast dye-induced kidney injury.
9. **Cocaine withdrawal** treatment: clonidine 0.1 mg tid, Ativan 1 mg q6h.
10. **Shiley catheter** for dialysis; side effects include clotting, infection, and kinking.
11. **Pseudomembranous colitis** (necrotic epithelial cells, mucus, fibrin, and neutrophils): frequently patchy with abrupt involvement of 2–10 or more crypts swelling and inflammation of the large intestine due to C. difficile infection. It is characterized by profuse, watery mucoid, and foul-smelling stools, especially common in patients with beta lactam or clindamycin use.
12. Bumex can be absorbed through a swollen gut; no beta-blocker use in spontaneous bacterial peritonitis.

9/9/2017

1. **Bladder scan** is unreliable in patients with **ascites**.
2. We may use **dexamethasone** (hydrocortisone still preferred) in acute adrenal deficiency while we can still order and get a relatively accurate **cortisol** test.
3. In sudden onset shortness of breath, we need to rule out **acute coronary syndrome (ACS) and acute pulmonary embolism**.
4. For low blood pressure, midodrine may be used (when IV fluid or pressor support is not appropriate) but can **precipitate bradycardia**. If bradycardia, may use fludrocortisone or intravenous hydrocortisone.
5. Anaerobic culture is preferred in the culture of tissue or aspirates. **Anaerobic flora** is prevalent in mucosal surfaces of the oral cavity, upper respiratory tract, gastrointestinal and genitourinary tracts. Specimens from these sites should not ordinarily be cultured for anaerobic bacteria but rather as **anaerobic culture**.
6. **Pyuria** is defined as the persistent findings of white blood cells in urine (10 WBC/cm^3 or >3 WBC/HPF or leukocyte esterase positive) in the absence of bacteria by culture. It is commonly seen in urethritis, nephritis, renal tuberculosis, and foreign bodies.
7. The following drug levels may require serum lab check: acetaminophen, amikacin, carbamazepine, chloramphenicol, digoxin, ethosuximide, flecainide, gentamicin, imipenem, lithium, phenobarbital, valproic acid, quinine.

8. **Urinary tract infection (UTI)**: upper UTI include pyelonephritis, renal and perinephric abscess, and prostatitis; lower UTI include urethritis and cystitis.
9. **Complicated versus non-complicated UTI**: underlying structural, neurological disease, bladder dysfunction, or immunocompromised is complicated UTI. UTI in males is automatically considered a complicated UTI.
10. Microbiology- **common bacteria in UTI**. Uncomplicated UTI: **E. coli (80%),** Proteus, Klebsiella, S. saprophyticus. Complicated UTI: E. coli (30%), **enterococcus (20%), Pseudomonas** aeruginosa, S. epidermidis, and other gram-negative rods. Catheter-associated UTI: yeast (30%), E. coli (25%), other Gram-negative rods, enterococci, S. epidermidis. Urethritis (can have discharge and usually pyuria only): chlamydia, gonorrhea, trichomonas, mycoplasma, HSV.
11. **Urine culture**: the isolation of organisms such as lactobacilli, enterococci, GBS, and coagulase-negative staphylococcus other than **S. saprophyticus** from voided urine may represent contamination of the specimen. However, if in voided midstream urine, found at high counts and pure growth, should be considered as a likely causative agent.
12. If there is a diagnostic uncertainty regarding cystitis versus early pyelonephritis. The use of **nitrofurantoin** 100 mg bid for 5 days, **fosfomycin**, and **pivmecillinam** should be avoided because they do not achieve adequate renal tissue levels while TMP-SMX may be used.
13. For acute cystitis, acceptable beta-lactam agents include amoxicillin-clavulanate, cefpodoxime, cefdinir, and cefadroxil for 5–7 days. Fluoroquinolone (leva, Cipro, ofloxacin) 3 days also works.
14. Inpatient **management of pyelonephritis** includes iv fluoroquinolones, aminoglycosides with or without ampicillin, an extended spectrum cephalosporins/penicillin, or a carbapenem.

9/10/2017

1. The majority of **pelvic inflammatory disease (PID)** causes are sexually transmitted infections or bacterial vaginosis-associated pathogens. They account for 85% of the causes.
2. PID during pregnancy is rare but can happen in **the first 12 weeks of gestation**, although mucus plugs from gestation supposedly decreases the risk. Diarrhea and lower abdominal symptoms may be common in PID.
3. **PID risk factors**: instrumentation of cervix, salpingitis (premenarcheal and adolescents not sexually active); in these situations, respiratory and enteric bacteria should be considered.
4. PID inflammatory process extending to the liver capsule to cause **perihepatitis** (Fitz-Hugh Curtis syndrome).
5. **PID signs and symptoms**: constant achy lower abdominal pain, tender abdomen, uterine bleeding, urinary frequency and abnormal vaginal discharge.
6. Acute cervical motion, and uterine and adnexal tenderness on bimanual pelvic examination are the defining characteristics of acute symptomatic PID.

7. **Lab works for PID**: pregnancy test, microscopic exam and gram stain of vaginal discharge, nucleic acid amplification for C. trachomatis and N. gonorrhoeae, HIV screening and syphilis serology.
8. **First line inpatient treatment for PID**: cefoxitin 2 g iv q6h or cefotetan 2 g iv q12h plus **doxycycline** 100 mg q12h; **ceftriaxone** plus **metronidazole** plus **doxycycline** 100 mg q12h; or clindamycin 900 mg q8h plus gentamicin loading dose 2 mg/kg of body weight followed by 1.5 mg/kg q8h. An alternative regimen is ampicillin-sulbactam 3 g q6h plus doxycycline 100 mg bid
9. **Outpatient treatment for PID**: ceftriaxone 250 mg im single dose plus doxycycline 100 mg po bid for 14 days and metronidazole 500 mg bid for 14 days. Cefoxitin 2 g im with probenecid 1 g plus doxycycline for 14 days and metronidazole 500 mg bid for 14 days. Other parental third generation cephalosporins, such as cefotaxime (1 g im in a single dose) or ceftriaxone 1 g in a single dose plus doxycycline 100 mg bid for 14 days and metronidazole 500 mg bid for 14 days.
10. **High potassium treatment**: D50 25–50 g iv, regular insulin 10 units, calcium gluconate if EKG changes, albuterol inhaler, Kayexalate 30 g or Lokelma (sodium zirconium cyclosilicate) 10 g tid for 6 doses (may stop early). Can also add bicarbonate drip or bolus.
11. **Ventricular tachycardia**, the transition from intravenous amiodarone to oral amiodarone should overlap 2–1 h, can do 400 mg tid for 3 days, 400 mg bid for 3 days, 400 mg daily for 3 days, then 200 mg daily forever. **Pulseless VT or VFib**: follows advanced cardiovascular life support protocol, after **third shock** if nonresponsive to shock, while continuing CPR and pressors, can give amiodarone 300 mg iv push, additional 150 mg iv if needed, upon return of spontaneous circulation, give 1 mg/min for 6 h, then 0.5 mg/min for 18 h. For stable ventricular tachycardia, can use amiodarone 150 mg iv once followed by the abovementioned drip. Mean daily amiodarone dosage >2.1 g can cause hypotension.
12. **Poor appetite**, may add Remeron 7.5 mg daily, or megestrol (has glucocorticoid and estrogen activities) 400 mg liquid bid.
13. **Antibiotics for bacteremia**: Gram-negative mostly treated for 7–14 days; gram-positive should be given antibiotics for 2–6 weeks depending on diagnoses. Patients with S. aureus bacteremia should be treated with 14 days of IV antibiotics from the first negative blood culture. All patients should undergo echocardiography to evaluate the presence of endocarditis; TEE may be warranted.

9/11/2017

1. **Esophagogastroduodenoscopy (EGD)** preparation: hold Plavix and Prasugrel for 7 days, Ticagrelor for 5 days, Eliquis for 2 days, and Pradaxa 1–2 days.
2. **Nothing per mouth (NPO) order** is necessary for anything requiring sedation including but not limited to transesophageal echocardiogram (TEE), upper GI studies like EGD, upper GI series, and stress test.
3. Only the presence of clear evidence of **volume depletion** (e.g., hypotension, decreased skin turgor, elevated hematocrit, possibly increased BUN/creatinine

ratio) despite a urine Na not low that suggests **cerebral salt wasting** rather than SIADH. By comparison, extracellular fluid volume is normal or increased in SIADH. Both have higher urine osmolarity as compared to serum osmolarity, **increased urine sodium of > 40 mEq/L, and decreased serum uric acid.**

4. **Gram-negative bacteremia** without sepsis: in immunocompetent patients, use ceftriaxone 2 g daily, ceftazidime 2 g q8h; in patients with hospital exposure or immunocompromised, will need Pseudomonas coverage with Zosyn or cefepime.
5. **Gram-negative bacteremia** with sepsis or septic shock: in immunosuppression, use gentamicin/tobramycin/amikacin (in reality, not commonly used) plus one of the following (cefepime, ceftazidime, Zosyn or meropenem). However, if there is no additional risk for drug-resistant bacteria, use only one of the following medications for pseudomonas coverage: cefepime, carbapenems, Zosyn, Levaquin. In septic shock, add vancomycin; may need to use vancomycin plus Zosyn and Levaquin if concerns for pseudomonas resistance.
6. For gram-negative bacteremia, initially give antibiotics parentally, but once the patient has effervesced and has remained **afebrile for 48 h** or longer, antibiotics can be switched to oral.
7. **Long-term catheter removal** is indicated in the setting of septic shock, suppurative thrombophlebitis, endocarditis, and bacteremia that continues despite greater than 72 h of appropriate antimicrobial therapy or infection due to Pseudomonas aeruginosa.
8. **Wernicke encephalopathy diagnosis** requires two of the following: dietary deficiency of thiamine, oculomotor abnormalities, cerebellar dysfunction, and either altered mental status or mild memory deficit. Treatment: thiamine 500 mg iv over 30 min tid for 2 days and 250 mg iv daily for 5 days and followed by oral thiamine 100 mg daily forever.
9. **Dysphagia (esophageal) etiologies**: diffuse esophageal spasm, nutcracker, and hypertensive lower esophagus sphincter. **Treatment**: diltiazem 180–240 mg daily for dysphagia patients. For primary symptoms of chest pain from dysphagia, give TCA (like imipramine 25–50 mg at bedtime) or calcium channel blocker (CCB) or trazodone 50 mg at night.
10. **Gastroesophageal reflux disease (GERD) symptoms treatment**: PPI once daily for 2 months first → if fail, switch to a different PPI → if fail, do PPI twice daily for 2 months. If fails, do esophageal impedance and pH studies.
11. Haloperidol should not be used in alcoholic Wernicke encephalopathy.
12. **Leukocyte larceny**: low PO_2 with ABG but normal pulse oximetry. It happens if the WBC count is > 50; it is due to excess oxygen consumption by leukocytes.
13. BiPAP will need to set EPAP and IPAP, and look at tidal volume, 200 cc is dead space (normal tidal volume is around 400 cc in females and 500 cc in males). **Minute ventilation** (tidal volume × respiratory rate) + 100% wall O_2.
14. Nasal cannula oxygen → venturimask → non-breather (Reservoir face mask) → high flow → BiPAP → PRVC ventilator.

9/12/2017

1. **Confusion**, check ammonia, ABG, CMP, mag, BNP, check telemetry. **Bleeding**, check INR, and LFTs, if fibrinogen less than 150 and bleeding consider transfuse cryoglobulin. **Seizure**, do Ativan 2 mg iv/im, Keppra load 2 g or 1 g, vitals, glucose check. **Syncope**, check tele, echo, rule out severe pulmonary hypertension, cerebrovascular accident.
2. No pulse, call **code blue**, may need to continue code until family arrival for young patients. **Chest compression, epinephrine 1 mg q3-5 min, bicarb, mag 4 mg, calcium gluconate 2 g**.
3. **Nifedipine** immediate release 10–20 mg tid; extended-release 60 mg daily. **Labetalol** 100–300 mg bid, maximum 2400 mg over 24 h. **Hydralazine** 10 mg qid for 2–4 days → 25 mg qid → 50 mg qid (maximum 300 mg over 24 h); use in combination with isosorbide dinitrate. **Lisinopril** 5–40 mg daily. **Isosorbide mononitrate** (Imdur) 5 mg, 10 mg, 20 mg bid for immediate release; extended-release 30–60 mg daily up to 120 or 240 mg daily. **Spironolactone** 50–100 mg daily, usually 12.5–25 mg daily for CHF.
4. **Ground glass opacity** on CT chest is a nonspecific finding; it indicates partial filling of airspaces and interstitial thickening or partial collapse of lung alveoli. **Differentials** include pulmonary edema, infection (like CMV, PCP, and other atypical pneumonia), interstitial lung disease (hypersensitivity pneumonitis), diffuse alveolar hemorrhage, and cryptogenic pneumonia.
5. **Hospital-acquired pneumonia** (HAP) or **ventilator-associated pneumonia** (VAP) is a clinical diagnosis based on a new lung infiltrate plus clinical evidence that the infiltrate is of infectious origin; symptoms includes fever, purulent sputum, leukocytosis, and a decrease in oxygenation.
6. **Blood pressure control** in ischemic stroke: blood pressure medications should be withheld unless systolic blood pressure greater than 220 mmHg or diastolic blood pressure greater than 120 mmHg. The first line treatment is labetalol (if no contraindications like bradycardia) 10–20 mg iv for 1–2 min, repeat every 10 min to a maximum dose of 300 mg; also, can use nicardipine 2.5 mg/h every 5 min or nicardipine drip. **Exceptions include end-organ damage like pulmonary edema, aortic dissection, and hypertensive encephalopathy which all require rapid blood pressure control to sBP <140 or lower**.

9/14/2017

1. **Glucose control** is acute stroke patients: insulin to achieve a glucose target of 140–180 mg. If fasting glucose is greater than 140 or random glucose is constantly >180, give additional or increase scheduled insulin dosage. A lower glucose target of <140 mg/mL may be appropriate for patients with well-controlled diabetes and stress hyperglycemia and no diabetes history before hospitalization.
2. **Hemolysis panel**: LDH, haptoglobin, hemoglobin, Coombs test, electrophoresis, iron, total iron binding capacity (TIBC), ferritin.
3. **Gastrointestinal (GI) bleed**: avoid volume overload, give fresh frozen plasma (FFP) if INR high, call gastroenterology consultation, iv proton pump inhibitor

(PPI), and stop or hold antihypertensive medications. Type and screen, packed red blood cell (PRBC) transfusion. Anemia kills patients by heart and thus it is often necessary to check troponin.

4. **Leukemoid reaction** (a reaction to stress or infection): leukocytosis exceeding 50,000/μL is referred to as a leukemoid reaction and is often characterized by a significant increase in early neutrophil precursors (e.g., promyelocytes, metamyelocytes, and myelocytes) in peripheral blood along with increased numbers of band forms, even less mature neutrophil precursors (promyelocytes, myeloblasts). Proliferation of the most immature elements (e.g., promyelocytes, myeloblasts) is specific for **acute leukemia** (defined as 20% or greater blasts [immature white blood cells] in the marrow or blood).
5. **White blood cell differentiation**: eosinophilic/basophilic/neutrophilic colony forming unit (CFU) → myeloblast → promyelocyte → myelocyte → eosinophil/basophil/neutrophil. Monocyte/lymphocyte colony forming unit (CFU) → monoblast/lymphoblast → promonocyte/prolymphocyte → monocyte/lymphocyte.
6. **Left shift** indicates an increase in the percentage of bands in peripheral blood, usually with some metamyelocytes and myelocytes.
7. Absolute neutrophil count = WBC (cells/μL) × % (PMN + bands)/100.
8. **Small bowel bacterial overgrowth**: altered mucosal defenses due to intestinal motility disorders and chronic pancreatitis.
9. **Hypertensive emergency** = severe hypertension with end-organ damage; **treatment**: decrease 15% BP in 24 h. Hypertensive urgency (no end organ damage): 25% BP decrease in 24 h.
10. **Treatment for bleeding from upper GI tract**: Vit K and fresh frozen plasma (FFP) if INR high and on warfarin, platelet transfusion if platelet <50; packed red blood cell (PRBC) transfusion and octreotide infusion after bolus if gastroesophageal varices.
11. Stroke imaging studies includes CT angiogram with contrast and perfusion study (code stroke CT scan), and brain MRI without contrast. **MRI with diffusion-weighted imaging (DWI), and fluid-attenuated inversion recovery (FLAIR) mismatch**: defined as the absence of a hyperintense lesion (yet to occur) on FLAIR images but restricted diffusion on DWI. Of note, **persistent hyperintensity in DWI** can also be seen in patients with previous stroke over 1 month ago or even earlier and some preexisting cerebral white matter disease.
12. **Hypertensive emergency** causes include seizure, TIA, CVA, status migraines, flash pulmonary edema (acute congestive heart failure), and heart attacks.
13. **Refeeding syndrome** refers to metabolic disturbances after reinstitution of nutrition to patients who are starved, severely malnourished or metabolically stressed due to severe illness. It is mainly characterized by **decreased potassium, magnesium, and phosphorus** in the initial 4–7 days of refeeding. **Treatment**: if phosphate drops below 0.65 mmol from a previously normal level within 3 days of reinstitution of nutrition, may need to decrease caloric intake to 480 Kcals/day for at least 2 days while replacing electrolytes. Additional treatments include thiamine, B complex, and a multivitamin and

mineral preparation. Electrolytes and metabolic panels should be monitored regularly.

9/16/2017

1. **Alcohol withdrawal syndrome**: may treat with thiamine 100–250 mg iv/im daily for 3–5 days followed by 100 mg po tid for 1–2 weeks then 100 mg daily oral.
2. **Wernicke encephalopathy treatment**: 500 mg iv tid for 2 days followed by 250 mg iv daily for 5 days followed by 100 mg tid for 2 weeks and then 100 mg daily.
3. **Indications for platelet (PLT) transfusions**: active bleeding with thrombocytopenia of <50,000 in most situations, and < 100,000 if disseminated intravascular coagulation (DIC) or central nervous system (CNS) bleeding; and preparation of invasive procedures.
4. **PLT transfusion in procedures**: neurosurgery or ocular surgery requires PLT > 100,000; most other surgery and endoscopic procedures require PLT > 50,000; bronchoalveolar lavage (BAL)/central line requires PLT > 20,000; LP requires 10,000–20,000 in hematologic malignancies and greater than 40,000–50,000 in patients without hematologic malignancies, but lower requirements in immune thrombocytopenic purpura (transfuse for bleeding rather than purely focusing on PLT count). Epidural requires PLT > 80,000; bone marrow biopsy requires PLT > 20,000.
5. **Causes of hypophosphatemia**: redistribution of phosphate into cells by insulin; decreased absorption; increased urinary excretion; removal by renal replacement therapies.
6. **Fasting/starvation and alcoholic ketoacidosis**: typically, happens in chronic alcohol abuse, malnutrition, and/or a recent episode of binge drinking. Diagnosis is suggested by an elevated anion gap and confirmed by detecting the **presence of ketone bodies**. Lactic acid is often elevated due to hypoperfusion and the altered balance of reduction and oxidation reactions in the liver. **Treatment** includes repleting K+, Mag++, PO_4 as needed, thiamine 100 mg iv first, and then D5 + NS.
7. **Heyde's syndrome** is a syndrome of GI bleeding from angiodysplasia in the presence of aortic stenosis.
8. Deficiency of ADAMTS13 in **thrombotic thrombocytopenic purpura (TTP)** is manifested by **fever, changes in mentation, thrombocytopenia, renal involvement, and hemolytic anemia**. **Treatment** includes fresh frozen plasma (FFP), steroids and plasmapheresis.
9. Treatment of **immune thrombocytopenia (ITP)** include steroids (prednisone 0.5–2 mg/kg/day) → anti-Rh(D) 50–75 μg/kg IV or IVIG → splenectomy, rituximab, romiplostim (Nplate), eltrombopag (Promacta), azathioprine, cyclophosphamide/danazol/vincristine
10. **Rituximab** targets CD20 (B cell protein marker) and is used in the following conditions: non-Hodgkin lymphoma, rheumatoid arthritis with methotrexate, and immune thrombocytopenia (ITP). **Side effects** include an increased risk of

progressive multifocal leukoencephalopathy (PML), a fatal demyelinating disease caused by the JC virus.

11. **Cameron lesions** are erosions or ulcers occurring in the sac of a hiatal hernia.
12. **Aortoenteric fistula** is caused by erosion of an atherosclerotic aneurysm into the duodenum. "**Herald bleed**"—hematemesis and or hematochezia, commonly seen after placement of a prosthetic abdominal aortic vascular graft. It is a medical emergency.
13. **Haemobilia or bleeding from the hepatobiliary tract** should be considered in any patients with acute upper gastrointestinal (GI) bleeding and a recent history of hepatic parenchymal or biliary tract instrumentation and/or injury. Triad: **biliary colic, obstructive jaundice, occult or acute GI bleeding**. It will require CT angiography, resuscitation, catheter angiography, and surgical consultation.

9/19/2017

1. For patients with an increased risk of suffering adverse events in the setting of significant anemia, such as those with unstable angina, or severe coronary artery disease, transfusing to **maintain hgb >8–9 rather than 7** may be necessary.
2. **For suspected esophagogastric variceal bleeding** and or cirrhosis, order somatostatin or an analog (e.g., octreotide 50 mg IV bolus, followed by 25 or 50 mg/h continuous IV infusion), also give an IV antibiotic infusion (ceftriaxone or fluoroquinolone) for spontaneous bacterial peritonitis prophylaxis.
3. **Trimethobenzamide** (Tigan) is an antiemetic used to prevent nausea and vomiting. It is believed to affect the chemoreceptor trigger zone (CTZ) of the medulla oblongata to suppress nausea and vomiting.
4. High heart rate in anxiety patients with heart rate 130 s = metoprolol tartrate 25 mg bid (caution: may mask symptoms, will need to identify the true cause of tachycardia); can check O_2, EKG, and troponin.
5. **Diet**: clear liquid → full liquid → (Pureed diet) → mechanical/dental soft → regular diet (cardiac, diabetic, renal diets). **Thickened liquids**: nectar thick, honey thick, and thin liquids.
6. **Dysphagia**: oropharyngeal- Zenker's diverticulum. Esophageal—rings (Schatzki ring), webs (Plummer-Vinson syndrome), peptic/radiation strictures, and tumors. **Infectious esophagitis**: odynophagia > dysphagia, often seen in immunosuppressed patients with candida, HSV, or CMV infection. **Pill esophagitis**: odynophagia > dysphagia, associated with NSAIDs, KCL, bisphosphonates, doxycycline, and tetracyclines.
7. **Eosinophilic esophagitis**: diagnosis requires > 15 eosinophils/hpf on biopsy with esophageal dysfunction (i.e., dysphagia, food impaction) and exclusion of GERD. Treatments include a modified diet (no milk, soy, eggs, wheat, nuts, and fish). Treatment is with **swallowed inhaled steroids** (swallowed fluticasone or oral viscous budesonide); if ongoing symptoms despite treatment and strictures, do dilatation.

8. **Neuromuscular (esophageal) dysphagia**: (1) **diffuse esophageal spasm**: treatment with calcium channel blocker (CCB) nifedipine sublingual 10–30 mg, isosorbide dinitrate 5 mg, or sublingual nitroglycerin before meals; (2) **achalasia**: treatment with CCB, nitrates, phosphodiesterase 5 (PDE-5) inhibitors (sildenafil, tadalafil, and vardenafil), and Botox. Also can be classified into hypermobility and hypomobility disorders (scleroderma, diabetes, alcoholism, amyloidosis, and others) of the esophagus. All dysphagia may be treated with proton pump inhibitors.
9. **GERD diagnosis** is based on symptoms and response to an empiric trial of proton pump inhibitor. **Refractory GERD**: if acidic symptoms correlate with reflux episodes, surgical fundoplication may be necessary. If there is no correlation or normal pH, it's called esophageal hypersensitivity and can be treated with tricyclic antidepressants (TCA), selective serotonin reuptake inhibitor (SSRI), or baclofen.
10. **Etiologies of upper gastrointestinal bleeding**: peptic ulcer disease, erosive gastropathy, erosive esophagitis, esophageal or gastric varices, portal hypertension gastropathy (needs octreotide and beta-blocker), vascular (angioectasia, AV malformation, hereditary hemorrhagic telangiectasia; treated with endoscopic procedures), Dieulafoy lesion, gastric antral vascular ectasia (GAVE), aortoenteric fistula, malignancy, Mallory-Weiss tear.
11. **Treatment of upper GI bleed**: pantoprazole 80 mg iv bolus → 8 mL/h = 40 mg iv bid. Esophageal varices treatment (on top of pantoprazole iv): octreotide 50 μg iv bolus → 50/25 μg/h continuous infusions + iv antibiotics (ceftriaxone, Cipro, or Levaquin) for 7 days. Endoscopic band ligation, sclerotherapy, arteriography with coiling, cyanoacrylate, stent placement, and balloon tamponade may also be necessary. For patients with gastric variceal bleed, TIPS or balloon retrograde transverse obliteration may be considered.
12. **Epiploic appendagitis** is an ischemic infarction of an epiploic appendage caused by torsion or spontaneous thrombosis of the epiploic appendage central draining vein. It is manifested by acute or subacute left lower quadrant pain and usually self-resolve in 3–4 days. It can be **treated with NSAIDs, ibuprofen 600 mg q8h**, or Norco q6h. WBC, ESR, CRP are usually normal or may be mildly elevated.

9/22/2017

1. **IV contrast dye allergy**, pretreatment for immediate hypersensitivity reaction or another type of action: 13 h before the procedure, give prednisone 50 mg orally at 13 h, 7 h, 1 h before, and diphenhydramine 50 mg oral or iv 1 h before contrast dye.
2. Platelet function test P2Y12 reaction units (PRU) level < 194 indicative of adequate P2Y12 receptor blockade.
3. TSH high while T4 normal → may need to increase levothyroxine vs subclinical hypothyroidism (no treatment necessary most often).
4. Lactic acidosis can be due to a **tourniquet**.

5. Lactic acid increase and acute abdominal pain = consider **acute bowel ischemia**. Call surgeon stat, order flat KUB or CT with contrast. Follow up with consultants to know the next step of the plan.
6. Rule in and rule out for a History of Present Illness while the Review Of Systems is shooting in the dark.
7. **Smallbore nasogastric** in the stomach, while **Dobhoff** in the duodenum for feeding.
8. Alcohol withdrawal or delirium tremens can be treated with valium 5 mg qid and lorazepam 2 mg iv q2h prn.
9. Consider palliative care consultation for patients in severe conditions, and keep family on board. What is the prognosis?
10. Sleep apnea → desaturation → lying on sides may provide relief.
11. Diabetic ketoacidosis patient not eating, glucose 130 s fasting, may add D5 + 1/2NS at 125 cc/h
12. **Familial hypercholesterolemia diagnosis**: high pretreatment cholesterol (total cholesterol > 290 or an LDL > 190) plus tendon xanthomas in patients or first and second-degree relatives or DNA-based evidence of an LDL receptor mutation or a familial defective apo B-100 or PCSK9 mutation.
13. For patients with familial hypercholesterolemia and uncontrolled LDL with statin, add **PCSK9 inhibitors** alirocumab or evolocumab.
14. In peptic ulcer disease bleeding, anticoagulants and anti-platelet medications can be resumed after hemostasis and a proton pump inhibitor are started.

9/23/2017

1. **Beta blockers** are indicated in all patients with acute coronary syndrome as they decrease myocardial demand, improve diastolic function, and have long-term effects on mortality. However, they are contraindicated in severe reactive airway disease, bradycardia, acute congestive heart failure, and high risk of cardiogenic shock.
2. **Tricyclic antidepressant (TCA)** intoxication: atropine-like presentation, convulsion, coma, cardiotoxicity. Treatment is $NaHCO_3$ and lidocaine.

9/24/2017

1. **Antibiotics for anaerobes**: **metronidazole** is inactive for microaerophilic streptococci (e.g., S. milleri), Cutibacterium (formerly Propionibacterium), and actinomyces; **carbapenems** is inactive for Bacteroides and metallo-beta-lactamases; **clindamycin** is inactive for B. fragilis, some clostridia other than C. perfringens; **cefoxitin** is inactive for B. fragilis; penicillins (Unasyn, Zosyn and tigecycline) is inactive for microorganisms with beta-lactamases.
2. **Anaerobes**: antibiotic selection empirically without benefits of in vitro susceptibility tests.
3. **Common anaerobic infections**: cerebral, epidural, and subdural empyema, pleuropulmonary infections arising from aspiration of oral and dental secretions → aspiration pneumonitis or lung abscess; infection from the female genital tract

other than sexually transmitted infections; skin infections (abscess, necrotizing fasciitis, pressures ulcers, and diabetic foot ulcers) from cutaneous flora like peptostreptococcus.

4. **Metabolic alkalosis** can only persist if the ability to excrete excess bicarb in the urine is impaired due to: hypovolemia, reduced effective arterial blood volume (like congestive heart failure or cirrhosis), chloride depletion, hypokalemia, decreased GFR, hyperaldosteronism, or combination of these factors.
5. **Batter** (loop diuretics with hypercalciuria), **Gitelman** (thiazide), **Liddle** (decreased aldosterone level causing increased Na reabsorption in the distal and collecting tubules): all have hypokalemia and metabolic alkalosis.
6. Other causes of **metabolic alkalosis**: loss of H+ from GI or kidneys, exogenic alkali, contraction alkalosis, post-hypercapnia (respiratory acidosis → renal compensation, rapid correction via intubation), and hyperaldosteronism. Classified as saline responsive (GI losses of H+, diuretics, post-hypercapnia, laxative, cystic fibrosis) and saline resistant metabolic alkalosis.
7. **Metabolic alkalosis** treatment: acetazolamide 250 mg po (not commonly used), stop Lasix, decrease respiratory rate, give normal saline 1 L bolus, and decrease tidal volume from 300 to 270 cc.
8. **Hypertensive urgency/emergency** definition: 180/120 or 160/100, will need to reduce MAP by 25% in 1 h, 2–6 h goal 160/100–110; 24–48 gradual normalization of blood pressure. Hypertensive urgency = hypertensive crisis; hypertensive emergency = malignant hypertension.

Takeaway Messages

1. Emphasis of progress notes on succinctness with a focus on diagnosis and plan of care while avoiding redundancy on reiteration of patient data already in the medical record system.
2. Understand the typical management for coronary artery disease, pneumonia, alcoholic cirrhosis and gastrointestinal bleeding, and COPD exacerbation.
3. Chest pain workups and medication precautions in stress test.
4. Try to understand the importance of goals of care discussions, especially in patients with possible poor prognosis.

Further Readings and References

1. Writing Committee Members, C.M. Otto, R.A. Nishimura, et al. 2021. 2020 ACC/AHA guideline for the management of patients with valvular heart disease: A report of the American College of Cardiology/American Heart Association Joint Committee on Clinical Practice Guidelines. *Journal of Thoracic and Cardiovascular Surgery* 162 (2): e183–e353.
2. Reeder, G.S., and H.L. Kennedy. *Overview of the nonacute management of ST-elevation myocardial infarction*, ed. C.P. Cannon and J. Hoekstra. Waltham: UpToDate. Accessed October 31, 2023.

3. Simons, M., and J.A. Breall. *Overview of the acute management of non-ST-elevation acute coronary syndromes*, ed. C.P. Cannon and J. Hoekstra. Waltham: UpToDate. Accessed October 31, 2023.
4. Connors, J.M. 2017. Thrombophilia testing and venous thrombosis. *New England Journal of Medicine* 377: 1177–1187.
5. Stern, R.S. *Overview of the treatment of hyponatremia in adults*, ed. M. Emmett. Waltham: UpToDate. Accessed October 31, 2023.

Chapter 3
A Brief Break at the Radiology Department

September 25th, 2017 Through October 22nd, 2017

Throughout residency training, a typical day as a trainee usually started around 5 a.m. and ended around 6–7 p.m. After 1-month ICU and 2 months of general medicine floor rotations, I had a relatively easy month at the radiology department where the work started at 8 a.m. or even 9 a.m. and ended around 2–3 p.m. I still remember the words my radiologist attending said when he informed me of the schedule of the day: "I will cut you loose after that". As such, compared to other rotations, the rotation at the radiology department was like a "semi-vacation" overall. Nonetheless, as a physician in training, besides more free time, learning remained my main goal despite minimal patient care responsibility.

While X-ray films are the foundation for the radiology rotation, understanding the benefits, side effects, and uniqueness of the available imaging modalities and gaining the basic skills for the interpretation of common imaging studies including X-ray, CT scan, and MRI were the goals of this rotation. Arguably, as an internal medicine trainee or even a practicing attending physician, we could rely on the readings by radiologists. The understanding of a disease and a patient's overall health (especially in critical conditions) change and can be remarkably different when you read the films/images yourself. As a practicing attending physician in internal medicine, I highly recommend reviewing the films ourselves and comparing the interpretation by us and the radiologist whenever possible.

Specific recommendations for the radiology rotation include familiarity with relevant anatomy, hands-on experiences with ultrasounds, fostering a systemic approach to interpreting X ray, CT scan, and MRI images, and understanding the utilities of nuclear medicine studies. Additional topics covered in the notes included transcranial Doppler, ileus versus small bowel obstruction, Cardiolite stress testing, aspiration pneumonitis/pneumonia, and plasmacytoma.

K. Zhou, *Internal Medicine Training Notes and Survival Guide*,
https://doi.org/10.1007/978-1-0716-4039-5_3

10/8/2017 Radiology Note

1. **Common bile duct** size normally <6–7 mm.
2. Pneumothorax can be diagnosed with **chest X-ray in expiration**.
3. **Adipose tissue** under ultrasound is bright.
4. **Lung nodules**: (1) ≥ 8 mm serial CT scans at 3, 6, 9 to 12 months, 18–24 months ⇒ consider PET → biopsy if increase in size. (2) For nodules ≤6 mm, routine follow-up CT is not required, but if suspicious morphology or upper lobe location or high risk, will need to repeat CT at 12 months. (3) Pure ground glass nodules ≥ 6 mm ⇒ continued surveillance by serial CT scan in 6–12 months. If <6 mm, repeat CT is not needed. Then every 2 years for a total of 5 years. Resection of Solitary pulmonary nodule at least 15–20 mm. (4) A part-solid (subsolid) nodule with a part-solid component likely to be malignant: if ≥6 mm, CT at 3–6 months, then at 5 years.
5. **Barium swallow test (also known as barium esophagram or esophagram):** done by radiologist and looks for etiologies of esophageal dysphagia. **Videofluoroscopic swallow study (VFSS) = modified barium swallow (MBS)**: done with speech pathologist to assess oropharyngeal dysphagia.
6. **Orbital X-ray** to detect grind metal before MRI.
7. In patients with ICD implantation or placement of a PICC line, will need to look for **pneumothorax** on chest X-ray.
8. **Esophagram**: look for esophageal web, stricture, and diverticulum but also motility disorders. **Three different waves**: primary peristalsis/waves (rapid wave opening sphincters followed by a slow wave of contraction moving the bolus), secondary waves (same radiographic appearance as primary waves but start at the point of retained barium bolus), tertiary waves (abnormal contractions of motility disorders). Look for pulsion at the C5–C6 level, assess soft tissue condition, and look for weakness, diverticulum, and traction diverticulum.
9. **Abdominal X-ray**: look for air, fluid level, free air, 2 positions needed.
10. **Knee**: look for distances between bones. Spur at the hip, acetabular impingement syndrome (pincer and Cam types).
11. Look for soft tissue swelling for ruling in/out fractures.
12. **Jones fracture** is a fracture in the meta-diaphyseal junction of the fifth metatarsal of the foot.
13. **Subcutaneous emphysema**: need CT to see tracheal patency. Dark is fat in CT scan → swelling of joint.
14. **Sniff test** for diaphragm paralysis → paradoxical elevation is abnormal.
15. **Boxer's sign**: fifth metacarpal fracture.
16. **Transcranial Doppler**: look at large arteries for vasospasm after subarachnoid hemorrhage.
17. Transcranial Doppler velocities above **120 cm/s** at the middle cerebral artery or Lindegaard ratio **(mean velocity MCA/ICA extracranial) ≥ 3** indicates vasospasm rather than hyperemia.
18. Thickening of colonic wall and colonic periwall tissue swelling = consider **diverticulitis**.

19. **Usual interstitial pneumonia (UIP)**: caudocranial gradient of peripheral septal thickening, bronchiectasis, and honeycombing. Life expectancy <5 years.
20. **Non-specific interstitial pneumonia**: ground glass opacities, reticular opacities, thickening of broncho-vascular bundles, traction bronchiectasis; responds to steroids, cessation of inciting drugs, and mycophenolate mofetil.
21. Sludge in gallbladder → **HIDA scan if no obvious wall thickening and edema**. HIDA scan can reveal functional abnormalities of the gallbladder.
22. Focal wall thickening of the intestine at hepatic flexure = consider **focal colitis**.

10/10/2017

1. Calcification patterns in CT chest scans: diffuse, central, popcorn, and laminated are usually **benign**. Potentially **malignant**: stippled, eccentric.
2. **Hiatal hernia**: retrocardiac mass with or without an air-fluid level on X ray. Paraoesophageal hernia accounts for 10% of hiatal hernia. Bladder suspension including **colposuspension** is a surgical treatment for stress urinary incontinence.
3. **Polyps versus stones** in gallbladder ultrasound: shadowing is typically seen with stones but not polyps.
4. Calcification in ultrasound: white with a shadow.
5. **Gallbladder wall thickening** can be seen in ascites. Lumpy and bumpy liver = cirrhosis.
6. Small bowel obstruction (SBO), order CT with IV contrast, if allergic to IV dye, do oral contrast. **CT criteria for SBO**: dilated fluid-filled bowel, small bowel dilation to ≥2.5 cm while colon not dilated (<6 cm).
7. A **phlebolith** is a small local, usually rounded calcification within a vein. It can be difficult to differentiate from kidney stones.
8. **Postoperative (paralytic) ileus** = possible obstipation and intolerance of oral intake due to nonmechanical factors causing disruption of the normal coordinated propulsive motor activity of the gastrointestinal tract after surgery.
9. **Gallstone ileus**: mechanical bowel obstruction by impaction of a gallstone in the ileum after being passed through a biliary enteric fistula. Treatment: removal of the obstructing stone after resuscitation.
10. Following abdominal surgery, “normal” **physiologic postoperative ileus** due to recovery of postoperative gut motility is 0–24 h in small intestines, 24–48 h in the stomach, and 48–72 h in the colon.
11. Prolonged and pathologic postoperative ileus = consider the occurrence of two or more of the following signs and symptoms on **postoperative day 4 or after:** nausea and vomiting, inability to tolerate an oral diet over the preceding 24 h, absence of flatus over the preceding 24 h, abdominal distension, and radiologic confirmation; will also needs to rule out postoperative complications.
12. **Gastrointestinal dysmotility** is related to inflammation, neural reflexes, and neurohumoral peptides.
13. **Symptoms of ileus**: abdominal distension, bloating, and gassiness; diffuse persistent abdominal pain; nausea and/or vomiting; delayed passage of or inability to pass flatus; inability to tolerate an oral diet.

14. **Differential diagnosis of ileus**: small bowel obstruction, intra-abdominal abscess, or retroperitoneal bleeding. Ileus does not have peritoneal signs of fever or tachycardia.
15. Nearly all patients with early postoperative **bowel obstruction** have an **initial return of bowel function and oral intake** which are followed by nausea and vomiting, abdominal pain, and distention. These do not happen in **ileus**.
16. Intense cramping pain, feculent emesis, or rapidly progressing pain or distention are more suggestive of bowel obstruction than prolonged postoperative ileus.
17. Localized tenderness, fever, tachycardia, and peritoneal signs suggestive of **bowel ischemia or perforation.** Suspicion → urgent surgery consult and get KUB → consider CT with oral contrast → consider upper GI contrast studies (Enteroclysis) and gastrografin (distinguishing ileus from partial small bowel obstruction). Treatment is emergent surgery.
18. **Ischemic bowel CT findings**: bowel wall thickening, mesenteric fat edema and/or fluid in the adjacent mesentery or peritoneal space, abnormal decreased bowel wall enhancement, and pneumatosis in mesenteric or portal vein.

10/11/2017

1. Upper GI exam in throat and esophagus only = Barium swallow.
2. Upper GI series evaluate for mouth to duodenum. **Fluoroscopy**: live radiographic images. **Videofluoroscopic swallowing exam** (by speech therapist) + esophagram (by radiologist) for dysphagia assessment.
3. **Enteroclysis** (similar to CT enterography) is an imaging of the small intestine, double contrast was infused via nasojejunal tube into the small bowel (barium and methylcellulose).
4. The **Mirizzi syndrome** refers to common hepatic duct obstruction caused by an impacted stone in the cystic duct or infundibulum of the gallbladder, which may present with cholecystoduodenal, cholecystocolonic, or cholecystogastric fistulas.
5. **Gallstone ileus** symptoms include episodic subacute obstruction. Signs include abdominal distension and decreased bowel sounds.
6. **Bowel obstruction symptoms** include abdominal pain, nausea and vomiting, abdominal distension, and obstipation.
7. Oral contrast only looks at the bowel. Ossific density at knee = consider old avulsion.
8. **Pellegrini-Stieda lesion** (ossifications of the medial collateral ligament (MCL) at or near its proximal insertion on the medial femoral condyle) treatment: steroid injection.
9. Bone density scan = Dexa scan.
10. **Concave humeral head underneath clavicle** = consider rotator cuff tear. Interstitial changes may indicate scarring of the lungs.
11. Thyroid nodules → hyperactive thyroid nodules (low TSH) → after ultrasound, do I131 reuptake → fine needle aspirations if decreased uptake of I131.

12. **Bladder wall thickening** refers to wall thickness of >3 mm when distended or > 5 mm when nondistended. **Diffuse:** outlet obstruction, neurogenic bladder, infection, and radiation treatment. **Focal:** cancer, artifact, cystitis, cystitis cystica and glandularis.
13. **Cardiolite test**: horizontal, sagittal, frontal images. **Gastric emptying study**: 30 min, 90 min, and 2 h.
14. V/Q scan needs chest X-ray prior for comparison purposes. Pulmonary embolism hints: **ventilation** is good, but **perfusion** is compromised.
15. **Lexiscan** also known as regadenoson, a pharmacological stressor for cardiac stress test. **Cardiolite (Technetium Tc-99m sestamibi)** is a radioactive tracer for the assessment of the blood flow during cardiac stress test. **Cardiolite 1-day protocol**: resting first with 10 mCi Tc99, then do 0.4 mg Lexiscan (regadenoson) + 30 mCi Tc99 test.
16. **Cardiolite 2-day protocol**: usually used for BMI >40, stress first, give Lexiscan and Cardiolite on day 1, and Cardiolite on day 2.
17. Black area decreases with stress in Cardiolite = normal study (anatomical structure without much blood supply).
18. **Lasix renal scan** (Lasix augmented renal flow and scan): look for a dilated collecting system or obstruction.
19. **Bone scan** for hip fracture after pining, look for nonhealing and other pathologies.
20. The gastric emptying study is a nuclear medicine study; the upper GI series is a barium study. **Two nuclear studies can't be done on the same day**.
21. **Radionuclide cisternogram** versus CSF leak: look for otorrhea and rhinorrhea, with pledgets for CSF leaks of the head or without for spinal leaks and normal-pressure hydrocephalus. It is a four day study and may simple just go ahead with blood patch treatment for CSF leak if concerns are high.
22. **Gastrointestinal (GI) bleeding scan** = RBC tag study. **CT angiography GI bleeding protocol** is better than tagged RBC scintigraphy in acute large bleeding.
23. **Parathyroid scan** (Technetium—only taken up by thyroid; Sestamibi—taken up by both parathyroid and thyroid): <0.5 cm will not be detected.
24. **Prostate cancer** needs a bone scan; the imaging study has to be clinically correlated.
25. **Hepatobiliary iminodiacetic acid (HIDA) scan** (biliary scan), use cholecystokinin (CCK) if no stone is found. Ejection fraction of gallbladder **35%–80%** is considered as normal. Biliary scan with CCK can help diagnose acalculous cholecystitis. **Hyperkinetic gallbladder** = biliary symptoms without gallstones (acalculous) + high gallbladder ejection fractions (>80%).
26. Chest wall pain in an old female, suspicious of facet arthritis, can order a total **body bone scan** to look at ribs.

10/13/2017

1. **Thyroid scan** using **I123** (10%–35% in 24 h is normal). Treat with **I131**, scan requires no pregnancy for 2 months and treatment requires no pregnancy for 6 months.

2. Patients with **sick euthyroid syndrome** can have low, normal, or only slightly elevated TSH.
3. Flushing and occasional upset stomach → neuroendocrine tumor, no biopsy. For carcinoid syndrome, do CT and ultrasound of the abdomen.
4. **Hip fracture with pins** develops pain, has pacer, cannot do MRI, looking for avascular necrosis of the femoral head, do bone scan.
5. I131 high dose ablation for thyroid cancer. Low dose for Graves' disease treatment. **Discontinue thyroid medications 1 week before I131 therapy**: bigger BMI, higher doses of radioactive substances.
6. **Honda sign** in bone scan = consider stress fracture of the sacrum.
7. **Renal flow and scan** to see whether the patient can pass tracers (delayed tracer excretion into the renal pelvis) into urination. If not, it is acute tubular necrosis which can have a residual cortical activity >97% (<30% is normal).
8. **Cholecystokinin (CCK) augmented biliary scan**: no biliary contraction with cholecystokinin and no gallstone = consider acalculous cholecystitis, cystic duct syndrome, or biliary dyskinesia.
9. **Cardiolite anatomy**: compare stress versus rest to get an idea of whether it is ischemia, look at color intensity.
10. **Radioactive tracer** takes 5 days to disappear in bone, but 24 h in the urinary bladder.
11. **For iodine contrast allergy**, give Benadryl and methylprednisolone orally before giving oral iodine (can follow specific protocols in UpToDate).
12. **Lasix renal scan and flow**: give Lasix to see whether the tracer disappears, if yes = no obstruction but can still have a dilated collecting duct system.
13. Physical finding of a **nodule over left thyroid** (ultrasound positive), TSH increased, decreased T4, decompensated thyroid gland →radioactive iodine uptake (RAIU) revealed decreased tracer uptake on the right and uniform tracer distribution of the left = cold nodule → fine needle aspiration (FNA).
14. **WBC scan = Tc99m WBC scan**. Hx of fracture at left inferior pubic ramus, recurrent bacteremia with MRSA, pressure ulcers bilaterally over buttocks, use WBC scan to rule out osteomyelitis.
15. **Thyrogen study**: D1 and D2 ingestion; D3 radioactive T131 (oral ablation dose)/T123 (diagnostic radioactive iodine), D4 scan whole body.
16. **Shunt patency study** to see whether CSF goes to the peritoneum without obstruction or leakage in ventriculoperitoneal shunts for hydrocephalus.
17. Normal ejection fraction of the gallbladder is **35%–80%**; normal radioactive iodine uptake (RAIU) of the thyroid gland is **10%–35% in 24 h (6%–18% in 4 h)**.
18. Cholelithiasis is a contraindication of CCK. Bone scan is a radionuclide test. The skeletal survey is X-ray.
19. High concentrations of **thyroglobulin antibodies** are found in 30% of Graves' disease and 80% of Hashimoto's disease. In virtually all Hashimoto's and the majority of Graves' disease, **thyroid peroxidase antibodies** (TPO-Ab) are elevated.

20. **Thyroid cancer** → surgery → I131 treated → 1 year follow up, whole body I 131 RAIU (post-thyroidectomy, post-thyroid ablation).
21. **Chest discomfort during pharmacological stress tests** can be relieved by IV aminophylline while some hospitals use caffeine beverages for treatment.
22. **Bone scan (if contraindication for MRI)**: post arthroplasty to look for infection and loosening, important to know the date of surgery. Increased tracer uptake around the prosthesis is abnormal if it happens 1 year after.
23. TSH low → RAIU → cold → FNA; TSH normal/high → FNA.

10/14/2017

1. **Risk factors for aspiration pneumonia**: decreased consciousness, dysphagia, mechanical disruption of glottic closure or cardiac sphincter due to tracheostomy, endotracheal intubation, bronchoscopy, and nasogastric feedings.
2. Dysphagia evaluation via bedside swallow test.
3. Three syndromes in the category of aspiration pneumonia: **chemical pneumonitis, bacterial infection, and airway obstruction** (distress and cyanosis ⇒ consider acute respiratory distress syndrome (ARDS): pulmonary edema, reduced surfactant activity, reflex airway closure, alveolar hemorrhage, and alveolar membrane formation). **Diagnosis**: chest X-ray in 2 h after aspiration; treat with immediate tracheal suction.
4. **Bacterial infection in aspiration pneumonia**: oral anaerobes and streptococci (hospital aspiration: S. aureus, P aeruginosa, G- bacilli)
5. **Major anaerobes** isolated from aspiration pneumonia infections are Peptostreptococcus, Fusobacterium nucleatum, Prevotella, Bacteroides melaninogenicus and other Bacteroides spp.
6. **Clinical features** of aspiration pneumonia: indolent symptoms, absence of rigors, failure to recover likely pulmonary pathogens with culture of expectorated sputum. The putrid odor of sputum or pleural fluid, concomitant periodontal disease, chest CT evidence of lung necrosis with abscess or empyema.
7. **Aspiration pneumonia (bacterial infection) treatment**: first line—ampicillin-sulbactam 1.5-3 g q6h if GFR is ok for mild symptoms, can give Augmentin 875 mg bid. Alternatives: metronidazole 500 mg tid + amoxicillin 500 mg tid or penicillin G.
8. If allergic to penicillins, do clindamycin 600 mg iv q8h. If Ok with cephalosporins, do ceftriaxone or cefotaxime + metronidazole. **Drugs that poorly work for aspiration pneumonia** include Bactrim, cipro, ceftazidime, and aminoglycosides.
9. For **hospital-acquired aspiration pneumonia**, treatment includes carbapenems or Zosyn with MRSA coverage if needed.
10. Duration of antibiotics in hospital acquired pneumonia: no cavitation or empyema, treat 7 days. Thoracentesis if pleural effusion. Patients with **lung abscesses** need a longer course of antibiotics, usually until there is radiographic clearance or significant improvements, likely 4–6 weeks.

11. Aspiration pneumonia may involve fluid or particulate matter (saline, Barium, water, gastric content pH > 2.5) which is not coherently toxic to the lung but can cause airway obstruction or reflex airway closure.
12. **Infiltrative hepatic liver disease** [only alkaline phosphatase (ALP) increase] can have mild hepatomegaly and ascites = consider metastases, lymphoma, hepatocellular carcinoma, sarcomas. An increase in ALP is commonly seen in **intra and extrahepatic cholestasis**.
13. **Autoimmune hepatitis**: elevated ALT and AST with a normal and near normal ALP and normal bilirubin. **GGT** helps differentiate ALP from liver versus bone.
14. Increased ALP + pruritus (hyperlipidemia) = consider **primary biliary cholangitis** → fibrosis and end-stage liver failure in 5–10 years after diagnosis (destruction of small and mid-sized bile ducts)

10/15/2017

1. **Myxedema coma** treatment: load with 5–8 μg/kg T4 IV, then 50–100 mg iv daily. If unstable with bradycardia and/or hypothermia (T3 more arrhythmogenic), because peripheral conversion is impaired, may also give 5–10 μg/kg T3 iv q8h. Additionally, give hydrocortisone 100 mg iv q8h until the exclusion of adrenal insufficiency.
2. **Antibiotics** (penicillins, cephalexin, azithromycin, or clindamycin) for pharyngitis if ≥2 of the following: T ≥ 38, tonsillar exudates, tender cervical adenopathy, no cough or rhinitis (Centor criteria for strep throat). In the ideal world, strep throat swab is necessary prior to antibiotics.
3. **Distinguishing bacterial from viral sinusitis includes** the presence of symptoms >7 days, maxillary tooth pain, unilateral sinus tenderness, fever, unilateral facial pain, purulent nasal discharge, and symptoms worsening after initial improvement. **Treatment** is amoxicillin, doxycycline, or TMP/SMX.
4. **The most common cause of bronchitis** (wheezing is common) is viral and rhinovirus, followed by other common causes of the "common cold". **The most common bacterial causes of bronchitis** are M. pneumonia and C. pneumonia. If fever, tachypnea, or dyspnea is present or pulmonary consolidation on physical examination, a chest X-ray is needed to rule out pneumonia.
5. **Adrenal suppression before surgery**: treat with hydrocortisone 100 mg iv q8h if hypotension from suppressed adrenal gland functions.
6. **ACEi/ARB** should be continued in CKD throughout CKD IV, even CKD V as long as tolerated without hyperkalemia (K < 5.5 mEq/L).
7. **Plasmacytoma** is a plasma cell dyscrasia: solitary plasmacytoma of bone, extramedullary plasmacytoma, or multiple plasmacytomas. **Solitary plasmacytoma** occurs as lytic lesions within the axial skeleton and extramedullary plasmacytomas often in the upper respiratory tract. Half of them produce paraproteinemia also known as monoclonal gammopathy. **Treatment**: radiotherapy. Solitary plasmacytoma of bone usually develops into multiple myeloma in 2–4 years.
8. Solitary plasmacytoma of bone and **extramedullary plasmacytomas**, in comparison with multiple myelomas, have one lesion either in the bone of soft tissue, but normal bone marrow (<5% plasma cells), normal skeletal survey, absent or

low paraprotein, and no end organ damage. **Multiple myeloma** diagnosis requires ≥10% bone marrow clonal plasma cells or biopsy evidence of a bony or extramedullary plasmacytoma together with disease specific signs and symptoms.

9. **Liothyronine (T3)** is not warranted for chronic treatment of hypothyroidism. T3 can be used for a short period to prevent symptoms of hypothyroidism in preparation of total radioactive iodine (RAI) uptake and scan in patients with thyroid cancer.

10/22/2017

1. Add prednisone 40 mg po qd after breakfast for community-acquired pneumonia (CAP).
2. **Resistant hypertension etiology workup**: ultrasound duplex Abd/pelvis limited (aorta), ultrasound renal-aorta limited, renin-aldosterone activity.
3. Ischemic stroke, keep sBP < 220/120 mmHg for the first 24 h. Hemorrhagic stroke: keep sBP < 140–160 mmHg.
4. Ranexa = ranolazine 1000 mg bid, Crestor = rosuvastatin, Isordil = isosorbide dinitrate 10–20 mg tid.
5. A fixed-dose combination of hydralazine (37.5–75 mg orally 3 times daily) plus isosorbide dinitrate (20–40 mg orally three times daily) for congestive heart failure with ejection fraction (CHFrEF) < 45%, especially in African American patients, provides mortality benefits.
6. **Angina status post stenting in 3 major vessels** (patent) medications: ranolazine 1000 mg bid, verapamil 240 mg qd (vasospasm), sublingual nitro 0.4 mg q5min × 3, prasugrel (Effient) 10 mg qd and aspirin, Isordil 20 mg tid.
7. **Benign prostate hyperplasia (BPH)**: tamsulosin (alpha antagonist) 0.8 mg qhs, Avodart (dutasteride) 0.5 mg qd. Finasteride is a 5a reductase inhibitor; flutamide is used for prostate cancer as an androgen blocker.
8. **Peripheral neuropathy treatment**: gabapentin, duloxetine, amitriptyline, or pregabalin.
9. **Amitiza (lubiprostone)** 24 mg bid: A chloride channel activator on the apical membrane of the gastrointestinal tract to increase intestinal fluid secretion and improve fecal transit.
10. **Atrial fibrillation (AFib)**: urgent treatment with medication or cardioversion if active ischemia, evidence of organ hypoperfusion, or severe manifestations of heart failure; explore causes/etiology: TSH, echocardiogram, BNP, and BMP. **Medication treatment**: verapamil, Cardizem, metoprolol, digoxin, and/or amiodarone, and keep serum K above 4 and Mag above 2.
11. Low risk for embolization if the **duration of AFib < 24–48 h** and no cardiac abnormalities (mitral valve disease, left ventricular enlargement on echo).
12. For patients with AFib ≥ 48 h or unknown duration, at least 3 weeks' oral anticoagulation before cardioversion and ≥4 weeks' anticoagulation after cardioversion. If **urgent restoration** is needed, do TEE to rule out left atrial thrombi. For patients with AFib < 48 h, order unfractionated heparin, or even without anticoagulation, can cardiovert. Rate control <85 at rest is reasonable.

Takeaway Messages

1. Understand normal anatomy and the uniqueness of nuclear medicine modalities like HIDA scan, Cardiolite, bone scan, and radioactive iodine uptake scan.
2. Wall edema and swelling in hollow organs usually indicate inflammation versus infection.
3. Besides detailed abdominal auscultation and palpation, imaging studies can be utilized to differentiate ileus and small bowel obstruction.
4. Be cautious of surgical emergencies like bowel perforation and ischemia.

Further Readings and References

1. Brant, W.E., and S. Moshiri. Pharynx and esophagus. In *Radiology key: fastest radiology insight engine*. https://radiologykey.com/pharynx-and-esophagus/. Accessed November 2, 2023.
2. Radswiki, T., R. Chieng, S. Iqbal, et al. *Adynamic ileus*. https://radiopaedia.org/articles/adynamic-ileus?lang=us. Accessed November 2, 2023. https://doi.org/10.53347/rID-12204
3. Recognizing bowel obstruction and ileus. *Radiology key: fastest radiology insight engine*. https://radiologykey.com/recognizing-bowel-obstruction-and-ileus/. Accessed November 2, 2023.
4. Klompas, M. *Treatment and prevention of Legionella infection*, ed. J.A. Ramirez. Waltham: UpToDate. Accessed November 2, 2023.
5. Morasch, M.D. *Aspiration pneumonia in adults*, ed. D.J. Sexton. Waltham: UpToDate. Accessed November 2, 2023.

Chapter 4
A Quick Dive into the General Medicine Floor with an Emphasis on Cardiology

October 23rd, 2017 Through November 19th, 2017
The majority of hospitalized patients, especially the aging baby boomers, have certain cardiac conditions, including but not limited to acute coronary syndrome, arrhythmias, congestive heart failure, valvular heart diseases, and/or pericarditis. The hospital of my rotation was a comprehensive cardiac care center and provides percutaneous coronary intervention (PCI), coronary artery bypass surgery (CABG), transcatheter aortic valve replacement, cardiac implants, and others on a routine basis. As a resident physician in this rotation, I was taking care of patients with mainly cardiac issues under the supervision of my hospitalist attending and cardiologist consultants. As a team member, I was involved in the decision-making process of many of the aforementioned procedures.

This rotation was thus the de facto cardiac care unit rotation, although the tedious workup for chest pain and its differentials were not mentioned in the notes of this chapter, congestive heart failure was discussed in Chap. 1, overall principles in the management of chest pain and acute coronary syndrome were covered in Chap. 2, and EKG was covered separately in a later chapter. The notes for this month mainly focused on areas a practicing general internist would otherwise be unfamiliar with, for example, percutaneous coronary stenting appropriateness and complications, indications for CABG, diagnosis and treatment of acute pericarditis.

Additional topics covered in this rotation/chapter included atrial fibrillation rate and rhythm control, venous thromboembolism (deep and superficial) and novel oral anticoagulants (NOACs), vertebral artery stenosis, cardiac resynchronization therapy, percutaneous coronary intervention, chylomicronemia, abdominal aortic aneurysm, cardioversion and cardiac ablation, and triple anticoagulation. Of note, this chapter and this book included no information on echocardiogram interpretation and minimal information on caring for heart transplant patients.

Knowledge and skills learned in this chapter together with the cardiac care knowledge in the first two chapters nonetheless serve as a major component of residency training and the foundation for the practice of internal medicine physicians. I

K. Zhou, *Internal Medicine Training Notes and Survival Guide*, https://doi.org/10.1007/978-1-0716-4039-5_4

recommend building a habit of detailed routine physical examination of jugular venous distension (hepatojugular reflux), pitting edema, skin color and contexture, cardiac auscultation, and pulmonary auscultation. This provides long-lasting benefits for us as clinicians and instant information for understanding a patient's conditions and diseases. Last but not least, always correlate the patient's symptoms and physical findings with laboratory data and EKG findings. During my years of practice and training, I came across multiple occasions that code STEMI was called on pericarditis or repolarization EKGs (please refer to the EKG section in a later chapter of the book), even though, undoubtedly, promptly recognizing and treating STEMI to minimize morbidity and mortality remains paramount.

10/23/2017

1. **Angina treatment**: beta blocker, calcium channel blocker (CCB), nitrate, ranolazine → angiography with PCI + aspirin
2. Anticoagulation for atrial fibrillation and atrial flutter is based on a CHA2DS2-VASc score ≥ 2.
3. Intermediate risk for coronary artery disease (CAD), may order C reactive protein (CRP); a high **CRP** predicts high risks for major cardiovascular events in the future.
4. An **unstable aortic aneurysm** is usually treated with beta blocker and nitroprusside while waiting for an urgent vascular surgery consultation.
5. **Radiocontrast nephropathy prevention**: (1) Among outpatients, give 3 mL/kg NS over 1 h pre-procedure and 1–1.5 mL/kg/h during and 4–6 h postprocedure with administration of at least 6 mL/kg postprocedure NS. (2) Among inpatients, give NS 1 mL/kg/h for 6–12 h preprocedure, intraprocedure and for 6–12 h postprocedure. (3) For all at-risk patients, acetylcysteine may be used (conflicting results in meta-analyses), 1200 mg po bid before and on the day of the procedure.
6. All **diastolic heart murmurs** are pathological and require investigation.
7. Disopyramide for patients with **vagally induced AFib**, especially in young athletes with slow heart rates during rest/sleep; flecainide and amiodarone are sequential alternatives.
8. For patients with **adrenally mediated AFib**, use a beta-blocker, followed by sotalol and amiodarone.
9. For patients **without structural heart disease**, use **flecainide or propafenone** as first line, alternatives include dofetilide, dronedarone, amiodarone, or sotalol if rhythm control is used for atrial fibrillation.
10. **Coronary artery disease (CAD)** but no advanced CHF, used **Multaq (dronedarone) or sotalol** for rhythm control in AFib.
11. For patients with **heart failure, amiodarone** is preferred to dofetilide if rhythm control is chosen in atrial fibrillation. Flecainide, propafenone, dronedarone, and sotalol are contraindicated in these patients.
12. **Left ventricular hypertrophy, use amiodarone or dronedarone** if rhythm control is chosen in atrial fibrillation

13. Unstable plaques in heart disease, do heparin drip. Isolated **distal DVT** (like peroneal vein DVT) = thromboses in the calf veins below the knee without involvement of the popliteal vein. Asymptomatic distal DVT usually requires no anticoagulation, but weekly ultrasound for 2 weeks. If the clot does not resolve but remains stable, longer periods of surveillance may be required. **Exceptions**: if risk factors like high d-dimer, extensive thrombosis involving >5 cm in length or 7 mm in diameter, or involvement of multiple veins, will need anticoagulation for at least 3 months unless contraindicated.
14. **The superficial femoral vein** is a misnomer; it is a deep vein.
15. Novel oral anticoagulant (NOAC) is **not recommended in valvular heart disease**: the DOAC pivotal trials excluded patients with **significant mitral stenosis**, prosthetic heart valves (nowadays, we do use NOAC for prosthetic valves with AFib), but not necessary others like aortic regurgitation, mild mitral stenosis, mitral regurgitation, tricuspid stenosis/regurgitation.

10/24/2017

1. **Pernicious anemia** does not produce acid and thus gastrin is increased.
2. **Treatment for dumping syndrome**: separate liquids from solids, frequent smaller meals, high protein high fiber, and low carbohydrate diet.
3. Status post gastrectomy has no parietal cells; PPI does not work.
4. **Small bowel bacterial overgrowth syndrome** (bloating, flatulence, abdominal discomfort, or chronic watery diarrhea): hydrogen predominant bacterial overgrowth treatment- **rifaximin 550 mg tid for 14 days**; methane predominant bacterial overgrowth treatment- **neomycin 500 mg bid + rifaximin 550 mg tid for 14 days**.
5. Diagnosis of small bowel bacterial overgrowth syndrome: a **positive carbohydrate breath test** or a bacterial concentration of $>10^3$ colony forming units/ml in a **jejunal aspirate culture**.
6. Nonsteroidal anti-inflammatory drugs (NSAIDs) worsen congestive heart failure (CHF) symptoms; **carvedilol** (Coreg) drops blood pressure more than metoprolol succinate; **metoprolol** decreases heart rate more than carvedilol. Metoprolol is a selective beta-1 blocker whereas carvedilol is a non-selective beta-blocker with alpha blockade effects.
7. Asthma and COPD exacerbations with supraventricular tachycardia (SVTs), **adenosine, and beta-blockers** may be contraindicated as they cause bronchoconstriction.
8. **Causes of iron deficiency anemia**: blood loss, reduced iron absorption in celiac disease, atrophic gastritis, H. pylori, bariatric surgery; redistribution after erythropoietin; pulmonary and urinary hemosiderosis.
9. Serum ferritin is an acute phase reactant. **Diagnosis of iron deficiency anemia**: ferritin <15 (<30 in pregnant women), ferritin <41 in a patient with anemia and comorbidities, transferrin saturation <16% or <20% in inflammatory conditions, anemia that resolves upon iron administration, absence of stainable iron in bone marrow.

10. **Iron sucrose 10 mL** (200 mg elemental iron) is routinely given 2–15 min in dialysis centers; a total of 5 doses during different dialysis sessions is common. For patients with cancer receiving erythropoietin stimulating agents, 10 mL may be infused over 60 min every 2–3 weeks.
11. **Ferric gluconate**: a typical dose is 10–15 mL as a 2-min bolus or diluted in NS and infused over 20–30 min.

10/27/2017

1. **Right vertebral artery stenosis**: angiogram and possible stent will require the patient to be off Coumadin and if a stent is placed, the patient would need dual antiplatelet therapy (DAPT) and Coumadin. The patient was placed on a full anticoagulation dose Lovenox in the interim with DAPT initiated after stent placement.
2. **Vertebral artery stenosis (evaluation via MRA) treatment indications**: hemodynamic symptoms and bilateral >60% stenosis, symptomatic vertebral origin embolism or aneurysm, asymptomatic vertebral artery aneurysm >1.5 cm.
3. **Dementia treatments**: donepezil 10 mg qam, memantine 5 mg bid.
4. Targeted BP control: hydralazine 25 mg tid, Imdur 60 mg qd, Coreg 25 bid to maintain sBP 160–180. Order platelet (PLT) function test, P2Y12, PLT function, aspirin function
5. Has contraindication for anticoagulation (i.e., GI bleed), therefore **cardioversion** may not be an option for the patient with atrial fibrillation.
6. AFib nonresponsive to medications treatment: consider **CRT** (cardiac resynchronization therapy pacemaker) also known as biventricular pacemaker (BIV PPM) and AV nodal ablation.
7. **Cardizem drip to metoprolol**: 10–25 mg IV Cardizem followed by Cardizem at 10 mg/day, transitioned to metoprolol 25 mg qid. If HR > 110, do metoprolol 5 mg IV push. Cardizem IV to oral: [IV rate × 3 + 3] × 10 mg qd
8. After **CRT pacemaker** placement, **metoprolol 100 mg** qd was added in AFib with **tachybrady syndrome**.
9. For high white count or fever, make sure to do a review of systems (ROS) to identify the cause, culture sputum, urine, blood, and stool as necessary.
10. **Steroid tapering** ≤ 20 mg qd: 10 mg for 3 days, 5 mg for 3 days, 2.5 mg for 3 days, and stop.

10/28/2017

1. **Four bacteria commonly contaminate blood culture**: coagulase-negative staph, Corynebacterium (G+ bacilli), Propionibacterium acnes (anaerobic G+ rods), and bacillus species (anaerobic G+ rod).
2. **Corynebacterium in the respiratory culture of pneumonia** treatment: Vanco for 2 weeks.
3. Lung cancer with high white blood cell (WBC) count: may need Vanco/Zosyn for 14 days.

4. **Supraventricular tachycardia (SVT)** treatment: adenosine to return to NSR; start metoprolol 25 mg bid, EP study, Echo, Cardiolite stress test in the setting of trop leak and diffuse ST depression (likely subendocardial).
5. **Dysphagia**—barium swallow. **Thoracentesis labs**: cell count, LDH, Pr, Glu, culture, pH, acid-fast smear, amylase.

10/29/2017

1. Acid base disorder **urine studies**: Urine Cl, Na, Cr, Pr, osmolarity (use urea if diuretics).
2. **Delta delta** = delta AG/delta HCO_3 = (calculated AG − [albumin] × 2.5)/(24-HCO_3): 1–2 HAGMA, <1 mixed, >2 metabolic alkalosis and acidosis.
3. **Symptoms of respiratory alkalosis**: paraesthesia, carpopedal spasm, and lightheadedness.
4. Chronic metabolic alkalosis should raise PCO_2 by about 7 mmHg for every 1 mEq/L elevation in HCO_3.
5. **Check urine Na for volume status in metabolic alkalosis**: if volume depletion, urine Na < 20 mEq/L except for diuresis; dialysis with low bicarbonate bath concentration will rapidly improve alkalosis.
6. Rarely severe metabolic alkalosis (HCO_3 > 50 mEq/L and/or pH > 7.55) can be treated with IV hydrochloric acid (HCl) or on HCL precursor ammonium chloride.
7. Workup for **anion gap (AG) metabolic acidosis**: look for ketonuria → renal function, lactate, toxic screen, osmolarity gap (>10). Workup for **non-AG metabolic acidosis**: check urine AG = (urine Na+ urine K) − Urine Cl.
8. **Fasting ketosis or alcoholic ketosis**, pay attention to K, P, Mg, combined acid base disease. Treatment with thiamine and D5 glucose.
9. **Pericarditis diagnosis** requires two of the following: Hx of chest pain, friction rub, ECG findings (**ST elevation and PR depression in most leads but reciprocal ST depression and PR elevation in lead aVR**), and effusion. **Causes of pericarditis** include infection (viral, bacterial, fungal); neoplastic (metastatic vs. primary serosal and cardiac tumors, mesothelioma); autoimmune [Rheumatoid arthritis, systemic lupus erythematosus (SLE), scleroderma, Sjogren's, polyarteritis nodosa (PAN), granulomatosis with polyangiitis (GPA = Wegener's granulomatosis), eosinophilic granulomatosis with polyangiitis (Churg-Strauss)]; drug-induced; uremia; cardiovascular disease (CVD); radiation; effusion without pericarditis, congestive heart failure (CHF), cirrhosis, and nephritic syndrome.
10. **Pericarditis**: Chest X-ray (CXR) ≥ 250 cc fluid = water bottle heart (pericardial effusion deserves cardiologist consultation); ECG of pericarditis = widespread concave **ST elevation and PR depression** throughout most of the limb leads (I, II, III, aVL, aVF) and precordial leads (V2-6), T wave inversions, CKMB/Tnl mildly elevated or normal, and CRP and ESR high.
11. **Pericardiocentesis labs**: total protein, LDH, Glu, culture and sensitivity, acid-fast stain, cytology, adenosine deaminase (ADA). ADA increases with bacterial

infections, granulomatous inflammation, malignancy, and autoimmune diseases. Pericardial biopsy for TB or malignancy.

12. **Treatment of pericarditis**: NSAIDs ibuprofen 600–800 mg tid or aspirin 750–1000 mg tid for 1–2 weeks or until resolution of symptoms followed by a taper, or colchicine 0.5 mg bid for 3 months; avoid steroids with anticoagulants.
13. **Recurrent pericarditis = relapsed pericarditis after 4–6 weeks' symptom free**. Risk factors for recurrent pericarditis include subacute onset, large effusion/tamponade, T > 38, lack of NSAID response after 7 days, and recurrent despite colchicine 0.5 mg bid × 6 m.
14. **Pericardial tamponade**, no y wave. **Beck's triad**: distant heart sounds, elevated jugular venous distension (JVD,) hypotension. Diastolic collapse. **Treatment**: pericardiocentesis, volume resuscitation, and + inotropes.
15. Differential diagnoses (DDx) of **pulsus paradoxus**: pulmonary embolism (PE), hypovolemia, severe COPD, right ventricular (RV) infarct, vs. cardiac tamponade. sBP ≥ 10 mg drop with inspiration = **Kussmaul sign**: The Kussmaul sign is seen in **constrictive pericarditis**, as well as with **restrictive cardiomyopathy**.
16. **Constrictive pericarditis**: TB, radiation therapy, bacterial, neoplastic. Adhesion of visceral parietal pericardial layers → increased systemic venous pressure. Point of maximal impulse is not palpable, but pericardial knock, and calcification on CXR are common in constrictive pericarditis. **Septal bounce** = abrupt displacement of septum during rapid filling in the early phase, prominent x and y descent, thickened pericardium with thickening.
17. **Constrictive cardiomyopathy** right ventricular systolic pressure (RVSP) < 55 mmHg, thickened pericardium; whereas **restrictive cardiomyopathy** only has RVSP > 55 mmHg.
18. Young patient with **SVT** management: adenosine → beta blocker 50 mg qd, EP study, stress test if trop leak.
19. **Trazodone** and **melatonin** for sleep. **Seroquel** may be appropriate for agitation or insomnia in senior patients.
20. Lasix low bioavailability 50% to variable; torsemide 70%–80% bioavailability; Bumex 90%–100% bioavailability.
21. Posterior circulation ischemia of vertebral arteries can cause significant vertigo from **cerebellar hypoperfusion or ischemia**. **Vertebral artery stenosis treatment**: DAPT to put P2Y12 around 100 therapeutic range, then do stenting; or DAPT 7–10 days before stenting.
22. **Downsloping ST** is bad indicating acute coronary syndrome or angina; **upsloping ST** elevation is Ok and may represent repolarization.
23. If Lexiscan, we do not need to stop beta-blocker, but in regular stress tests, we may have to stop beta blocker (debatable).

10/30/2017

1. **Gastric bypass vitamin supplementation:** vitamin complex (Vit B1, thiamine is most important), extra dose thiamine 100 mg iv × 2 weeks, 250 mg po qd.

2. The **Thrombolysis in Myocardial Infarction (TIMI)** score for unstable angina (UA) and non-STEMI risk stratification: ≥65 yo, ≥3 risk factors for CAD, coronary stenosis ≥50% stenosis, presence of ST segment deviation on admission EKG, at least three angina episodes in prior 24 h, increased serum cardiac enzymes, use of aspirin in prior 7 days.
3. Seven **diagnostic criteria** in classic beriberi: three or more months of thiamine deficiency diet; enlarged heart with normal sinus rhythm; dependent edema; signs of neuritis, pellagra, or both; minor electrocardiogram changes such as nonspecific ST-T wave changes; no identifiable cause for heart disease; response to thiamine therapy. **Treatment**: up to 100 mg of thiamine IV for a few days followed by oral 25 mg/day for 2 weeks.
4. In **orthostatic hypotension**, heart rate (HR) should go up; however, if **autonomic dysfunction**, HR will have no change with position change.
5. **Fluid restriction and diet recommendation** for congestive heart failure (CHF) and chronic kidney disease (CKD).

10/31/2017

1. **Fascicular tachycardia**, which mimics both VTach and SVT on EKG, is the most common idiopathic ventricular tachycardia (VT) of the left ventricle. It's a re-entrant tachycardia due to ectopic focus in the left ventricle seen in young patients without structural heart disease. **Treatment**: verapamil
2. **P wave**: morphology- monophasic in lead II, biphasic in lead V1; axis P wave should be upright in leads I&II, inverted in aVR. Left atrial enlargement (LAE) = P mitrale; right atrial enlargement (RAE) = P pulmonale (VII > 2.5 mm).
3. **Inverted u wave** = consider coronary artery disease (CAD), hypertension (HTN), vascular heart disease, congenital heart disease, cardiomyopathy, and hypothyroidism.

10/31/2017

1. **Angiography/percutaneous coronary intervention (PCI) complications**: hematoma with retroperitoneal extension, arteriovenous fistula, pseudoaneurysm, ventricular perforation, contrast-induced nephropathy, stroke, dissection of the aorta or coronary arteries.
2. **Atrioventricular (AV) block Mobitz Type II** can progress to complete heart block, stop AV nodal blocking agents, permanent pacemaker probably is needed as well.
3. **Bradycardia** treatment: 0.5 mg **atropine** IV q5 min up to 3 mg. The second line of treatment in symptomatic bradycardia is **dopamine** drip at 5–20 μg/kg/min infusion or **epinephrine** at 2–10 μg/min. Additionally, **transcutaneous pacing can be applied after atropine when available** before permanent pacemaker placement.
4. **Brugada syndrome**: "coved" ST elevations and RBBB in V1-V3. Treatment: implantable cardioverter-defibrillators (ICDs).
5. **Cardiac device infections**: pocket infection, deep infections (transvenous portion of the leads), usually caused by Staph aureus, Strep, Corynebacterium,

Propionibacterium, G-rods, or candida. Around **30%–70%** of patients with staph bacteremia with any hardware will have device infection; **treatment**: device explantation; 50% of patients with device-related endocarditis have valve vegetation (others include pneumonia, lung abscess, or septic emboli).

6. Cardiac risk assessment before surgery: **Modified Revised Cardiac Risk Index**.
7. Modified barium swallow (done by speech therapist) vs. barium swallow (esophagram, done by radiologist only).
8. **Elevated troponins**: Type I NSTEMI (major cardiac muscle damage due to coronary artery stenosis), Type II NSTEMI (significant cardiac muscle damage due to demand supply mismatch rather than coronary artery stenosis), acute myocardial injury (insignificant cardiac muscle damage due to demand ischemia), vs. demand ischemia (no troponin elevation but supply-demand mismatch).
9. For acute congestive heart failure (CHF), **B-type natriuretic peptide (BNP) can be normal in obese patients.**
10. **Pulmonary embolism (PE) and deep vein thrombosis (DVT)** need loading doses Xarelto 15 mg bid for 3 weeks then 20 mg qd; or Eliquis 10 mg bid for 7 days, and then 5 mg bid; or dabigatran 150 mg bid after heparin/Lovenox for 5–10 days.
11. Limited data for using direct oral anticoagulants (DOACs) in **left atrial appendage thrombus**. Caution the use of DOAC (except Eliquis) for **BMI** greater than **40** or weight greater than **120 kg** due to concerns of under-dosing and limited data in this population.
12. **Amiodarone** is the second-line option in patients with high risk for thrombus with AFib as it cardioverts. May cardiovert patients if symptomatic hypotension or worsening congestive heart failure (CHF) with rate control.
13. **RIMA and LIMA** are the right and left internal mammary arteries.
14. **Cardiac dysfunction in HIV**: myocarditis, dilated cardiomyopathy, pulmonary hypertension.
15. **Cardiac resynchronization therapy** with pacing both the LV and RV (biventricular pacing) or LV alone by either a CRT-pacemaker (CRT-P) or by a combined CRT-implantable cardioverter-defibrillator (CRT-D) is indicated for despite maximal medical therapy for 3 months or at **least 40 days** after myocardial infarction, **LVEF ≤ 35%** (NYHA Class II, III/IV) and intraventricular conduction delay with **QRS ≥150 ms** (QRS 120–150 ms needs discussions and referrals for CRT). In addition to the standard pacing lead in the right ventricle (RV), another lead is placed through the coronary sinus into the left ventricle (LV) in CRT.
16. **Carotid dissection**: unilateral headache; ipsilateral Horner syndrome; contralateral hemispheric findings. Treatment: patients with ischemic stroke or TIA and extracranial carotid or vertebral arterial dissection, need antithrombotic treatment with **either antiplatelet or anticoagulation for at least 3–6 months**. Aspirin 81 mg (ASA) should be started 24 h after thrombolysis. ASA in the acute phase within 48 h of stroke onset and antiplatelet therapy (ASA, Plavix,

ASA-dipyridamole, or cilostazol) for secondary prevention. If recurrent stroke or contraindications for antiplatelet therapy, do **endovascular stenting** for carotid dissection (**stenting** if contraindications to anticoagulation or if medical management fails).

17. **Intravenous alteplase** (tenecteplase is now more commonly used) should be started within 3–4.5 h of clearly defined symptom onset of ischemic stroke.
18. **Spectrum of congestive heart failure (CHF)**: congestion and perfusion (wet vs dry & warm vs. cold)
19. Patients with **diastolic dysfunction** do not tolerate tachycardia/arrhythmia due to loss of the atrial kick, hypertension due to increased left ventricular (LV) wall stress, and ischemia from increased LV stiffness. These will lead to pulmonary edema from sympathetic responses.
20. The **mainstay of treatment of diastolic dysfunction** is blood pressure control to stop and reverse left ventricular hyperplasia (LVH), optimize volume, rate control of AFib, and re-vascularization.
21. **Treatment of cardiogenic shock**: norepinephrine (first line treatment), if unable to maintain pressure, add dobutamine to norepinephrine or switch to epinephrine. Additional options for cardiogenic shock treatment: epinephrine, dobutamine (beta 1 and 2 agonists) → dopamine → milrinone → epinephrine, especially in dry/wet and cold CHF.
22. **Intra-aortic balloon pump indications**: cardiogenic shock not quickly reversed with pharmacologic therapy; hypotension unresponsive to other interventions; a low output state; acute mitral regurgitation (MR) from papillary muscle rupture or ventricular septum ruptures; recurrent ischemic chest pain with signs of hemodynamic instability.

11/2/2017

1. **Acute gout treatment**: indomethacin 50 mg tid for 3 weeks, start allopurinol 2 weeks after acute attack. Alternative treatments include prednisone or prednisolone, at an initial dose of 30–40 mg once daily until flare resolution begins, then taper over 7–10 days; oral NSAIDs may also be used. Colchicine: 0.6 mg 3 times on the first day or taken as 1.2 mg for the first dose followed by 0.6 mg an hour later and then 0.6 mg once or twice daily is also commonly used in acute gout attack.
2. **DOACs (also referred to as NOACs)**: are absolutely not used in metal valves, but may be used in AFib with Factor V Leiden, moderate to severe aortic stenosis, moderate to severe mitral stenosis, bioprosthetic valves (3 months after valve placement).
3. Two consecutive LDL < 40, need to **decrease statin** dose.
4. **Pretreatment of IV dye allergy**: three doses of 50 mg oral prednisone administered 13, 7, and 1 h before contrast administration, plus 50 mg oral or IV diphenhydramine 1 h before contrast administration.
5. Convert IV Cardizem to po: oral dose in mg/d = [rate (mL/h) × 3 + 3] × 10.

6. The patient became incredibly agitated requiring **Precedex and fentanyl** for sedation which caused hypotension, requiring central line and vasopressor therapy. Can switch sedation medication to **versed**.

11/3/2017

1. Every patient with a newly implanted automatic implantable cardioverter defibrillator (**AICD**) should have it interrogated. The same for each new admission, especially for patients with syncope and dizziness.
2. In congestive heart failure (CHF) patients, **metformin increases the risk of lactic acidosis (debatable)**.
3. Stroke/transient ischemic attack (TIA) patients, order MRI brain without contrast, MRA brain, MRA with and without contrast neck. Code stroke head and neck CT angio may suffice the need for head and neck MRA.
4. Nicotine dependence: nicotine patch 21 mg qd for 6 weeks, 14 mg for 4 weeks, and 7 mg for 2 weeks.
5. **HEART score** for chest pain: History, ECG, Age, Risk factors, and Troponin. Score 0–3 discharge (0.7%–0.9% MACE); score > 4–6 admit (12%–16.6%); score ≥ 7 (50%–65% MACE). MACE is an abbreviation for major adverse cardiovascular events; higher MACE risks warrant early invasive measures.
6. Hard to control AFib treatment: metoprolol succinate 150 mg qd, Cardizem 30 mg q6h, metoprolol tartrate 5 mg IV q6h prn. May consider amiodarone and/or digoxin.
7. Stenting became the standard of care for percutaneous coronary interventions (PCIs), with **balloon angioplasty** alone being used only in situations where a stent could not be delivered to the target lesion or if contraindications for dual antiplatelet therapy.
8. Target vessel revascularization was defined as any repeat PCI in the target vessel.
9. Vessels **smaller than 2 mm, tortuous, angulated, and calcified arterial segments** are not suitable for stenting.
10. **Suboptimal stenting** = residual stenosis ≥10%, evidence of stent thrombosis, dissection or abrupt closure, absence of TIMI 3 flow, or need for three or more stents.
11. **Angiographic predictors of inability to predilate** include moderate to severe coronary calcifications, heavy plaque burden, or diffuse coronary artery disease.
12. **Appropriateness considerations for direct stenting**: vessel diameter >2.5 mm, proximal lesion location, no severe calcifications, no bifurcation lesions, absence of very severe lesions and bifurcation lesions, ST-elevation myocardial infarction (STEMI).
13. **High-pressure balloon dilation stents** are deployed with a high-pressure technique utilizing ≥12–16 atm (atmospheric pressure).
14. The presence of a myocardial **fractional flow rate reserve (FFR)** >0.05 (ratio of distal coronary to aortic pressure during IV adenosine infusion) correlates with a large stent cross-sectional area and a reduced risk of subsequent restenosis.
15. **Periprocedural complications of percutaneous coronary interventions**. **Coronary A complications**: (1) dissection and abrupt closure after percutane-

ous transluminal coronary angioplasty (PTCA), not common after stenting, (2) intramural hematoma, (3) perforation (PTCA balloon or perfusion balloon catheter), (4) distal embolism (CKMB increase supporting microembolization and periprocedural necrosis), (5) side branch occlusion (myonecrosis, stent jail treated with ostium dilated through stent struts). **Complications of stenting**: failure of stent deployment, stent thrombosis/infection, increased risk of mycotic aneurysms, and spontaneous coronary artery perforation. Myocardial ischemia and infarction are treated with **percutaneous coronary intervention**. **Emergency coronary artery bypass grafting (CABG)** is used for failed percutaneous coronary intervention (PCI).

16. **Vascular complications at femoral artery access site**: minor or major hematomas, pseudoaneurysm, arterial laceration, retroperitoneal hematoma, AV fistula, arterial occlusion, and local infection with/without sepsis. Radial artery access is more commonly used with less side effects.
17. **Non-cardiac surgery after PCI**: wait after DAPT for at least 1 month after bare metal stents, at least 6 months for drug-eluting stents, and at least 14 days for prior balloon angioplasty.
18. **Indications for revascularization with CABG or PCI**: (A) patients with activity-limiting symptoms despite maximum medical therapy; (B) active patients who want PCI for improved QoL compared to medical therapy; (C) patients with anatomy for which revascularization has a proven survival benefit such as significant left main CAD (>50% luminal narrowing) or multivessel disease with a reduction of LVEF <50% and a large area of potentially ischemic myocardium.
19. **Single vessel coronary artery disease** = greater than 70% diameter stenosis or a 50%–70% diameter stenosis with a positive fraction flow reserve (<0.8) in either the proximal or mid portion of the artery.
20. **Fractional flow reserve (FFR)** measurement = the ratio between the mean coronary pressure distal to a coronary stenosis and the mean aortic pressure proximal to the stenosis. An FFR of 1.0 is considered normal. An FFR lower than 0.75–0.80 correlates with myocardial ischemia (MI).
21. **ST elevation myocardial infarction (STEMI) treatment**: (A) radial as opposed to a femoral approach for PCI; (B) undergoing PCI, perform non-culprit vessel PCI as well; (C) direct stenting after aspiration thrombectomy; (D) DAPT, IV heparin (start 4 h later after PCI if no stent but need CABG), beta-blocker should be used; (E) discharge after 72 h.
22. Mild Stage II and moderate Stage III chronic kidney disease (CKD) may benefit from PCI/CABG in CAD and should be strongly recommended.

1. **Indications for CABG**: (A) 50% left main stenosis; (B) 70% stenosis of proximal left anterior descending (LAD) and proximal circumflex artery; (C) triple vessel disease in asymptomatic or mild/stable angina; (D) triple vessel disease with proximal LAD stenosis and poor LVEF; (E) one or two vessel disease and a large area of viable myocardium in high-risk area in patients with stable angina; or (F) 70% left proximal LAD stenosis with LVEF <50% or ischemia on noninvasive testing.

2. **Coronary artery bypass grafting (CABG) preop**: vein mapping, echo, carotid Doppler, and pulmonary function test.
3. **Multivessel coronary artery disease (MVD)** = greater than 70% stenosis in at least two major coronary arteries with a diameter of ≥2.5 mm or in one coronary artery in addition to greater than 50% stenosis of the left main trunk.

11/6/2017

1. **Vitamin B12 deficiency treatment**: cyanocobalamin 1000 μg subcutaneously qd for 7 days then qweek for 4 weeks then qd for 90 days and then monthly.
2. Indications for primary prevention using **automated implantable cardioverter defibrillator (AICD)**: prior myocardial infarction with LVEF ≤30%, Class II and III CHF with LVEF <35% after 40 days to 3 months of guideline-directed medical therapy; prior MI with nonsustained VT and LVEF ≤40% (if VF or sustained VT-induced during electrophysiology study). Consider **life vest upon discharge** prior to AICD placement in these patients.
3. Consider **Cardiac Resynch Therapy** with if EF < 35%, LBBB (QRS > 120 ms), and symptomatic heart failure ⇒ CRT-D with biventricular pacer.
4. **Iron supplementation** if ferritin <100 or ferritin 100–200 and transferrin saturation <20%.
5. **Aortic regurgitation treatment**: nifedipine, hydralazine, and ACEi.
6. For development delay patients, we will need to work with the case manager and social worker to arrange for group homes.
7. **Obstructive sleep apnea (OSA)** concerns will need an outpatient sleep study.
8. If the digoxin level is high, may do digoxin dosing qod.
9. **Superficial thrombophlebitis**: initial management of uncomplicated, less extensive thrombosis at low risk for VTE, i.e., affected vein segment <5 cm, remote from saphenofemoral or saphenopopliteal junction, no medical risk factors, is supportive and consists of extremity elevation, warm and cool compression, NSAIDs.
10. **Isolated distal DVT** (peroneal, posterior, anterior tibial, and muscular veins) encompasses thromboses located below the knee in the calf veins (ie, the popliteal vein is not involved): a select minority can avoid anticoagulation. If no anticoagulation: survey patients every week for 2 weeks with proximal compression ultrasound (CUS) for clot extension or resolution.
11. Antibiotic treatment is not indicated unless there are signs of infection (i.e., high fever, purulent drainage) in superficial thrombophlebitis. Aortic stenosis is very sensitive to fluids and requires extreme caution with fluid status.
12. **Acute kidney injury (AKI)** treatment: usually can be treated with IV fluid at the beginning; GFR < 30, do heparin, otherwise Lovenox is Ok.
13. **Lovenox (enoxaparin)** has not been FDA-approved for use in dialysis patients. Lopressor hold is necessary if HR < 55 or sBP < 100.
14. If a **mass** is discovered in imaging studies, may need an interventional radiologist to do a **biopsy**.
15. Enalapril 20–40 mg qd and Lisinopril 5–10 mg for heart.

11/7/2017

1. **Diagnosis of syphilis**: standard contact isolation, order Chlamydia and gonorrhea, HBV/HCV screening. **Treatment**: doxycycline 100 mg bid for 14 days if penicillin allergy.
2. **AFib with RVR** treatment: Cardizem drip (5–25 mg/h) and Lopressor 5 mg IV q6h
3. Respiratory failure: $SO_2 < 88\%$ or increase in O_2 use to >5 lpm nasal cannula.
4. In **long QT syndrome**, avoid Zofran, and Seroquel, can give Tigan (Trimethobenzamide) for nausea, and Zolpidem for sleep.
5. Plavix loading is necessary for stenting. If CABG, do only aspirin in NSTEMI/STEMI and heparin drip or full anticoagulation dose Lovenox but no Plavix.
6. Cardizem maximum dose is 90 mg q6h; IV drip to po transition: first give oral, 2 h later, stop IV drip.

11/8/2017

1. **Occam's razor**: the simpler one the better
2. **Na correction in hyperglycemia**: corrected Na = measured Na + [2.4 × (measured glucose − 100)/100] or 1.6 for glucose 100–400 and 4 for glu >400.
3. Infusion of large volumes of solutions containing NaCl and no alkali can cause **hyperchloremic metabolic acidosis**.
4. **PTH** inhibits Na+/H+ antiporter activity and bicarbonate reabsorption, causing hyperchloremic metabolic acidosis.
5. Lactic acid should be ordered as STAT.
6. Biopsy with local anesthetic no NPO; systemic anesthesia, need NPO order.
7. **Keep family on board** for decision-making with the patient's permission, especially when consulting palliative care or hospice.

11/9/2017

1. **Chylomicronemia syndrome** occurs when serum triglyceride level >1000 mg/dL, is represented by excess **very low-density lipoprotein (VLDL)**, turbid infranatant, can cause recent memory loss, abdominal pain or/and pancreatitis, dyspnea, eruptive xanthoma, flushing with alcohol and lipemia retinalis. Acute treatment of chylomicronemia syndrome is insulin drip.
2. **Three major categories of chylomicronemia syndrome**: familial chylomicronemia syndrome (caused by **lipoprotein lipase or apo CII mutations**), multifactorial chylomicronemia syndrome (**MFCS**), and familial partial lipodystrophy (**FPLD**).
3. Most patients with chylomicronemia syndrome have a secondary cause such as the administration of exogenous triglyceride (TG)-elevating therapies such as estrogen, tamoxifen, glucocorticoids, tacrolimus, cyclosporine, protease inhibitors, or poorly controlled diabetes.
4. **High-intensity statin therapy** is more effective than low-intensity statin therapy for lowering TG levels. Among patients with TG 200–880, atorvastatin 80 and rosuvastatin 20 mg qd reduce fasting TG 43%–44%. Additionally, add a **fibrate** and/or **omega-3** fatty acid.

5. For recurrent pancreatitis due to high TG, treatment with a very low-fat diet with a strict reduction in refined carbohydrates, complete avoidance of alcohol, and caloric restriction is necessary.
6. CYP3A4 is responsible for the metabolism of both statins and fibrates. **Fenofibrate is the preferred fibrate** that requires combined therapy with a statin and fibrate to minimize statin-induced muscle toxicity.

11/10/2017

1. Lopressor 200 mg bid is the maximal dose.
2. Use BiPAP/CPAP to replace nasal cannula if persistent respiratory acidosis. Effient (prasugrel) causes low PLT.
3. Order **care management consultation** for social worker and case manager assistance for difficult financial situations with no insurance or poor living conditions.
4. Cardizem drip at 20 mg/h can be replaced with Cardizem 90 mg q6h or Lopressor 25 mg bid.
5. **Hyponatremia**: check urine and serum osmolarity, urine Na and Cl. In SIADH, serum osmolarity is lower than urine osmolarity. Target Na in SIADH is around 127–128 (patients may be discharged if serum Na is maintained at 127–128 or above).

11/11/2017

1. **Workup for hyponatremia**: serum osmolarity, urine random sodium, urine osmolarity, morning cortisol, and TSH. Syndrome of inappropriate antidiuretic hormone (SIADH) is common.
2. Seizure: **elevated prolactin essay** when measured in the appropriate setting at 10–20 min after a suspected seizure is a useful adjunct test for the differentiation of generalized tonic-clonic or complex partial seizure from psychogenic nonepileptic seizures; however, serum prolactin assay is elevated in both epilepsy and syncope. **Repeat 6 h later** which is usually the patient's baseline prolactin level.
3. No insurance, make sure the patient has medications upon discharge. If not, talk to the case manager; if not possible, no discharge.
4. **Diabetes supplies**: Insulin Lantus solar star pen, test strips, glucometer and lancet needles, BD ultra fine pen needles 4 mm 32-gauge needles.
5. **Supraventricular tachycardia (SVT)** treatment: keep K+ above 4 and mag above 2.
6. CPAP with auto-titration set at 5–10 cmH_2O
7. **Chest pain**: nitro drip at 10 cc/min and heparin drip for 2 days for UA; can add Imdur, nitro sublingual, Ranexa.
8. **Metformin in low ejection fraction (EF) and hemodynamically unstable patients causes lethal lactic acidosis.**

11/13/2017

1. For **asymptomatic abdominal aortic aneurysm** (AAA), elective repair thresholds are **5.5 cm in males** and **5 cm in females** to prevent rupture. Elective repair

is not recommended until the risk of rupture exceeds the risks associated with repair (≥5.5 cm in males and ≥5 cm in females).

2. An abdominal aorta with a maximal diameter of **>3.0 cm** is considered **aneurysmal** in most adult patients between **renal-inferior mesenteric arteries** (IMA).
3. Timing of elective AAA repair is affected by other factors: coexistent peripheral artery disease (PAD) or peripheral aneurysm (iliac aneurysm, femoral aneurysm) and other factors increasing the risk of ruptures like advanced age and rapid aneurysm expansion (5 mm in half year).
4. Repair of suprarenal and/or thoracoabdominal aneurysm, threshold 5.5–6 cm.
5. AAA is a coronary heart disease equivalent and should be treated with **anti-platelet therapy, statin, and anti-hypertensive therapy to reduce cardiovascular (CV) risks, smoking cessation, and high levels of physical activity**.
6. **Aneurysm surveillance**: annual ultrasound (U/S) for <4.5 cm; annual or more frequent for larger ones: ultrasound every 6–12 m for 4.5–4.9 cm; ultrasound every 3 m for 5–5.4 cm. CT may be used as an alternative to ultrasound.
7. **Endovascular repair** is preferred in favorable anatomy and no high surgical risks. Open surgical repair in young and low perioperative risk to limit radiation exposure from stent-graft surveillance (**CTA at 1–6 months** to look for sac expansion and endoleak) after endovascular repair, or the need for secondary procedures.
8. For patients with **ruptured AAA or aortic dissection** (stat vascular surgery consultation is necessary), systolic blood pressure should be lowered to between 80 and 100 mmHg (permissive hypotension) using: "**esmolol** (250–500 μg/kg IV loading dose, then infuse at 25–50 μg/kg/min; titrate to maximum dose of 300 μg/kg/min) or **labetalol** (20 mg IV initially, followed by either 20–80 mg IV boluses every 10 min to a maximal dose of 300 mg, or an infusion of 0.5–2 mg/min IV)". Alternatives are verapamil or diltiazem. Once the heart rates consistently <60 BPM, give vasodilator therapy with **nitroprusside** infusion (0.25–0.5 μg/kg/min titrated to a maximum of 10 μg/kg/min) or **nicardipine** infusion (2.5–5 mg/h titrated to a maximum of 15 mg/h).
9. Nitroglycerin may also be used in AAA rupture, but it produces relatively greater venodilation than arteriolar dilation. Consider **nitroglycerin drip in patients with symptomatic coronary disease and those with hypertension** following coronary bypass. Prolonged infusions may cause tachyphylaxis.
10. Treatment of acute aortic dissection depends on the type/location. **Aortic dissection of the ascending aorta is a cardiac surgical emergency**. Aortic dissection below the ascending aorta (the descending thoracic and/or the abdominal aorta) can often be managed medically unless there is evidence of end-organ ischemia, progression, or rupture.
11. Poor candidate for anticoagulation due to alcoholism.
12. Anticoagulation of AFib depends on **CHA2DS2-VASc** score; S2 for stroke or TIA or VTE; V is vascular disease like peripheral arterial disease (PAD), myocardial infarction (MI), and aortic plaque.

13. **Sulfasalazine** causes oligospermia; Vit B12 deficiency can cause seizures; lisinopril causes high K.
14. **Keppra 1500 mg** bid is the maximal dose. Aldosterone preserves Na and Cl and excretes K and H.
15. **Refractory AFib** treatment: Cardizem 60 mg q6h, Lopressor 75 mg tid, amio drip starts after 150 mg in 10 min.
16. Low-dose aspirin is recommended for individuals **aged 50–59 years of age who have a 10% or greater 10-year risk of CVD risk** for primary prevention. Evidence to recommend aspirin in populations aged 60–69 as primary prevention is less robust and should be individualized.
17. **Glycopyrrolate**: used for excessive secretions and to reverse bradycardia; it is a muscarinic anticholinergic that does not cross blood-brain barrier (BBB).
18. **Paroxysmal AFib** = spontaneous termination <7 days usually <48 h; **persistent AFib** ≥ 7 days or prior cardioversion; **permanent AFib** = sinus rhythm (SR) can't be restored (terminated but relapsed); **long-standing AFib** ≥ 12 months.
19. **HAS-BLED** score: hypertension (HTN), abnormal liver or kidney function (2), stroke Hx, bleeding Hx or predisposition to bleeding, labile INR, elderly >65 yo, prior drug (2) (alcohol usage + medication predisposing to bleeding). Total 9 points, **≥3 pts indicating high risk for bleeding**.

11/14/2017

1. **Legionella treatments**: antibiotics (ABX) with intracellular penetration include macrolide, quinolones, tetracycline, and rifampin. Duration: A minimum of 5 days and do not stop therapy until the patient is clinically stable and afebrile for at least 48 h.
2. Severe pneumonia or chronic comorbidities may be slow to respond and often require **7–10 days** of treatment in Legionella pneumonia. Immunocompromised, treat for a **minimum of 14 days,** and consider reducing immunosuppression (when feasible) in Legionella pneumonia.
3. Combination therapy using both a fluoroquinolone and a macrolide does not appear to improve outcomes for legionella infection. Adding rifampin (an agent that achieves high intracellular concentrations and can penetrate biofilms) to either fluoroquinolone or macrolide monotherapy does not appear to improve outcomes but may increase adverse events for legionella infection.
4. For legionella infections, other drugs have been used successfully **include tetracycline, doxycycline, tigecycline, and TMP-SMX**.
5. Levofloxacin 500 mg IV qd for 10–14 days or 750 mg for 5 days was effective for mild, moderate and severe legionella infection. Azithromycin 500 mg qd for 5–7 days in mild legionella infection and 7–10 days for severe legionella infection. No fever for 24 h, can switch iv to po.
6. **Transplant patients** with legionella, only use Cipro or levofloxacin as macrolide interacts with cyclosporine and tacrolimus.
7. Stroke patients concerning **embolic/thrombotic**, may need transesophageal echocardiogram (TEE), telemetry, loop recorder, and thrombophilia workup.

8. **Multifocal atrial tachycardia (MAT)** does not require anticoagulation, may be treated with calcium channel blocker (CCB), beta blocker, Magnesium, Amio, digitalis, ibutilide, or flecainide if concerned.
9. AFib can have tachycardia-induced cardiomyopathy ⇒ congestive heart failure
10. AFib <7 days = paroxysmal; >7 days = persistent; >1 year = long-standing, failed cardioversion = permanent.
11. **Cardioversion**: chemical or electrical, needs a minimum of 3 weeks' anticoagulation no matter what the CHA2DS2VASc score. The TEE approach shortens the pre-cardioversion anticoagulation duration; however, patients still require **4 weeks of anticoagulation after cardioversion** or the need to be therapeutically anticoagulated at the time of the cardioversion.
12. If only the female gender is the risk factor, the CHA2DS2VASc score is 0.
13. **Emergent cardioversion** if chest pain, hemodynamically unstable, or acute congestive heart failure (CHF).
14. Congestive heart failure (CHF) AFib—use amiodarone or dofetilide for Afib rhythm control. CAD—use dofetilide, dronedarone, or sotalol or amiodarone for Afib rhythm control. No structural heart disease—uses dofetilide, dronedarone, flecainide, propafenone or sotalol for Afib rhythm control.
15. **Central sleep apnea** can be related to congestive heart failure, stroke, or renal failure, use of opioids and other CNS depressants, CNS disorders, and high altitude. **Potomania** also known as beer potomania, beer drinker's potomania, and beer drinker's hyponatremia is a specific hypo-osmolality syndrome related to massive consumption of beer (poor in electrolytes).
16. **For AFib with low BP**, use digoxin or amiodarone rather than beta blocker or calcium channel blocker (anticoagulation first when possible); cardioversion is the reserved option.
17. **Radioablation at pulmonary veins and left atrium** for AFib; side effects include AV fistula and pulmonary hypertension in the lungs. MAZE procedure is used to treat atrial fibrillation.
18. For atrial flutter, **radioablation at the right atrium**.
19. **Idarucizumab** is an antidote for dabigatran; **Andexanet alfa** (Andexxa, Portola) is an antidote for patients treated with rivaroxaban (Xarelto, Janssen) or apixaban (Eliquis) who require anticoagulation reversal due to uncontrolled or life-threatening bleeding.
20. For **severe mitral stenosis** or mitral valve area $\leq$1.5 cm^2 and bioprosthetic valve [surgical or transcatheter] **within the first 3–6 months after implantation**, and a mechanical heart valve, will need to use warfarin rather than novel oral anticoagulants (NOACs).
21. **Orthostatic positive →** tilt table testing and then start midodrine
22. **Euthyroid sick syndrome** has elevated rT3 except in renal failure.

11/15/2017

1. The patient is on l**ong-term large amounts of opioids**, upon admission, we need to place her back on the same pain medication to prevent withdrawal. The same for baclofen.

2. Eye drops: artificial tears. Voiding trial → catheter removal.
3. **Dronabinol** is an anti-nausea medication, brand name Marinol. It is a tetrahydrocannabinol, made from cannabis also known as marijuana. It does not cause **QTc prolongation**.

11/17/2017

1. In diabetes mellitus (**DM**), gastroesophageal reflux disease (**GERD**) can be caused by autonomic neuropathy with decreased esophageal sphincter pressure; increased number of transient lower esophageal sphincter (LES) relaxations due to hyperglycemia, impaired clearance function of the tubular esophagus, or delayed gastric emptying.
2. For **diabetic gastroparesis**, initial treatment with **metoclopramide** (long-term use of metoclopramide can cause tardive dyskinesia). In patients who fail to respond to metoclopramide, do a trial of **domperidone** and oral **erythromycin** → cisapride (serotonin-4 receptor agonistic properties) → venting gastrostomy tube and decompression.
3. **Erythromycin** can increase serum **tacrolimus** levels.
4. VTach, order EKG. Mechanical valve and risk factors (atrial fibrillation, MI, left atrial enlargement, low ejection fraction (EF), endocardial damage) should be treated with both **warfarin and aspirin**. Aortic stenosis + AFib INR target is 2–3.
5. To minimize fluid intake, a more predictable/effective anticoagulation than IV heparin for DVT is Lovenox.
6. **Penile bleeding** after Foley, use Flomax. For stress tests, no caffeine, a light breakfast is Ok.
7. No major bleeding, Hgb stable, ulcerative colitis, Ok to restart anticoagulation.
8. Low blood pressure (BP), AFib with RVR, trial beta blocker if blood pressure is able to maintain, digoxin if already on full anticoagulation and concerns for drop in blood pressure, may give amiodarone if soft blood pressure or hypotension.
9. **Tumor lysis syndrome (TLS)** is an oncologic emergency with the release of large amounts of potassium (K), phosphorus (P), and nucleic acid (uric acid) into systemic circulation leading to acute kidney injury (AKI), mostly in high-grade lymphoma (Burkitt especially) and acute lymphocytic leukemia (ALL) and other tumors that have a high proliferative rate, large tumor burden, or high sensitivity to cytotoxic therapy. Labs show hyperkalemia, hyperphosphatemia, secondary hypocalcemia, hyperuricemia, and AKI.
10. **Hyperuricemia treatment**: prophylaxis with allopurinol or rasburicase and IV fluid hydrations in TLS. **Hyperphosphatemia** causes deposits of calcium phosphate throughout the body leading to calcification, arteriosclerosis, and acute kidney injury (AKI).

11/19/2017

1. **Crushing chest pain** = consider aortic dissection, myocardial infarction, pulmonary embolism?
2. **Triple antithrombotic therapy** may be needed in patients taking long-term oral anticoagulation who require dual antiplatelet therapy (DAPT) after intracoronary stent placement and patients on DAPT subsequently require initiation of oral anticoagulation like new onset of atrial fibrillation.
3. For most patients with atrial fibrillation who require an oral anticoagulant and who undergo percutaneous coronary intervention (PCI), triple therapy for the first month (even after the first week, then **drop aspirin**) → then continue antithrombotic therapy with a novel oral anticoagulant **(NOAC) plus clopidogrel** rather than with triple anticoagulation therapy during the first 6–12 months after percutaneous coronary intervention (PCI). After 12 months, long-term antithrombotic therapy with either **NOAC monotherapy** or NOAC plus an antiplatelet agent is reasonable.
4. For a bare metal stent (BMS), **1 month of triple therapy** irrespective of ischemic or bleeding risk (if AFib) is necessary.
5. For patients undergoing urgent PCI, may load Plavix 600 mg at diagnosis and continue 75 mg daily. For patients stable with unknown coronary anatomy and who are scheduled for coronary angiography with possible PCI, **do not give P2Y12** inhibitor as many patients either do not have coronary artery disease that needs revascularization or have severe coronary artery disease that requires coronary artery bypass grafting (CABG). Patients with prior diagnostic coronary angiography who are scheduled for PCI should receive **clopidogrel 600 mg at least 2 h before PCI**.
6. Patients are at high thrombotic risk if **prosthetic mitral valve** (3–6 months after valve placement) or **high CHA_2DS_2VASc score** (5 and above).
7. For patients taking NOAC, continue therapy until **24–48 h** before the procedure. In patients with chronic kidney disease (CKD), hold NOAC at least **36–48 h** before the procedure, especially for dabigatran.
8. For patients on warfarin, measure INR for at least 2 days to make sure INR is at the lower end of the target range in the morning of the procedure, especially if a large sheath is placed in the femoral artery. No **bridge** is necessary for patients taking warfarin unless **mechanical heart valves or AFib with CHA2DS2VASc score ≥5, ischemic stroke within 3 months, or recent VTE within 3 months**.
9. Intraprocedural anticoagulation for PCI, **use unfractionated heparin, if INR < 2, give full dose heparin**, and delay PCI if INR > 2.5 if possible.
10. For patients who did not take oral anticoagulation in the morning of PCI, start **NOAC** in the **evening**. If the femoral artery approaches, start the **next morning**.
11. **Lisinopril** at bedtime if morning (AM) blood pressure is low. Premature atrial contraction (**PAC**) can cause **irregular heart sounds** in auscultation.
12. Planning for PCI, **make sure to check if the patient can lie flat**. Claustrophobia to MRI, may order Xanax or Ativan if the patient is anxious or unable to lie still.
13. Dry nose: nasal spray Ocean blue.

14. **Wernicke-Korsakoff syndrome treatment**: thiamine 500 mg iv tid for 3 days then reassess for improvement. If improved symptoms, continue 250 mg IV qd for 5 days then 100 mg qd.
15. **Hepatic encephalopathy treatment**: lactulose titrate to have 2–3 or 4 bowel movements daily, can add rifaximin 550 mg tid.

Takeaway Messages

1. Pericarditis has reciprocal ST depression and PR elevation in lead aVR and can be treated with ibuprofen 600–800 mg tid or aspirin 750–1000 mg tid until resolution of symptoms with taper.
2. Understands the differentials of troponin elevation (different types of troponin elevation): only Type I NSTEMI has major coronary artery stenosis.
3. Cardiac resynchronization therapy is recommended for LVEF $\leq$ 35% and QRS $\geq$ 150 ms despite maximal medical therapy for 3 months or 40 days after myocardial infarction.
4. Low QRS wave on EKG together with soft blood pressure and distant heart sounds, make sure to get a stat echocardiogram and consider pericardiocentesis if pericardial (cardiac) tamponade.

Vacation time November 20th, 2017 through December 17th, 2017.

Further Readings and References

1. Murdoch, D., and S.T. Chambers. *Treatment and prevention of Legionella infection*, ed. J.A. Ramirez. Waltham, MA: UpToDate. Accessed November 3, 2023.
2. Adelstein, E., and S. Saba. *Cardiac resynchronization therapy in heart failure: Indications and choice of system*, ed. F. Masoudi. Waltham, MA: UpToDate. Accessed November 2, 2023.
3. Carrozza, J.P., and T. Levin. *Periprocedural complications of percutaneous coronary intervention*, ed. D. Cutlip. Waltham, MA: UpToDate. Accessed November 2, 2023.
4. Dalman, R.L., and M. Mell. *Management of asymptomatic abdominal aortic aneurysm*, ed. J.L. Mills, D.L. Clement, and M.A. Creager. Waltham, MA: UpToDate. Accessed November 2, 2023.
5. Chait, A., and R.H. Eckel. 2019. The Chylomicronemia syndrome is most often multifactorial: A narrative review of causes and treatment. *Annals of Internal Medicine* 170 (9): 626–634.
6. Kapa, S., P. Gaba, C.V. DeSimone, and S.J. Asirvatham. 2017. Fascicular ventricular arrhythmias: Pathophysiologic mechanisms, anatomical constructs, and advances in approaches to management. *Circulation: Arrhythmia and Electrophysiology* 10 (1): e002476.
7. Daskalov, I., and T. Valova-Ilieva. 2017. Management of acute pericarditis: Treatment and follow-up. *ESC*. https://www.escardio.org/Journals/E-Journal-of-Cardiology-Practice/Volume-15/Management-of-acute-pericarditis-treatment-and-follow-up. Accessed November 2, 2023.
8. Burns, E., and R. Buttner. 2021. Pericarditis. In *Life in the Fastlane*. https://litfl.com/pericarditis-ecg-library/. Accessed November 2, 2023.

Chapter 5
First Taste of Being a Nocturnist Followed by a General Medicine Floor Rotation

December 18th, 2017 Through February 11th, 2018

The training of internal medicine physicians included medical practices covering the hospital on nights. We have a formal specialty name for the internal medicine physicians who work solely night shifts. We call them nocturnists. In the current job markets, nocturnists are physicians who take care of general internal medicine floor patients and do admissions during the night, and sometimes, nocturnists are also responsible for taking care of patients in the ICU (open ICU). It is worth noting that as critical care has its own specialty, large hospitals usually have designated intensivists covering the ICU during both days and nights (closed ICU).

Being a full-time nocturnist is a tough job, not only because of the job duty itself but also the long-term health consequences as a night owl. The job duty mainly involves admitting patients from the emergency department and cross-covering patients' care on the general medicine floor and, at times, ICU (if open ICU). The night can become quite stressful, especially when the day team leaves you with multiple patients in the ER to see and hands you unstable patients on the floor right at the beginning of your shift. At times, the night can be even busier when a couple of rapid responses or codes are called.

My first night shift month in residency training involved caring for patients on both the general medicine floor and ICU (open ICU). The focus of an intern for this month was no longer only data gathering but also taking care of patients, prescribing medications (for agitation, insomnia, and other patient symptoms during the night), answering floor pages, running rapid responses or even codes. Admitting sick patients to the general medicine floor and ICU was the other major job duty of this rotation. When the night got quiet, my senior resident and I usually sat in front of the computers next to the ICU nursing station and reviewed the labs and vitals of the ICU patients in anticipation of any expected and unexpected events.

This was a daunting even intimidating task and experience as it sounded and it was also a difficult one. With the guidance of my senior resident and the close supervision of the attending physician, I not only survived the rotation but thrived.

K. Zhou, *Internal Medicine Training Notes and Survival Guide*, https://doi.org/10.1007/978-1-0716-4039-5_5

I still remember as part of the daily routine of night shifts, my participation in the early morning rounding (usually started at 4–5 a.m.) in the ICU with the chair physician of critical care medicine. During the rounds, we residents were often grilled on questions related to patient care and medicine in general. This experience helped identify knowledge gaps, foster a culture of learning, improve knowledge retention, enhance critical thinking skills, and, lastly, build up confidence levels.

Topics covered in this chapter included sepsis and septic shock, myasthenic crisis, diabetic ketoacidosis, bradycardia, rapid response, gastrointestinal bleeding, acute respiratory distress syndrome, ventilator management, acute chest syndrome, lithium toxicity, periprocedural anticoagulation, and tube feeding. As you will soon read, the notes in this section began with one psychiatry lecture and the review of hyperphosphatemia during my 4-week vacation before the night shift rotation. Additionally, I also merged my one-month rotation of the general medicine floor to this chapter. Topics thus additionally included pancreatitis, H. pylori infection and treatment, disseminated intravascular coagulation, normal pressure hydrocephalus, diabetes control in hospitalized patients, chronic kidney disease, and ischemic stroke.

12/11/2017

1. **Major depressive disorder (MDD)**: both selective serotonin reuptake inhibitors (SSRIs) and serotonin–norepinephrine reuptake inhibitors (SNRI) take 4–6 weeks to work and 4–6 weeks to be metabolized.

   SSRI: **fluoxetine (Prozac)** has a long half-life, but still has risks for withdrawal symptoms if sudden discontinuation and suicidal ideation risks in young adults; caution use in the elderly and abnormal liver function test (LFT). **Sertraline (Zoloft)** has a half-life between Prozac and Paxil. **Paroxetine (Paxil)** has a short half-life, can have withdrawal if sudden discontinuation, and has suicidal risk in young patients. **Escitalopram (Lexapro)** is highly selective and has high bioavailability; it is used in multi-comorbidity and has minimal to no interaction with other drugs.

   SNRI: **venlafaxine (Effexor)** can be used in neuropathy; **duloxetine (Cymbalta)** 20, 40, 60 mg qd can be used in fibromyalgia and neuropathic pain. **When Effexor < 150 mg qd = SSRI; if >150 mg qd = SNRI**.
2. **Generalized anxiety disorder (GAD)**: because both SSRI and SNRI take 4–6 weeks to work, benzodiazepines (GABAa binding, can cause addiction) are commonly used in the interim. **Alprazolam (Xanax)** has a half-life of 11.2 h, Ativan (lorazepam) has a half-life of 12–18 h, **clonazepam (Klonopin)** has a half-life of 30–40 h, **diazepam (Valium)** has a half-life of 48 h.
3. **Bipolar I** is characterized by at least one manic episode. **Bipolar II** has at least one hypomanic episode and one major depressive episode, but no mania. **The cyclothymic disorder** has numerous periods of hypomanic symptoms that fall short of meeting the criteria for hypomanic and numerous periods of depressive symptoms that fall short of meeting criteria for mild depression for at least 2 years. Treatment: mood stabilizers which include lithium, carbamazepine, valproic acid, and lamotrigine.

Lithium: takes weeks to work, excessive amounts are lethal and requires dialysis; the therapeutic window is small.

Carbamazepine: is an inducer of CYP3A4. The therapeutic reference range of carbamazepine is 4–12 mg/L. The minimum toxic level is **15 mg/L**. Critical level is **30 mg/L**.

Oxcarbazepine (Trileptal): isomer of carbamazepine, weak inducer of CYP3A4, no need to monitor concentration.

4. **Antipsychotics** for schizophrenia: Haloperidol 1st generation; second generation includes risperidone (Risperdal), ziprasidone (Geodon, Zeldox), olanzapine (Zyprexa), Aripiprazole (Abilify), and quetiapine (Seroquel).
5. **Olanzapine (Zyprexa) and risperidone**: rapid effects, extrapyramidal symptoms (EPS) side effects, can cause metabolic syndrome.
6. EPS side effects are less in second generation than in first generation antipsychotics. Zyprexa causes obesity. **Aripiprazole (Abilify)** is a partial D2 agonist and antagonist; it has suicidal risks for young patients.
7. **Bupropion (Wellbutrin)** can be used in smoking cessation but increases risks for suicidal ideation in young adults and seizures. **Amphetamine** causes seizures.
8. **Somatoform disorder** treatment: behavioral therapy, live with the disease.

   Xanax withdrawal, treated with Klonopin or diazepam, may add buspirone, or gabapentin.
9. Some antidepressants can be used in terminal disease or amyotrophic lateral sclerosis (ALS) to increase sleep and appetite together with psychological counseling, i.e., **mirtazapine** which activates 5-HT2 and 5-HT3 receptors.
10. **All patients with a history of suicide should document discussions of suicidal ideation**. In these patients, if SSRI is used, we can choose **sertraline and fluoxetine**. The benefits and potential side effects will have to be discussed in detail with the patient.
11. **Tricyclic antidepressants (TCAs) are only used per patients' preference due to cost**. For anxiety and pain, may use **venlafaxine and duloxetine.**
12. Seniors have a slow metabolism and high risks for falls. Depression in children is characterized by **irritability**, usually treated with SSRI.
13. Bipolar depression, use lithium or Lamictal. **Forced treatment** is only used in patients with the potential to self-harm or the potential to harm other people; legal authorities like the police department will have to be involved to place the patient on a hold.
14. **Monoamine oxidase inhibitors** (MAOIs): selegiline, isocarboxazid, phenelzine, and tranylcypromine. MAOIs are only used in conditions where SSRI and SNRI do not work. Defensive medicine, **suicidal risk** → admit, place on one-on-one, and get psychiatrist clearance before discharge.
15. Bipolar is treated with valproic acid (slow onset) or **risperidone/olanzapine (rapid onset).**
16. Schizophrenia is diagnosed only if the patient develops **hallucinations when not in depression**.

17. Gabapentin and pregabalin can be used to treat anxiety. **Wellbutrin** has no sexual side effects; Wellbutrin inhibits norepinephrine (NE) and dopamine (DA) neurotransmitter reuptake.
18. In patients with opioid abuse, **SNRI** can be used but BZDs should be avoided.
19. Anxiety or depression attack once, treat with antidepressants for **9–12 months**. If three attacks or more, the patient should be treated lifelong.
20. Patient denial should ask why. **Depression becomes anxiety after treatment with Cymbalta, can add olanzapine or valproic acid.**
21. Antidepressants should not be used in pregnancy, recommend electroconvulsive therapy (ECT). Use **SSRI** if absolutely cannot be avoided in pregnancy; defer to the obstetrician and gynecologist who might prescribe it.
22. Seniors with mild depression and insomnia can be treated with mirtazapine. Risk of fall, and hallucination in seniors: treat with **risperidone**. For behavioral control or agitation, use **Seroquel.**

12/12/2017

1. **Hyperphosphatemia etiology**: (1) acute increase in phosphate load, e.g., tumor lysis syndrome (TLS), exogenous phosphate from laxatives, rhabdomyolysis, hemolysis, transfusion of red blood cell (RBC)/stored blood; (2) acute extracellular shift of phosphate, e.g., lactic acidosis, diabetic ketoacidosis (DKA); (3) acute kidney injury (AKI) or chronic kidney disease (CKD); (4) a primary increase in tubular phosphate reabsorption, acromegaly, bisphosphonates, Vitamin D toxicity, hyperphosphatemic familial tumoral calcinosis. **Physiological regulation of phosphate**: serum phosphate concentration, parathyroid hormone (PTH), phosphatonins (FGF23, sFRP-4).
2. **Pseudohyperphosphatemia**: spurious hyperphosphatemia due to interference with analytical methods in hyperglobulinemia, e.g., multiple myeloma (MM), Waldenstrom macroglobulinemia, or monoclonal gammopathy, high dose liposomal amphotericin B use, hyperlipidemia, and hemolysis hyperbilirubinemia.
3. **Acute severe hyperphosphatemia** can cause symptomatic hypocalcemia. Treatments include normal saline and hemodialysis, especially common in CKD or AKI.
4. If $P > 6$ mg/dL, give **phosphate binders** (calcium carbonate/acetate, sevelamer, lanthanum).
5. In refractory hyperphosphatemia to dietary restrictions, phosphate binders, treatment of hyperparathyroidism using **calcimimetics** [like cinacalcet (Sensipar)] instead of calcitriol or vitamin D analogs or by **parathyroidectomy** is necessary.
6. Other phosphate binders: (1) **sucroferric oxyhydroxide** 2.5 g tid with meals for patients with eGFR < 15; (2) **ferric citrate and calcium citrate** may increase aluminum toxicity.
7. **Tumor lysis syndrome (TLS)**: the use of allopurinol in TLS can cause xanthinuria → xanthine nephropathy or xanthine stone formation, and will need high rate IV hydration. **Rasburicase** degrades uric acid to the much more water-soluble compound allantoin without the risk of xanthinuria, but should not be

used in G6PD deficiency. **Febuxostat (Uloric) and rasburicase** can be used in kidney failure patients.

8. **Cairo-Bishop definition of TLS**: **laboratory TLS** is defined as 2 or 3 abnormal serum values (uric acid, P, K, Ca) ≥25% increase from baseline; present with 3 days before or 7 days after instituting chemo in the setting of adequate hydration with or without alkalization and use of a hypouricemic agent.

   Clinical TLS was defined as laboratory TLS plus one or more of the following: increases Cr ≥1.5 ULN, cardiac arrhythmia, sudden cardiac death, or seizures.
9. TLS can be seen in patients on **effective targeted therapy** for colon cancer and other solid tumors as well as CLL treated with **fludarabine, rituximab, lenalidomide, or venetoclax**.

12/15/2017

1. **Cocaine abuse treatment**: diazepam 10 mg q3–5 min, nitroglycerin, nitroprusside 0.3–0.5 mg/kg/min (maximal dose 10 mg/kg/min), phentolamine (usually reserved as the last resort for hypertension) 1–2.5 mg q5–15 min, or give valium 5 mg q3–5 min or lorazepam 1 mg IV q5–10 min. Give aspirin and heparin if acute chest pain with troponin elevation until percutaneous coronary intervention. Aspirin use should be avoided in aortic dissection.

Night Rotation

12/18/2017

1. **Polymicrobial bacteremia** with G+ cocci in chains and G-rods: Pep/Tazo 3.375/100 mL treatment.
2. Base excess >3 = metabolic alkalosis; base excess ≤ −3 = metabolic acidosis
3. Patient hypotensive on Levophed, bandemia, together with respiratory acidosis with high Cl, treatment: cefepime, metronidazole, vancomycin, pan culture.
4. **Seizure** → EEG; **pulmonary embolism** (PE) → do echocardiogram to assess cardiac stress if any abnormal vital sign(s) or elevated troponins.
5. **Fluid resuscitation** in sepsis: hypovolemia is an important factor contributing to shock and tissue hypoxia.
6. **Sepsis and septic shock** management: (1) Administer 30 cc/kg crystalloid (lactate ringers may be preferred) for hypotension or lactate ≥2 mmol/L in 3 h, use capillary refill time to guide resuscitation; (2) obtain blood culture before starting broad-spectrum antibiotics; (3) prompt removal of intravascular devices as a possible source of infection; (4) timely initiation of pressor support; (5) add albumin if a large amount of fluid resuscitation; (6) additional treatments include stress ulcer prophylaxis and Lovenox alone (not with sequential compression devices) over heparin subu for deep vein thrombosis prophylaxis; (7) goals of care discussions and adoption of palliative care principles; (8) enteral tube feeding within 72 h.
7. **Pneumonia**, on high flow treatment, if still desaturation, start BiPAP while the patient on meropenem.

8. **Chronic obstructive pulmonary disease (COPD) usually causes upper lobe changes**. Fever, acidosis, pleural effusion ⇒ consider empyema. Do chest CT scan or U/S and start antibiotics. Will need **thoracentesis** with fluid analysis for pleural effusion and **chest tube** placement for empyema or complicated parapneumonic pleural effusion.
9. Drop in hemoglobin and hematocrit (H&H), need to look for etiologies: bleeding, retroperitoneal?
10. **Quinolones are contraindicated** in myasthenia gravis (MG). Propofol has a shorter half-life than midazolam (Versed). **Minute ventilation** (respiratory rate × tidal volume) target <10 L/min (normal 5–8 L/min).
11. Dexmedetomidine (Precedex) drip for sedation. **MG crisis** treatment: IVIG then dexamethasone (Decadron) 4 mg IV q6h.
12. **Progressive bulbar palsy** includes difficulty swallowing, weak jaw and facial muscles, progressive loss of speech, and weakening of the tongue
13. **Myasthenic crisis = consider** respiratory insufficiency requiring support from invasive or non-invasive ventilation. It is usually preceded by generalized weakness (76% of patients), bulbar symptoms (19% of patients), or weakness of respiratory muscles (5% of patients). **Treatment**: rapid therapy with plasma exchange or intravenous immune globulin, immunomodulating therapy with high-dose glucocorticoids; consider azathioprine, mycophenolate mofetil, or cyclosporine if glucocorticoids are contraindicated or previously ineffective.
14. **Elective intubation** should be considered any one of the following: vital capacity (VC) falls below 15–20 mL/kg; maximal inspiratory pressure (MIP) is less negative than −25 to −30 cmH_2O (i.e., between 0 and −30 cmH_2O).
15. **Trachea shifts to the left**, concerns for hemothorax, and bronchoscopy showed a mass in the left main bronchus.
16. Metabolic acidosis → respiratory acidosis; may treat with BiPAP prior to intubation.
17. **Non-anion gap (AG) metabolic acidosis** related to high ostomy output (diarrhea, loss of bicarbonate within the intestines); treatment: D5 + NS at 100 cc/h.
18. **Hepatorenal**: albumin 50 mL → Bumex, additional treatments include midodrine and octreotide. Renal metabolic acidosis treatment: bicarb 650 mg bid; in unstable patients, consider bicarb drip 8.4% at 100 cc/h IV if pH ≤ 7.2.
19. **Hemophilia A** (congenital deficiency of factor VIII) is X-linked and shows heavier bleeding; whereas **hemophilia B** (deficiency in factor IX) is mild, usually mucocutaneous surface bleeding.

12/19/2017

1. Stable angina + positive troponins without ST elevation in EKG = consider non-ST elevation myocardial infarction (**NSTEMI**) → needs angiogram and heparin drip. If you doubt whether or not to start anticoagulation, do echo for wall motion abnormalities. **Unstable angina** is typical chest pain at rest; treatment for unstable angina is the same as NSTEMI.
2. If hypertension (HTN) at night, can give Lisinopril 2.5 mg qhs.

3. **Presyncope**: very obvious orthostatic, give midodrine 2.5 mg (can uptitrate to 10 mg) po q8h, normal saline bolus, discontinue inciting medications. Fludrocortisone is rarely necessary and is associated with increased all-cause hospitalizations.
4. **Subclinical hypothyroidism** if AFib, may need treatment.
5. High BP > 170 mmHg, temporary management: hydralazine 25 mg po or hydralazine 5 mg/10 mg IV or labetalol if heart rate >60 bpm. May also start amlodipine 10 mg qd and Lisinopril 10 mg qd.
6. **Angioedema, anaphylaxis**: order C3, C4 complement; C1 esterase inhibitor function. Treatment with **Benadryl** 25 mg IV q8h, **Solu-Medrol** 40 mg IV q8h, and **DuoNeb** for breathing, can also give **famotidine** 20 mg iv bid. **Epinephrine** 0.5 mg im in the anterolateral aspect of the middle third of the thigh if the patient crashes.
7. **Erythropoietin** increases the risks for seizures.
8. High troponin → calculate Thrombolysis In Myocardial Infarction Risk Score (**TIMI**) score, CV risk factors → heparin drip if no contraindications and echo → contact cardiologist or cardiac catheterization centers for transfer.
9. Morphine sulfate oral solutions, highly concentrated, brand name **Roxanol**, used for terminally ill patients.
10. **Pleural fluid analysis**: albumin, gram stain, culture, glucose, pH, LDH, cell count and differentiation. Questran = cholestyramine. Ursodiol = ursodeoxycholic acid.
11. High ammonia, a sharp increase in LFTs. Treatment: lactulose 20 mg po, and/or rifaximin 550 mg tid. **Hepatitis workup**: HCV ab, HBV surface Ag, antinuclear antibody (ANA), smooth muscle antibody, alpha fetoprotein (AFP). **Ursodiol** 600 mg tid is used in cholithiasis and PSC and PBC.
12. **Urinary tract infection treatment**: Klebsiella is usually sensitive to ceftriaxone 1 g IV. Enterococcus faecium is usually sensitive to Zyvox 600 mg q12h and penicillins.
13. Cocaine abuser, not awake after treatment of diabetic ketoacidosis (DKA), concerns for hemorrhagic stroke, CT head needed.
14. **Diabetic ketoacidosis (DKA), pH 6.9**, treatment: 1 amp bicarb, 10u insulin, 2-L normal saline, 3 mg Ativan for cocaine users, add bicarb drip after rapid fluid resuscitation.
15. **Etiology of 5Is for DKA**: infection, infarction, no Insulin, idiopathic, inflammation.
16. Aneurysm of thoracic aorta status post TEVAR (transthoracic endovascular aortic repair). During the procedure, the patient had **cold limbs**. DVT was found and underwent femoral endarterectomy and embolectomy with iliac stents. EBL (estimated blood loss) 250 mL, then was started on **ASA, Plavix, and heparin drip**.
17. Heparin half-life is 4 h; lumbar drain can be removed while patient on heparin gtt.
18. For deep vein thrombosis (DVT) or pulmonary embolism (PE), we need to **assess risk factors**, smoking, stationery? Travel? Family history? Provoked or unprovoked?

19. **Chronic low Na** 105, we should not raise Na by 6–8 mEq/L over 24 h; monitor Na q2-4h. If over-correction, give D5 IV at 40 cc or 20 cc/h, desmopressin acetate (DDAVP) (1 to 2 μg iv or subcu q8h for 24–48 hours) may also be given for over-correction.
20. **Bleeding rapid management**: PT/INR, PRBCs after blood type and cross-match, surgery consult STAT if needed, O_2, NS wide open.
21. **Seizure and sepsis rapid response,** check Airways, Breathing, Circulation, and vitals. Order labs: lactic acid, CBC, troponin, BMP, ABG, Mg, EKG, CT brain, EEG.
22. **Rapid shallow breathing index** = RR/tidal volume in liters, ≤105 indicates 80% chance of extubation.

12/20/2017

1. **Case presentation in ICU**, needs to pay attention to tests and exams; ICU admission focuses on **etiology, diagnosis, and treatment**. Start thinking of these when history is taking.
2. Be calm, low blood pressure and bradycardia, Treatment: **dopamine** 800 mg titrate, NS at 250 cc/h; consider addition of Neo-Synephrine (phenylephrine) 40 mg IV (alpha-1 adrenergic receptor agonist with minimal to no beta-adrenergic activity).
3. **ACLS protocol for symptomatic bradycardia**: 0.5 mg **atropine** IV q5min up to 3 mg. Second line of treatment in symptomatic bradycardia is **dopamine** drip at 5–20 μg/kg/min infusion or **epinephrine** at 2–10 μg/min. Additionally, if possible **transcutaneous pacing can be applied after atropine** before permanent pacemaker placement.
4. Nutrition for a patient with **necrotizing fasciitis** involving the perineal space and labia majora: multivitamin, Floranex (lactobacilli), may check vitamin A, C, D, Zn, and repletion prn. Treatment: Vanco, cefepime 2 g q8h, and Flagyl 500 mg q8h.
5. Ventilator weaning, transition to **pressure support ventilation**, if tolerated, may extubate.
6. Chronic hyponatremia <105, **may start nothing per mouth (NPO) until Na stabilizes**.
7. **BiPAP** in patients with altered mental status (AMS): 16/8. Caution beta-blocker (BB) in lung disease.
8. **Multifocal atrial tachycardia (MAT)** treatment: usually no treatment necessary; may consider verapamil 1 mg IV, then if needed 4 mg over 5 min, 5 mg over 5 min for up to 3 doses. Maintenance 120-480 mg qd po. Metoprolol 5 mg IV over 5 min, 5 mg IV over 5 min at 10 min intervals for 2–3 additional doses, maintenance 50–100 mg bid po.
9. **Hospital-acquired pneumonia (HAP)** = pneumonia that occurred 48 h or more after admission and does not appear to be incubating at the time of admission. Ventilator-associated pneumonia (VAP) is a type of HAP that develops more than 48–72 h after intubation.

10. **Extensively drug-resistant (XDR) G-bacilli** = resistance to all commonly used systemic antibiotics except colistin, tigecycline, and aminoglycosides. **Panresistance** refers to G-bacilli with diminished susceptibility to all antibiotics for the empiric treatment of HAP and CAP, including cefepime, ceftazidime, imipenem, meropenem, piperacillin-tazobactam, Cipro and Levaquin.
11. **Gastrointestinal percutaneous endoscopic gastrostomy (PEG) tube placement requires platelet (PLT) > 16,000 and no ascites.**
12. **Essential tremor treatment**: propranolol 120 mg qd, primidone 250 mg qd (may cause altered mental status, has to be tapered slowly), or topiramate 100 mg qd.
13. **IV iron**: iron sucrose 200 mg IV qd for 5 days.
14. **Rapid response**: SO_2 87%, RR50, HR 140 s, **Management**: O_2, STAT EKG, and chest X-ray (CXR), IV Lopressor 5 mg, Lasix 40 mg IV, Ativan 1 mg IV, morphine 1 mg IV. Check labs STAT CBC, CMP, Mag, lactic acid, ABG, troponin, and d-dimer (if concerns of venous thromboembolisms).
15. **Pulmonary edema**: cardiogenic versus noncardiogenic (seizures, kidney failure, blood transfusion reaction, high altitude). **Treatment** usually includes ventilation support, supplementary oxygen, and diuretics.
16. In Na correction, may discontinue hypertonic saline, transition to or decrease (if already on) salt tablets after **Na ≥ 125**.
17. Effexor = venlafaxine. 100 cc–200 cc/h urine is Ok, should not raise Na > 0.5–1 mmol/h in hyponatremia; if yes, give D5W.
18. **Risks for osmotic demyelination syndrome**: serum sodium <105, concurrent hypokalemia, alcoholic, malnourished, and liver disease.
19. **Symptoms of hyponatremia**: headache (HA), fatigue, nausea and vomiting (N&V), dizziness, gait disturbance, forgetfulness, confusion, and muscle cramps.
20. The goal of **initial Na correction** should be 4–6 mEq/L in 24 h period, maximal 8 mEq/L. **Treatment**: 3% NS at 15–30 cc/h plus Lasix (DDAVP if overcorrection).
21. **Severe symptoms of hyponatremia**: coma, respiratory arrest. Treatment: bolus 3% NS to reach 4–6 mmol/24 h increase in Na.
22. CPAP: FiO_2 30%, PEEP at 5. **Lactate Ringer (LR) has K inside**, avoid its use if K+ > 5.5 mEq/L.
23. **Recurrence of anion gap in DKA with high glucose**, give high dose sliding scale insulin (SSI), then ½ normal saline (NS) bolus and 1/2NS at 150 cc/h.

12/21/2017

1. **Whiteout of 1 lung**: get CT chest, usually due to mucus plug versus progressive pneumonia if acute; patient on ventilator, will need to adjust ventilator setting (possibly the depth of endotracheal tube) for presumed single lung intubation, set tidal volume at 300 cc.
2. **Purified protein derivative** (PPD) is not reliable in patients with massive use of steroids. For tuberculosis diagnosis, will need to check acid-fast stain, culture, and QuantiFERON.
3. Protonix drops platelet (PLT).

4. Patients who had a fall and were on the ground or sitting for a prolonged time → order creatinine phosphokinase (**CPK**) to rule out **rhabdomyolysis**.
5. **Differential diagnoses (DDx) for AFib**: cardiac event, electrolyte abnormality, thyroid stimulating hormone (TSH), medication noncompliance, viral infection, and congestive heart failure (CHF).
6. Continuous EEG to rule out status epilepticus versus postictal. If with dopamine, heart rate increases to 130 s, replace dopamine with Levophed.
7. Stroke on Plavix and ASA, order **platelet function, aspirin, C2Y12 tests**; low blood pressure (BP) in stroke (neurologist even orders phenylephrine at times), order normal saline to maintain sBP 130–160 s.
8. **Sedation during ventilation**: propofol 1% + midazolam 100 mg IV.
9. **Autoimmune disease screening**: QuantiFERON-TB, antineutrophil cytoplasmic antibodies [ANCA = pANCA (myeloperoxidase (MPO) antibody) + cANCA (proteinase 3 (PR3) antibody)], extractable nuclear antigen (ENA) panel [also known as Antibodies to Saline-extracted Antigens including Anti-RNP, Anti-Ribonucleoprotein, Anti-U(1)RNP, Anti-SmRNP, Anti-SSA, SSA (Ro), Anti-Sjögren Syndrome A, Anti-SSB, SSB (La), Anti-Sjögren Syndrome B, Anti-Sm (Sm), Smith Antibody, Scl-70, Anti-Topoisomerase, Scleroderma Antibodies, Anti-Jo-1, Antihistidyl Transfer RNA Synthetase Antibodies], antiphospholipid syndrome screening (anticardiolipin, beta-2-glycoprotein antibody, lupus antibody), rheumatic factor, anti-cyclic citrullinated peptide (anti-CCP) antibodies, ESR, CRP, protein electrophoresis, and ANA with reflex.
10. **Acute respiratory distress syndrome (ARDS)** diagnoses require all of the following: (1) respiratory symptoms started within 1 week; (2) bilateral opacities consistent with pulmonary edema on CT or chest X-ray (CXR) not fully explained by pleural effusion, lobar collapse, lung collapse, or pulmonary nodules; (3) no cardiac failure or fluid overload; (4) $PaO_2/FiO_2 \leq 300$.
11. **ARDS** severity depends on PaO_2/FiO_2 ratio: severe <100; 100 < moderate <200; 200 < mild <300.
12. **Differential diagnoses (DDx) of ARDS**: (1) cardiogenic pulmonary edema; (2) acute exacerbation of pulmonary fibrosis/fibrosis/another chronic interstitial lung disease (ILD); (3) diffuse alveolar hemorrhage; (4) idiopathic acute eosinophilic pneumonia; (5) cryptogenic organizing pneumonia; (6) acute interstitial pneumonia (Hamman-Rich syndrome) in patients without preexisting lung disease.

12/22/2017

1. **Midline** can be used for <29 days; **central lines** (peripherally inserted central catheter (PICC), triple lumen catheter (TLC), Hohn catheter, Medi port) can be used for months.
2. **Platelet (PLT) transfusion indications**: PLT < 10, PLT < 20 with risks of bleeding, or PLT < 50 with active bleeding. 1-unit PLT transfusion increases serum platelet by 50,000/uL.
3. Hgb drop, platelet decrease, stop aspirin (ASA), Plavix, heparin, start PPI and sucralfate 1 g po qid before meals if concerns for upper GI bleed. PLT transfusion 2 units if <20 with risk of bleeding. Low PLT and heparin-induced throm-

bocytopenia (HIT) panel negative, do not need to check PLT function aspirin/C2Y12 response units or venous Doppler of lower extremities (the results are likely obvious).

4. **NSAIDs** should not be used in chronic kidney disease (CKD). Na correction in hyponatremia should be no more than **0.5 mmol/h**.
5. **Scopolamine** (hyoscine) is a medication for motion sickness and postoperative nausea and vomiting. It is also used before surgery to decrease saliva.
6. Eating, please decrease or even stop (back off) **fluids**. Stop IV vancomycin whenever appropriate. Check brain dead with a neurologist.
7. JP (Jackson-Pratt) drain is commonly used in surgery. Tuberculosis (TB) and malignancy can have large amounts of pleural effusions.
8. **Pleural effusion amylase** is increased in ruptured esophagus, pancreatitis, pancreatic pleural fistula, and lung adenocarcinoma.
9. Patient on tube feeds with nothing per mouth: may need **400 cc** free water flush through Dobbhoff tube q4h in **hypernatremia**.
10. Klebsiella pneumonia treatment: third generation cephalosporin, carbapenem, aminoglycoside, and quinolones.
11. **Pancreatitis treatment**: if left ventricular ejection fraction (LVEF) ok, do Lactate Ringer (LR) at 250–300 cc/h for first 48 h.
12. **Asthma exacerbation**: low dose inhaled corticosteroid (ICS)/leukotriene receptor antagonist (LTRA) → ICS + long-acting beta-agonist (LABA)—increase ICS to medium or high dose maintenance ICS-LABA before adding long-acting muscarinic antagonist (LAMA) → oral steroids. Patient with asthma exacerbation with home medications: loratadine, **mometasone 200 mg**, and albuterol for asthma episodes. Pulmonary consult: add montelukast 10 mg, mometasone 200 mg, benzonatate 100 mg, methylprednisolone 4 mg qd. Additional options for severe and refractory asthma include omalizumab (anti-IgE antibody), mepolizumab and reslizumab (anti-IL-5 antibodies), benralizumab (IL-5 receptor alpha antagonist), dupilumab (IL-4 receptor alpha antagonist), and tezepelumab (anti-thymic stromal lymphopoietin antibody).
13. **Preparations for transfer out of ICU**: off pressors, feeding plans, Foley removed, IV drip minimal, central line removal if peripheral iv established.
14. **Excessive secretion**: consider ordering cultures and antibiotics!
15. **Tube feeding**: start tube feeding at 20 cc/h, advance by 10 cc increment q4h to goal (maximal 125 cc/h after a few days), check residual q4h, head of bed at 30°.
16. Head of bed at 30°, **copious amount of secretion from trach, treatment**: glycopyrrolate, thorough trach site care, keep the area dry, keep trach tight and support trach tube with any movements of the patient.
17. Senior patients with potentially poor outcomes, will need to consult palliative care/goals of care discussions.
18. **Rapid response for altered mental status (AMS)**: found to have low blood pressure. Subjective, Objective, order labs, Glasgow Coma Scale (E2V3M6), start normal saline (NS) bolus 1 L, make NPO, repeat SLP, discontinue (D/C) Seroquel 25 mg qhs and other mentation altering meds, change Cardizem to withholding parameters.

19. **Acute GI bleed**: EGD, colonoscopy (revealed arteriovenous malformation (AVM)) → bleeding scan (if patient stable and slow bleed), CT angiogram abd/pelvis (if concerns possible large bleed) → capsule enteroscopy.
20. NPO for emergent EGD, after EGD, can order clear liquid as diet.
21. Rapid response with too much fentanyl, treat with Narcan 0.4–2 mg, q2–3 min, and may start IV drip if recurrent symptoms.

12/24/2017

1. **Periprocedural anticoagulation**: half-life of low molecular weight heparin (LMWH) is 3–5 h, unfractionated heparin is 45 min; half-life of warfarin is 36–48 h, fondaparinux 17–21 h. The last dose before the procedure for heparin is 4 h, LMWH 24 h, and fondaparinux 2–4 days.
2. **Decision making bridging in anticoagulation**: estimated thromboembolic risk, and bleeding risk (HAS-BLED), determine the timing of anticoagulant interruption, whether to use bridging (mechanical heart valve and CHA2DS2-VASc score ≥ 5 will need bridging).
3. **Increased risks for thromboembolic events**: atrial fibrillation (Afib), prosthetic heart valves, and recent venous or arterial thromboembolism (in 3 months).
4. **Etiologies of arterial embolism**: AFib, paradoxical embolism, nonbacterial thrombotic endocarditis in a patient with malignancy, dilated or poorly controlled left ventricle or left ventricle aneurysm, thrombophilia.
5. Estimates of procedural bleeding risk: **high bleeding risks for neuraxial (epidural/spinal) anesthesia, intracranial, and cardiac procedures**.
6. **Temporary IVC filters** are indicated in recent (prior 3–4 weeks) acute venous thromboembolism (VTE) who require interruption of anticoagulation because of surgery or contraindications (like brain bleeding and gastrointestinal bleeding) in which full dose anticoagulation will need to be delayed for **12 or more hours or stopped for an extended period**.
7. Settings in which **continuing anticoagulation** may be preferable: (a) dental procedures; (b) cutaneous procedures; (c) selected cardiac procedures (cardiac implantable devices, endovascular procedures, and catheter ablation).
8. **Bridging** at high or very high risks of thromboembolism including recent stroke, mechanical heart valve, CHA2DS2-VASc score of 7 or 8 (if bleeding risk acceptable, can bridge at CHA2DS2-VASc score of ≥5). Stop warfarin 3–5 days before surgery. Resume warfarin 12–24 h after surgery, typically on the evening of surgery. Unfractionated heparin, LMWH, Eliquis, or Xarelto may be resumed 24 h after the procedure. Hold these meds 1–2 days before the procedure.
9. **Bridging indications:** (a) embolic stroke or systemic embolic event within the previous 3 months; (b) mechanical heart valve, especially mitral valve; (c) mechanical aortic valve with additional stroke risk factors; (d) AFib with CHA2D2VASc score of 5–6; (e) VTE in the past 3 months; (f) stenting of coronary artery in previous 12 weeks; (g) previous VTE in interruption of chronic anticoagulation.

10. **Periprocedural anticoagulation and DVT prophylaxis**: skip LMWH or unfractionated heparin one dose before surgery. Resume heparin and LMWH or warfarin 24 h after surgery. Resume heparin drip 4 h after cath if the patient is a candidate for CABG). If therapeutic anticoagulation dose LMWH, wait at least 24 h after the last dose of LMWH before a spinal or epidural catheter is placed.
11. OSA can cause a pH of 7.17 while off BiPAP 20/8.

12/25/2017

1. Fecal occult blood test positive, may need gastrointestinal expert consultation. Low molecular weight heparin including dalteparin and enoxaparin may not be appropriate and requires dosage adjustment to once daily in chronic kidney disease with eGFR ≤30. **Steroids may suppress fever.**
2. In patients with possible hypothalamic-pituitary-adrenal (HPA) suppression (**hypotension is the key criteria**), **random serum cortisol level** should be checked if unexplained nausea, vomiting, hypotension, orthostasis, change in mentation, hyponatremia, or hypokalemia. Stress dose **intravenous corticosteroids** should be considered and even started in the presence of postoperative stressors, e.g., infection, myocardial infarction, bleeding, or other complications.
3. Random cortisol secretion rate greater than 200 mg/day in 24 h after surgery is rare.
4. Indications for evaluation of **inhaled glucocorticoids** perioperatively for hypothalamic-pituitary-adrenal (HPA) axis suppression: if on ≥750 μg/day inhaled steroids for ≥3 weeks, ≥2 g/day of high potency or super high potency of glucocorticoids for over 3 weeks, cushingoid appearance. Again, check only if concerns for hypotension together with other aforementioned symptoms.
5. Evaluation of HPA axis suppression: morning cortisol **<3-5 μg/dL** 24 h off glucocorticoid replacement dose = probable impaired hypothalamic-pituitary-adrenal axis. Between 5 and 10 μg/dL, do ACTH (Cosyntropin) stimulation testing, if cortisol level > 18μg/dL 30 min after 250 μg ACTH, it is considered normal. An insulin tolerance test ("gold standard" for HPA axis evaluation) or metyrapone stimulation test in acute ACTH deficiency is usually not necessary.
6. Use **meropenem** for diffuse chorioamnionitis history.
7. If PLT > 50, do aspirin, significant concerns for VTE/Stroke, may even transfuse PLT, then give ASA. If PLT < 50, hold pharmaceutical DVT prophylaxis heparin or Lovenox.
8. **Large ischemic stroke** with atrial fibrillation treatment: maintain blood pressure, and **hold anticoagulation for 7–10 days** to minimize hemorrhagic transformation.
9. **Anticoagulation after acute ischemic stroke**: small- or moderate-sized infarct with no intracranial bleeding, warfarin can be resumed/initiated after 24 h (NOAC after 48 h). **Withholding anticoagulation for 2 weeks** if large ischemic strokes, symptomatic hemorrhagic transformation, or poorly controlled hypertension. Aspirin may be beneficial until therapeutic anticoagulation with warfarin.
10. **Immune thrombocytopenic purpura (ITP)** treatment: Decadron 60 mg qd, wean off in 3 weeks: 60-40-20-10-5-2 mg daily -2 mg every other day.

11. Concerns for pulmonary embolism, do CT angio chest and ultrasound for DVT of lower extremities.
12. Propofol + versed can cause a drop in blood pressure.
13. ARDS treatment: **low tidal volume** ventilation 4–8 cc/kg of ideal body weight, **increased constant PEEP**, decreased tidal volume ⇒ consider pressure support with sufficient sedation and anesthesia during **intermittent neuromuscular blockade** with Nimbex (cisatracurium besylate); **prone ventilation** ≥ 12 h/day and keep patient dry in a negative fluid balance using fluid restriction, diuresis, albumin with furosemide in selected patients with hypoproteinemia and acute lung injury.
14. **Septic shock low blood pressure** but adequate preload, add norepinephrine to increase blood pressure then add Lasix → add albumin → goal in patients with anasarca or heart failure.

12/26/2017

1. **Diverticulitis**- complicated patients can have abscess, obstruction, perforation, fistula. Diagnosis: lower abdominal pain and abdominal tenderness on physical examination. Order a CT scan with oral or without oral contrast; either is ok; water-soluble contrast does not harm the body.
2. **Differential diagnosis (DDx)** of diverticulitis: colorectal cancer, acute appendicitis, inflammatory bowel disease, infectious colitis causing diarrhea, ischemic colitis. Others include tubo-ovarian abscess, ovarian cyst torsion, ectopic pregnancy, cystitis, and nephrolithiasis.
3. **CT**: wall thickening (>5 mm) = consider neoplastic, inflammatory, infectious, or ischemic conditions colitis. Colonic wall thickening plus additional **peridiverticular inflammation** = consider diverticulitis or infectious colitis.
4. Colonoscopy should not be performed in acute colitis, but **6 months after recovery**.
5. **Antibiotics for diverticulitis** should cover G-rods and anaerobes, particularly E. coli and B. fragilis. Outpatient treatment with Cipro 500 mg q12h+ Flagyl; TMP-SMX+ Flagyl, or Augmentin or moxi for 7–10 days.
6. **Diet**: clear liquid, full liquid, soft low residue, mechanical soft, general diet.
7. Inpatient treatment of uncomplicated **acute colonic diverticulitis** typically begins with administration of IV antibiotics, fluids, and pain meds. IV antibiotics single agent: ertapenem 1 g IV qd; Zosyn 3.375 q6h, ticarcillin-clavulanate. Combined regimen includes metronidazole with Cipro, Levaquin, cefazolin, or Rocephin. Inpatient, **NPO** for bowel rest in acute diverticulitis, **clear liquid** may be ok in mild diverticulitis.
8. Diverticulitis in patients during hospitalization: also known as healthcare-associated intra-abdominal infection, treat with a single agent like above, or cefepime, ceftazidime with Flagyl plus ampicillin or vancomycin. Diet: NPO or clear liquids for bowel rest.
9. Recommendations for diverticulitis: diet modifiers to include fiber intake, and use mesalamine. Recurrent diverticulitis may need surgery.

10. **Ischemic colitis** and colonic ischemia usually happen at **watershed areas**, splenic flexure, and the rectosigmoid junction. Etiology: nonocclusive colonic ischemia, embolic and thrombotic arterial occlusion, mesenteric vein thrombosis (distal small intestine and proximal colon).
11. **Phlebosclerotic colitis** is a rare form of ischemic colitis from venous obstruction by **fibrotic sclerosis and calcification** of the colon wall. Symptoms include recurrent diarrhea, chronic severe lower abdominal pain, nausea, vomiting, and tarry stool with tests positive for fecal occult blood. Treatment is surgery versus a wait-and-watch approach.
12. **Acute ischemia of large bowel** CT images demonstrating: pneumatosis coli, lack of formed stool, thickening of the peritoneum and lateral colonal fascia, and ascites.
13. All patients with suspected colonic ischemia should receive supportive care, including **fluid resuscitation, cessation of inciting factors, bowel rest**, and possibly broad-spectrum **antibiotics and stat surgery consultation**.
14. **Risk factors for ischemic colitis**: atherosclerosis, atrial fibrillation, peripheral arterial disease, aortoiliac instrumentation/surgery, cardiopulmonary bypass, myocardial infarction, hemodialysis, drugs, constipation and diarrhea, mesenteric fistula or AV malformation.
15. Compared with ischemia affecting the small intestines, the cramping pain that accompanies **colonic ischemia** is usually not severe, is felt laterally rather than periumbilically, and is often associated with hematochezia.
16. Ischemic colitis: **hyperactive phase → paralytic phase → shock phase**; labs and workups for bowel ischemia: serum lactic acid, LDH, CPK, amylase, CBC, CMP, coagulation studies; stool Cx, ova, and parasite testing, C. diff toxin study, CT with contrast, lower endoscopy.
17. Colonic ischemia + peritonitis ⇒ stat surgery consult. If no peritonitis, order **CT abdomen with contrast**; if no risk factors of thrombosis, order **sigmoidoscopy or colonoscopy with biopsy**. If vascular occlusions, order **systemic anticoagulation** for mesenteric arterial or venous occlusion.
18. **Nonocclusive mesenteric ischemia treatment**: stat vascular surgery consult, fluid resuscitation, initiation of broad-spectrum antibiotics, and placement of nasogastric tube for gastric decompression. Pressors for mesenteric ischemia should be **dobutamine (beta-1 receptor activation with negated alpha-1 activation from beta-2 activities)**, low-dose dopamine, or milrinone as they can improve cardiac output with lower risks for worsening mesenteric perfusion. Heparin drip may be useful.
19. **Diagnostic criteria for disseminated intravascular coagulation (DIC)**: thrombocytopenia, low fibrinogen, elevated D-dimer, and FDP ≥40 mg/mL. Septic shock needs pan culture and monitoring for shock liver.
20. **Pressors**: NS0.9% + Levophed 32 mg for MAP >65; D5 + vasopressin 20u for MAP >65; or Neo-Synephrine 160 mg in NS 0.9% start at 1 mg/kg/min titrate to a max of 3 mg/kg/min.
21. **Sedation medications**: propofol 1%; fentanyl 2500 μg start at 50 μg/h, max 200 μg/h; midazolam 100 mg, start 2 mg/h, max 15 mg/h.

22. Young patients, do not take risks; weird EKG rhythms (**peak T waves and PR prolongation**) may have hyperkalemia.
23. Not responding → rapid response → urgent labs and Rx.
24. HCO_3 10 or lower, may need to give **bicarb drip** if very sick. CO3 < 22 in CKD, give **bicarb tablet** po.
25. **TSH 11**, patient crashing with septic shock, considering **myxedema coma**, order Synthroid 50 µg IV, stress dose steroids Solu-Cortef 100 mg iv q8h.
26. **Septic shock treatment** example: NS 125 cc/h, Levophed 50 mg IV, NS bolus 4 L, meropenem/azithromycin, Solu-Cortef 100 mg IV once.
27. **Anasarca** treatment: albumin 50 mL IV + 40 mg IV Lasix once.
28. Mild increase of trop 0.08, but **wall motion abnormality or anteroseptal hypokinesis** in echo, order stat heparin drip, then call cardiologist or transfer for cardiac cath.

12/27/2017

1. **Severe C. diff**-associated diarrhea criteria include any of the following: >12 BM/day; T > 103; WBC >25, hypotension, ICU care, ileus. Treatment: Vanco 125 po q6h + Flagyl 500 mg IV q8h for 10–14 days. IDSA only recommends combined **oral vancomycin and intravenous flagyl for fulminant disease** (hypotension, shock, ileus, or megacolon). Recurrent infection: fidaxomicin is the first line treatment option.
2. Vancomycin in **a tapered** (125 mg orally 4 times daily for 10–14 days, then 125 mg orally 2 times daily for 7 days, then 125 mg orally once daily for 7 days, then 125 mg orally every 2–3 days for 2–8 weeks) and pulsed regimen **or vancomycin as a standard course** are acceptable alternatives for **a first C. diff infection recurrence**. For patients with multiple recurrences, vancomycin in a tapered and pulsed regimen, vancomycin followed by rifaximin, and fecal microbiota transplantation are alternatives.
3. **Hypertensive emergency and NSTEMI**: metoprolol 50 mg bid, nitroglycerin paste q6h; amlodipine 10 mg qd, hydralazine 10 mg iv q2h or 5 mg IV q1h. Update: will recommend **nitroglycerin intravenous** drip in such situations.
4. Recurrent hypertensive emergency with runs of VTach discharge home meds: hydralazine 25 mg tid, Imdur 30 mg qhs (or 20 mg isosorbide dinitrate with 37.5 mg hydralazine 3 times daily), amlodipine 10 mg qd, clonidine patch 0.2 mg qwk.
5. Sepsis in ICU: if line flushes do not draw, can use **alteplase** (Cathflo® Activase®) protocol to salvage it; if unsuccessful, call IR to replace.
6. **ICU adrenal crisis treatment**: hydrocortisone 100 mg IV q8h; fludrocortisone 0.1 mg (later increased to 0.2 mg) po qam (not needed on the second day), normal saline 2-L bolus, followed by normal saline at 150 cc/h.
7. Speed of Na correction: a. hypernatremia: acute hypernatremia: 3–6 mL D5/kg/h (not commonly used), q4h BMP, speed of lowering <1 mEq/L/h, normalization in 24 h. For **chronic hypernatremia, rate D5 at 1.35 mL/kg/h (commonly used)**, goal is around Na decrease by 10 mEq/L/day, correction less than 0.5 mEq/L/h. Hyponatremia: Na increase should be less than 6-8 mEq/L/day, rate < 0.5 mEq/L/h.

8. Admission: **may need to hold home meds** upon admission.
9. **Hypertensive urgency**: Cardene (Nicardipine) drip, labetalol, or hydralazine 10 mg iv q2h prn.
10. **Post craniotomy**: Decadron 10 mg IV once then Decadron 4 mg every 6 h, can taper over weeks after 7 days (update: **Decadron offers no benefits but potential harm; whereas hypertonic saline or mannitol can be beneficial in decreasing intracranial pressure or cerebral edema in subarachnoid hemorrhage, traumatic brain injury, acute ischemic stroke, intracerebral hemorrhage**). Keppra 500 mg IV bid for the prevention of seizures (duration will be decided by whether seizure attack inside the hospital; if no post-traumatic seizure, **duration of anti-epileptic drug is 1 week**). Try to avoid opioids to minimize the risks of confusion.
11. Butalbital/acetaminophen/caffeine (Fioricet) 1 tablet q4h prn is used for headaches.
12. Diagnostic criteria for **rhabdomyolysis**: creatinine kinase at least 5× above normal, usually >5000 with clinical findings.
13. **Altered mental status**: will need to think of **lumbar puncture STAT**, stop meds causing altered mentation. Always think of **lumbar puncture and brain MRI** as additional workups for altered mentation.
14. **Midline** only works for **24–48 h for blood draws**.

12/28/2017

1. Proper signout from ICU to the general medicine floor; keep checking meds interfering with blood pressure. Greenfield inferior vena cava filter. **FDA recommends the removal of IVC filters within 25–54 days of their implantation**.
2. Keep checking meds interfering with mentation changes.
3. **Pancreatitis**: exact Ins and Outs; trend CBC, LFT, lipase [**Ranson's criteria for mortality**]. If dialysis, cautiously replete K or Mg.
4. Fluctuating blood pressure → pheochromocytoma (**24 h urine fractionated metanephrines or plasma-free metanephrines**).
5. For acute kidney injury, may need to order a US renal aorta retro (renal ultrasound) or CT scan to rule out **obstruction/hydronephrosis**. Check for **acute tubular necrosis (ATN)** with urinalysis (muddy brown casts or renal tubular epithelial cells), FENa >2%.
6. **Linezolid** causes serotonin syndrome, may need to hold **duloxetine with the use of linezolid**.

Ventilator

7. **Types of breaths** in ventilator support: volume control/assist, pressure control/assist, and pressure support. Trigger, target (peak inspiratory flow rate, pressure limit, etc.), termination (volume, time, flow).
8. **Volume control/assist**: volume-limited assist control and volume-limited synchronized intermittent mandatory ventilation. **Pressure control/assist**: pressure-limited assist control and pressure-limited synchronized intermittent ventilation.

9. **Pressure support**: The patient-initiated breaths with a pressure limit, ventilator provides driving pressure for each breath/maximal air flow rate.
10. **Modes**: assist control (volume/pressure limited), synchronized intermittent mandatory ventilation, and pressure support. **Pressure-regulated volume control (PRVC)** = the ventilator attempts to achieve set tidal volume at the lowest possible airway pressure.
11. Bad ventilator setting consequences: **respiratory alkalosis** with subsequent intracranial hypertension, decreased oxygen delivery with **resultant ischemia**, and **atrophy of respiratory muscles**.
12. Trigger: pressure triggering or flow-by triggering (2 L/min). Tidal volume in ARDS uses less than 6 cc/kg of predicted body weight (PBW).
13. Tidal volume: rarely should be >10 mL/kg of PBW. Return to the previous tidal volume is indicated for patients who develop auto-PEEP >5 cmH_2O or a **plateau airway pressure >30 cmH_2O** following an increased tidal volume. High peak pressure = consider elevated airway resistance. High airway pressure = consider decreased lung compliance.
14. **Respiratory rate**: initially at 12–16/min. For assist control, set **4 breaths per minute below the patient's native rate (if patient's RR above 12–16)**. For synchronized intermittent mandatory ventilation, the rate is set to ensure that at **least 80% of the patient's total minute ventilation** is delivered by the ventilator.
15. In ARDS, the **required RR is higher** (up to 35 breaths per minute) to facilitate low tidal volume ventilation.
16. PEEP is usually at 5 cm H_2O, but up to 20 cm H_2O may be used in patients undergoing low tidal volume ventilation for ARDS.
17. **High peak flow rate** shortens inspiratory time and increases expiratory time (decreased I:E ratio) to facilitate CO_2 elimination.
18. FiO_2 adjusted to maintain SO_2 94%–98% as default. Target SO_2 in ischemic heart disease is higher (**SpO_2 92%–96%** as in most patients), 90% (**SpO_2 88%–92%** is appropriate) in lung disease due to COPD/chronic hypoxia; **88%–95%** for ARDS as tradeoff to avoid high plateau pressures.
19. **Asynchrony** causes dyspnea, increases the work of breathing, and prolongs the duration of mechanical ventilation. Common causes include ineffective triggering of a ventilator-delivered breath, double triggering, and prolonged inspiratory time.
20. **Flow pattern**: square wave (constant flow), ramp wave (decelerating flow), sinusoidal wave ramp-provides even flow.
21. **Adjustable settings of ventilator**: RR, FiO_2, tidal volume, PEEP. Inspiratory flow rate, trigger sensitivity. Indirectly inspiratory/expiratory duration.
22. Persistent breath-to-breath peak pressures greater than 45 cmH_2O are a risk factor for barotrauma. **Peak airway pressure should be <35–45 cmH_2O. Driving pressure = Pplat − PEEP, and should be < 15 cmH_2O. $P_{peak} = P_{plat} + P_{resistance}$**
.
23. Pplat is determined by an **inspiratory hold** maneuver in which the patient is given a fixed volume of air.

1/1/2018

1. **Feeding assessment**: assess residual, bowel movements.
2. **Sore throat**: look at the throat to see whether there are exudates/pus, consider CT neck if the neck is swelling. Calculate **Centor scores**: 1 point for each- no cough, tender/swollen anterior cervical lymph nodes, tonsillar swelling or exudates, age 3–14 (−1 point if age ≥ 45). The higher the score, the more probable the patient has Strep throat.
3. Abnormal CXR, not the typical pneumonia, get chest CT or CT angio PE study. Look at **CXR** to decide whether to use diuretics.
4. **Altered mental status (agitation)** in Bipolar treatment: Ativan 1 mg (can go up to 2 mg) prn, Haldol 1 mg im q4h, Seroquel 20 mg po bid.
5. **Indications for hemodialysis in lithium toxicity** if lithium concentration **≥4 mmol/L**, or if **≥2.5 mmol/L** and significant symptoms (seizure, depressed mental status), renal insufficiency, or other conditions that limit lithium excretion (like congestive heart failure).
6. **Initial treatment for lithium toxicity**: 2× maintenance fluid hydration rate for 2–3 L, use D5 if hypernatremia at 100 cc/h.
7. **Lithium toxicity** can happen/get worse from the concomitant use of NSAIDs, hydrochlorothiazide, and ACEi.
8. In **hypernatremia but hypervolemic**: ok to use thiazide and D5 at the same time.
9. **Zosyn** is first-line coverage for anaerobes (meropenem is reserved for ESBL infections).
10. **ARDS treatment**: low tidal volume ventilation increases PEEP to decrease tidal volume. Target the recommended tidal volume of 6–8 mL/kg predicted body weight (PBW).
11. Concerns for **pulmonary embolism**, order CT angiogram pulmonary embolism study and venous doppler for bilateral lower extremities.
12. **Small-bore feeding rates**: at 30–50–60 cc/h. Trickle feeds rate: 10–20 cc/h or a maximum of 500–1000 kcal per day.
13. **Rhabdomyolysis needs to check statin use**.
14. **Switch from PSV to PRVC**, try to maintain minute ventilation and backup rate.
15. Breathing above the vent, we need to increase FiO_2.
16. **Severe sepsis** diagnostic criteria: sepsis with tissue hypoperfusion (increased lactate, oliguria), or organ dysfunction like increase in Cr, PT/INR, etc.
17. If the patient is already on dialysis, ok to get CT angio to rule out pulmonary embolism or other contrast studies then dialysis. However, the patient should get **dialysis within 24–48 h after contrast dye use** to reduce the intravascular volume load.
18. **Criteria for fresh frozen plasma (FFP) use**: management or prevention of bleeding; coagulation factors replacement; thrombotic thrombocytopenic purpura; warfarin reversal.
19. Check **bowel sounds, bowel movements, and whether the patient is passing gas** in a surgical patient.

20. **Pleurodesis medication** examples: doxycycline, minocycline, tetracycline, bleomycin, cisplatin, doxorubicin, etoposide, and talc.
21. **Flash pulmonary edema**: start echo, Doppler lower extremities, CXR, ABG. Treatment: diuretics, oxygen, Duonebs.
22. **Hypernatremia** while on nasogastric tube feeds: increase free water flush, usually 100–450 cc q6h.
23. **Pressure support ventilator settings**: FiO_2, PEEP, pressure above PEEP; may transition to high flow.
24. **Pressors**: Levophed → Neo-Synephrine → dopamine → vasopressin. Vasopressin causes vascular vasoconstriction, no central effect for vascular pressure. Dobutamine is used for cardiogenic shock with low CO.
25. **Propofol (quick) → Versed (suppressive, mild sedative, long half-life, cleared by the liver) → Precedex (short-acting) is prn for awake and not anxious.** Richmond Anxiety Sedation Scale (RAS 0- -3) drowsy but arousable is used for a target level of consciousness while on a ventilator. **Fentanyl for pain and sedation.**
26. Kidney or liver issue: can prescribe Dilaudid, and fentanyl, but not **morphine as its metabolism depends on liver function and its clearance depends on kidney function.**

1/2/2018

1. Discussion of **palliative measures** indications: (A) poor prognosis and imminent hypoxic respiratory failure; (B) poor mental status and no improvement with treatment; (C) poor quality of life with progressively declining. **Comfort care** means withdrawal of all care including no dialysis, BiPAP, intravenous antibiotics, fluid, artificial feeds, no lab draws; remove central line and dialysis catheter. **Comfort care differs from hospice care** in that there are no time limitations with comfort care. Hospice usually means that a patient has a life expectancy of less than 6 months.
2. Answer to life expectancy during hospice discussions: "**But based on how it looks, does not seem like it would be long.**"
3. Old cultures were positive for yeast, VRE, and clostridium. **Treatment for spiking fever of 104**: start micafungin, linezolid, and meropenem; remove CVP, IJ cath, and place a new PICC line; reculture and CXR. I would also check for Beta-D-glucan study, and consult infectious disease.
4. Procedure or surgery, **order PT/INR** prior. **Tamiflu** is typically prescribed for 5 days. PCA **hydromorphone pump** setting: at 0.2 mg/h continuous rate, lockout interval 10 min, limit 1.2 mg/h, loading 0.4 mg.
5. **Extreme metabolic acidosis**: ventilator settings- 30%/36RR/PEEP5/tidal volume 450.
6. BiPAP orders 10/6 after extubation if appropriate.
7. **High-dose diuretics** can interfere with thoracentesis results. Intraabdominal pressure goes up → Ppeak also goes up.
8. Wide-spectrum antibiotics for sick patients in ICU. Vent management likely is not working if the patient is agitated.

9. In mild **pancreatitis**, in the absence of ileus, nausea, or vomiting, oral feeds can be initiated as soon as the pain is decreasing and markers are improving. Low residual, low fat, soft diet is recommended.
10. Keep checking meds interfering with BP, liver failure.
11. **Video-assisted thoracic surgery (VATS)**: The cardiothoracic surgeon decides when to restart warfarin, usually a couple of days later after chest tube removal or even when the chest tube is still in. DVT prophylaxis can be started sooner, like the day after surgery.

1/3/2018

1. **IV contrast allergy**: Regimen 1: Three doses of 50 mg oral prednisone administered 13, 7, and 1 h before contrast administration, plus 50 mg oral or IV diphenhydramine administered 1 h before contrast administration. Regimen 2: Two doses of 32 mg oral methylprednisolone were administered 12 and 2 h before contrast material administration.
2. **Lithium intoxication**: treat with normal saline. **Nephrogenic diabetes insipitus** (can be from lithium toxicity) treatment: hydrochlorothiazide and indomethacin (NSAIDs). **Central diabetes insipidus treatment**: Desmopressin can be administered intranasally, orally, subcutaneously, or intravenously.
3. **Asynchrony ARDS** etiologies: increased dead space, and has to increase RR to maintain PO_2, thus, treatment is increasing PEEP or FiO_2, inspiratory duration, triggering sensitivity.
4. Unexpected COPD/emphysema: test for **alpha 1 antitrypsin**.
5. Lethargic, concerns for aspiration → NPO, speech eval.
6. For hip fracture, usually recommends **LMWH 40 mg subcu for 4–6 weeks** after hip fracture surgery; some orthopedic surgeons use **aspirin 81 mg bid** for 6 weeks.
7. **Incentive spirometry** for post-surgery; lung congestion → repeat CXR.

1/5/2018

1. **Low flow nasal cannula** 1–6 lpm provides 24%–40% FiO_2; 1-L O_2 adds approximately 3% FiO_2.
2. **Standard face mask** 5–10 lpm provides 35%–40% FiO_2. **A partial rebreather** at 6–10 lpm provides only 40%–70% FiO_2. **Non-rebreather mask** at 10–15 lpm, 60%–80% (not 100% due to air leak).
3. **Air-entrainment mask** (venturi mask) 4–15 lpm, 24%–60% FiO_2 stays constant, depending on color.
4. **High-flow nasal cannula** up to 60 lpm in non-hypercapnic acute hypoxic respiratory failure.
5. **BiPAP settings**: 18/4 → 20/8 (EPAP maximum of 20–25 cm H_2O), respiratory therapist consult, used in both types of respiratory failure. The primary problem is hypoventilation, not good for pneumonia.
6. CPAP can pressure support for breathing = PEEP. A patient can breathe on its own while the machine provides PEEP; use only if hypoxemia in OSA or CHF.

7. **Tumor lysis syndrome**: increase in K, uric acid, and phosphorus; decrease in calcium and occurrence of renal failure. **Treatment**: avoid IV contrast and NSAIDs, allopurinol, aggressive hydration +/– diuretics to increase urine output to 80–100 cc/h; consider alkalization; rasburicase, or febuxostat. **Do not replace calcium as it can potentiate calcium phosphate crystal deposition in soft tissues.**
8. **Angioinvasive fungi**: **aspergillus and mucormycosis and Rhizopus**. Aggressive treatment with an infectious disease consult is needed.
9. High respiratory rate (RR) above the vent, treatment: increase PEEP pressure/RR/tidal volume.
10. Check bowel sounds and whether or not passing gas in surgery patients.
11. **JVP forms**: a atrial contraction; c tricuspid contraction; v venous filling; x atrial relaxation; x' right ventricle pulls tricuspid down; y atrium emptying.

1/7/2018

1. **Pirfenidone** for lung fibrosis. Diamox = acetazolamide; minute ventilation ideally 6–10, if >10 indicating too much dead space.
2. **No 2 nuclear tests on the same day**; i.e., no V/Q scan and Cardiolite on the same day (should be 24–48 h apart).
3. Pressure control: set PEEP + pressure above PEEP; RR. PRVC = set PEEP, tidal volume, RR.
4. NG tube for free water flushes at **400 cc, q6h.**
5. **BNP increases** with diastolic HF, ACS, HTN with LVH, valvular heart disease, AFib, pulmonary embolism, pulmonary hypertension, sepsis, COPD, and hyperthyroidism.
6. **Multigated acquisition (MUGA)** provides a more accurate ejection fraction assessment.
7. Daily assessments: lines, drips, tubes, KUB for nasogastric (NG) tube, and gastrointestinal (GI) issues.
8. **Pulmonary edema**: morphine in asthmatics worsens symptoms because it releases histamines.
9. Liver failure with hgb 5 with acute bleeding: **octreotide** 50 μg for an hour then 25 μg/h for 72 h, **albumin**, **vit K** 10 mg IV, **FFP**, **ceftriaxone**, **PPI** iv; add metronidazole 500 mg, PPI even PLT < 52; vasopressin 50u IV prn for maintaining MAP >65, rifaximin 550 mg bid → tid, pyridoxine 100 mg IV qd.

1/8/2018

1. **Rapid response**, always consider pulmonary embolism (PE), acute myocardial infarction (AMI), stroke, bowel obstruction/ischemia, aortic dissection, and meningitis. Typically order d-dimer, troponin, lactic acid, arterial blood gas, and all necessary tests and exams appropriate. Find the root cause, then treat it.
2. Concerns for ST elevation myocardial infarction (**STEMI**), give aspirin, get serial EKG, call cardiologist, and activate STEMI protocol (caution ticagrelor).

3. **Uncontrolled severe hypertension in ESRD** on hemodialysis (HD) treatment: lisinopril 40 mg qd, amlodipine 10 mg qd, labetalol 400 mg tid, clonidine 0.3 mg tid, minoxidil 5 mg bid.
4. **Alcohol withdrawal delirium tremens treatment**: lorazepam (Ativan), diazepam (Valium), or midazolam (Versed); additional treatment include thiamine, folic acid, and pantoprazole (Protonix). Diazepam (Valium), lorazepam (Ativan), and chlordiazepoxide (Librium) are used most frequently to treat or prevent alcohol withdrawal, but other benzodiazepines may also be used.
5. **Metabolic acidosis**: we may push bicarb or use BiPAP to maintain a normal pH in severe conditions.
6. **Bacteremia**: check for endocarditis with echocardiogram in patients with G+ bacteremia. Bacteremia: not a candidate for percutaneous coronary intervention (PCI).
7. Tachycardia and pulmonary edema: may order **morphine** IV (**anxiolytic** and **vasodilatory** properties).
8. **Atrial fibrillation** treatment: metoprolol (Lopressor) 5 mg IV q2min × 1–2 doses → if not effective, Cardizem 0.25 mg/kg (actual body weight, typically 15–20 mg) IV over 2 min → if not effective, amiodarone 150 mg over 10 min then 1 mg/h for 6 h, then 0.5 mg/min for 18 additional hours or until switched to oral therapy. Alternative is digoxin 0.25 mg IV bolus then 0.125 mg every 6 h to a maximum of 1.5 mg over 24 h especially if soft blood pressure.
9. **Beta blockers are contraindicated in acute systolic HF** in pulmonary edema and signs of cardiogenic shock, severe bradycardia, hypotension, or wheezing related to asthma.
10. Chronic obstructive pulmonary disease (COPD) patients with atrial fibrillation (AFib) and ischemic heart disease: congestive heart failure and hypertension can be treated as usual with beta-blockers; **cardioselective blockers** like atenolol and metoprolol may help avoid increasing risks for COPD exacerbation.
11. Cardioselective beta-blockers (**atenolol and metoprolol**) are at least 20× more potent at **blocking beta 1 than beta 2 receptors**, the risk of bronchoconstriction via beta 2 blocking is negligible. Only 3 beta blockers have mortality benefits in congestive heart failure: the cardioselective agents **metoprolol XL** and **bisoprolol**, and then noncardioselective **carvedilol.**
12. Tachycardia of atrial fibrillation with rapid ventricular rate (RVR) + low blood pressure Treatment: amiodarone 150 mg IV stat+ amio-D5W 360 mg for 2 days. **Atrial flutter** typically is difficult to treat and may require a **combination of metoprolol and diltiazem and even cardioversion and amiodarone** treatment.
13. Sepsis with **metabolic acidosis**: may use BiPAP at 12/6 if difficulties breathing.
14. **Precedex has anti-anxiety effects**; difficulty extubating due to high respiratory rate. Treatment: decrease sedation with propofol, add and transition to Precedex.
15. **Solu-Medrol** dosing for COPD exacerbation (wheezing): 125 mg iv once, followed by 40 mg iv q6h or q8h, or 60 mg iv q6h or q8h → prednisone 40 mg qd.
16. Maximal body temperature (Tmax) overnight 99 on high dose steroid (Solu-Medrol 80 mg IV q8h) is concerning (steroids suppress fever).

17. Add cefazolin if surgical wound. SVT → QTc issue → stop Levaquin. Minoxidil use, then no hydralazine. Both **minoxidil and hydralazine** are peripheral vasodilators and can cause reflex tachycardia and are not recommended for use together.
18. **Prealbumin**: if high, indicates chronic kidney disease, steroid use, alcoholism, or Hodgkin lymphoma. If low, it may indicate malnutrition, chronic disease, and liver disease.

1/9/2018

1. **Dobhoff, also known as small bore feeding tube;** can be used for feeding and medication administration: make sure to get a KUB after its placement.
2. **McConnell's sign**: echo pattern of RV dysfunction consisting of akinesia of mid-free wall but normal motion at the apex (D-sign caused by bowing of the septum into the left ventricle. It is a specific finding for pulmonary embolism with **acute or chronic right heart strain**.
3. Echo feature of **right ventricle dysfunction in pulmonary embolism**: (A) right ventricular wall hypokinesis; (B) right ventricular dilatation; (C) pulmonary artery hypertension.
4. **Indications for thrombolysis in pulmonary embolism with cor pulmonale:** cardiac arrest or hemodynamic instability, as well as high risks for mortality.
5. High HR → CXR → **pneumothorax**; can be a cause of high BP/high HR/high RR.
6. **Pressure support ventilator setting**: PEEP 5, pressure above PEEP 12, FiO_2 40%.
7. Had seizure → order EEG to capture encephalopathy and possible status epilepticus.

1/10/2018

1. Check **home meds** on patients as home medications may be held at admission.
2. Vomiting → **ileus** (listen to the abdomen, no or minimal bowel sounds) → treatments of ileus include daily bisacodyl suppository, scheduled Reglan, and Compazine; hold feeds or NPO.
3. Had medical clearance for transmetatarsal amputation (TMA), but still developed STEMI.
4. **Reverse INR from warfarin use criteria**: INR $\geq$ 10 or active bleeding. Labetalol for HTN in pregnancy.
5. **Single chamber pacing** has one lead in the **right atrium** (used for asystole of any etiology in isolated sinus node dysfunction with intact AV conduction) or **right ventricle** (prevents ventricular bradyarrhythmia like AFib) vs. dual chamber vs. triple chamber (biventricular pacemaker). **Dual-chamber pacing (DDD)** device (2 leads to the right atrium and right ventricle, used in heart block) is appropriate for patients with sinus rhythm and intact, delayed, or absent atrioventricular conduction. It provides sensing and pacing capabilities in both the atrium and the ventricle. **The biventricular pacemaker** has three

leads to the right atrium, right ventricle, and left ventricle; it is also known as **cardiac resynchronization therapy**.

6. **Pacemaker syndrome** = loss of AV synchrony, especially common in single-chamber VVI pacing, causing acute congestive heart failure symptoms (fatigue, dyspnea, cough, dizziness, atypical chest discomfort, hypotension, crackles, edema, murmur, and presyncope or syncope). Diagnosis via pacemaker interrogation. **Treatment**: upgrade to a dual-chamber.
7. **Biventricular pacing** (also known as cardiac resynchronization therapy) indications: left ventricular ejection fraction ≤35% (at least 3 months after goal-directed medical optimization after the initial diagnosis of HFrEF or at least 40 days after myocardial infarction); LVEF 35%–50% but the anticipation of requiring frequent ventricular pacing (≥40% of the time); QRS ≥ 150 ms with LBBB; refractory symptoms attributable to heart failure.
8. Increased **cTn** seen in sepsis, AFib, congestive heart failure, pulmonary embolism, myocarditis, myocardial contusions, and renal failure. **Mechanism of troponin increase**: (A) myocyte necrosis; (B) increased myocyte membrane permeability; (C) normal turnover of myocardiocytes.
9. **Enalapril and captopril** are OK during breastfeeding, but not lisinopril. Labetalol is good for HTN in pregnancy.
10. pH ok, but the patient remains to have altered mental status (AMS), look for other causes of AMS → **CT head, check for infections** (lumbar puncture and brain MRI may be necessary).
11. No response or improvement to treatments → Seek expert opinion first, and have patient and family discussions for goals of care, palliative care, or hospice consult (cardiogenic shock). Check **postdialysis CXR** in CHF.

1/11/2018

1. **Altered mental status**: EEG for seizure activity → nonconvulsive status epilepticus: Dilantin 1 g IV STAT and Keppra 1 g q12h (alternative: If the patient has a second episode of witnessed seizure, please start Keppra 3000 mg intravenous loading dose and maintenance dose of 1500 mg intravenous twice a day). Changed to Dilantin 100 mg IV q6h (increased to 200 mg iv q6h) + Vimpat 200 mg bid.
2. **COPD exacerbation**: taper prednisone from 40 mg qd, add Pulmicort and arformoterol (Brovana) 15 mg. Trilogy BiPAP/CPAP for home discharge.
3. **Aa gradient** = $PAO_2 - PaO_2 = FiO_2 \times 713 - (4/5)\ PCO_2\text{-}PaO_2$. Normal <4 + age/4 or 2.5 + (0.2 × age)
4. Pulmonary manifestation of rheumatoid arthritis: pulmonary parenchymal disease (**interstitial lung disease**) and **inflammation of the pleura** (pleural thickening and effusion), airway, and pulmonary vasculature (**vasculitis and pulmonary hypertension**).
5. Agitation: Versed 1 mg IV q6h; morphine for wound vac change, Seroquel.

1/13/2018

1. **Sudden drop in blood pressure (BP)**, unable to get BP and drop in SO_2, Treatment: call rapid response, BiPAP, 2 L NS, Bicarb × 2 amp, Levophed.
2. **Indications for Bicarb drip treatment**: pH < 7.2 and HCO_3 < 10; or pH < 6.9. In reality: lactic acid = 6.1, pH = 7.14, HCO_3 = 16.6. Treatment: $NaHCO_3$ 8.4% SYR 50 mEq IV × 4.
3. Shock (BP low) in ICU, Treatment: Neo-Synephrine (phenylephrine) 160 mg in NS, double concentration 320 mg/mL + 0.9NS Levophed 32 mg + D5W vasopressin (Pitressin) 20 units
4. **Shock**: (1) Distribution (septic vs. nonseptic: SIRS, neurogenic, anaphylactic, others); (2) Cardiogenic (arrhythmogenic, cardiomyopathic, mechanic); (3) Hypovolemic (hemorrhagic vs. non-hemorrhagic); (4) Obstructive (pulmonary embolism, cardiac tamponade, and tension pneumothorax).
5. **Mixed shock or unknown cause shock**: endocrine, metabolic (acidosis, hypothermia), polytrauma.
6. Diagnosis of **rhabdomyolysis**: CK 5 times upper limit normal. **Preop steroid stress dose**: hydrocortisone succinate 25 mg IV q8h for 2 days.
7. Pressure support trial 10/6, 10 is pressure support, 6 is PEEP. **Wheezing needs bronchodilator and steroids.**
8. **Dobutamine** improves hemodynamics in pulmonary hypertension **at liver transplantation and after RV infarction**.
9. **Acute chest syndrome = new radiodensity on CXR** accompanied by fever and/or respiratory symptoms in sickle cell disease. Pathophysiology: vaso-occlusion within the pulmonary microvasculature. Etiology (infection, asthma, hypoventilation), bone marrow fat emboli.
10. **Diagnosis of acute chest syndrome**: radiographic consolidation and at least one of the following: (1) > 38°; (2) 2% decrease of baseline SO_2; (3) PaO_2 < 60 mmHg; (4) tachypnea; (5) use of accessory muscle; F. chest pain; G. wheezing; F. rales.
11. **Differential diagnosis of acute chest syndrome**: pulmonary embolism, acute coronary syndrome, pneumonia. **Treatment:** pain control, fluid management, O_2 and spirometry, blood transfusion to keep Hgb > 10; antibiotics, venous thromboembolism prophylaxis, D5 + 1/2NS at 120 cc/h. For severe acute chest syndrome, can proceed with an **exchange transfusion**.
12. Chronic transfusion in adults with ≥2 episodes of moderate to severe acute chest syndrome in 24 months: Exchange transfusion to **maintain Hgb S percentage ≤ 50%; erythrocytapheresis q4-6m for 1–2 years**.
13. Acute painful episodes, also known as "**sickle cell crisis**" = consider vaso-occlusive events in sickle cell disease and resulting tissue ischemia and inflammation.
14. **Hydroxyurea → l-glutamine → chronic transfusion** decreases the frequency of painful vaso-occlusive episodes of acute chest syndrome.

General Medicine Floor

1/16/2018

1. **Non-alcoholic fatty liver disease (NAFLD)** is subdivided into nonalcoholic fatty liver (NAFL) or nonalcoholic steatohepatitis (NASH). Spider angioma; caput medusa.
2. **NAFLD activity score** (NAS): steatosis (0–3), lobular inflammation (0–2), hepatocellular ballooning (0–2), and fibrosis (0–4). ≥7 indicates NASH.
3. Steatosis → steatohepatitis → cirrhosis → fibrosis → hepatocellular carcinoma.
4. **Treatment for NAFLD**: weight loss, HAV&HBV vaccination, treatment of risk factors for CVD, Vit E/pioglitazone for selected patients, no alcohol use.
5. Patients who develop **cirrhosis** and have **complications** (**ascites, variceal bleeding**) or the model for **end-stage liver disease (MELD) score ≥10** should be referred for liver transplantation evaluation.
6. **Decompensated cirrhosis** presentations: jaundice, pruritus, signs of upper gastrointestinal bleeding (hematemesis, melana, hematochezia), abdominal distension from ascites, or confusion from encephalopathy.
7. **Acute non-alcoholic liver failure** workup: hep B surface Ag, anti-hep B core IgG, Ab to HCV, serum ferritin and transferrin saturation, total IgG or gammaglobulin level, ANA, anti-smooth muscle Ab, anti-liver/kidney microsomal Ab.
8. **Alcoholism** causes nutritional deficiency including protein-calorie malnutrition and deficiencies of vitamin A, D, thiamine, folate, pyridoxine, and zinc.
9. For upper quadrant pain, do an ultrasound to rule out gallstones/pancreatitis, **po contrast for diverticulitis**. Bowel ischemia → X-ray → CTA.
10. Besides STEMI, **ST elevation** can be seen in LBBB, acute pericarditis, myocarditis, hyperkalemia, Brugada syndrome, arrhythmogenic right ventricular cardiomyopathy, pulmonary embolism (S1Q3T3), transthoracic cardioversion, Prinzmetal angina.
11. **Causes of dominant R wave in V1**: RVH (PE), RBBB, post-myocardial infarction, V1 and V3 reversed (WPW Type A), hypertrophic cardiomyopathy, dystrophy (myotonic, Duchene)

1/17/2018

1. **Nuplazid (pimavanserin)** is used for the treatment of hallucinations and delusions associated with Parkinson disease psychosis.
2. **ADHD medications**: Evekeo (amphetamine), Adderall (amphetamine + dextroamphetamine), Dexedrine (dextroamphetamine), Vyvanse (lisdexamfetamine), Ritalin (methylphenidate).
3. **Antipsychotics**: Abilify (aripiprazole), Thorazine (chlorpromazine), Zyprexa (olanzapine)
4. **Thorazine** increases mortality in elderly patients with dementia-related psychosis. Indications for Thorazine: (A) bipolar schizophrenia: 30-–800 mg qd in 2–4 doses; (B) intractable hiccups: 25–50 mg tid-qid; (C) N/V: 10–25 mg q4-6h prn po or im, no IV, IV only 2 mg in surgery.
5. **Pancreatic panniculitis**: inflammatory nodules on the distal legs, commonly seen in pancreatitis or pancreatic malignancy.

1/18/2018

1. **Pancreatitis**: mild acute pancreatitis; **moderately severe acute** pancreatitis (transient organ failure <48 h and/or local systemic complications >48 h); **severe acute** pancreatitis (persistent organ failure that may involve one or multiple organs).
2. Patients with **severe pancreatitis** may have fever, tachypnea, hypoxemia, and/or hypotension.
3. Pancreatitis can have leukocytosis, elevated hematocrit, increased BUN, hypocalcemia, and hypoglycemia.
4. **Diagnosis of pancreatitis** requires two out of the following: acute onset of persistent severe epigastric pain radiating to the back; elevated serum lipase or amylase to **>3× upper limit normal** (ULN); characteristic findings of acute pancreatitis on imaging.
5. **Local complications of pancreatitis:** acute peripancreatic fluid collection (7–10 days), pancreatic pseudocyst (≥4 days), acute necrotic collection and walled-off necrosis (>10 days).
6. Acute pancreatitis categories: **interstitial edematous** acute pancreatitis; **necrotizing** acute pancreatitis.
7. **Initial treatment**: Fluid replacement at 5–10 cc/kg/h for the first 12–24 h; pain control with opioids; monitor SO_2, urine output (ideally 0.5–1 cc/kg/h), electrolytes, glucose; monitor for abdominal compartment syndrome.
8. In **mild pancreatitis**, in the absence of ileus, nor vomiting, oral feeds can be initiated as soon as the pain is decreasing and inflammatory markers are improving, usually in 24–48 h after onset.
9. **Peripancreatic vascular complications**: (A) splanchnic venous thrombosis; (B) pseudoaneurysm- unexplained bleeding, drop in Hgb, sudden expansion of fluid collections; (C) abdominal compartment syndrome.
10. ERCP should be performed early in the course (within 24 h of admission) for patients with **gallstone pancreatitis and cholangitis**. Other indications for ERCP include patients with **common bile duct obstruction, dilated common bile duct, or drainage of symptomatic pancreatic pseudocysts.**
11. After bariatric surgery, recommend a diet with all essential nutrients: My Plate, DASH diet (fruits, vegetables, whole grains, and low-fat dairy foods), The Vegetarian Resource Group. **Types of bariatric surgeries**: Roux-en-y gastric bypass (early satiety), sleeve gastrectomy, biliopancreatic diversion with duodenal switch.
12. **Chronic myelogenous leukemia (CML)** is characterized by uncontrolled production of mature and maturing granulocytes, predominantly neutrophil, also basophil and eosinophil. **Symptoms of CML** include fatigue (34%), malaise (3%), weight loss (20%), excessive sweating (15%), abdominal fullness (15%), and bleeding episodes due to platelet dysfunction (21%) while 50% are asymptomatic.

1/20/2018

1. **Pack year**: its calculated by multiplying the number of packs of cigarettes smoked per day by the number of years
2. **Annual low-dose CT** for high-risk adults 50–80 years old with 20 pack-year smoking history and current smoker or have quit within the past 15 years with discontinuation of screening once the individual has not smoked for 15 years or has limited life expectancy.
3. Low-dose CT refers to a non-contrast study obtained with a multidetector CT scanning during **a single maximal inspiratory breath hold with a scanning time of <25 s**.
4. National lung screening trial found that annual lung cancer screening with low-dose CT **reduces all-cause mortality by 6.7%**, and prevents 3–9 deaths over 6 years per 1000 persons.
5. **Drugs causing thrombocytopenia**: (A) abciximab, amiodarone, Tylenol, alemtuzumab (for CLL and MS); (B) beta-lactams; (C) carbapenems, ceftriaxone; (D) daptomycin; (E) eptifibatide, ethambutol, furosemide; (F) gold compounds; (G) Haldol, ibuprofen, Levaquin, linezolid, MMR vaccine, mirtazapine, naproxen, oxaliplatin, penicillin, phenytoin, piperacillin, quinine, ranitidine, rifampin, simvastatin, sulfonamides, suramin, tirofiban, TMP-SMX, valproic acid, vancomycin.
6. **H. pylori treatments (either one of them)**: Clarithromycin-based therapy (Triple therapy, concomitant therapy, sequential therapy, hybrid therapy); levofloxacin-based therapy; bismuth quadruple therapy (bismuth subsalicylate, metronidazole, tetracycline, PPI for 14 days).
7. **Confirmation of eradication of H. pylori**: urea breath test, fecal Ag test, or upper endoscopy performed 4 weeks after completion of treatment. **PPI should be withheld 1–2 weeks prior to testing.** Endoscopy with biopsy for culture and sensitivity should be performed in patients with persistent H. pylori infection after **two courses of antibiotic treatment**.
8. **H. pylori** is naturally resistant to several commonly used antibiotics including vancomycin, trimethoprim, and sulfonamides.
9. **Salvage regimens** (used when failed other treatments): **Bismuth quadruple therapy**; levofloxacin triple therapy (levo 500 mg qd, amoxicillin 1 g bid, PPI bid); **high dose dual therapy** (high dose PPI and amoxicillin for 14 days); **clarithromycin based concomitant therapy** (clarithromycin, amoxicillin, a nitroimidazole, PPI), rifabutin triple therapy (rifabutin, amoxicillin, PPI).
10. Treatment **during pregnancy for H. pylori** is typically acid suppression. If H. pylori is present, treatment is typically deferred after delivery.

1/21/2018

1. **Disseminated intravascular coagulation** (DIC) is also known as consumption coagulopathy and defibrination syndrome. DIC: procoagulant exposure → coagulation- fibrinolysis → organ damage. **Procoagulants**: tissue factor, lipopolysaccharide (LPS), meningococcal sepsis, microparticles containing tissue factor, and cancer procoagulant.

2. In severe intravascular hemolysis, such as **acute hemolytic transfusion reaction (AHTR)** caused by ABO mismatch, coagulation is activated by a combination of processes including tissue factor (TF) release by monocytes, generation of cytokines including TNF and IL-1 and reduced NO.
3. **Damage-associated pattern molecules** (DAPM, AKA alarmins) including cell-free DNA (cfDNA), extracellular histones, and DNA-binding proteins, play a critical role in the pathogenesis of DIC.
4. Alarmin → neutrophil extracellular traps (NETs): nuclear chromatin becomes decondensed and released into the cytoplasm (NETosis), followed by rupture of the plasma membrane and expulsion of cellular contents into the extracellular space.
5. **NETosis** is highly procoagulant: activating clotting cascades via: (A) delivery of TF, (B) activation of contact phase of DNA (cfDNA), (C) cytotoxicity of cfDNA activating TLR9, (D) induction of PLT aggregation of cfDNA.
6. In **chronic DIC**, the liver can cleave FDPs, clotting time may thus be normal and thrombocytopenia may be present or absent. Thrombosis generally predominates over bleeding with only lab evidence of **increased thrombin generation and fibrinolysis**. Seen in malignancy.
7. DIC versus other thrombotic microangiopathies (TMAs): Thrombotic Thrombocytopenic Purpura (TTP)—**accumulation of very long vWF**; hemolytic uremic syndrome (HUS)- **complement-induced damage**.
8. **Causes of DIC**: sepsis, malignancy, trauma, obstetrical complication, intravascular hemolysis like acute hemolytic transfusion reaction (AHTR).
9. **An FDP level of more than 40 mg/mL** is considered critical.
10. **Acute DIC**: lab evidence of thrombocytopenia, coagulation factor consumption (prolonged PT, PTT, low fibrinogen), and fibrinolysis (increased FDPs) with increased D-dimer without another etiology.
11. **Chronic DIC**: evidence of fibrinolysis (increased D-dimer) in the absence of other etiology like VTE in appropriate clinical settings.
12. **Differential diagnosis of DIC**: liver disease, TTP, HUS. Purpura fulminans-protein C deficiency.
13. Patients with serious bleeding and a prolonged PT or PTT, or fibrinogen <50 and serious bleeding. Treatment: **FFP or cryoprecipitate** or Plasma Frozen within 24 h of Collection (**PF24**) or coagulation factor replacement. If **fibrinogen < 100, give cryoprecipitate**; if **fibrinogen > 100 and PT and PTT increase, do FFP or PF 24**.
14. **Initial procoagulants** include TF, bacterial products, microparticles, and cfDNA and DNA binding protein for NETs.
15. Sepsis, lung clear, urine antigen negative, likely UTI, **stop azithromycin** (azithromycin is mainly used fr legionella pneumonia concerns).

1/23/2018

1. **Droplet precautions:** suspected influenza for 7 days after illness onset or until 24 h after the resolution of fever and respiratory symptoms, whichever is longer while a patient is in a healthcare facility.

2. **C. diff precautions**: continue contact precautions for a minimum of 48 h after the resolution of diarrhea.
3. Patients with **VRE** can remain colonized for long periods after discharge from the hospital and should be placed in isolation when readmission to hospitals.
4. **MRSA** new admission, nasal swab for MRSA, if negative, no isolation.
5. Proximal DVT (popliteal, femoral, iliac), anticoagulated for ≥3 months.
6. Isolated distal DVT has no proximal components, located below the knee, confined to calf veins like peroneal V., post/ant. tibial V., or muscular V., no anticoagulation.
7. For asymptomatic distal DVT, we can elect observation with proximal vein compressive ultrasound weekly for 2 weeks. If extension toward proximal veins, do anticoagulation for 3 months.
8. **Contraindications for anticoagulation**: active hemorrhage, PLT < 50,000, or prior intracranial hemorrhage (not an absolute contraindication).
9. **Sudden unexpected death in epilepsy (SUDEP)**: a fatal complication of epilepsy defined as sudden and unexpected nontraumatic and non-drowning death of a person with epilepsy, without toxicological or anatomical cause of death.
10. **Sudden cardiac death/arrest treatment**: electrophysiology study, cardiac MRI, catheterization, life vest/ICD, ASA, metoprolol, Lipitor.
11. Factors favor the use of anticoagulation: extensive superficial venous thrombosis (SVT) above the knee, close to the saphenofemoral junction, severe symptoms, involvement of the greater saphenous vein, history of venous thromboembolism (VTE) or SVT, active cancer, recent surgery.
12. SVT of >5 cm in length in lower extremities will need a **prophylactic dose of fondaparinux or LMWH or Xaretlo 10 mg daily** for 45 days over no anticoagulation.
13. **Paget–Schroetter disease**, is a form of upper extremity deep vein thrombosis (DVT), a medical condition in which blood clots form in the deep veins of the arms. These DVTs typically occur in the axillary and/or subclavian veins. LMWH has anti-cancer properties and thus is commonly used in cancer.
14. Currently **prostate cancer imaging (staging CT and bone scan) only** if PSA > 20 ng/mL or a PSA level of >10 ng/mL with a T2-4 tumor, or Gleason score > 8.
15. The **post-thrombolysis protocol for post-tPA stroke care** includes: (A) avoid antiplatelet and anticoagulant agent for 24 h until a repeat CT scan shows no hemorrhage; (B) frequent neurological and vital sign evaluations; (C) maintain BP < 180/105 mmHg.
16. **Prevention of VTE in orthopedic surgery patients**: (A) THA and TKA and hip fracture surgery: antithrombotic ppx for ≥10–14 days to 35 days; LMWH should be given 12 h before and after surgery. (B) for patients undergoing major orthopedic surgery, expand thromboprophylaxis in the outpatient period for up to 35 days. (C) At clinical practices, some surgeons prefer aspirin 325 mg twice a day for 6 weeks upon discharge to rehabilitation facilities. In patients during hospitalization, do dual prophylaxis with anti-thrombotic agents and intermittent pneumatic compression (IPC) devices (IPCD) during hospital stay.

1/24/2018

1. In one episode of blood loss, 4–6 h later, hemoglobin should be stabilized.
2. **Analgesic nephropathy** is characterized by papillary necrosis and chronic interstitial nephritis and caused by long-term consumption of **analgesic agents** (2 or 3 or more analgesic agents and usually codeine or caffeine, ASA + NSAIDs).
3. Radiographic manifestation of analgesic nephropathy: **small kidneys, calcification involving the renal papilla; indented/irregular contour**.

1/25/2018

1. **Normal pressure hydrocephalus (NPH)**: pathologically enlarged ventricular size with normal pressures on lumbar puncture (**normal CSF opening pressure between 18 and 20 cmH_2O**). NPH symptoms include dementia, gait disturbance, and incontinence. Treatment: ventriculoperitoneal shunt.
2. **Causes of NPH**: intraventricular/subarachnoid hemorrhage and prior acute or ongoing chronic meningitis from infection, cancer, inflammatory diseases, Paget's disease at the skull base, and mucopolysaccharidosis of the meninges can also cause NPH in rare cases.
3. **Cognitive disturbances of NPH** have prominent subcortical and frontal features with **psychomotor impairments** showing decreased attention and concentration and apathy, and impaired **executive function** (ability to **conceptualize** all facets of activity and **translate** that into behaviors). Cortical features including aphasia, agnosia, and apraxia are less prominent.
4. MRI of NPH: ventriculomegaly; white matter lesions (transependymal egress of fluid); aqueduct flow void.
5. **Confirmatory test of NPH**: removal of CSF (lumbar tap test/lumbar drainage); intracranial pressure monitoring; CSF infusion test; cisternography
6. **NPH treatment**: ventricular shunting → repeated high-volume taps
7. **Lewy body dementia**: cognitive fluctuation, visual hallucination, Parkinsonism, and rapid eye movements.
8. BPH **storage symptoms**: increased daytime frequency, nocturia, urgency, and urinary incontinence. **Voiding symptoms**: slow urinary flow, splitting or spraying; intermittent urinary stream, hesitancy, straining, and terminal dribbling.
9. **Diagnosis of BPH** requires the presence of storage, voiding, and/or irritative urinary **symptoms** in conjunction with a **diffusely enlarged firm and nontender prostate** on physical examination.
10. **Toxicology screening**: urine toxicology, urine methadone, buprenorphine, salicylate level, ethanol level, and acetaminophen level.
11. **Severe sepsis** defines tissue **hypoperfusion** (increased lactic acid, oliguria) and/or organ dysfunction (increased Cr, coagulopathy) in sepsis.
12. **Pelvocaliectasis**: dilatation of the renal pelvis and the renal calyx from obstruction of urine flow.
13. **Brain mass**, likely GBM, is treated with Decadron 10 mg IV once, followed by 4 mg q6h, +/− Keppra for seizures if any. Will also need neurosurgery and oncology consults.

14. **Metabolic alkalosis causes**: loop/thiazide diuretics, vomiting, antacids, hyperaldosteronism. Pathophysiology: bicarbonate not being excreted in urine from reduced effective arterial blood flow, associated with chloride depletion or inadequate distal tubal chloride delivery, hypokalemia, and AKI.
15. **Treatment of metabolic alkalosis**: (A) if vomiting/gastric suctioning treatment—H_2 blockers and PPIs; (B) increase renal bicarb excretion [if reduced blood flow, treat with NS (third spacing in CHF and cirrhosis) at 100 cc/h; potassium-sparing diuretics like amiloride, spironolactone, eplerenone, acetazolamide]; (C) chronic respiratory acidosis- post-hypercapnic metabolic alkalosis treatment- NS or acetazolamide.
16. **Non-anion gap metabolic acidosis**: HARDASS: Hyperalimentation, Addison's disease, RTA, Diarrhea, Acetazolamide, Spironolactone, and Saline infusion
17. In patients with high-risk stigmata of recent hemorrhage, the high dose bid PPI may be switched to a similar oral dose **72 h after endoscopy** provided there is no recurrent bleeding.

1/30/2018

1. **Anticoagulation in catheter ablation to prevent recurrent AFib**: (1) continue VKA in the periprocedural period; (2) for once-a-day NOACs, hold the dose the day before and the morning of the procedure; (3) for twice a day NOAC, hold both doses the day before. Post-procedure: (1) if INR < 2 in VKA, restart UFH without bolus 6 h after sheath pull. Increase oral warfarin on the night of the procedure and continue UFH until INR reaches (2) If NOAC, restart 6 h after the procedure.
2. **Neutropenia** is defined as ANC < 1500 (WHO uses 1800). ANC = WBC × (PMN + bands percentages)/100. Mild neutropenia 1000–1500, moderate 500–1000, severe <500. Agranulocytosis ANC < 200.
3. **Glucose control**: in ICU target 140–180 mg/dL; insulin infusion should be started for persistent serum glucose >180 mg/dL (10 mmol/L) with diabetic ketoacidosis.
4. For most not critically ill hospitalized patients with DM, goal **preprandial blood glucose < 140 with all random glucose < 180** with fasting blood glucose no lower than 90–100.
5. In the course of giving an IV regular insulin infusion, start **approximately half of the patient's usual total daily insulin dose**, divided into increments until the trend of blood glucose value is known.
6. Yale ICU protocol for glucose >180, blood glucose (BG)/100, then round it to near 0.5 units for bolus and initial infusion rate, POC q4h. i.e., initial BG 325 mg/dL, 325/100 = 3.25, IV bolus 3.5u + start insulin infection 3.5u/h
7. **Chronic UTI increases risks for prostatitis. Acyclovir especially IV needs hydration using 1/2 NS or NS.**
8. **Multiple sclerosis** patients: order vit D, ESR, CRP, check for double vision (optic neuritis)
9. High BNP, bilateral infiltrate, pleural effusion → echo needed, Lasix 40 mg if shortness of breath, add Duoneb scheduled dosing.

10. **Cirrhosis with high protein and low albumin** → hypergammaglobulinemia (IgG and IgA) which may be caused by **multiple myeloma (MM)**.
11. **Arcus senilis**: an old age syndrome where there is a white, grey or blue opaque ring in the corneal margin.
12. **Hydroxyurea** causes marked fluctuation in WBC and PLT, it can also cause fever.
13. 10 mg morphine = 1 mg Dilaudid (6 × stronger than morphine).
14. AFib treatment: Cardizem 10–20 mg IV bolus → 30 mg po, 3 h later. Or 15–20 mg IV once, repeat after 15 min.
15. **SVT/AFib**: digoxin 500 mg loading (24 h no higher than 1 g), then 125 mg at 6–8 h intervals until rate controlled.
16. No need to trend lactic acid in GI bleed. Valacyclovir (Valtrex) prophylaxis may be necessary in renal transplant patient or patients on certain chemotherapy.
17. **LVAD**: left ventricular assistive device.

1/31/2018

1. **PPI can cause low Mag → low K. Heparin** interacts with adrenal angiotensin II receptors inhibiting aldosterone production and causing **increased serum K**. No NOAC use, if weight > 120 kg (update: NOAC has now been used more and more in obese patients with weight > 120 kg).
2. Avoid antipsychotic use in Parkinson's disease (PD), use BZDs. Seroquel can be used in Parkinson's disease for agitation. **Bleeding**: use SCDs for DVT prophylaxis.
3. **Shiley catheter**: inserted via the brachiocephalic veins for temporary hemodialysis (HD), can be used for less than 3 weeks. **Permacath**: a tunneled central venous catheter of HD for an extended period (weeks to months). **Double lumen pigtail Shiley** catheter is a non-tunneled catheter for both short-term (usually < 1 week) dialysis and IV access.
4. **Ischemic stroke**: eligible for thrombolysis/thrombectomy → withhold DAPT but not thrombolysis if eligible. No bleeding, start ASA within 48 h of stroke after thrombolysis while determining the cause of stroke.
5. For AFib in TIA × 3, start anticoagulation right away, otherwise look for hemorrhagic transformation and **resume oral anticoagulation after 1–2 weeks** if hemorrhagic transformation or large ischemic stroke.
6. If extracranial ICA stenosis → carotid revascularization: ASA before CEA and long-term antiplatelet therapy; stenting for carotid artery stenosis (**CAS),** prescribe **DAPT for 30 days then long-term single agent antiplatelet therapy.**
7. If large artery atherosclerosis inside the brain: **DAPT for 90 days** then single agent antiplatelet therapy.
8. **If small vessel disease or cryptogenic, start long-term antiplatelet therapy**.
9. The screening threshold for hemochromatosis is **a fasting transferrin saturation of 45%–50%**. If transferrin saturation is greater than 45%, the presence of C282Y or H63D mutation may be evaluated to confirm the diagnosis of hemochromatosis.

2/1/2018

1. **Toxic epidermal** (mucous membrane is typically involved) **necrolysis**: ≥30% of the skin is involved. **Stevens-Johnson syndrome:** <10% of skin is involved.
2. **Severe adverse cutaneous drug reactions** [toxic epidermal necrolysis (TEN) and Stevens-Johnson Syndrome (SJS)]: early symptoms include fever and flu-like symptoms. A few days later, the skin begins to blister and peel, forming painful raw areas.
3. **Complications** include dehydration, sepsis, pneumonia, and multiple organ failure. The most common cause is medications including lamotrigine, carbamazepine, allopurinol, sulfonamides, antibiotics, and nevirapine, mycoplasma pneumonia.
4. **Treatment** includes care at the burn unit and ICU. Efforts include stopping the cause, pain meds, and antihistamines, antibiotics, IVIGs, and corticosteroids may be used. TEN mortality 25%–30%; severity score (SCORTEN).
5. **Wernicke's encephalopathy diagnosis** requires two of the following: dietary deficiency, oculomotor abnormalities, cerebellar dysfunction, and either AMS or mild memory impairment. **Treatment**: thiamine 500 iv tid for 2 days + 250 mg iv qd for 5 days then 100 mg po daily.
6. **APCHEII score for acute pancreatitis**: a score of <8 equals <4% mortality; **>8** equals mortality rates of 11%–18%.
7. **Hemoglobin Koln**, an unstable Hgb variant, is characterized by mild anemia, reticulocytosis, splenomegaly, and pigmenturia. It comprises 10%–25% of total Hgb; Hgb Koln has a high affinity for O_2 in the absence of compensatory erythrocytosis and easy heme dissociation.
8. **Management for an unstable hemoglobin variant**: supportive, avoidance of oxidant drugs, prevention and prompt treatment of infections, and folic acid supplementation.
9. **Hepatopulmonary syndrome** (HPS) = **abnormal arterial oxygenation** from **intrapulmonary vascular dilation** (IPVDs) in a patient with liver disease, portal hypertension, or congenital portosystemic shunts.
10. HPS should be suspected in patients with chronic liver disease who have **dyspnea, platypnea/orthopnea, spider nevi**, and/or oxygenation dysfunction ($SO_2 < 96\%$), confirmed by **A-a ≥ 15 or PO_2 < 80 mHg**.
11. Lindsay nails in chronic kidney disease (CKD): half-half nails, it is edema of the nail bed.

2/2/2018

1. The best estimate of GFR is the **CKD-EPI equation**, NOT the Cockcroft and Gault equation or MDRD equation. Normal values: albumin/Cr ratio < **30 mg**/g; protein/Cr ratio < **200 mg**/g, 24 urine protein **<150 mg**/d.
2. **EPO** should be initiated when hemoglobin falls below 10 g/dL. Patients with CKD not on hemodialysis should maintain a daily protein intake of **0.6–0.8 g/kg** of body weight. Patients on peritoneal dialysis and hemodialysis should target daily protein intake of **1.0–1.2 g/kg** of body weight.

3. **ACEi, ARB, and non-dihydropyridine calcium channel** blockers like **verapamil, and diltiazem** can reduce proteinuria and progression of CKD. Patients on diuretics who are elderly, or who take aspirin, should avoid NSAIDs.
4. **Genetic diseases** associated with CKD include **polycystic disease, Alport syndrome, medullary cystic disease** (hyperuricemia/gout, tubular basement membrane disintegration leads to fibrosis, ESRD)
5. HIV may cause collapsing **focal glomerulosclerosis and tubulointerstitial injury**, especially in individuals of African descent.
6. AKI is associated with increased risk for **CKD development, progression to ESRD, and death**.
7. **Analgesic nephropathy** results from chronic ingestions (typically >5 years of 2 antipyretic analgesics, like acetaminophen and ASA, often with caffeine and codeine included), which slowly leads to **renal papillary necrosis and interstitial nephritis**, and progressive renal failure later on.
8. **Obtain spot urine Pr/Cr ratio if non-albumin proteinuria is suspected** (e.g., Bence Jones proteinuria). Detection of **Bence Jones protein** may be suggestive of multiple myeloma or Waldenström's macroglobulinemia.
9. Urine sediment: RBC > 3–5/HF abnormal; RBC cast = consider glomerulonephropathy. Urine WBC leukocytes + eosinophils (UTI, pyelonephritis, interstitial nephritis).
10. **Goal blood pressure** in CKD is <140/90 and < 130/80 if albuminuria.
11. **Diagnosis of anemia** if Hgb < 13.5 in males and < 12 in females. **EPO increases the risk of cardiovascular events, stroke, and death**.
12. **Phosphorus restriction** starts when P > 4.6. **Sodium bicarb** (0.5–1 mg/kg/day) should be initiated when bicarb is less than 22 in serum to preserve acid-base balance and potentially slow CKD progression.
13. **25-OH Vit D** is a good reflection of total body Vit D stores due to its long half-life. 1,25-OH Vit D (**calcitriol**) and its analogs are useful for treating CKD-related secondary hyperparathyroidism in dialysis.
14. To differentiate Vit D and CKD-induced PTH elevation, we need to check **serum P** and Vit D levels.
15. **Stage 3b CKD**: screen for bone/mineral metabolism disorder, check serum calcium, phosphorus, 25 OH Vit D, and iPTH levels.
16. **High phosphate in CKD**, check calcium → give calcium-based or non-calcium-based phosphate binders depending on serum calcium level: calcium-based – aluminum hydroxide, calcium carbonate/acetate; non-calcium based- sevelamer carbonate (Renvela), lanthanum carbonate (Fosrenol).
17. **Thiazide is not effective in GFR < 30**, use loop diuretics.

2/3/2018

1. **Hospital-acquired pneumonia occurs** 48 h or more after hospitalization and does not appear to be incubating at the time of admission.
2. Stop **chlorhexidine** once the patient is off the ventilator.

3. **Heparin-induced thrombocytopenia (HIT)** diagnosis can be based on 4Ts: thrombocytopenia-fall ≥50% and nadir ≥ 20; timing 5–10 days or <1 day with prior exposure; thrombosis; no other alternative cause.
4. **Ischemic stroke/TIA etiology**: atherothrombotic (atherosclerotic plaque disruption with superimposed thrombosis), cardioembolic, lacunar (commonly from small vessel disease related to hypertension and diabetes), cryptogenic (carotid plaques, aortic arch atheroma may be present). Cryptogenic strokes sometimes can be due to thrombophilia, right to left shunt, or cardioembolic.
5. **Ischemic stroke workup**: MRI, MRA, CT, Echo, telemetry, carotid Doppler, EKG.
6. **Intracranial hemorrhage** workup: STAT CT head/angio if suspicious for vascular source? LP for xanthochromia if no evidence of ICH but suspicious for subarachnoid hemorrhage (SAH). Coagulation profile. **Treatment**: reverse coagulation, keep INR < 1.4, PLT > 100 K, give DDAVP if uremic; strict BP control, BP goal <140 mmHg, can use nicardipine/labetalol drip.
7. **SAH treatment**: endovascular coiling vs. surgical clipping, **nimodipine** (60 mg every 4 h for 21 consecutive days within 96 h of SAH onset) to decrease risk of vasospasm (monitor with transcranial Doppler) in **aneurysmal (may also be beneficial in traumatic) SAH**; seizure prophylaxis with Keppra (duration 1–2 weeks or longer depending on actual seizure or not); no heparin but use SCDs.
8. Zosyn, Unasyn, and Augmentin have excellent anaerobic coverage.
9. Diagnosis of HIT begins with HIT panel: **heparin-induced Ab** (PLT factor 4 Ab), is confirmed by **serotonin release assay**.
10. **Light's criteria have to be met by all three to confirm exudate fluid analyses**: pleural fluid/serum LDH > 0.6, protein >0.5, LDH > 2/3.
11. **Valproate taper**: 20%–25% of the original taper every week.

2/4/2018

1. **Non-responsiveness with very low Glasgow Coma Scale or rapid difficulty breathing** management: intubation, call critical care and update family.
2. **The vibration (chest physical therapy) system**: indicated for the mobilization of secretions, lung expansion therapy, the treatment and prevention of pulmonary atelectasis, and can provide supplemental O_2 when used with compressed O_2. Can add **3% NaCl nebulizing treatment** for mucus plug.
3. **J tube blockage treatment**: try cola for 30 min and then flush or use CREON (pancrelipase).
4. **Chloraseptic spray** for sore throat for nasogastric tube.
5. H_2 blocker **famotidine** and proton pump inhibitor **pantoprazole** can cause **thrombocytopenia**.
6. Abdominal gas and pain, nausea, and vomiting, treatment: **nasogastric tube intermittent wall suction** to relieve bowel obstruction or ileus.

2/6/2018

1. Januvia = **sitagliptin**; it is a **dipeptidyl-peptidase-4 inhibitor**, common dosage 100 mg qd; 50 mg qd in CKD. Victoza = liraglutide; it is a glucagon-like peptide-1 receptor agonist that decreases weight and cardiovascular events. Tresiba = insulin degludec (long acting). Toujeo = insulin glargine (other brand names include Lantus, Basaglar).
2. **J-tube**: a feeding pump is needed when feeding, no bolus feeding. **G tube**: no feeding pump is necessary; bolus feeding is ok.
3. Proximal DVT, may **need CT chest angiogram to rule out PE**.
4. **Causes of thrombocytosis**: infection, cancer, anemia, renal failure, abdominal surgery, removal of spleen, and essential thrombocythemia.
5. Change PO to IV ratio for **levothyroxine** = 2:1
6. **Always talk to the patient's family after approval of the patient**.
7. **Tilt table testing → drop in HR or symptoms of dizziness or fainting** (abnormal results = vasovagal syncope, may need pacemaker if major bradycardia or AV block).
8. **Dyspnea management**: order ABG, chest X-ray, BNP, if respiratory acidosis, start BiPAP.

2/9/2018

1. First seizure: ask for previous subtler events, ie, auras, changes in awareness, and periods of inattention. **Deja vu** mostly represents an epileptic aura in a **partial simple seizure** from temporal lobe epilepsy.
2. Unilateral shaking and subjective aura before the onset of convulsion suggest progression to a secondarily generalized seizure is typical of **focal epilepsy**.
3. **Provoked seizure** is reserved for isolated events in patients without epilepsy by alcohol or sleep deprivation. Provoked seizures usually do not require antiepileptic medication treatment.
4. Patients with **cholangitis** (abdominal pain, elevated liver function test, and possible altered mentation) should receive immediate broad-spectrum antimicrobial therapy. Meanwhile, **urgent ERCP** should be considered.
5. Diastolic function of the left ventricle: diastolic dysfunction is **impaired ventricular relaxation with increased stiffness** of the left ventricle and increased filling pressure.
6. Mitral inflow signal: diastolic dysfunction alters the relationship between early and late filling (E wave and A wave), how rapidly flow velocity declines **in early diastole** (E wave deceleration time = DT), and how long it takes for filling the ventricle to start after the ventricle relaxes (length of isovolumetric relaxation time = IVRT).
7. Normal values: **E/A ≤ 0.8 or > 2, DT 140–240 ms**, IVRT ≤70–100 mm/s, **peak E velocity < 50 mm/s (denotes normal filling pressure)**, left atrium maximum volume index (normally should be less than) 34 mL/m^2, peak tricuspid regurgitation velocity < 2.8 m/s, pulmonary venous S (systolic deflections)/D (diastolic deflections) ratio < 1.
8. Grade 1 **diastolic dysfunction**: impaired **relaxation** and decreased **suction** of LV. Grade II: increased **stiffness**, elevated left atrial pressure (**LAP**). Grade III,

restrictive filling-reversible, high LAP, non-compliant LV, maybe reversible with reduction of preload, i.e., diuretics. Grade IV, **restrictive filling, nonreversible, no benefit from diuretics**.

9. Supranormal filling in young adults and athletes E/A > 2. **Grade 1** diastolic dysfunction **E/A ≤ 0.8**. **Grade 2 E/A > 2**, but the Valsalva maneuver causes E/A to drop below 1. **Grade 3&4 E/A > 2.**
10. **Treatment of diastolic congestive heart failure**: Lasix 40 mg IV bid. Strict I and O, daily weight and fluid restriction, keep K > 4 and Mg > 2, metoprolol succinate, add ACEi, keep HA1c < 7%.
11. **General treatments for diastolic CHF**: sodium restriction and moderate EtOH consumption is recommended. Use **mineralocorticoid receptor antagonists** in patients with congestive heart failure with preserved ejection fraction while cautioning volume depletion. **SGLT2 inhibitors** now are the only group of medications recommended for congestive heart failure with preserved ejection fraction. Continue routine treatment for comorbidities of HTN, AFib, myocardial ischemia (**epicardial atherosclerosis, high coronary wall shear stress, or coronary microvascular disease**), and hyperlipidemia.
12. **Exercise training or cardiac rehab** is the only intervention shown to consistently improve exercise capacity and quality of life in congestive heart failure with preserved ejection fraction.

Takeaway Messages

1. Rapid response usually focuses on ruling in/out acute medical emergencies including pulmonary embolism, acute coronary syndrome, stroke, acute gastrointestinal bleeding, acute abdomen, aortic dissection, and sometimes meningitis.
2. Order blood culture before antibiotics and broad-spectrum antibiotics if the source of infection is unknown.
3. Check for etiologies for diabetic ketoacidosis: the 5 Is.
4. Familiarity with ACLS protocol for code blue also known as cardiac arrest and bradycardia. Understand the etiology of 5Hs and 5Ts for code blue. Symptomatic bradycardia treatment includes atropine 1 mg bolus q3-5h, dopamine at 5–20 μg/min, and epinephrine 2–10 μg/min if no transcutaneous pacing is available.
5. Pressors (preference from high to low) used in ICU include norepinephrine, epinephrine, and vasopressin for septic shock, norepinephrine, dobutamine, and epinephrine for cardiogenic shock.
6. Low tidal volume breathing, prone, and neuromuscular blockade decreases mortality in ARDS.

Further Readings and References

1. Evans, L., A. Rhodes, W. Alhazzani, et al. 2021. Surviving sepsis campaign: international guidelines for management of sepsis and septic shock 2021. *Critical Care Medicine* 49 (11): e1063–e1143.
2. Stubbs, J.R., and A.S. Yu. *Overview of the causes and treatment of hyperphosphatemia*, ed. M. Emmett and R.H. Sterns. Waltham, MA: UpToDate. Accessed November 3, 2023.

3. Douketis, J.D., and G.Y.H. Lip. *Perioperative management of patients receiving anticoagulants*, ed. L.L.K. Leung. Waltham, MA: UpToDate Accessed November 3, 2023.
4. Holanda, M.A. Basic modes of mechanical ventilation. *Xlung* https://xlung.net/en/mv-manual/basic-modes-of-mechanical-ventilation. Accessed November 3, 2023.
5. Holanda, M.A. Formulas and parameters of mechanical ventilation. *Xlung* https://xlung.net/en/mv-manual/formulas-and-parameters-of-mechanical-ventilation. Accessed November 3, 2023.
6. Vege, S.S. 2019. In *Management of acute pancreatitis*, ed. D.G. Adler. Waltham, MA: UpToDate. Accessed November 3, 2023.
7. Lamont, J.T. *Treatment regimens for Helicobacter pylori in adults*, ed. M. Feldman. Waltham, MA: UpToDate. Accessed November 3, 2023.
8. Leung, L.L.K. *Evaluation and management of disseminated intravascular coagulation (DIC) in adults*, ed. P.M. Mannucci. Waltham, MA: UpToDate. Accessed November 3, 2023.
9. Flevas, D.A., P.D. Megaloikonomos, L. Dimopoulos, et al. 2018. Thromboembolism prophylaxis in orthopaedics: an update. *EFORT Open Reviews* 3 (4): 136–148.
10. Passman, R. *Catheter ablation to prevent recurrent atrial fibrillation: Anticoagulation*, ed. B.P. Knight and N.A.M. Estes. Waltham, MA: UpToDate. Accessed November 3, 2023.
11. Fuentes, B., R. Gutiérrez-Zúñiga, and E. Díez-Tejedor. 2020. It's time to say goodbye to the ESUS Construct. *Frontiers in Neurology* 11: 653.
12. Altersberger, M., and T. Binder. *Diastolic function & diastolic dysfunction*. https://123sonography.com/diastolic-function-and-diastolic-dysfunction. Accessed February 29, 2024.

Chapter 6
Immersion in the Infectious Disease World

February 12th, 2018 Through March 11th, 2018

Infectious diseases are major causes of morbidity and mortality in patients both inside and outside of the hospital. Minor infections in otherwise healthy adults can be treated with oral antibiotics as an outpatient. Infections in senior adults and adults with immunocompromised conditions and severe infections or infections from invasive pathogens usually require inpatient treatments and sometimes prolonged intravenous antibiotics.

Although the training in infectious disease management starts with medical school, it cultivates into clinical application and refinement during residency training and actual clinical practices. Although broad-spectrum antibiotic use may be appropriate in patients with critical and severe infections from unknown pathogens, tailored antibiotic(s) targeting specific pathogen(s) is usually the preferred treatment upon discharge or whenever more data are available. This is of paramount importance in the practice of medicine as antibiotic resistance and "superbugs" become more and more common. To decrease unnecessary antibiotic exposure and minimize the development of antibiotic resistance, notes in this chapter provided the foundation for the treatment of infectious diseases as an internal medicine physician with an advanced level of knowledge in infectious diseases in later chapters of this book.

Cellulitis, Strep throat, pneumonia, urinary tract infections, influenza, and wound infections are the common causes of outpatient office visits, but also major reasons for hospitalization. Persistent fevers and respiratory failure, especially in patients with multiple comorbidities and immunocompromised conditions almost universally require hospitalization. The treatment of infection usually begins with culture and identifying and controlling the source of infection and eventually fosters the development of a tailored antibiotic regimen. It is a complicated process that requires consideration of comorbidities, past surgical and medical history, environmental exposures, animal contacts, travel history, and social history. The occupation of infectious disease is one of the most respected specialties; infectious disease

K. Zhou, *Internal Medicine Training Notes and Survival Guide*,
https://doi.org/10.1007/978-1-0716-4039-5_6

physicians are among the smartest physicians. They do not only help the treatments for infections but also diagnose complicated systemic presentations such as vasculitis and rare neurological diseases.

As a resident or attending physician, we have to always rule out or diagnose infections with high mortality and morbidity risks at the earliest possible time. These infections include but are not limited to endocarditis, meningoencephalitis, necrotizing fasciitis, and necrotizing cellulitis (discussed in previous and later chapters). This chapter provided some preliminary knowledge about these infections, but it is far too short to help us become a competent physician for infectious diseases, even though I did spend another month at a large teaching hospital for infectious disease training and compiled additional notes in later chapters. Prompt recognition, diagnosis, and treatment of infections with high mortality and morbidity risks require clinical vigilance, and this book will provide you some foundation for such vigilance while you grow your clinical experiences.

2/12/2018

1. **Post-op fever etiologies:** pneumonia and atelectasis at the first 24–48 h; urinary tract infection (UTI) at day 2 and after; wound infection at day 5; drug fever (anesthetic drugs or blood transfusion) at any time; deep vein thrombosis (DVT)/pulmonary embolism (PE) at postoperative day 5 (POD 5).
2. **Strep pyogenes (Group A strep) and C. perfringens** cause rapid deterioration after surgery.
3. **Mouth Kote** solution for dry mouth.

2/13/2018

1. **Complicated urinary tract infection (UTI)** = acute UTI with any of the following: fever, signs and symptoms of systemic illness including chills and rigors, flank pain, CVA tenderness, pelvic or perineal pain in men (accompanying prostatitis). Male UTI is automatically a complicated UTI.
2. **Acute pyelonephritis** can be the progression of upper UTI to renal corticomedullary abscess, perinephric abscess, emphysematous pyelonephritis, or papillary necrosis.
3. For urinary tract infection (UTI), imaging is necessary for **persistent symptoms despite 48–72 h treatments, obstruction, and recurrent symptoms within a few weeks**.
4. **CT without contrast** is the standard radiographic study for demonstrating calculi, gas-forming infections, hemorrhage, obstruction, and abscess.
5. CT without contrast is used **for kidney stone, retroperitoneal bleeds**. **Resistance to aztreonam and ceftriaxone = ESBL**, usually treated with carbapenem (diminished susceptibility for cefepime, tazobactam, Augmentin) and rarely quinolones.
6. No nitrofurantoin for pyelonephritis, as it only accumulates in the bladder.
7. Recurrent UTI, differential diagnoses: **anatomical, neurological, or medication use causing urinary retention.**

8. **Asymptomatic bacteriuria** does not need treatment except during pregnancy or going through urological procedures.
9. Joint infection (**septic joints**), treat for 4 weeks.
10. Flank pain and/or costovertebral angle tenderness in the setting of pyuria and bacteriuria = consider **pyelonephritis**. Diagnosis of pyelonephritis does not necessarily need a CT scan. CT findings of pyelonephritis may include **low attenuation extending to the renal capsule** on contrast enhancement with or without swelling.
11. **Pyelonephritis** outpatient treatment: Fluoroquinolones × 7 days or TMP-SMX × 14 days. Inpatient: Ceftriaxone, amp/sulbactam or aminoglycoside for 7 days is sufficient if the patient responds.
12. For **bacterial endocarditis**, oral ampicillin has poor absorption, Do Not Use.
13. **Enterococcus faecalis** has penicillin-binding proteins (PBPs); it is resistant to cephalosporins, indolent, and responds poorly to many antibiotics. Ampicillin causes bacterial cell wall leaks. **Ampicillin iv plus gentamicin or ceftriaxone** (high concentration) is the treatment for enterococcus faecalis endocarditis.
14. Ampicillin reduces net positive bacterial surface charge of vancomycin-resistant enterococcus (VRE). **Ampicillin IV is used together with daptomycin** to kill VRE.
15. **Ampicillin iv 2 g q4h + daptomycin 10 mg/kg** IV qd for VRE or enterococcus faecalis nonresponsive to antibiotics.
16. Enterococcus faecalis vs. faecium: **E. faecalis** is more virulent but **susceptible to ampicillin** whereas **E. faecium** is less virulent but non-susceptible to ampicillin. Enterococcus faecalis treated with daptomycin for 3 days, blood culture remains positive, antibiotics should be changed to **ampicillin + daptomycin**.
17. **Daptomycin** is the only antibiotic with in vitro bactericidal activity against VRE that is approved by the FDA.
18. **Enterococcus faecalis can usually be treated with penicillins (like ampicillin) or linezolid**, however, occasionally, it can be bacteriostatic with ampicillin/penicillins. Enterococcus usually has no response to gentamicin alone.
19. **Large numbers of Enterococcal organisms**, i.e., due to vegetation, can confer resistance to **penicillins**.
20. All E. faecium are resistant to synergism with tobramycin. The majority of E faecium and E faecalis do not respond to synergism with amikacin.
21. Combinations of ampicillin or **penicillin with gentamicin or streptomycin** are preferable to vancomycin-aminoglycoside combinations for E. faecalis endocarditis because of concerns of nephrotoxicity.
22. High-level penicillin resistance in Enterococcus infection: use vancomycin or daptomycin + aminoglycoside. **If concerns for nephrotoxicity, use 10–12 mg/kg IV daptomycin.**
23. **Enterococcal bacteremia**: If only one single positive blood culture positive but no sepsis signs or symptoms or in a polymicrobial infection on appropriate therapy for a more virulent organism, it may be contaminant if repeat blood culture negative. If febrile, then should be treated for 5–7 days (if symptoms have resolved and no valvular abnormality is found).

24. **Common bugs in endocarditis**: native valve endocarditis (NVE): S. viridans 36% > **S. aureus** 28% > enterococcus 11% > S. epidermidis > gram-negative rods (GNR). Early prosthetic valve endocarditis (PVE): **S. aureus** > **S. epidermidis** > enterococcus > other GNR. Late PVE: **S. viridans = S aureus**/epidermidis (10%–20% by coagulase negative staphylococci) > enterococcus.
25. **HACEK endocarditis** is caused by a group of slow-growing (culture requires ≥5 days) fastidious bacteria including G negative bacteria of **Haemophilus** aphrophilus (new name: Aggregatibacter aphrophilus), **Actinobacillus** actinomycetemcomitans, **Cardiobacterium** hominis, **Eikenella** corrodens, **Kingella** kingae. HACEK bacteria are normal flora of the mouth and upper respiratory tract in humans, can cause endocarditis (accounts for 1%–3% of infectious endocarditis) in patients with heart disease or artificial valves, which can take 1 –3 months for diagnoses after symptom onset. Treatment for HACEK endocarditis is **ceftriaxone 2 g daily**.
26. A 65-year-old female with **mechanical mitral valve** (no fever, but mute with altered mentation upon presentation) was transferred to the hospital for **intracranial hemorrhage** from warfarin use and later was found to also have ischemic stroke at the same time. Blood culture later revealed **Cardiobacterium** and the patient was started on **ceftriaxone** but still developed **mycotic aneurysms** requiring urgent stat **neurosurgical clipping**.
27. **Blood culture-negative infective endocarditis categories:** (1) blood culture negative due to previous antibiotic use; (2) fastidious microorganism-induced endocarditis (HACEK plus nutritionally variant Streptococci, Pasteurella spp., mycobacteria, and fungal organisms); (3) infection with intra-cellular organisms possibly requiring diagnosis with serology [Coxiella burnetii (Q fever), Bartonella spp., Brucella spp., Tropheryma whipplei, Mycobacteria species and non-candidal fungi].
28. **Diagnosis of infective endocarditis** is established if (1) 2 Major Criteria or (2) 1 Major Criterion and 3 Minor Criteria or (3) 5 Minor Criteria are met. **Generalized symptoms** in infective endocarditis include fever, chills, weight loss, cough, weakness, and/or malaise.
29. **Duke 2023 criteria for endocarditis**: (1) Major criteria: **positive blood culture**, positive lab test (PCR or other nucleic acid-based technique for Coxiella burnetti, Bartonella, or Tropheryma whipplei from blood), indirect immunofluorescence assays of IgM and IgG ab against Bartonella henselae or Bartonella Quintana with IgG ≥ 1:800)**; imaging criteria**- Echo, cardiac CT, PET showing vegetation, new or worsening regurgitation or new partial dehiscence of prosthetic valve; surgical major criteria via **direct inspection during heart surgery**. (2) minor criteria: predisposition (history of infectious endocarditis, prothetic valve or valvular repair or more than mild stenosis or regurgitation, hypertrophic obstructive cardiomyopathy, injection drug abuse, endovascular intracardiac device); fever; vascular phenomena (positive rheumatoid factor, Osler nodes, Roth spots, immune complex-mediated glomerulonephritis).
30. **Indications for cardiothoracic surgery in patients with left-sided native valve infective endocarditis**: infection-related valvular dysfunction and wors-

ening heart failure, paravalvular extension of infection, difficult infection like MRSA and fungal endocarditis, persistent infection, large vegetation (>10 mm), septic embolization and microhemorrhage in the brain (need timely surgery).

2/14/2018

1. **Soft tissue infections**: animal exposure, usually strep (Group A streptococcus like Streptococcus pyogenes)/Staph, treat with **vancomycin** (**cefazolin** is preferred if no concerns for MRSA), **reimage if no response**. In diabetes and immunocompromised, may include GNR and thus additional coverage may be needed.
2. **Phlegmon** = acute inflammation of the soft tissues yet to become pus. **Group B strep (GBS)** also known as Streptococcus agalactiae (S. agalactiae) are almost all sensitive to penicillins, but highly resistant to clindamycin (but clindamycin may be used as an adjunct treatment for toxin suppression); **Staphylococcus** are almost all resistant to penicillins.
3. Ask for skin conditions during routine history taking, and explore possible causes of soft tissue infections.
4. **Perinephric stranding, fat stranding**, refers to edema within the fat of the perirenal space on CT/MRI.
5. **Flu isolation** should start from **symptom onset to day 7 or until 24 h after the resolution of symptoms**, whichever is longer,
6. **Endocarditis**: watch for a drop in cardiac function, look for echo test.
7. **Erysipelas** is a well-defined erythema with a raised edge reflecting more superficial involvement. It indicates **Group A Strep infection**.
8. **Levaquin** can cause nausea and high risk for C. diff infection and tendon rupture in the elderly. **Vancomycin** needs to monitor kidney function.
9. **Uncomplicated** (exudative characteristics, but normal pH and glucose and no bacterium in pleural fluid) versus **complicated** (bacterial invasion of the pleural space, increased LDH, and low pH) parapneumonic effusions versus **empyema** (a subcategory of complicated parapneumonic effusion with frank pus).
10. **Thoracic empyema** develops when there is an evident bacterial infection of the pleural fluid, resulting in either **pus or the presence of bacterial organisms on the G stain**. A positive culture is not required for diagnosis (anaerobics, antibiotics use, inoculations).
11. Treatment for osteomyelitis or joint infection requires antibiotics, usually IV, for **4 weeks**.
12. In general, a **pH < 7.2 or a glucose < 60 mg/dL** = complicated parapneumonic effusion. Low glucose in thoracentesis = consider empyema, malignancy, TB, rheumatoid pleurisy, and lupus pleuritic.
13. **Soft tissue infection** = cellulitis, if **non-purulent** = consider probability of infection from beta hemolytic **Strep** > S. aureus. If **purulent** = consider probability of infection from **S. aureus** > Strep.
14. Saltwater or raw oyster fish causes bullous skin lesions due to infection of **Vibrio vulnificus**: **hemorrhagic bullae and sepsis**, especially in patients with cirrhosis; treatment with either minocycline or doxycycline (100 mg orally

twice daily), plus either cefotaxime (2 g intravenously every 8 h) or ceftriaxone (1 g intravenously daily).

15. **Ceftriaxone** dosing for bacterial meningitis is **2 g q12h for 7–21 days**.

2/15/2018

1. **History taking for refractory pneumonia**: smoking history, contact with animals, vaccination, and previous hospitalization for pneumonia or respiratory disease, difficulty swallowing. **Differential diagnoses**: viral versus fungal pneumonia, bronchiectasis, MRSA, aspiration pneumonia, malignancy, interstitial lung diseases, empyema. **Lab orders**: RSV PCR, nasal swab for MRSA, check immunoglobulins, chest CT scan. **Treatment** with linezolid and Zosyn to cover G+, G−, and anaerobes. If procalcitonin is minimally elevated or normal, need order extensive workup for **fungal pneumonia** and to rule out interstitial lung disease. Consider **pulmonologist consultation for bronchoscopy**.
2. If **sputum or nares culture is negative for MRSA**, may stop linezolid/vancomycin, especially true for pneumonia.
3. **No nasal MRSA, unlikely MRSA in the lung**. Bactrim is not good for Streptococcus but good for proteus/MRSA.
4. **Empyema treatment**: repeat blood culture, continue Zosyn, consult CT surgery for VATS/chest tube, pleural fluid.
5. **Empyema**: pus accumulates in the pleural space. The pus is seen after thoracentesis or any drainage procedure of the pleural space and is generally characterized as thick, viscous, and opaque. A positive culture is not needed for diagnosis.
6. Common **bacteria/virus** in pneumonia: **RSV, pneumococcus, Hemophilus, oral flora.**
7. **Atypical pneumonia** is usually less common in adults: **Legionella** accounts for **1%–5%** of community-acquired pneumonia but up to **30%** of hospital-acquired pneumonia, esp. in patients with **emphysema and COPD**.
8. Consider **inhaled ribavirin for RSV** infection in immunosuppressed patients. **Prophylaxis for high-risk contacts of confirmed flu: oseltamivir 75 mg po bid for 5–10 days**.
9. **ESR > 70** greatly increases the likelihood of osteomyelitis.

2/17/2018

1. **Gram + bacilli**: bacillus, **Clostridium, Corynebacterium, Listeria, Nocardia**, Actinomyces, Erysipelothrix.
2. **G- bacilli**: Campylobacter bacilli, E coli, H. pylori, Klebsiella, Pseudomonas, Enterobacter.
3. **G- rods**: Klebsiella, E. coli, Pseudomonas, and Acinetobacter baumannii.
4. Renal adjustment of Xarelto: PE/DVT if CrCl >30 no adjustment needed; **if CrCl < 30, avoid use**. AFib if CrCl <50, prescribe 15 mg qd; if CrCl <30, do not use.
5. Vancomycin causes kidney issues; **in AKI/CKD, use linezolid or daptomycin**.
6. **Atypical pathogens (legionella, mycoplasma, chlamydia, virus)**: nothing grows on routine culture. Presentations vary from insidious onset to acute;

imaging features vary from interstitial infiltrates to tree-in-bud opacities to dense consolidation.

7. **Reasons for failure to improve in infection**: insufficient time for antibiotics to work, which may take up to 72 h; insufficient drug levels for lung penetration. Resistant bug → may need bronchoscopy; wrong diagnosis → may order CT; parapneumonic process → may need chest tube or VATS; metastatic infections.
8. **Chest tube placement** is necessary for empyema treatment.
9. **Vancomycin-resistant enterococcus (VRE) positive urine culture** but asymptomatic, negative UA, no need for isolation or treatment.
10. Diarrhea can be due to GI bleed. Mild abdominal pain, concerns for **acute cholecystitis → HIDA scan.**
11. **Native valve endocarditis**: S. viridans > S. aureus > Enterococcus > S. epidermidis.
12. HAP or HCAP: **Tamiflu** for 5 days with droplet precautions if flu +; **Vanco** for MRSA; **meropenem** for aspiration and pseudomonas.

2/18/2018

1. **Meropenem** antibacterial spectrum: G+, G−, Pseudomonas, anaerobic (Peptostreptococcus) spp., Bacteroides, Fusobacterium.
2. **Tough C. diff infection**: vancomycin 250 mg po q6h + metronidazole 500 iv q8h → septic encephalopathy, do vanco 250 mg po q6h. Not tolerating po → discontinue metronidazole and vancomycin, start fidaxomicin 200 mg po q12h, no response, re-add metronidazole 500 mg iv q12h.
3. **Stool lactoferrin** is a marker for fecal leukocytes and an **indicator of intestinal inflammation.**
4. **Pneumonia with possible cholangitis** treatment: Levaquin and Flagyl. Aztreonam does not have anaerobic or gram-positive coverage.

2/20/2018

1. Deep respiratory culture to rule out MRSA; PO_2 is usually 5× FiO_2. Differential diagnoses (DDx) of **ARDS include congestive heart failure (CHF) and bilateral pneumonia**.
2. Symptoms unresponsive to Zosyn? → Culture of sputum for the common viruses (rarely performed) and to rule out other non-bacterial causes of pneumonia.
3. Outpatient setting, flu symptoms, clean chest X-ray (CXR), normal WBC, just typical flu symptoms, but flu PCR -, may just treat with Tamiflu for 5 days in flu season.
4. **Procalcitonin serial level** for bacterial infection may be useful but not required for deciding the duration of antibiotics.

2/21/2018

1. **Clavulanic acid** can cause kidney damage.
2. **Klebsiella** is resistant to ampicillin and amoxicillin. **Tigecycline** causes liver failure.
3. **Primary influenza pneumonia** manifests as persistent symptoms of cough, sore throat, headache, myalgia, and malaise for >3–5 days.

4. **RSV pneumonia** is the most common in infants and children and the second most common viral cause of pneumonia in adults—may benefit from treatment with **Ribavirin if immunocompromised**.
5. Fluconazole and amiodarone interaction lead to **QTc prolongation**.

2/22/2018

1. **Fungal infections**: mucocutaneous (oral, esophageal, vulvovaginal, balanitis), skin and soft tissue infections (blastomycosis, **aspergillus, mucormycosis, and Rhizopus**), candiduria, candidemia.
2. **Cryptococcus diagnosis**: CSF Cryptococcus Ag, Indian ink stain, fungal culture, cell counts vary, serum Cryptococcus Ag > 1:8. **Treatment** for cryptococcal meningitis: induction therapy with **amphotericin B and flucytosine for 8 weeks**; consolidation and maintenance therapy with **fluconazole for a year**.
3. Central nervous system (CNS) infection symptoms: meningitis, **altered mentation, headache**, fever, meningismus, increased intracranial pressure (common for all CNS infections, not only Cryptococcus).
4. **Histoplasmosis**: severe to mild pneumonia (PNA) and/or cavitary and hilar lymphadenopathy (LAN) for chronic pulmonary infections, disseminated treatment: **itraconazole; or amphotericin** if severe; steroid may be used.
5. Some G- bacilli produce broad-spectrum beta-lactamase that can hydrolyze penicillins and cephalosporins. The common classes are **ESBLs and amp C (beta-lactamase)** produced by **SPICE** (Serratia, Providencia, "Indole-positive" Proteus species, Citrobacter, and Enterobacter species).
6. Empiric choices for ESBL and SPICE: No penicillin or cephalosporins; may use **nitrofurantoin for cystitis only**; TMP-SMX, carbapenem, aminoglycosides and fluoroquinolones (FQ) for severe or life-threatening illness; meropenem 1 g iv q8h for CNS infections **or ertapenem 1 g IV q24h if not treating pseudomonas, Acinetobacter or CNS infections**. Oral options of TMP-SMX or FQ may be ok for stable improving patients.
7. **Augmentin** does not cover pseudomonas or other SPICE organisms. Caution the use of ampicillin-sulbactam (**Unasyn**) for polymicrobial intra-abdominal infections due to the high rate of resistance of E coli.
8. Piperacillin/tazobactam (Zosyn) has similar coverage in G+, G-, and anaerobic coverage, but is better than Unasyn in overall G- coverage including **pseudomonas and most SPICE**. Zosyn does not cover MRSA, VRE, atypicals, ESBLs. The typical dosage for Zosyn in patients with good kidney function is **4.5q q6h for pseudomonas**.

2/24/2018

1. **Mycoplasma** does not increase blood WBC and patients with mycoplasma infection typically will get better by themselves, thus if urine Legionella Ag-, can stop azithromycin. Regardless, the duration of **azithromycin** treatment is usually 3 days for 500 mg daily and 5 days if 500 mg the first day and 250 mg for the rest 4 days.

2. Pneumonia does not transmit between people; **RSV/flu does and thus requires droplet isolation**.
3. **Ampicillin for listeria**, and ceftriaxone may cause abnormal liver function tests. Ceftriaxone for pneumonia (PNA), the duration of treatment is 5 days.
4. **Downgrading antibiotics in pneumonia**: vancomycin + meropenem → discontinue vancomycin (if MRSA nares negative), continue meropenem for 7 days (the typical duration of antibiotics for hospital-acquired pneumonia).
5. Many yeasts on top of other bacteria: Vanco/Zosyn, add **micafungin**, inappropriate to use fluconazole if concerns of QTc prolongation or bacteremia (due to high resistance rate).
6. **Flu A + pneumonia (PNA) with bilateral infiltrate**: Vanco/cefepime and Tamiflu (5-day course) → ceftriaxone → Vantin.
7. **Cellulitis** with **lymphangitis** treatment: cefazolin 2 g q8h.
8. **Klebsiella, lung abscess**: Zosyn → discontinue Zosyn once we know Klebsiella ESBL → continue ertapenem for **35 days**.
9. **Flu A+ PNA extensive infiltrates + ARDS** on ventilation: Vanco/Zosyn/Tamiflu → stop vancomycin if respiratory culture negative → Zosyn for 5 days then stop; **Tamiflu for 10–14 days.**
10. **Anaerobes** can be the main cause of infection in the pleural space and lungs, intra-abdominal, gynecological, CNS, upper respiratory tract, and cutaneous disease. **Bacteremia** can be associated with anaerobic cellulitis, aspiration pneumonia, Bartholin gland infection, and brain abscess.
11. **Anaerobic infection** in oropharyngeal and lung abscesses treatment: clindamycin or a beta-lactamase inhibitor like Augmentin. In patients allergic to penicillin, clindamycin or metronidazole plus a drug against aerobes and microaerophiles is useful.
12. **Anaerobic gastrointestinal (GI)/pelvic infections**: metronidazole, carbapenems (imipenem/cisplatin, meropenem, ertapenem), beta-lactamase inhibitors (Zosyn, Unasyn, Augmentin), tigecycline, or moxifloxacin.

2/25/2018

1. **Screen for DVT** in swelling limbs.
2. **CSF analysis normal values**: appearance-clear; opening pressure-10–20 cmH_2O; WBC-0–5 cells/μL (<2PMN); normal cell counts do not rule out infection; glucose level **>60%** of serum glucose; protein level **<45** mg/dL.
3. **Bacterial meningitis**: appearance-clear, cloudy or purulent; opening pressure > 25 cmH_2O; WBC > 5–100 cells/μL; If partially treated, CSF can have as low as 1 WBC/μL, glucose <40% of serum glucose, protein elevated >50 mg/dL in CSF studies.
4. **Common bacteria in meningitis**: S pneumonia, G− rods, and listeria. **Antibiotics for bacterial meningitis**: vancomycin, ceftriaxone, ampicillin, acyclovir. Give dexamethasone 10 mg iv once before antibiotics if concerns for Strep pneumonia meningitis to lower residual neurological sequela.
5. **Viral meningitis**: appearance-clear, normal opening pressure or elevated; WBC 10–1000 (lymph but PMN early), glucose normal or >60% (may be low in HSV), protein >50 mg/dL in CSF studies.

6. In viral meningitis, common pathogens include enteroviruses (esp., coxsackie virus), HSV2 (HSS-1 encephalitis), HIV, west Nile virus, and VZV. In HIV, **Cryptococcus, CMV, toxoplasmosis, and JC virus-PML** are all possible pathogens. **Only herpes encephalitis or meningitis** has medication treatment (acyclovir) in viral CNS infection.
7. **Predicted WBC count after traumatic tap**: a good rule of thumb is subtracting 1 WBC for every 500–1500 RBCs measured in cerebrospinal fluid (CSF).
8. **Guillain-Barré syndrome (GBS)**: albuminocytologic dissociation- increased protein but normal CSF cell count, is a hallmark in acute and chronic inflammatory demyelinating polymyopathies. **Protein levels may be normal in the first week of symptoms.**
9. **Herpes encephalitis**: spikes in EEG, focal periodic spikes over the **temporal lobe**, hallucinations.
10. **Vasodilators**: nitroprusside, nitroglycerin; **inotropic drugs**: dobutamine and milrinone.
11. **Acute conjunctivitis**: **infections**-bacterial/viral, often adenovirus; **noninfectiou**s-allergic/nonallergic; **bacterial conjunctivitis** is caused by S. aureus (most common), S. pneumonia, H. influenzae and Moraxella catarrhalis.
12. **Hyperacute bacterial conjunctivitis**: due to Neisseria species-striking discharge, treatment with Ceftriaxone 250 mg im once + Azithromycin 1 g oral once; **epidemic keratoconjunctivitis**, treatment with steroids. Both should be referred to see an **ophthalmologist** as they are vision-threatening.
13. Soft contact lens wearers have a high risk of **pseudomonal keratitis** → ulcerative keratitis, corneal opacity with a pen light.

2/26/2018

1. **Continuous fever** after 10 days Tamiflu, 5-day Vanco/Zosyn, ordered meropenem for pseudomonas coverage for another 7–8 days.
2. For patients with **AICD/pacemaker**, we need to interrogate the pacemaker especially if concerns for syncope, dizziness, or arrhythmias.
3. Gastrointestinal (GI) bleed: EGD/colonoscopy → CT angiogram GI bleeding protocol if quick drop in hemoglobin to detect rates of bleeding as low as 0.5 mL/min: **mesenteric angiogram with coil embolization if diverticular origin non-stop**. If there is a slow drop in hemoglobin, can order an **RBC tag study** for low rates of bleeding (0.1–0.5 mL/min).
4. We should **avoid iron supplementation** in patients at high risk for infection, such as neutropenia or posttransplant patients, and during active or resistant infection because iron may promote microbial growth and disrupt the body's neutrophil and immune response.
5. **Leukocytosis in multiorgan failure plus UA positive for fungi**: ordered Zosyn for 5 days and micafungin 100 mg iv for 7 days.
6. Abdominal abscess with **Klebsiella bacteremia**. **Treatment**: Zosyn + linezolid for 1 month

7. Cellulitis with wound culture for **MRSA and Pasteurella**: treatment with IV Vanco for 2–3 days, do **amoxicillin** 500 mg po q8h for 7 days for Pasteurella.
8. Altered mental status (AMS) with fever, WBC 33 concerning for encephalitis/meningoencephalitis. **Treatment**: Vanco/ceftriaxone/ampicillin/acyclovir. Later, blood culture positive for GBS on 2/21, S. agalactiae confirmed on 2/22 → Discontinue acyclovir and ampicillin, **keep Vanco/ceftriaxone, add clindamycin for toxin suppression**, suspected epidural abscess, septic encephalopathy. On 2/23 blood culture positive for G+ cocci → lumbar puncture and echo → meningitis diagnosed. Treatment: **dexamethasone** (may not be necessary as steroid only was only proven beneficial for Pneumococcal meningitis) **7 mg iv q6h + penicillin G 4 million units q4h for 13 days**, stop other antibiotics.

2/27/2018

1. **Flagyl should not be used for >4 weeks** as it can cause significant neuropathy if >4 weeks' use. Bactrim increases serum K in patients.
2. **Fluconazole** is better than micafungin in UTI/kidney fungal infection.
3. Osteomyelitis should be treated for 6 weeks. **Precedex causes fevers, hypertension/hypotension.**
4. Concerns for meningitis/encephalitis: CSF studies should include **HSV1, HSV2, PCR, VZV PCR, and Cryptococcus** Ag.
5. **Penicillin causes seizures**. If seizures, change penicillin to ceftriaxone.
6. **Hemoptysis differential diagnoses**: bronchitis, bronchiectasis, lung cancer, use of blood thinners, pneumonia, pulmonary embolism, pulmonary edema from congestive heart failure, tuberculosis, autoimmune (like **vasculitis**).
7. **Aspiration:** start antibiotics 2 days after the event if fever persists as aspiration usually only causes aspiration pneumonitis. **Fulguration**- the destruction of small growths or areas of tissue using diathermy.
8. **Xanthochromia in CSF = 2–4 h after bleeding**, subdural hematoma, or increased CSF concentration of protein (>150 mg/dL) or systemic hyperbilirubinemia (serum bilirubin >10–15 mg/dL).
9. **H. influenza** can cause meningitis, cellulitis (buccal and periorbital regions), epiglottitis, pneumonia (insidious onset), pericarditis, arthritis, and fever, cough, and purulent sputum production.
10. The usual pattern of bacterial infection post influenza is that the **patient improves and 2 weeks later develops bacterial superinfection**. The usual pathogens are **Staph and Strep** leading to pos-viral pneumonia.

2/28/2018

1. Concerns of osteomyelitis, also has urinary tract infection, if vitals stable, hold antibiotics, **order MRI then biopsy of the bone, then antibiotics**. Check ESR and CRP periodically.
2. Absorption of **oral Flagyl** is almost entirely in the small bowel of healthy individuals; however, in patients with acute C. diff infection, significant Flagyl concentrations exist in the stool due to decreased absorption associated with

diarrhea and due to excretion into the colon in the setting of inflammation. As diarrhea decreases, stool concentration of C. diff decreases.

3. **Vancomycin** is not absorbed and achieves very high concentration in the gastrointestinal tract during therapy.
4. ESBL UTI isolation, **stop 48 h after last incontinence**. Once diarrhea has resolved/settled (formed stool) in C. diff for **a minimum of 48 h**, the patient is no longer considered infectious. However, stool carriage can persist for over 3–6 weeks post-cessation of symptoms while no treatment is needed.
5. **Severe C. diff colitis** treatment: vancomycin 250 mg po q6h + Flagyl 500 mg iv q8h. If worsening (ileus, increased WBC, increased lactate, shock, toxic megacolon, peritonitis), order abdominal CT and urgent surgical consult. **Treatment**: fidaxomicin, or fecal transplant vs subtotal colectomy (? Possible role for diverting loop ileostomy or colonic lavage, may also consider Vanco per rectum)
6. **Loop ileostomy is better than loop colostomy** because of better blood supply in the former.
7. **Ileo-anal pouches** are constructed for people who have had the large intestine removed for ulcerative colitis and Crohn's disease in selected cases, familial adenomatous polyps, colon cancer, and toxic megacolon.
8. **End ileostomy**: when the large intestine is removed and the end of the ileum is brought out as a stoma. This can be a temporary or permanent procedure.
9. **Loop ileostomy**: when the large intestine is removed and the two ends are joined together via anastomosis. The ileostomy is formed to allow the joint in the bowel to heal for a few months and is only a temporary measure.
10. Total proctocolectomy with an **end ileostomy, ileorectal anastomosis, continent ileostomy** (K pouch)**, J pouch**.
11. **Penicillin decreases seizure** threshold; Levaquin **750 mg** daily is used for legionella, pneumonia, and bacteremia; Levaquin **500 mg** daily is for UTI.
12. Tazobactam does not cover anaerobes. **If use metronidazole, we need to decrease Coumadin by 30%–35%.**
13. **Cytochrome 450** CYP2C9 **inhibitors**: amiodarone, fluconazole, fluoxetine, Flagyl, ritonavir, Bactrim.
14. Meningitis, encephalitis, broad coverage: vancomycin, ceftriaxone, ampicillin, acyclovir (micafungin). Consider the **addition of dexamethasone** if concerns of Strep pneumoniae meningitis are high or cannot be ruled out.

3/1/2018

1. **Cefepime has no MRSA or anaerobic coverage**. Treatment of infections, tough ones, adjust one antibiotic at a time.
2. For MRSA pneumonia, **change Vanco to linezolid** for its better penetration/absorption in the lungs and no renal toxicity.
3. **Vancomycin trough (the lowest level) 15–20: do not draw specimen until steady state is achieved i.e., fourth dose**. Draw trough specimen immediately before (<30 min) next dose; draw peak specimen 1–2 h after completion of IV dose. Steady-state usually after 4 half-lives.

4. **MRSA pneumonia** treatment duration is **10 days**; linezolid is better than vancomycin for pneumonia.
5. **Hemoptysis with CHF and lung infiltrates** treatment: meropenem 2 g q8h iv, Lasix 40 mg iv bid.
6. Patient nonresponsive, if remains unresponsive for the next 24 h off sedation, **consider repeat LP and CSF analysis** if concerns for infection. Send fluid for additional CSF studies, CSF PCR for HSV1, HSV2, HSV6, VZV, and West Nile (unlikely in winter).

3/2/2018

1. Antibiotic treatment for patients with **symptomatic pharyngitis or tonsillopharyngitis** who have a positive rapid Ag test or positive culture for Group A streptococcus. For adults: **penicillin V 500 mg 2–3 × /day for 10 days**. For children, we use either **penicillin V or amoxicillin for 10 days**. Intramuscular penicillin is better than oral penicillin. Alternatives include cephalosporins, clindamycin, and macrolides.
2. **Cordis catheter** is a double or single-lumen introducer that allows for large and rapid infusion or swan Ganz (pulmonary artery catheter or right heart catheter) catheterization.
3. **Shiley catheter** is a non-tunneled catheter that can be used for dialysis up to less than 3 weeks. **Perm-Cath, Hickman, and Groshong** catheters are long-term tunneled dialysis catheters.
4. Mitral valve replacement → CHF with pericardial effusion → pericardial window → multiorgan failure, septic shock, develops shingles. The patient also has LLL pneumonia with a negative culture. Cannot rule out fungemia together with known adrenal insufficiency, DM, AKI on CKD; **Treatment**: micafungin, Valtrex 500 mg qd, linezolid, and Zosyn. Remove Cordis, repeat cx positive for E. coli, plus C. diff positive treatment: Vanco oral 250 mg q6h + iv Flagyl 500 mg iv q8h.
5. **UTI with enterococcus**, VRE high risk and critically ill patients, order iv synergy treatment with **ampicillin and ceftriaxone**.
6. Pacemaker change → SOB and nonproductive cough → DVT/PE, leukocytosis. Treatment: **Vanco/meropenem** (of note, carbapenems are reserved for ESBLs).
7. **Conjunctivitis** → eye drops for 5 days. Male UTI with E coli treatment: ceftriaxone inpatient and was changed to Vantin oral for 7 days antibiotic in total.
8. **E. coli bacteremia**: stop meropenem, add aztreonam, then do Levaquin for a total of 7–14 days.
9. **Fever with altered mental status**: concerns for CNS encephalitis, like herpes encephalitis on top of left lower lobe pneumonia, possible aspiration. Treatment: discontinue Vantin, **start Unasysn 500 mg q8h, acyclovir 500 mg iv q8h**. Lumbar puncture needed, done no WBC, glucose normal, discontinue acyclovir.
10. **Oral candida** in the setting of lymphocytes of 520,000, oral dysphagia. **Treatment**: fluconazole 100 mg po qd for 10 days.
11. **Encephalitis, brain abscess with Propionibacterium (contamination), MSSA bacteremia**. Treatment: Vanco 1 g iv q12h, meropenem 2 g iv q8h, acy-

clovir 10 mg/kg iv q8h, send fluid for viral cx HSV1, HSV2, VZV. Propionibacterium is a contaminant, thus only keep Vanco if viral studies are negative.

12. After neurosurgery, **prescribe dexamethasone 4 mg iv q6h** to prevent edema. Keppra 1000 mg bid for seizure prophylaxis.
13. **Decadron 4 mg q6h** iv for brain mass/edema.

3/3/2018

1. **Genital herpes**: Herpes simplex virus (HSV)-2, sometimes HSV-1, associated symptoms in the primary episode of HSV included **fever, malaise, and headache** on top of the painful genital lesion and dysuria, lasting 2–4 weeks if not treated. If no suppressive therapy, the median recurrence rate for HSV-2 is **4 times per year with 40% having at least six** recurrences and 20% having ten recurrences per year. HSV-1 usually recurs once a year. Antiviral therapy does not eradicate latent HSV infection. Treatment: **initiation of oral antiviral therapy within 72 h of lesion appearance can decrease duration and severity and avoid complications**.
2. Treatment of **primary genital HSV**: acyclovir 400 mg tid or 200 mg 5×/day for 7–10 days, famciclovir 250 mg tid, or valacyclovir 1000 mg bid for 7–10 days. **Treatment for episodic (<4×/year) herpes infection**: acyclovir 800 mg tid for 2 days or 800 mg bid or 400 mg tid for 5 days, or famciclovir 1000 mg bid for 1 day, 125 mg bid for 5 days, valacyclovir 500 mg bid for 3 days, 1000 mg qd for 5 days, or 2 g once. **Treatment for suppressive therapy (>4×/year) herpes infection**: acyclovir 400 mg bid, famciclovir 250 mg bid, valacyclovir 500–1000 mg qd.
3. **Complicated HSV infections** include aseptic meningitis, encephalitis, transverse myelitis, end-organ disease including hepatitis, pneumonitis, and disseminated HSV. For complicated HSV infection, do IV **acyclovir** 5–10 mg/kg q8h for 2–7 days until improvement then oral for **a total of 10 days**.
4. For patients with genital HSV-2 infection and an uninfected partner, the patients should take **chronic suppressive therapy, valacyclovir 500 mg qd** with acyclovir as alternative.
5. **E. coli urinary tract infection (UTI)** with altered mentation can be treated with ceftriaxone for 7 days.
6. In the absence of suspected endocarditis or critical illness, **enterococcal bacteremia can be treated with monotherapy**.

3/4/2018

1. **Darifenacin (Enablex)** 7.5 mg po qd is used for overactive bladder (OAB).
2. **Angioedema** (intubation if necessary): (A) **associated urticarial symptoms treatment**- antihistamine (iv Benadryl, famotidine iv), glucocorticoids, epinephrine im if angioedema affecting airway. (B) **no associated urticarial symptoms treatment** -icatibant, ecallantide first line; FFP and solvent detergent plasma are second line treatment.

3. **Plasma cell dyscrasia** is characterized by clonal protein accumulation. Symptoms are due to clonal expansion, but also due to abnormal protein effects (amyloid deposition, renal failure). Order serum protein electrophoresis (**SPEP**), urine protein electrophoresis (**UPEP**), and serum immunofixation (**IFE**). M protein <3 g/dL and no end organ damage = consider MGUS. **Plasma cell dyscrasia** usually has an elevated gamma gap (>4 g/dL) which is defined as the difference between serum total protein and albumin.
4. **Discontinuation of isolation** when MRSA off antibiotics for 72 h, VER off antibiotics for 72 h, C. diff resolution of symptoms for 48 h, flu after 5-day treatment of Tamiflu (correction: **Flu isolation** should start from **symptom onset to day 7 or until 24 h after the resolution of symptoms**, whichever is longer). Check with infection prevention at the local hospital as policies may vary.
5. **Streptococcal bacteremia** treatment: penicillin 3 million units IV q4h for 10–14 days.
6. **Persistent MRSA pneumonia** treatment: continue linezolid for 14 days, add vancomycin iv, and monitor Vanco trough. Need extensive workup to identify the source of infection and then source control.

3/5/2018

1. **Culture of Propionibacterium** will need to hold in culture for 2 weeks (very slow growing). **Sites of infection** include pockets (oral cavity, large intestine), stent, and wound.
2. **Cellulitis by Streptococcus**, ok to use cefazolin or oxacillin, but if bacteremia, may be better to prescribe penicillin q4h. Penicillin does not cover staph.
3. **Ceftolozane/tazobactam (Zerbaxa)** for pan-resistant pseudomonas.
4. Small bowel obstruction patient received surgery; postoperatively was afebrile but WBC went up, differential diagnoses: AICD-related hematoma, rule out infected hematoma; indwelling PICC line and TPN, rule out fungemia/bacteremia; s/p bowel resection, rule out abdominal wall abscess; lower extremity edema, rule out leukocytosis due to CHF exacerbation or cellulitis. Final diagnosis: **abdominal abscess positive for enterococcus faecium**. **Treatment:** discontinue Zosyn, do amoxicillin 500 mg pot id for 7 days after improvement with iv antibiotics.
5. **Acute respiratory distress syndrome (ARDS) from Legionella community-acquired pneumonia (CAP)**: Levaquin 750 mg IV qd, later changed to doxycycline 100 mg q12h for 2–3 weeks. Later admitted to ICU for ARDS, restarted Levaquin 750 mg, and also started on Vanco and cefepime.

3/6/2018

1. Infectious disease (ID) specific questions and hints: **pets, prostheses, stents, valve replacements, travels, and lines.**
2. **Intravenous drug user (IVDU) source of infection**: oral/skin flora, bacteria from skin flora, water for dilution, and possible sexually transmitted infections (including HIV, HBV, HCV, syphilis, gonorrhea).

3. **Septic shock** is defined as: arterial hypotension (sBP < 90, mean BP < 65, or reduction in systolic blood pressure (sBP) > 40 mmHg from baseline) persisting for 1 h despite adequate fluid resuscitation (30 cc/kg in the first 3 h following presentation) or lactate >2 mmol/L after adequate fluid resuscitation. The use of vasopressors to correct hypotension does not exclude shock.
4. **Panculture**: blood, urine, and sputum cultures for aerobic and anaerobic microorganisms, routine, fungal, Acid-Fast Bacilli (AFB) culture and stain.
5. High suspicion for infection or abscess, if interventional radiologist (IR) biopsy culture is negative, **do an open biopsy.**
6. Murmurs at tricuspid are usually not easy to hear. Anaerobic culture causes **lysis of polymorphonuclear neutrophils (PMNs)** thus easy to grow certain bacteria.
7. Approximately, **half** of all patients with prosthetic valves who developed S. aureus bacteremia had **definitive endocarditis**.
8. In patients with community-acquired S. aureus bacteremia, any prior swelling in a prosthetic joint should lead to consideration of arthrocentesis to assess for infection (**40% of risk for prosthetic joint infection in staph bacteremia**).
9. Cellulitis in non-ST elevation myocardial infarction (NSTEMI): blood culture × 2, **start cefazolin 2 g IV q8h for 7–14 days.** If Streptococcus bacteremia, do penicillin G 25mu divided in q4h. If severe, prescribe intravenous vancomycin, daptomycin, or linezolid if pustulous. May need Vanco + Zosyn.
10. IV to po antibiotics switch timing: **if a patient has defervesced and remains afebrile for 48 h.**
11. Zosyn or Vanco/Zosyn does not cover **atypical pneumonia** and needs to add macrolides (azithromycin or doxycycline).
12. **ESBL coverage**: carbapenems, or Levaquin.
13. **Productive pneumonia on Zosyn + azithromycin non-responsive** → ID discontinued both, added Vancomycin and Ertapenem for ESBL.
14. **Mild Legionella pneumonia** treatment: 3–7 days levofloxacin or azithromycin. **Moderate to severe Legionella pneumonia** treatment: Levofloxacin or azithromycin for 7–10 days. In immunocompromised patients and patients with complications (e.g., empyema, or extrapulmonary infection), consider **10–14 days of antibiotics** or a **21-day course of levofloxacin** or a 10-day course of azithromycin.
15. **Gallstone cholangitis**, give Zosyn for 7 days but also need ERCP.
16. **Bacterial peritonitis categories**: spontaneous bacterial peritonitis (**SBP**, with positive peritoneal fluid culture), culture-negative neutrocytic ascites (**CNNA**); nonneutrocytic bacterial ascites (**NNBA**, polymorphonuclear leukocytes count below 250/μL, also known as monomicrobial non-neutrocytic bacterial ascites); **secondary bacterial peritonitis** (infection of the peritoneum by organisms from disruption of the integrity of the gastrointestinal or urogenital tracts or associated organs); **peritoneal dialysis associated bacterial peritonitis**.

3/7/2018

1. Extensive lung infiltrate in otherwise healthy adults, concerns for empyema, immunosuppression, also ask for previous pneumonia, sickness, sinusitis, antibiotic use history, lymph node enlargement (**if recurrent pneumonia, check immunoglobulin levels**). Prescribe 7-day antibiotic treatment.
2. Extensive pneumonia, will need to think about HIV defining disease; **COPD is at high risk for legionella**.
3. Bacteremia from S. pyogenes, may prescribe **penicillin G** for 7–10 days.
4. Order antibiotics, first think about where the infection comes from; ideally **perform relevant culture first** unless emergent conditions, like meningitis.
5. **Cellulitis, well-demarcated redness**: prescribe Vanco/Zosyn if stents/grafts (update: without pus or abscess, Strep is likely the cause and thus cefazolin usually is sufficient).
6. **Duration of lines**: groin (femoral vein) central line to be removed in **24 h**; central lines including internal jugular lines or subclavian lines to be removed or exchanged in **14 days**. Peripheral intravenous (PIV) line should be changed in **1–14 days**; midline can be used for **15–30 days**; peripherally inserted central catheter (PICC) and tunneled catheter can be used for **31–90 days to >90 days**; PICC and tunneled catheter and port **>90 days**.
7. Oral antibiotics: **penicillin VK 500 q6h for 7 days for S. pyogenes bacteremia** after iv antibiotics to 48 h after fever defervescence with good source control. Cefadroxil and cephalexin (Keflex) are both first generation cephalosporins. **Cefoxitin and cefotetan** are second generation cephalosporins with **anaerobic coverages**.
8. If debridement for osteomyelitis, make sure the pathology to **look at the wound margin**. This determines the duration of antibiotics. If **clean margin, antibiotics may be stopped** right away after amputation/debridement otherwise antibiotics should be continued for 4–8 weeks.
9. **ESRD increases tuberculosis (TB) risks**.
10. Hospital medicine **consult for aspiration pneumonitis** in permanent pacer implantation: Ok to implant/place pacemaker, order chest X-ray and single organism at nares for MRSA; Ok to give Unasyn.
11. **Denture but no teeth, the chance of oral flora infection is less likely.**
12. Amoxicillin 1000 mg q8h for 7 days can be used as a treatment for **community-acquired pneumonia.**

3/8/2018

1. Levaquin **750 mg** for legionella; Levaquin 750 mg daily dosing for pneumonia and bacteremia; **500 mg** daily dosing for urinary tract infections (UTI).
2. Tazobactam does not cover anaerobes. Flagyl increases INR.
3. **Oral flora**: actinomyces, Bacteroides, Bifidobacterium, eubacterium, fusobacterium, lactobacillus, peptococcus, peptostreptococcus, Propionibacterium, treponemal (all are anaerobes). **General fungi** include candida, Cladosporium, aspergillus, Cryptococcus.
4. **Ventilator-associated pneumonia (VAP)** treatments: micafungin, ertapenem, linezolid.

5. **Community-acquired pneumonia** usually is not contagious and does not transmit between people but some virus infections including respiratory syncytial virus and influenza virus are contagious (requires droplet isolation).
6. **Amp C. beta-lactamases** are cephalosporinases encoded on **the chromosomes and plasmids** of many of the Enterobacteriaceae and a few other organisms together abbreviated as SPICE organisms (Serratia, Providencia, "Indole-positive" Proteus species, Citrobacter, and Enterobacter species). Amp C. beta-lactamases mediate resistance to cephalosporins, most penicillins, and beta-lactamase inhibitor beta-lactam combinations. AmpC beta-lactamases are inducible in many bacteria. For those AmpC bacteria, use **carbapenem**, but carbapenem resistance can arise by mutations that reduce influx (outer membrane porin loss) or enhance efflux. Fluoroquinolones provide an alternative treatment option for infections with organisms producing **Amp C. beta-lactamases.**
7. Enterobacter aerogenes (now known as **Klebsiella aerogenes**) in respiratory culture causes **nosocomial opportunistic infections**: if Zosyn MIC 85, only do ertapenem.
8. A negative ESBL-confirmation test after a positive ESBL screening test is caused by **plasmid born amp C** in E. coli, K. pneumoniae, and proteus mirabilis.
9. **Carbapenem** is used for ESBL, but cephamycin (Cefoxitin, Cefotetan, and Cefmetazole), cefepime, Zosyn, ceftolozane-tazobactam (Zerbaxa), and ceftazidime-avibactam are alternatives for ESBL. Occasionally, fluoroquinolones may also be used for ESBLs.
10. **Prednisone long-term side effects**: Pneumocystis jirovecii pneumonia (PCP) precaution, bacteremia, abscess concerns if long-term use. May require PCP prophylaxis.
11. **Cefepime** does not cover anaerobes. **Ertapenem** does not cover pseudomonas; Zosyn and meropenem cover G- and anaerobes and pseudomonas, but **Amp C**. beta-lactamase-positive bacteria usually is resistant to Zosyn.
12. **G+ bacteremia**, if not staph or enterococcus, may use penicillin.
13. For Staph bacteremia or bacterial infection, use **oxacillin**.
14. Enterococcus infection: use ampicillin, amoxicillin, daptomycin, vancomycin, or linezolid. If **enterococcus bacteremia**, we need to think of combined synergies of antibiotics in patients with endocarditis, like **ampicillin plus ceftriaxone**: ampicillin 12 g/day (could be divided every 4 h or continuous infusion) plus ceftriaxone 2 g every 12 h for 6 weeks for endocarditis.
15. Be cautious if the clinical exam does not match the diagnosis or lab; something could be hidden.
16. A 48-year-old female presented with 5 days' watery diarrhea: colitis in CT, stool lactoferrin, ova, and parasites, check ANA, ANCA, CRP, ESR, ASCA. Came back positive for **salmonella colitis ➔ Use ceftriaxone/Vantin for 5 days**, check HIV, Ig G, Ig A.
17. ESBL urinary tract infection (UTI) is treated for a total of **3 days with ertapenem**, and contact isolations.

18. Complicated UTI is treated with 7-day antibiotics; pneumonia can be treated with antibiotics for 7 days if complicated.
19. Osteomyelitis after wound debridement: **cefepime iv for 6 weeks**.

3/9/2018

1. High suspicion for osteomyelitis: CT/MRI/pathology all confirmed osteomyelitis; if biopsy negative, next pursue further studies vs. empiric treatment. Tissue culture later grew **Streptococcus salivarius**.
2. Osteomyelitis is usually treated with antibiotics for 6 weeks.
3. **Corynebacterium** genus are catalase + , aerobic or facultative anaerobic non-motile G+ rods: C. diphtheria and the non-diphtherial corynebacteria are known as **diphtheroids**.
4. **Infected graft**: culture grew MRSA, do vancomycin for a total of 31 days after surgical removal. Need to monitor **weekly vancomycin trough, basic metabolic panel, and CBC weekly. Goal trough 15–20 mg/L**.
5. **Vancomycin iv as outpatient**: decrease hospital dosing from 1.5 g to 1 g q12h as 1.5 g q12h is likely to become toxic next week.
6. Add **metronidazole** if on cephalosporins for concerns of polymicrobial (including anaerobes) infection.
7. **Sepsis patient with liver failure and ascites**: differential diagnoses (DDx) include hospital-acquired pneumonia (HAP), spontaneous bacterial peritonitis (SBP), line infection, urinary tract infection (UTI), C. difficile infection. Order (workups): blood culture (routine and anaerobic), urinalysis plus urine culture, lactic acid, nares MRSA screen, and C. diff toxin. Follow blood cultures. If positive, will have to remove lines. Empirical antibiotic coverage: Vanco, micafungin, cefepime, Flagyl. Recommend paracentesis with fluid analyses and culture.
8. **Micafungin does not treat UTI and has no activity against Cryptococcus**. Micafungin is the preferred antifungal medication for concerns of **fungemia**. Total parenteral nutrition (TPN) increases the risk of fungal infection.
9. **Cirrhosis patients have a high risk for cryptococcal meningitis**. Line infection does not have outside redness or pain; the most often source of infection is the **tip of the line**.
10. Sepsis (antibiotics, fluid, diagnosis, control of source of infection) targets end-organ damage from bacterial infection: (A) **antibiotics** in 1 h, blood culture, tissue culture before antibiotics; (B) screen for **organ dysfunction** (liver, kidney, lung, and heart)

3/11/2018

1. Syncope in an old female, low glucose→ **Somogyi effect**. Combative behavior-increase Lamictal from 100 mg bid to 100 mg qam and 125 qpm.
2. For procedures the next day will require (A) **stop/hold** anticoagulation/aspirin overnight; (B) **NPO** after midnight; (C) check PT/INR (and CBC and BMP).
3. **Severe headache**: on butalbital/acetaminophen/caffeine (Fioricet), can add magnesium sulfate 1 g intravenous piggyback bolus (IVPB). Meclizine Antivert

25 mg tid for vertigo. Symptomatic management with antiemetics may be beneficial as well.

4. **Subarachnoid hemorrhage (SAH)** status post ruptured right superior cerebellar artery (SCA) aneurysm sp. coiling, seizures, hydrocephalus sp. EVA (external ventricular drain). Recommendations for headache: **continue nimodipine 60 mg q4h for a total of 21 days**. Continue transcranial Doppler for a total of 21 days. **Seizures**: continue carbamazepine (Tegretol) 200 mg tid (from 300 mg tid) and Lamictal 150 mg bid. Continue **bromocriptine 5 mg tid for altered mental status and agitation secondary to autonomic dysregulation**. Continue aspirin 325 mg for SCA aneurysm.
5. **Traumatic brain injury (TBI) medications: levodopa/carbidopa** may improve consciousness; **propranolol** and **pindolol** may reduce post-TBI agitation; **prazosin** may reduce daytime sleepiness, improve headaches and improve cognition; **bromocriptine** may improve arousal; **amantadine** may improve functional recover; **lamotrigine** may reduce aggressive behavior; **modafinil** and **methylphenidate** may improve day time arousal and attention; **melatonin** may improve daytime sleepiness and **Ramelteon** may improve total sleep time and thus cognition.
6. The most common etiology for aortic stenosis is rheumatic heart disease, **congenital bicuspid valve, and senile calcific aortic valve disease**. Severe aortic valve stenosis = aortic valve area **$\leq$1 cm^2**, and gradient (peak resting) pressure approaching **50 mmHg (mean 40 mmHg)** cutpoint. Size matters, thus critical aortic stenosis is usually defined as an aortic valve area of **0.7 cm^2** or less.
7. **Classic triad of aortic stenosis (AS)**: **syncope**, **angina**, and heart failure with symptoms of orthopnea, paroxysmal nocturnal dyspnea (**PND**), and dyspnea on exertion (**DOE**).
8. Patients with severe AS are relatively afterload fixed and preload dependent, meaning cardiac output does not increase with after-load reduction. Thus, all afterload reducing agents ACEi, CCB, and beta blockers are contraindicated. However, in patients with mild to moderate AS, vasodilators and nitrates like hydralazine can increase CO.
9. **Aortic valve replacement (AVR)** is indicated if symptomatic (Stage D1); asymptomatic severe AS plus left ventricular ejection fraction (LVEF) < 50% (Stage C2); or asymptomatic severe AS with decreased exercise tolerance or fall in systemic blood pressure with exercise (exercise testing is recommended to uncover symptoms, do not exercises if symptomatic); asymptomatic moderate AS undergoing other cardiac surgeries.
10. Transcatheter aortic valve (AoV) replacement (**TAVR**); medical management with careful **diuretics** as needed, control hypertension (HTN), maintain sinus rhythm (**SR**), digoxin if congestive heart failure (**CHF**) and decreased LVEF or if atrial fibrillation (AF); avoid vasodilators and negative inotropes like beta-blocker (BB) or CCB if severe AS. **Avoid physical exertion** once AS moderate to severe. Intra-aortic balloon pump (IABP) bridge to surgery. Balloon **AoV valvotomy (BAV)**: 50% increases aortic valve area and decreases peak pres-

sure, but 50% restenosis by 6–12 months and increased risk of periprocedural stroke and aortic regurgitation (AR).

11. Concerns for **disseminated intravascular coagulation** (DIC): order PT, PTT, INR, d-dimer, fibrin degradation products (FDPs), and fibrinogen.
12. **Hepatic encephalopathy grade**: Grade I-changes in behavior, mild confusion, slurred speech, disordered sleep; Grade II-lethargy, moderate confusion; Grade III- marked confusion (stupor), incoherent speech, sleeping but arousable. Grade IV—coma, unresponsive to pain.

Takeaway Messages

1. Enterococcus faecalis and faecium should be treated with IV or oral penicillin for urinary infections and IV penicillin with or without combined ceftriaxone or gentamicin for blood infections.
2. Gram positive bacteremia requires echocardiogram to rule out endocarditis. The diagnosis of infective endocarditis requires 2 major or 1 major plus 3 minor or 5 minor (2, 1 + 3, 5) criteria. Septic embolic in the brain or lungs, mycotic aneurysm, intracranial hemorrhage, and Janeway lesions are minor criteria.
3. Clindamycin can be added for cellulitis due to Strep pyogenes infections for toxin suppression.
4. If a patient has defervesced and remains afebrile for 48 h, we may switch IV antibiotics to oral.
5. Uncomplicated (exudative characteristics, but normal pH and glucose and no bacterium in pleural fluid) versus complicated (bacterial invasion of the pleural space, increased LDH, low pH) parapneumonic effusions versus empyema (a subcategory of complicated parapneumonic effusion with frank pus). Empyema should be treated with a chest tube and IV antibiotics for 4 weeks.
6. Headache, fever, confusion (2 or all three symptoms) with or without meningismus signs require lumbar puncture to rule out meningitis and encephalitis.

Further Readings and References

1. Murray, B.E., and W.R. Miller. *Treatment of enterococcal infections*, ed. D.J. Sexton. Waltham, MA: UpToDate. Accessed November 14, 2023.
2. Chu, V.H. *Antimicrobial therapy of left-sided native valve endocarditis*, ed. S.B. Calderwood. Waltham, MA: UpToDate. Accessed November 14, 2023.
3. McHugh, J., and O.A. Saleh. 2023. Updates in culture-negative endocarditis. *Pathogens* 12 (8): 1027.
4. Fowler, V.G., D.T. Durack, C. Selton-Suty, et al. 2023. The 2023 Duke-International Society for cardiovascular infectious diseases criteria for infective endocarditis: updating the modified Duke criteria. *Clinical Infectious Diseases* 77 (4): 518–526.
5. Albrecht, M.A. *Treatment of genital herpes simplex virus infection*, ed. M.S. Hirsch. Waltham, MA: UpToDate. Accessed November 14, 2023.
6. Wang, A., and J. Gaca. *Surgery for left-side native valve infective endocarditis*, ed. S.E. Kasner, D.J. Sexton, and A. Bolger. Waltham, MA: UpToDate. Accessed November 14, 2023.
7. Sabatine, M.S. 2017. *Pocket Medicine: The Massachusetts General Hospital Handbook of Internal Medicine*. 6th ed. Philadelphia: Lippincott Williams & Wilkins.

Chapter 7
Deja Vu ICU Rotation Followed by a Miscellaneous Learning Rotation

March 12th, 2018 Through May 6th, 2018

Life in the medical intensive care unit (ICU) is almost always intimidating and stressful. Patients are usually very sick and require close monitoring and patient families deserve frequent updates and family meetings. Patients in the ICU are usually on pressor support, ventilator support, or close monitoring for blood pressure management and/or nursing staff support. Life-or-death situations happen all the time in the ICU. As an intern, resident, or attending physician, our job is to stabilize the patient while persistently trying to identify the cause for the patient's declining health and to prevent its further deterioration.

Patients in the ICU usually have multiple critical conditions including but not limited to severe sepsis, septic shock, acute respiratory failure requiring invasive and noninvasive ventilator support, status epilepticus, and diabetic ketoacidosis (DKA). Stabilization of vitals in ICU patients utilizing pressors, ventilator support, and various medication drips is the major component for the care of these patients; meanwhile, identifying and treatment of the etiology or etiologies are of the same significance but may be passed over to the general medicine floor physicians when appropriate. While focusing on stabilizing patient conditions, identifying the source of infection can have long-lasting effects and can aid the decision of duration of antibiotics, understanding the etiologies for respiratory failure and starting corresponding treatment can facilitate the weaning of ventilation support, and correction of the etiologies of DKA will prevent its recurrence after DKA resolution.

Additionally, recognizing the limitations of us residents or even attending physicians as an individual during clinical practices and timely consulting of specialists is of foremost importance and usually can expedite patient recovery and even be lifesaving. Talking to nursing staff, respiratory therapists, speech therapists, registered dietitians, and other allied health professionals as well as case managers and social workers is also of great benefit as they usually provide additional valuable information for patient care. Meanwhile, for the use of uncommon or unfamiliar medications, pharmacists in the hospital are a great resource from which to seek

K. Zhou, *Internal Medicine Training Notes and Survival Guide*,
https://doi.org/10.1007/978-1-0716-4039-5_7

help. The practice of medicine is teamwork, especially for patients with critical and/or unstable conditions. We as interns, residents, or attending physicians are limited in our understanding of diseases and patients, despite the extensive training during medical school, residency training, and clinical practices.

Lastly, we need to understand the limitations of modern medicine and initiate goals of care discussions with patients and their families, especially when expecting poor outcomes. Although significant advancement has been made in patient care in the past decades, and as residents or attending physicians we try our best to help patients get better and live longer and healthier while minimizing patient suffering and preventing health deterioration, much of the time we are limited in our capabilities of controlling the uncontrollable, such as the progression of cardiorenal syndrome in a patient who does not want dialysis, progression of respiratory failure unresponsive to noninvasive ventilation support in a patient with a clear wish of no intubation, or continuous decline in mobility and worsening of functional status of a patient with incurable cancer. Many times, in such situations, I try to tell my patient and the patient's family that we will continue to try our best, but at the same time, at least sometimes, we do need to prepare for the worst.

Admittedly, the notes of this chapter focus more on patient management, but data gathering (for example, detailed history taking and thorough medical record review) and analyses are equally important. Topics in this chapter include sedation for ventilation, extubation, Parkinson's disease, status epilepticus, ventilator settings, gastrointestinal bleeding, and intravenous lines and flushes.

3/12/2018 ICU

1. **Herpes encephalitis treatment**: acyclovir 10 mg/kg IV q8h for 14–21 days.
2. **Upper gastroesophageal variceal bleed**: IV bolus octreotide at 25–50 μg followed by continuous IV octreotide at 25–50 μg/h for 72 h. May repeat bolus in the first hour if bleeding is not controlled. Pantoprazole 80 mg iv once followed by 40 mg iv bid.
3. **Sedation and anesthesia in the mechanically ventilated patients**: pain assessment and if pain, prescribe analgesic (morphine, hydromorphone, fentanyl) → decide a sedation strategy (daily interruption of sedation, sedation scale-based protocol, or no sedation) and choose sedatives: midazolam (caution use in renal failure), propofol (rapid wake-up), and dexmedetomidine (decreased sedation needs and rapid wake-up, used if brief sedation is needed).
4. **Cisatracurium (neuromuscular blockers)** does not have amnestic properties (it paralyzes the patient while the patient remains awake) and sedation to the point of amnesia is required with propofol or midazolam.

3/14/2018

1. If **supraventricular tachycardia**: may give adenosine for diagnostic purposes.
2. **COPD is an upper lobe disease**.
3. **Indications for urgent dialysis**: AEIOU—intractable **A**cidosis, **E**lectrolyte disarray (K, Ca, Na), **I**ntoxicants (Li, ASA), **O**-intractable fluid **O**verload, **U**remic symptoms (nausea, seizures, pericarditis, bleeding)

3/17/2018

1. **Indications for cuff leak test before extubation**: excessive airway manipulation; traumatic intubation; prolonged intubation attempt (>10 min); large tubes; patients with difficulty intubation, laryngeal edema, mucosal swelling from intubation. **Post-intubation factors** for cuff leak test: intubation >36 h, agitation while intubated, high cuff pressures, recurrent intubation. **Patient factors** for cuff leak test: female, short neck, trauma patients, known airway pathology (tracheal stenosis, tracheomalacia), children's small height to internal diameter ETT ratio.
2. Management for the above high-risk extubation. **Before extubation**: (1) attend to reversible risk factors; (2) perform cuff leak test; (3) pretreatment with IV steroids, dexamethasone at 0.15 mg/kg q6h for 4 doses of methylprednisolone 20 mg q4h for 4 doses preceding extubation; (4) high flow O_2 right after extubation. **Post extubation**: high flow O_2, close observation and morning VBG, ABG, consider noninvasive ventilation CPAP/BiPAP, reintubation if develops airway obstruction or respiratory failure (Racemic epinephrine nebulization: epi 1 mg/5 mL NaCl inhaled by nebulizer every 20 min as needed, Helium 40%).
3. **Syncope**: the most important part is history, prodrome, carotid stenosis does not cause syncope. **Common causes of syncope** include structural heart disease (like aortic stenosis, hypertrophic obstructive cardiomyopathy), functional heart disease (like second and third-degree AV block), seizure, stroke, vasovagal syncope, and orthostatic hypotension.
4. **Agitation in Parkinson's disease (PD) treatment**: assessment for precipitant or underlying causes (infection, delirium, dementia, adverse events of PD drug or other drugs) → treat infection, manage delirium/dementia if present → reduce and stop sedatives, anxiolytics, and antidepressants. If still not responding → reduce/stop PD meds (anticholinergics, amantadine, monoamine oxidase b (MAO-B) inhibitors, catechol-o-methyltransferase (COMT) inhibitors, dopamine agonist, levodopa in sequence for discontinuation) → initiate antipsychotic therapy with quetiapine, clozapine, and/or pimavanserin (Nuplazid).
5. The prevalence of **deep vein thrombosis** following decannulation from **extracorporeal membrane oxygenation (ECMO)** is high at 8.1 episodes/1000 cannula days, and **routine venous Doppler ultrasound** following decannulation is warranted in this population.
6. A 66-year-old female became **mute after an MCA infarct**. EEG revealed **complex partial seizure** (EEG report: This is a mildly abnormal EEG during an awake state. The intermittent generalized slowing can support the presence of a mild diffuse dysrhythmia. No definite epileptiform activity was seen. Sleep recording was however not obtained). Treatment: Continue Keppra 500 mg bid po or iv. One day later, since the mental status was not back to baseline, added fosphenytoin 1 g IVPB was followed by Dilantin 100 mg po tid (or fosphenytoin IVPB if unable to take oral for any reason). Three days later, Dilantin level

was therapeutic. Will try to taper off of Keppra over 24 h, to see if mental status improves. Six days later, AMS resolved, and checked the Dilantin level.

7. **Rounding on patients, always think**: telemetry, Foley, eating/bowel movement/urination, dysphagia/swallow, fluid (iv fluid infusion vs. lasix).
8. **Status epilepticus**: pay attention to vitals, respiratory and circulatory status. (1) In the first IV: **lorazepam 2–4 mg IV** (max rate 2 mg/min, may repeat another 2 mg), diazepam (max 5 mg/min) up to 10 mg per dose; wait for 1 min for additional dose. If no IV, do midazolam 10 mg IM if weight >40 kg. (2) In the second IV: **fosphenytoin 20 mg/kg PE** (phenytoin sodium equivalents) at 100–150 PE/min or phenytoin 20 mg/kg (max 1.2 g) at 25–50 mg/min or **valproic acid** 30 mg/kg at 10 mg/kg/min or **Keppra 40–60 mg/kg** (max 4.5 g) over 15 min. (3) Refractory status epilepticus: start continuous EEG after intubation, midazolam, propofol, or phenobarbital. Use **Versed first**, if seizure persists after 45–60 min, change to **propofol or phenobarbital**. PE is the abbreviation for phenytoin sodium equivalents (PE).
9. **Phenytoin** (not fosphenytoin) and any of the **benzodiazepines** (BZDs) are incompatible and will precipitate if infused through the same IV line. The same applies to phenytoin and any fluid with **glucose or dextrose**.
10. **Propofol-related infusion syndrome:** a rare lethal multiorgan failure related to probable mitochondrial injury, characterized by **lactic acidosis, rhabdomyolysis, hyperlipidemia, and cardiac failure**. Risk factors include a high rate of propofol infusion over prolonged periods.
11. **Status epilepticus**: in the first IV, lorazepam or versed or valium; in second dose IV, fosphenytoin 20 mg/kg PE at 100–150 mg/min or phenytoin at 20 mg to 50 mg/min OR valproic acid 30 mg/kg at 10 mg/kg/min or Keppra 40–60 mg/kg (max 4500 mg) over 15 min.
12. **Keppra** 1 g load then 500 mg bid ⇒ intubate, propofol sedation ⇒ midazolam at 100 mg/100 ml max 10 mg/h → phenytoin (Dilantin) 1200 mg iv once, max dose 50 mg/h.

3/18/2018

1. **Parkinson's disease (PD) treatment**: levodopa can cause **bradykinesia**, intrusive/troublesome or akinetic symptoms; dopamine agonist (bromocriptine, pramipexole, ropinirole, rotigotine, injectable apomorphine) can cause **impulse control disorders**; monoamine oxidase inhibitors (MAOIs) **selegiline and rasagiline** may be useful in patients with early PD but only provide mild symptomatic benefit as monotherapy; **anticholinergics** (procyclidine, trihexyphenidyl) are most usual as monotherapy in patients under age 70 with **disturbing tremor** but no significant bradykinesia or gait disturbance; **amantadine useful in young patients** with mild PD or perhaps later when dyskinesia becomes problematic.
2. Dopamine agonist is associated with fewer motor fluctuations than levodopa, levodopa is associated with a higher incidence of levodopa-related dyskinesia in young onset PD. **Use dopamine agonist for age < 65, and levodopa for age > 65.**

3. **Thiamine** supplementation should be considered in all patients with delirium, use Haldol (0.5–1 mg po/1 min) and benzodiazepines for agitation delirium in the hospital.
4. **Neuroleptic malignant syndrome**: mental status change, **rigidity**, fever, and dysautonomia. Seen in neuroleptic agents, and antiparkinsonian medication withdrawal. Lab test: increased K, leukocytosis, mild elevation of LDH, ALP, liver function tests (LFTs); electrolyte abnormalities, myoglobinuria, acute renal failure; a low serum iron concentration (highly sensitive).
5. Differential diagnosis of neuroleptic malignant syndrome (NMS): **serotonin syndrome (shivering, hyperreflexia, ataxia, nausea, and vomiting)**, malignant hyperthermia; malignant catatonia (psychosis, agitation, and catatonic excitement, improvement with lorazepam). **Treatment of NMS**: lorazepam, dantrolene, bromocriptine, amantadine.
6. **Motor fluctuation and dyskinesia** of levodopa side effects: off, on, wearing off, freezing of gait, failure of on, off.
7. **For endotracheal tube size 6 (size 7.5–8 is needed for bronchoscopy),** more pressure is needed for pressure support ventilation (12/5) for extubation, 30 min later, do venous blood gas (VBG) before extubation.
8. Swallow evaluation, excessive secretion: **chest physical therapy, vibrating vest, decrease sedation to wake patient up, pressure support trial.**
9. **Forme fruste**: an atypical usually incomplete manifestation of a disease.
10. **Causes of hyperchloremia**: loss of body fluid; high sodium; **Ringerfundin (RF) fluid** or chronic kidney disease (CKD); diabetes insipidus; fever, diabetic coma; drugs-androgens, estrogens, corticosteroids, and diuretics.
11. **Hyperchloremic metabolic acidosis** etiologies: diarrhea, renal tubular acidosis (RTA), defective renal acidification, normal saline (NS) infusion.
12. **Duoneb** causes tachycardia and urinary retention.
13. **Do Not use Precedex (dexmedetomidine) > 24 h** as it causes hypertension, hypotension, nausea, bradycardia, fever, vomiting, hypoxia, tachycardia, and anemia.
14. **Metabolic acidosis management**: decrease pain meds, avoid benzos, and check causes, BiPAP can be used. If intubated, may push bicarb, add sedation while intubation. If compensated (normal pH), no BiPAP is needed.
15. **Amlodipine edema does not respond to Lasix**.
16. **Status epilepticus**: Keppra and phenytoin loading dose and maintenance dose → intubate to protect the airway, **add Vimpat to prevent the patient from going back to status epilepticus**, and add Versed for sedation. **Nonconvulsive status epilepticus**: typical seizure activity on EEG with the absence of any clinically obvious convulsions.
17. **Intubation medications**: The patient was given 2 mg iv Versed, followed by etomidate 10 mg iv and rocuronium 70 mg iv, intubated with ETT size 7.5.
18. **Dilantin** crystalizes immediately with D5W, it is recommended diluting Dilantin with normal saline (NS).

19. Troponin **rise and fall** indicate cardiac cause and possible acute myocardial infarction, **use BNP** to differentiate congestive heart failure (CHF) from chronic obstructive pulmonary disease (COPD).
20. **Moderate aortic stenosis (AS)** and shortness of breath (SOB) due to congestive heart failure (CHF) with left ventricular ejection fraction (LVEF) 50%, treatment: Coreg 6.25 mg bid, hydralazine 50 mg tid, Imdur 60 mg qd, Aldactone 50 mg qd. (**37.5 mg of hydralazine hydrochloride and 20 mg of isosorbide dinitrate three times daily** is used for congestive heart failure patients who cannot tolerate angiotensin-converting enzyme inhibitors; the combination provides mortality benefits in African American population)
21. **Automated implantable cardioverter defibrillator (AICD) for primary prevention**: structural heart disease, sustained VT; syncope of undetermined origin, inducible ventricular tachycardia (VT) or ventricular fibrillation (VF) at electrophysiology (EP) study; LVEF <35% due to prior MI, at least 40 days post-myocardial infarction (MI), NYHA CHF class II/III; LVEF <30% due to prior MI, at least 40 days post-MI; LVEF ≤40% due to prior MI, inducible VT or VF at EP study.
22. **Pericardial rub sounds** are characterized by 1 systolic + 2 diastolic sounds (atrial contraction, ventricular contraction, and relaxation); it usually indicates pericarditis; treatment: ASA, ibuprofen, indomethacin, or colchicine.
23. **CT angiogram (CTA)** positive for calcification of coronary arteries, should get a stress test = consider calcification of coronary artery.
24. Do not combine fibrate (**if absolutely necessary, use fenofibrate**) with statin as they increase myopathy risks. If typical angina, give aspirin (ASA), statin, and beta-blocker.
25. **Endotracheal tube (ETT) size**: 7.5 mm for adult females, 8.5 mm for adult males, larger tube for bronchoscopy, **small tubes need greater pressure**. Endotracheal tube (ETT) size 8, PSV 10/5; at least size 7.5–8 ETT for bronchoscopy.
26. Elective intubation is better than urgent intubation.
27. **No PICC line/midline in end-stage renal failure/HD patients. Do Hohn's catheter (tunneled small-bore catheters) in these patients**, because the forearm veins, upper arm veins, and subclavian veins are of critical importance for the creation of fistula. The **internal jugular vein** is the preferred vessel for central venous access in these patients.
28. Rapid shallow breathing (Tobin) index is **reliable when pressure support ventilation (PSV) is used during ventilation**. Angiogram tomorrow: NS at 80 cc/h for 8 h before and after to prevent or minimize contrast dye injury. Lovenox morning dose is on hold for procedures during the day; prophylactic DVT anticoagulation usually can start 24 h after the procedure.
29. **Iron supplementation**: iron sucrose 300 mg IV qd for 5 days.
30. **Acute myocardial infarction (AMI) and unstable angina are contraindications for stress tests. For the stress test, if on a beta-blocker, keep the beta-blocker during the stress test. If not on a beta-blocker, do not start until after the stress test.**

3/18/2018

1. Allergy cross-reactivity occurs between **tropical fruits and latex allergy**, **peanuts and Atrovent (ipratropium)**, and **sulfa drugs and diuretics**.
2. Sudden increase in proteinuria: **membranous glomerulonephropathy** (GN) (check antiphosphatase A2 Ab+, HBV, HCV, and SLE), **focal segmental** GN (HIV), and minimal change disease.
3. HA1c 8.5% requires a **Glucagon-like peptide 1 (GLP-1) agonist with sodium-glucose transport protein 2 (SGLT-2) inhibitor and metformin. Glimepiride** has a lower incidence of hypoglycemia than glyburide, especially in chronic kidney disease (CKD). Syncope patients should avoid glyburide.
4. **Herpes encephalitis** treatment in hospital: acyclovir 10 mg/kg q8h for 14–21 days, Keppra 1000 mg bid IV. Decadron at 4 mg q6h for 4 days is only useful if **S. pneumoniae meningitis** (may decrease hearing deficits in Haemophilus influenzae meningitis and neurological deficits in meningococcal meningitis).
5. **Invasive fungi**: Pneumocystis jirovecii Pneumonia (PCP), aspergillus, Cryptococcus, candida, histoplasmosis, and mucormycosis.
6. **Respiratory acidosis** = consider pulmonary embolism (PE), congestive heart failure (CHF)? Long-term steroid use is not recommended for COPD/asthma unless needed.
7. **Eosinophilia**: asthma, air pollen allergy, asbestosis. **Wheezing = narrowed airway entry**.
8. Haloperidol, fluphenazine, and trifluoperazine are associated with a low risk of seizure induction; **clozapine increases seizure**.
9. **Air bronchogram** refers to air-containing bronchi or bronchioles in lung cancer, bronchiectasis, lymphoma, and pneumonia.
10. **Screening for lung cancer**: annual low dose CT in adults aged 50–80 who have a 20-pack-year smoking history and actively smoke or have quit in the past 15 years.
11. Woman aged 50–74 with average risk: **biennial mammography**. Women with higher than average risk, begin biennial mammograms at age 40.
12. Selective estrogen receptor modulators (SERMs) tamoxifen and raloxifene reduce risk for estrogen receptor-positive (ER+) invasive breast cancer; **tamoxifen increases endometrial cancer** and venous thromboembolism (VTE) in women >50. Raloxifene increases VTE risk but not endometrial cancer risk.
13. **Colorectal cancer screening** is recommended in people 45–75 years of age. Based on screening colonoscopy findings, surveillance colonoscopy is recommended: no polyp or <20 small <10 mm **hyperplastic** polyps, q10y; 1–2 small <10 mm **tubular adenomas q5-10y**; 3–10 tubular adenomas or $\geq$ 10 mm or **villous adenoma q3y**; sessile serrated polyps <10 mm q5y; >10 mm q3y.
14. Tegretol = carbamazepine; Rituxan = rituximab.
15. **Autoimmune hemolytic anemia treatments**: Solu-Cortef (hydrocortisone sodium succinate injection), prednisone, methylprednisolone, or Rituxan 1 dose.

3/19/2018

1. Echo is more reliable than stress test; Lexiscan is not that reliable in wall motion abnormalities.
2. **Clubbing** is seen in colitis, GI cancer, COPD, endocarditis, left to right cardiac shunt, malformation, and hyperthyroidism.
3. Autoimmune diabetes, **latent autoimmune diabetes in adults (LADA)**: check for islet cell autoantibodies (ICA), autoantibodies to glutamic acid decarboxylase (GAD), tyrosine phosphatase–related islet antigen 2 (IA-2), and insulin autoantibodies (IAA), and C-peptide. **LADA is a subtype of T1DM**.

3/20/2018

1. **Rapid response**: look for myocardial infarction (MI), stroke or cerebrovascular accidents, pulmonary embolism (PE), acute abdomen, meningitis, and seizure.
2. Low K causes atrioventricular (AV) block, and bradycardia, should not be on beta blockers. Bradycardia patients for breast reconstruction may be pretreated with **atropine IV 0.5 mg** right before the procedure.

3/25/2018

1. **Central venous pressure (CVP)** = right atrial (RA) pressure, does not correlate with pulmonary wedge pressure. **Pulmonary wedge pressure** = left atrium pressure, between 4 and 12 mmHg is normal. B-type natriuretic peptide (BNP) indicates atrial dilation.
2. Acute dyspnea from allergic reaction. Treatment: **IV Benadryl** 50 mg IV and **solumedrol 125 mg** IV, then if not responding, order 1 mg vial of epi to be given **0.3 mg IM q5min for 4–5 doses**. Meanwhile, start nasal cannula for oxygen, and contact anesthesia for possible intubation if not responding. **Then order respiratory treatment with racemic epinephrine.**
3. **Endotracheal tube (ET) tube size 8**, pressure support trial 10/5 before extubation.
4. Overlap warfarin and heparin for 48 h, **stop heparin 24 h after INR therapeutic**; linezolid covers vancomycin-resistant enterococcus (VRE). High risk for pulmonary embolism (PE) in **Tetralogy of Fallot (TOF)** with pacemaker in AFib.
5. Pulmonary hypertension, ventricular enlargement, and left ventricular dysfunction require diuresis.
6. ARDS management example: increase FiO_2, PEEP $5 > 8 > 10 > 15$
7. **Second hypertension workup**: serum aldosterone, renin activity, fractional metanephrine, TSH, cortisol, renal artery duplex ultrasound.
8. Bradycardia for Endoscopic Retrograde Cholangiopancreatography (ERCP): **premedication with atropine 0.5 mg IV prior to procedure and repeat during procedure prn up to a total of 2 mg IV**.
9. Protonix iv 40 mg/100 ml q5h for acute GI bleed (such use not common in actual practice).

3/26/2018

1. We may need to order **CT chest** to differentiate CHF with EF 25% exacerbation from pneumonia, and shortness of breath. Procalcitonin >0.3–0.5 is an alternative to confirm pneumonia as well.
2. **Whispered pectoriloquy** = an increased loudness upon auscultation with whispering. This indicates **lung consolidation**.
3. Lactic acid high → ischemic bowel. **Ischemic bowel** is a surgical emergency. Check venous leg Doppler before sequential compression device/pump. Start **trickle feeds** for tube feeding at the beginning.
4. **Ceftriaxone** causes gallbladder sludge.
5. **Acute respiratory distress syndrome (ARDS)** needs negative fluid balance, increased respiratory rate (RR), increased positive end-expiratory pressure (PEEP), and low tidal volume ventilation.
6. **Use micafungin for fungemia**, not fluconazole.
7. Nausea and vomiting, may need to give Reglan and Zofran around the clock.
8. Scopolamine and **N-acetylcysteine (Mucomyst) inhalation**, if sticky sputum.
9. **Definity** (perflutren lipid microsphere), a diagnostic ultrasound-enhancing agent, is added if the ventricle cannot be seen with echo.
10. Pacemakers usually **set rate at 70–80 s**; defibrillators usually set to **fire at 140 s**.
11. Atrial fibrillation originates from the right upper atrial or **pulmonary veins**. Atrial flutter originates from the right **atrium**, and responds to ablation. Antiarrhythmic drugs, rate control meds, and cardioversion are options for treatments of atrial fibrillation and flutter.
12. For sinus tachycardia, we can use metoprolol but have to treat the cause. **The reentrant circuit has narrow QRS tachycardia.**

3/28/2018

1. **Iron overload** = multiple PRBC transfusion, eg. Thalassemia, sickle cell anemia (SCA), inherited bone marrow failure syndrome, myelodysplastic syndrome (MDS); increased absorption from hereditary hemochromatosis (HFE gene C282Y); ineffective erythropoiesis (thalassemia, sideroblastic anemia, Vit B12, and folate deficiency); liver disease, gestational alloimmune liver disease (GALD) also known as (AKA) neonatal hemochromatosis (maternal Ab crosses the placenta and causes liver failure and cirrhosis); alcoholic liver disease, chronic non-alcoholic fatty liver disease (NAFLD), chronic viral hepatitis, porphyria cutanea tarda (PCT).
2. **Effects of iron overload**: liver function tests (LFTs) abnormalities, cardiac involvement, diabetes, hypogonadism, hyperpigmentation, and arthropathy.
3. **Hemochromatosis diagnosis**: **≥300** μg/L ferritin in males, 200 in females without significant inflammation or infection with increased transferrin saturation of **≥45%**; iron overload by MRI of the liver and heart; iron overload by liver biopsy. Treatment: iron removal via **phlebotomy** in the range of 1.5–2 g (**5–6 phlebotomies**) with normalization of ferritin.
4. **Intubation ventilator settings**: Tidal volume 480, respiratory rate (RR) 14, FiO_2 100%, PEEP 5, I/E ratio 1/3: 2/3.

5. BiPAP can decompensate patients, especially **drop blood pressure**. If decompensated, take off BiPAP, do breathing treatment and diuretics.
6. Respiratory distress, identify etiology if no lung involvement otherwise, **no intubation except for protecting airways** in decreased **Glasgow Coma Scale of 8 or lower.**

3/29/2018

1. **Henoch-Schoenlein purpura (HSP)** is self-limited and is characterized by a tetrad of clinical manifestations including **palpable purpura** in patients with neither thrombocytopenia nor coagulopathy, **arthralgia and/or arthritis, abdominal pain, renal disease**. Patients with HCP (IgA vasculitis) can have GI involvement including **bowel wall edema**.
2. HSP pain management: mild to moderate pain, use **naproxen** 10–20 mg/kg in 2 doses, maximal 1 g daily, **ibuprofen**; severe pain, use **glucocorticoids**, prednisone 1–2 mg/kg/day, maximal dose 60–80 mg/day or methylprednisolone 0.8–1.6 mg/kg/day.
3. **Hospitalization in HSP** if: (A) inability to maintain hydration with oral intake; (B) severe abdominal pain; (C) significant gastrointestinal (GI) bleed; (D) change in mentation; (E) severe joint involvement limiting ambulation or self-care; (F) renal insufficiency, hypertension (HTN), nephrotic syndrome.
4. **Chart review** in general provides excellent information for patient care. It is important to get records from a primary care doctor (PCP), cardiologist, and oncologist.
5. In the intensive care unit (ICU), every patient should have a **central line and IV access**.
6. Signs of elevated intracranial pressure (ICP) include **cranial nerve VI (CNVI) palsies**, **papilledema** secondary to impaired axonal transport and congestion, spontaneous periorbital bruising, and a triad of **bradycardia, respiratory depression, and hypertension** (Cushing's triad, AKA Cushing's reflex/response). Normal intraocular pressure is **10–21 mmHg**. Normal intracranial pressure in adults is 7–**15 mmHg**. Normal CSF opening pressure is **6–25 mmHg**.
7. Acute respiratory distress syndrome (ARDS) needs to **increase RR, PEEP, and diuretics** as appropriate, if **PEAK pressure is too high, consider pressure support ventilation (PSV)**.
8. **Non-typeable Haemophilus influenzae** is the most common cause of bacteria-induced **COPD exacerbation**.
9. **Osler-Weber-Rendu** = Hereditary hemorrhagic telangiectasia- vascular dysplasia.
10. Alcoholic liver disease, **platelet likely not functional**, be cautious of heparin and Lovenox.
11. **Shortness of breath (SOB), cardiomegaly, and troponin leak** are indications for ordering an echocardiogram.
12. PEEP can be up to 12–14 cmH_2O (usually 5–12 cmH_2O), judge **PEEP based on compliance**.

13. **Foster Kennedy Syndrome** = mass in the frontal lobe, leading to a constellation of visual and smell changes: optic atrophy of the ipsilateral eye, disc edema in the contralateral eye, central scotoma ipsilateral, and ipsilateral anosmia.

3/31/2018

1. Increased excretion of **albumin** is a marker of chronic kidney disease (CKD) due to diabetes mellitus (DM), glomerular disease, and hypertension (HTN). Increased excretion of **low molecular weight (LMW) globulins** is a marker for some types of **tubulointerstitial** disease.
2. When monitoring proteinuria in adults with chronic kidney disease (CKD), total protein to creatinine ratio in spot urine samples should be measured using **albumin to creatinine ratio except concerns for non-albumin proteinuria** or albumin to creatinine ratio > **500—1000 mg/L** (the actual total protein to creatinine ratio in spot urine should be measured).
3. Benzodiazepines (BZDs) in alcohol withdrawal have the risk of **behavioral disinhibition (social dysdecorum or loss of implicit social knowledge)** in liver failure and thus require caution in their use.
4. **Antipsychotics** in alcohol withdrawal lower the threshold for **seizures**, and thus are second line agents. Antipsychotics may be used when hemodynamic stability and alcohol withdrawal are controlled with BZDs (BZDs also prevent seizures). Typical antipsychotics like **haloperidol** can effectively treat psychosis with acute agitation. **Olanzapine** can be used for both **psychosis and agitation**.
5. For psychosis without acute agitation, the atypical antipsychotics of **risperidone, olanzapine, and quetiapine** can be used. Use **disulfiram for enforced abstinence**, **naltrexone or topiramate to dampen craving**, and **naloxone if opiate overdose is suspected**.
6. **Haldol and chlorpromazine (Thorazine**) provide rapid tranquilization. They should be administered with a BZD to prevent a lowered threshold of seizures.
7. Alcohol related psychosis = severe alcohol abuse = poor prognosis = severe alcoholism.
8. Swelling not responding to diuretics, check **prealbumin and albumin**. If albumin is low, do 25% albumin bid for 3 days, and add bumetanide as well. May benefit from Lasix or Bumex drip if anasarca.
9. Always talk to patients/family to get the full story.
10. Hemorrhagic stroke needs to get **INR back to normal**. If INR is elevated, check DIC panel and correct INR meanwhile.
11. Ativan for alcohol withdrawal. **If the patient requires > 25 mg/day Ativan, think of psychosis**. May need to use **atypical antipsychotics**.
12. Alcohol withdrawal for over 2 days not eating treatment: place **nasogastric tube** and start tube feeds.
13. Acute respiratory distress syndrome (ARDS), **adjust FiO_2 first then PEEP** to achieve goal oxygen saturation.
14. Pressure support trials in ventilation 10/5, trickle tube feeds.

15. Steroids in urgent conditions, also known as **stress-dosing steroids**, may be appropriate in septic shock.
16. Always discuss with patient **code status** and sign DNR/DNI per patient wishes; in some facilities partial code (DNR only or DNI only) is allowed while in others DNR and DNI have to come together.
17. Pay attention to differentiate chronic obstructive pulmonary disease (COPD) exacerbation from congestive heart failure (CHF) exacerbation. **In CHF exacerbation, the patient may not need BiPAP**.
18. **Evaluation of hypothalamic–pituitary–adrenal axis (HPA)** axis suppression: in patients with chronic glucocorticoid therapy, a morning earlier than 8 a.m. cortisol level < **3–5 mg/dL (24 h off glucocorticoid replacement dose**) is highly suggestive of an impaired HPA axis, will need additional glucocorticoid intake perioperatively (100 mg IV hydrocortisone before induction of anesthesia and 50 mg q8h for 24 h, then taper dose by half per day to maintenance dose); an early morning cortisol level **> 10 mg/dL**, no need for additional glucocorticoid intake perioperatively; between **5 and 10 mg/dL**, do adrenocorticotropic hormone (ACTH) stimulation test also known as Coysntropin test -30 min after 250 μg corticotropin (ACTH) stimulation for preoperative evaluation of the HPA axis. A **cortisol level > 18 μg 30 min after ACTH stimulation test** = consider an adequate adrenal reserve and no need for stress dose steroids. If stopping glucocorticoid for 24 h is not possible, check Cosyntropin stimulation test to target 18 μg.
19. **Glucocorticoid therapy in septic shock**: administer a glucocorticoid like hydrocortisone with or without fludrocortisone to patients with **refractory septic shock with going requirement for vasopressor** can lead to a faster resolution of shock and a possible mortality benefit in sicker patients. **Typically administer 200–300 mg per day of hydrocortisone IV in divided doses (50 μg q6h or 100 q8h) for at least 3 days (up to 5–7 days)** and taper the dose as guided by clinical response.
20. Drugs such as **azoles antifungal agents and ritonavir** that inhibit cytochrome P450 can cause increased serum levels of glucocorticoids.
21. Anesthetic agent **etomidate** should be avoided in patients with risk for adrenal suppression and crisis as it inhibits steroid synthesis.
22. The **low-dose dexamethasone suppression test** (1 mg dexamethasone overnight and measure serum cortisol in the morning) for differentiating patients with Cushing disease of any cause from patients who do not have Cushing's syndrome. **Suppressed** = consider **no Cushing** disease but could be hypercortisolism from alcohol use disorder, obesity, insulin resistance, neuropsychiatric disorders, or others.
23. The **high-dose dexamethasone suppression tests** help distinguish patients with **Cushing disease** (Cushing syndrome by pituitary hypersecretion of ACTH) from patients with ectopic ACTH syndrome. It is performed with a baseline cortisol measured on the morning of the test, then 8 mg of dexamethasone given overnight with measurement of cortisol in the following morning.

4/1/2018 Mechanical Ventilation

1. **Indications for mechanical ventilation**: protect the airway, can't breathe, requires sedation.
2. **Mode**: **Assist control (AC)** = continuous mandatory ventilation. The patient triggers the ventilator to deliver a specific volume (8 ml/ideal body weight (IBW), 500–600 cc). Set the backup respiratory rate to 12. Compliance = delta V/delta P.

   Pressure control (PC) = patient or time triggering a set of changes in pressure. Alarm: output read—AC (pressure), PC (volume). **Ventilator settings**: volume, pressure, respiratory rate, flow rate, O_2, patient vs. ventilator control.
3. CPAP or PEEP (5–20 cmH_2O): **pressure support only occurs on inspiration**. The patient initiates each breath, high pressure, bigger breath, 5–15 cmH_2O.
4. **Orders for vent**: mode, AC, 16 as backup RR; tidal volume 550 mL; Fraction of Inspired Oxygen (FiO_2), PEEP 5.
5. Air goes into the lung, resistance from airways = compliance of lungs; **peak pressure** = airflow-airways resistance. **Plateau pressure** = air stops (inspiratory hold), represents compliance.
6. Plateau pressure vs. peak pressure = compliance vs. airway pressure. **Plateau pressure** increases in pneumothorax (PTX), pulmonary edema, acute respiratory distress syndrome (ARDS), and pneumonia (PNA). **Peak pressure** increases with bronchospasm, secretions, mucous plug, and tip of endotracheal tube occluded.
7. ARDS should use low tidal volume, increase respiratory rate (RR) → increase ventilation → increase dead space. **Tidal Volume is** more reliable as it measures 100% air in without the influence of dead space.
8. **PEEP** opens more alveoli, more lung recruitment, intrathoracic pressure increase → decreases venous return → decreases cardiac output (CO) → **low BP**.
9. In congestive heart failure (CHF), increased PEEP, may improve lung aeration as it decreases venous return.
10. If blood pressure (BP) is marginal or soft, do not increase PEEP. If congestive heart failure, we can **increase PEEP to push alveolar fluid** out of the alveoli if blood pressure tolerates.
11. **ARDS**: compliance of lung drops due to inflammation and hyaline membrane. Increase tidal volume (TV) = consider increased inflammation → death, thus may **increase PEEP to 12 or 14**, but keep low tidal volume 6-6 mL/kg ideal body weight (IBW).
12. **COPD**: good compliance but obstructed airways, trapped air → need very long expiratory phase. Increased CO_2, may increase respiratory rate (RR) and tidal volume (TV) for ventilator adjustment. CO_2 retention, **set I:E = 1:2**. Inspiratory flow rate 60 L/min, thus expiratory flow rate should be 80–100 L/min in COPD make sure flow back to 0 before next breath, and good bronchodilators. **Be careful of breath stacking!!**
13. **Liberation from ventilation**: (A) lifting sedation; (B) weaning trial. Begin liberation from ventilation when $FiO_2 < 45\%$ and off vasopressors, may start

SBT (spontaneous breathing trial) → pressure support (PS), PEEP, tube compensation, get support as low as physiological. ABG pH > 7.35, $PCO_2 < 45$, PO_2 60–70. RSBT (Tobin) index = RR/Vt < 105, NIF (negative inspiratory force) < −30, and minute Ventilation <15 L/min are good predictors for successful extubation.

14. Additional predictors for **successful weaning of ventilator**: mechanisms of ventilation good; arterial blood gas (ABG) good; mental status appropriate, able to protect airways; secretions controlled; air leak heard.
15. Septic patient, before intubation: IV access, central line first, get ready to use pressors.
16. **Metabolic acidosis**: 7.2/20/60/15 (ABG readings) pure metabolic acidosis; look at RR and TV. RR 30, TV 400. IF use AC 12/450/5/100%, may drop pH to 6.9 → cardiac arrest, thus set RR 20 and TV 550.
17. Chronic obstructive pulmonary disease (COPD) stage IV with FEV1 < 30; PCO2 > 45, ABG 7.34/60/55/30; **only target pH, not CO_2, can keep CO_2 high in COPD**.
18. Causes of asthma: air irritant, gastroesophageal reflux disease (GERD), postnasal drip, solvents, and wood dusts. **Sampler's triad**: **aspirin sensitivity, asthma, nasal polyps → respond well to leukotriene inhibitors.**
19. Obstructive: FEV1/FVC < 0.7; methacholine challenge test. Intermittent asthma = symptoms in 2 days or less per week; **persistent asthma** symptoms in **≥ 2 days/week** (mild not daily, moderate daily, severe throughout the day).
20. SABA- albuterol (ProAir, Ventolin MDI-Neb), levalbuterol AKA Xopenex. **Omalizumab** is effective in severe persistent allergic (IgE-mediated) asthma → add oral corticosteroids.
21. **Forced vital capacity < 80% of predicted** = consider restrictive lung disease. Functional residual capacity (FRC) = expiratory reserve volume (ERV) + residual volume (RV). Vital capacity (VC) = inspiratory reserve capacity (IRC) + tidal volume (TV) + expiratory reserve capacity (ERC).
22. **Functional reserve capacity (FRC)** is determined by the interaction between the chest wall and lungs.
23. **Lung diffusion test** also known as the diffusing capacity for carbon monoxide (DLCO) is affected by architectural destruction and extrinsic constructure.
24. Hypothalamic–pituitary–adrenal axis (**HPA**) **suppression** and thus **steroid taper needed** in (A) ≥20 mg prednisone qd for 3 weeks; (B) ≥5 mg prednisone qhs for a few weeks; (C) any patient with cushingoid appearance.

4/2/2018

1. Gastrointestinal (GI) bleed treatment example: fresh frozen plasma (FFP) 2 units; vit K 10 mg IV, Stat PRBC.
2. **Kayexalate for hyperkalemia**: change K for Na, not good for CHF.
3. In outpatient practice, if a critical lab and patient not responding to phone calls when emergent labs or conditions, may call the police.

4. **Calcium chloride** is preferentially to be given via **central line** (peripheral venous catheters may be acceptable). **Calcium gluconate** can be given via peripheral venous catheters for EKG changes in hyperkalemia.
5. Albuterol may need to be given at **least 5 × (20 mg) usual dose** for hyperkalemia.
6. **Calcium gluconate** is the treatment for hyperkalemia, **hypermagnesemia (calcium antagonizes neuromuscular and cardiovascular effects of magnesium**), hypocalcemia, and calcium channel blocker overdose.
7. **HCO_3** for salicylic acid poisoning. **Plasma lytes** have the same pH as blood for trauma patients and are used for fluid replacement.
8. **BiPAP** setting 20/6 for COPD exacerbation.
9. **Care management** for a visiting nurse, home care, skilled nursing facility, and assisted living facility discharge arrangements.
10. **Hypertensive emergencies**: For adults with compelling conditions (i.e., aortic dissection, severe pre-eclampsia or eclampsia, or pheochromocytoma crisis), lower sBP to below **140 mmHg** during the first hour and to **below 120 mmHg in aortic dissection**. Otherwise, reduce the systolic blood pressure (sBP) to a maximum of 25% within the first hour, then if the patient is stable, lower the BP to 160/100–110 mmHg over the next 2–6 h, and cautiously to normal blood pressure over the following 24–48 h.
11. **Hypertensive encephalopathy**: reduce mean arterial pressure (MAP) by 25% over 8 h with labetalol, nicardipine, and esmolol. Acute ischemic stroke: withhold antihypertensives unless sBP > 220 mmHg or DBP >120 mmHg. If tissue-type plasminogen activator (tPA) use, keep sBP < 185 and dBP < 110 before tPA. After initiating drug therapy with tPA, keep SBP < 180 and dBP < 105 for 24 h. **Tenecteplase (TNK)** is now preferred over tPA for thrombolysis in stroke patients in many hospitals.
12. Acute intracranial hemorrhage in the first 24 h: if signs or symptoms of increased intracranial pressure (ICP), goal mean arterial pressure (MAP) < 130 (or **sBP < 180**) mmHg with **goal cerebral perfusion pressure (MAP–ICP) of 50–70 mmHg**; if no ICP increase then MAP <110 or **sBP < 160** mmHg.
13. For acute heart failure, **use IV nitroglycerin, sublingual nitroglycerin, or IV enalapril** to lower BP or relieve chest pain in cardiac ischemia.
14. Preeclampsia/eclampsia: **hydralazine, labetalol, nicardipine**, lower sBP <140 in the first hour.
15. Preoperative HTN: defined as blood pressure of 160/90 or higher or systolic blood pressure (sBP) >20% preoperative value for ≥15 min, **use nitroprusside, nitroglycerin, clevidipine, nicardipine, and esmolol** if necessary.

4/3/2018

1. **24 h within non-ST elevation myocardial infarction (NSTEMI), arrhythmia** chances are high, if unstable vitals, may need ICU care otherwise can be admitted on a cardiac telemetry floor.
2. Check with **all the specialties** plan of care for patients in the ICU.
3. **Seizure emergent treatment**: Ativan 1–2 mg for a maximum 4 mg (recommended to give 4 mg all at once during a seizure); or **valium 5–10 mg for a**

maximum of 10 mg, risks for respiratory depression if more than 2 doses. If seizure continuous with concerns for status epilepticus after at least 2 doses of Ativan or valium, begin **fosphenytoin at a dose of 20 mg phenytoin equivalent (PE)/kg IV and a rate of 3 mg PE/kg/min** (no more than 150 mg/min). If seizure is present, an **additional 5–10 mgPE/kg IV of fosphenytoi**n can be given at 10 min after loading dose. Also, may administer weight-based doses of IV valproate, phenobarbital, levetiracetam, versed, propofol, or phenobarbital.

4. **ICU care pearl**: ask the charge nurse in the morning for OR patients; have a plan for all the patients; know who can be transferred to the floor; look at previous admission/Healthlink look for social history, heart conditions, echo, antibiotic use; if conditions do not change in second day, ask why and change the way of thinking needed (wrong diagnosis, progressing disease?..); X-ray chest/abdomen of patients as necessary; may send the patient to the floor on BiPAP, make sure VBG at 8 p.m. and 4 a.m.; diabetic ketoacidosis (DKA) patient may need to be on Zofran/Reglan around the clock for short term upon transferring out of ICU; **Compazine and Tigan if QTc prolongation**; keep patient on fluids as necessary.

4/4/2018

1. **CPAP settings**: 8 cm H_2O with autotitration to maintain $SO_2 > 92\%$.
2. **Mild metabolic alkalosis** is acceptable if kidney function is good, HCO_3 can be peed out thus no action is needed.
3. Kidney failure workup includes **renal ultrasound/abdominal and pelvis CT, urinalysis, urine lytes, FENA, and urine creatinine albumin ratio, addition of vasculitis workup if hematuria**.
4. **Altered mental status (AMS)** causes include drugs/ethanol use or withdrawal/infection/metabolic derangement/brain disorders/seizures/systemic organ failure/physical disorders. Will need to rule out meningitis and encephalitis. Workup may require **EEG, lumbar puncture, and brain MRI**.
5. **Status epilepticus**: Ativan 2 mg IV, Keppra 1 g load, phenytoin 150 mg IV, EEG continuous → add lacosamide 200 mg bid on top of **phenytoin 800 mg q8h, Keppra 1500 mg bid**. If no IV access, do midazolam 10 mg IM or buccal or nasal midazolam.
6. Lactic acid is usually high in the ischemic **bowel** which is a surgical emergency.
7. Sepsis and diabetic ketoacidosis (DKA), if beta-hydroxybutyrate **<1, ketone may not be from DKA, may bridge with long acting insulin even when anion gap (AG) exists**.
8. Use **central venous pressure (CVP)** to gauge fluid condition, goal 8–12 cmH_2O.
9. If PT/PTT, INR grossly normal or mildly elevated, but **large bleeding, give recombinant factor VIIa (especially if within 4 h of intracranial hemorrhage, alveolar hemorrhage)**.
10. Status epilepticus is defined as **5 min of continuous seizing or ≥ 2 discrete seizures between which there is incomplete recovery of consciousness**.
11. Use of, or overdose with **drugs that lower seizure threshold**: theophylline, imipenem, high dose penicillin G, cefepime, quinolones, metronidazole, isonia-

zid, tricyclic antidepressants (TCAs), bupropion, lithium, clozapine, flumazenil, cyclosporine, lidocaine, bupivacaine etc.

12. **Classification of status epilepticus**: **generalized convulsive** status epilepticus (GCSE); **focal motor** status epilepticus; **myoclonic** status epilepticus (MSE); **absence** status epilepticus.
13. In cases with focal onset seizure, a causative lesion must be sought. In primary generalized epilepsies, certain anti-seizure drugs, like **phenytoin, carbamazepine, and oxcarbazepine** should be avoided if the patient is having **myoclonic or absence seizure**.
14. A particularly focal motor status epilepticus with very prolonged and very regular jerking activity is called **epilepsia partialis continua** (EPC). **Rasmussen encephalitis** is a common cause of EPC in children and adolescents—refractory, unremitting focal seizures, progressive cerebral hemiatrophy in EEG.
15. **Myoclonic** status epilepticus (**MSE**): the EEG demonstrates rapid epileptiform discharges time-locked to movement- pervasive for an epileptic origin of the myoclonus. MSE is divided into epilepsy syndrome-related causes and symptomatic causes, examples of MSE: **Juvenile myoclonic epilepsy, and Lennox-Gastaut syndrome**. EEG usually shows the often-severe encephalopathy and frequent brief sometimes regular epileptiform discharges.
16. **Tonic status epilepticus** is rare in adults; it consists of maintenance of a tonic posture, particularly of axial musculature, rather than frank convulsions-Lennox-Gastaut syndrome. Time-frequency analysis (TSE) EEG shows widespread fast activity or very rapid spikes but may also include background suppression or attenuation.
17. The primary drugs used for refractory status epilepticus are **midazolam, propofol, and pentobarbital.**
18. **Respiratory distress**, agonal breathing: make sure to start **BiPAP** or even if compensated metabolic acidosis.
19. **Necrotizing infection**: bad, bad, bad, bad, broad-spectrum antibiotics and stat general surgery consult.

4/6/2018

1. Cardiomegaly, make sure to do echocardiogram.
2. **Kidney failure**, urinalysis with micro also needs complement levels, renal flow, and scan (renal ultrasound). **Vasculitis workup** if suspicion of systemic inflammatory disease as the cause for renal failure: C3, C4, CH50, ESR, P-ANCA, C-ANCA.
3. **Basic principles of diuretic dosing**: determine the effective dose.
4. A patient resistant to IV furosemide is not likely to respond to an equivalent IV dose of another loop diuretic, such as Bumex or torsemide. **Ototoxicity can be minimized** with continuous infusion of high-dose Lasix when higher doses of diuretics are needed.
5. Loop diuretics are highly protein-bound; **severe hypoalbuminemia (<2 g/day) reduces the delivery of diuretics to the renal tubule**. Maximal single IV diuretic doses: 160–200 mg furosemide; 8–10 mg bumetanide; 50–100 mg

torsemide. Can add **hydrochlorothiazide (HCTZ) or metolazone** to loop diuretics for refractory edema.

6. The **central venous pressure (CVP)** catheter is an important tool to assess right ventricular function and systemic fluid status. Normal CVP is 2–6 mm H_2O. CVP is elevated by: overhydration which increases venous return; heart failure or PA stenosis which limits venous outflow and leads to venous congestions; positive pressure breathing, and straining.
7. **Positive pressure breathing** like BiPAP and CPAP provides help to congestive heart failure (CHF) by decreasing preload.

4/7/2018

1. **Vocal cord dysfunction**, also known as (AKA) **paradoxical vocal fold motion disorder**, is characterized by adduction of the vocal cords during inspiration. **Symptoms** include mid-chest tightness, dyspnea, and lack of symptom relief with asthma treatment. It can happen in asthma, or related to performances (athletes) or exposure to certain irritants, such as smoke or perfume.
2. **Vocal cord dysfunction** treatment consists of **laryngeal control techniques, biofeedback, and relaxation techniques**, usually under the direction of a **speech pathologist**.
3. **Complicated parapneumonic effusion and empyema** should be suspected if no response to appropriate antibiotic therapy for pneumonia → Treatment with a small bore (10–14 Fr, 3.3–4.7 cm) thoracostomy tube.
4. Focal calcification anterior to the spine may represent **splenic venous thrombosis**.
5. **Post-intensive care syndrome**: new or worsening function in one or more physical cognitive or mental domains that continues after discharge following a critical illness.
6. **Critical illness neuromyopathy** refers to generalized **axonal sensorineural polyneuropathy** associated with severe illness and treatment in the ICU.
7. **High peak pressure** → indicates high airway resistance or low lung compliance. If it is from auto PEEP, may disconnect the ET tube for a few seconds.
8. In patients with hypoxemic respiratory failure due to **heart failure**, **noninvasive positive pressure ventilation** decreases the need for mechanical ventilation, improves respiratory parameters, and may decrease mortality.
9. **High-altitude pulmonary edema** is believed to be noncardiogenic and exaggerated hypoxic vasoconstriction of the pulmonary vasculature. **Symptoms and Signs**: dyspnea at rest, nausea and vomiting (N&V) disturbed sleep, tachycardia and tachypnea, crackles and wheezing, pink frothy sputum or front hemoptysis. Treatment: **O_2, rest, and consideration of descent from high altitude**. Vasodilators (nifedipine, phosphodiesterase-5 inhibitors, sildenafil, or tadalafil) can be used. **Diuretics besides acetazolamide** may be necessary.
10. **Acetazolamide** is the preferred drug for preventing acute mountain sickness and high-altitude cerebral edema.
11. **Ibuprofen** is reasonably the first choice for symptoms of mild acute mountain sickness, like headache (HA) and nausea.

12. **Isopropyl alcohol** does not increase the anion gap (AG). **Salicylate and acetaminophen** don't increase serum osmolarity but increase AG.
13. A normal A-a gradient is less than age in years divided by 4 + 4.
14. The chance of an effusion with a pleural fluid **adenosine deaminase (ADA) < 35 IU/L being tuberculosis (TB) is negligible**.

4/8/2018

1. AFib with rapid ventricular rate (RVR): if not responding to metoprolol 5 mg, may give **Cardizem 15 mg IV** then Cardizem drip (**contraindicated if decreased left ventricular ejection fraction**). If soft or low blood pressure, may give **amiodarone 150 mg IV** stat, which may be followed by drip (the only concern is cardioversion-induced blood clot, but if running out of options, this is the right intervention) → or **digoxin 0.5 mg iv** (followed by 0.25 mg every 6 h to a maximum of 1.5 mg over 24 h)
2. **Digoxin loading** 0.5 mg → 6 h later 0.25 mg → 12 h later 0.25 mg → then 0.125 mg qd.
3. **Pressure support ventilation** for pressure support 10/5 in weaning. BiPAP 16/6 for hypercapnia hypoxic respiratory failure.
4. **Tardive dyskinesia**: avoid dopamine antagonists.
5. **Cryptogenic stroke**: arrange for a 30-day event monitor as an outpatient; if unremarkable, arrange for a loop recorder.
6. **Antithrombin deficiency**: Type 1-**decreased** functional and immunological antithrombin level; Type II-decreased **functional antithrombin activity** when concentration is normal.
7. Intention to start the patient on warfarin, because of delay in factor II (prothrombin) suppression: **heparin is given concomitantly for 4–5 days to prevent thrombus propagation**.
8. **Isosorbide dinitrate** is short-acting whereas **isosorbide mononitrate** is long-acting.
9. If left ventricular ejection fraction (LVEF) < 40%, start angiotensin-converting enzyme inhibitor (ACEI), spironolactone, beta-blocker (BB), hydralazine, and Lasix. If the patient is allergies to ACEI, do **hydralazine 25 mg tid plus isosorbide dinitrate 20 mg tid** at the same time.
10. EKG ST elevation shape matters: **Convex** = consider ST elevation myocardial infarction (STEMI); **Concave** = consider non-ST elevation myocardial infarction (NSTEMI) and others. **LVEF** low will need workup to understand the cause, so does wall motion abnormalities under echocardiogram → may need **left cardiac catheterization**.
11. After 1–2 days with intracranial hemorrhage (ICH), we can consider adding anticoagulation therapy, weighing the competing risk of venous thromboembolism VTE (degree of immobility) versus the risk of hematoma expansion (BP control <140/90 mmHg, **spot sign**, hematoma volume). **The spot sign** is focal accumulation/pooling/extravasation of contrast-containing blood within the hematoma with CT angiogram of the head; it indicates a poor outcome.

12. Only patients (ICH survivors) with an exceptionally **high risk for atherothrombotic events should be treated with antiplatelet therapy**, and only those with high risk for cardioembolic stroke should be treated with **anticoagulation, but likely weeks later**.
13. The risk of ICH expansion and recurrence is highest in the first days after intracranial hemorrhage (ICH), while the risk of thromboembolism continues to accumulate over time. **The majority of patients who require anticoagulation can initiate the treatment between 7 and 14 days following an intracerebral hemorrhage (ICH).**
14. If **smoking history (Hx) and respiratory symptoms**, order DuoNeb. If tachycardia, give ipratropium bromide (Atrovent) and levosalbutamol (Xopenex).
15. **Post-surgical ileus**: Ok to give bethanechol (M1 parasympathetic receptor agonist) 10 mg × 3. **Neostigmine** IV inhibits acetylcholinesterase in smooth muscles of the intestines; may also be used in ileus but benefits may be very transient.
16. **Metabolic alkalosis**: treat with normal saline drip. **Metabolic acidosis** may be treated with diuresis or Lactate Ringers
17. **Chest X-ray (CXR)** for fluid status; pleural effusion may require **thoracentesis** to rule out **empyema**. An **extubation bundle** should be ordered upon extubation.
18. **Seizure rapid** management: Ativan 4 mg IV × 1; valium 5 mg IV; Keppra 1 g; or phenytoin 150 mg IV (may be used in combination). Continuous EEG and lactic acid may not need to be monitored in the ischemic bowel.

4/11/2018

1. Patients admitted for chronic obstructive pulmonary disease (COPD) exacerbation with good oxygen saturation, venous blood gas (VBG) revealed pH 7.2. Treatment: **BiPAP** 16/6 or 18/6.
2. If chronic kidney injury (CKD) or kidney insufficiency, **Enoxaparin sodium (Lovenox)** dosing will need adjustment as it is excreted through the kidney only.
3. **Moxifloxacin** does not need renal adjustment whereas Levaquin does.
4. **Combivent** cross-reacts with peanut allergy. **Latex** cross-reacts with papaya/tropical fruits.
5. Watch **Ins/Outs** as many patients benefit from negative fluid balance.
6. Allergies to fish = consider **iodine** contrast allergy. **Metabolic acidosis**: BiCarb 50 mg in 1/2NS at 60 cc/h (used mainly in hyperkalemia, serum $HCO_3 < 10$, or $pH < 7.1$).
7. A-a gradient essentially documents a high respiratory effort, and low arterial PCO_2 relative to the achieved level of oxygenation (arterial O_2). **Normal A-a gradient**: patient's age/4 + 4. **Corrected calcium** = 0.8× (normal albumin—measured albumin) + serum calcium.
8. **Seashore sign**: normal lung slide (physiological ultrasound appearance); **barcode/stratosphere sign**: pneumothorax/bullae.

4/12/2018

1. **Dexmedetomidine (Precedex)** is only used for sedation if no hemodynamical instability and extubation in 24 h.
2. **Fentanyl** is used for pain with sedation. **Versed** for sedation and anxiety. **Propofol** patients feel but have amnesia; **Precedex** only calms the patient. **Suboptimal sedation** can cause physical stress such as unplanned extubations or catheter removal, and psychological stress such as anxiety.
3. High temperature but normal or low heart rate = consider **typhoid fever**, a life-threatening infection of Salmonella Typhi.
4. Acute patients may order troponin to assess severity.
5. **Upper gastrointestinal (GI) bleed in liver failure**: Esophagogastroduodenoscopy (EGD) with banding urgently; transjugular intrahepatic portosystemic shunt (TIPS) from interventional radiology (IR); packed red blood cells (PRBC) and fresh frozen plasma (FFP); pantoprazole (Protonix); octreotide 50 ug bolus and the drip; ceftriaxone, cipro, or Levaquin for 7 days. May also give IV Vit K.
6. Concerns for **decompensating if continuous desaturation even after BiPAP** or on a ventilator, consider the next step of care or goals of care discussions.
7. **Mass transfusion protocol**: If transfuse ≥6 units of PRBC, will need to transfuse 4–6 u FFP and 6 u pooled donor platelets (PLTs). 30 μg/kg vitamin K to reverse INR
8. **Large volume paracentesis** (>5 L ascites fluid removal): Supplementing **5–8 g of albumin per liter** over 5 L of ascitic fluid removed to decrease complications associated with paracentesis. Potential complications from large volume paracentesis include **electrolyte imbalances** and **increases in serum creatinine** levels secondary to large shifts of intravascular volume.

4/16/2018

1. **Warfarin reversal**: clinically significant bleeding treatment with vit K 5–10 mg IV, and **Prothrombinex-VF** (a three-factor prothrombin complex concentrate, **PCC**, also known as **Kcentra**) 50 iu/kg iv and fresh frozen plasma (FFP) 150–300 mL. If PCC unavailable, administer FFP at **15 cc/kg**; INR greater than therapeutic range but <4.5 and no bleeding, lower or omit the next dose of warfarin; INR 4.5–10 and no bleeding, cease warfarin if bleeding risk is high, consider K 1–2 mg orally or 0.5 mg to 1 mg IV; INR > 10 and no bleeding, iv vit K 3–5 mg IV, if bleeding risk high, do PCC 15–30 mg/kg.
2. **Prothrombinex VF (PCC)** completely reverses INR in **15 min**. **Vit K is essential for sustaining the reversal**.
3. Management for patients on warfarin undergoing procedures: if necessary, warfarin can be **held for 5 days before surgery**. Or **iv vit k** can be given the night before surgery.
4. High risk for thrombosis, bridge when INR < 2 with low molecular weight heparin (LMWH) or unfractionated heparin (UFH). If LMWH, hold it **24 h** before surgery; if UFH, hold it **4–6 h** before surgery. After surgery, start LMWH/UFH 12–24 h postoperatively. **If LMWH, begin with prophylactic dose; if UFH,**

avoid bolus. Delay resumption of therapeutic dose LMWH 48–72 h after surgery if high bleeding risk. Continue LMWH/UFH for a minimum of 5 days and cease 48 h after target INR is achieved.

5. **Cefepime virtually has no anaerobic coverage**.

4/21/2018

1. Seizing: head foot trembling/tremors.
2. "We will try ...this/that if not working, then we try comfort care." **Common treatments for dyspnea**: diuretics if concerns for fluid overload, nebulizer, O_2, steroids like iv Solu-Medrol if smoking history or known chronic obstructive lung disease, BiPAP if known CO_2 retention.
3. **VFib and VTach** → shock/epi → × 2 shocks then amiodarone → bicarb, Mag++ stabilizer.
4. Rapid, if the patient seizes, call an anesthesiologist for **intubation** if the patient is unable to protect the airway, **ACLS** (**code blue**) anesthesiologist comes in automatically.
5. Consider giving fluid or diuretics in urgent conditions.
6. **Sinus tachycardia** if above 150, give calcium channel blocker (CCB)/beta blocker. If fluid overload, caution CCB is used as the patient may have decreased left ventricular ejection fraction.
7. **Syncope etiologies:** reflex syncope (**vasovagal, reflex syncope**); **orthostatic** syncope; **cardiac arrhythmia; structural cardiopulmonary disease**; if the total loss of consciousness, has to rule out **seizures**, sleep disturbances; accidental falls; some psychiatric conditions like psychogenic pseudosyncope or **pseudo-seizure**.

4/22/2018

1. **Mitochondrial disease treatments**: **CoQ 10**, lipoic acid, folic acid, vit D2, B12 injection, creatine, **levocarnitine**, ribose for glycogen storage disorder.
2. No spironolactone if chronic kidney disease (CKD) or acute kidney injury (AKI).
3. **Prednisolone** is not metabolized in the liver; prescribe **nadolol** only if EGD notices variceal bleeding and the patient is not in acute liver decompensation.
4. **Acetaminophen intoxication**: liver dysfunction may not present for 2–6 days. Treatment: **Nasogastric lavage**, activated charcoal if within 4 h of ingestion, **N-acetylcysteine (NAC)**, administered **up to 72 h after ingestion**. If the time of ingestion is unknown or chronic ingestion >4 g/day, low threshold to start NAC with low or undetectable acetaminophen (APAP) levels. Oral NAc is preferred, loading dose **140 mg/kg -> 70 mg/kg q4h × 17** additional doses. IV NAc (if unable to tolerate po, GIB, pregnancy, ALF): 150 mg/kg × 1 h → 50 mg/kg in total over 4 h → 100 mg/kg over 16 h. **Labs**: CMP 2 h before NAC (antidote), repeat LFT, INR, acetaminophen level, mag, phosphate level.
5. **Therapeutic misadventure**: injury or an adverse event caused by medical management rather than an underlying disease.
6. **Crohn's flareup**: IV Solu-Medrol 40 mg iv q12h; mild disease, treat with 5-aminosalicylic acid (5-ASA) like sulfasalazine 4–6 g/day. **Mild-moderate**

disease: budesonide oral. **Moderate-severe disease**: oral prednisone, 5-aminosalicylic acid (5-ASA), 6-mercaptopurine (6-MP), or methotrexate (MTX) 15–20 mg/week. **Severe or refractory**: anti-tumor necrosis factor (TNF) agents, vedolizumab (Entyvio), or ustekinumab (Stelara). May need to **add fluoroquinolone and Flagyl** for perianal disease, strictures, fistulas, and abscesses.

7. **Dwelling time (duration for use) for catheters**: peripheral catheter 96 h; midline 1–4 weeks; PICC 2–4 weeks; central tunneled catheter >6 months; central non-tunneled catheter 5–10 days; central implanted port can stay as long as it needs to be (accessed through a **non-coring Huber needle inserted through the skin which should be changed q7d**).
8. Total parenteral nutrition (TPN), vasopressors, chemo meds, amiodarone, and nicardipine should be **infused through a central line.**
9. Peripheral line administration of **IV amiodarone is associated with a great risk of thrombophlebitis**.
10. **Nicardipine** should be administered via a central or large vein to decrease the risk of extravasation, venous thrombosis, phlebitis, local irritation, swelling, and rarely vascular impairment. **Peripheral infusion sites for nicardipine infusion should be changed q12h to minimize the risk of venous irritation**.
11. **Flushes:** peripheral intravenous (PIV) line should be flushed q12h, midline and peripherally inserted central catheter (PICC) line q24h with saline; **central tunneled catheter q24h with 2.5 ml heparin**; central non-tunneled, flush q8h with 10 ml saline. Also, flush after a blood draw or administration of blood products.
12. "I'm not sure whether I have explained this well. So, if you don't mind, please tell me what you think I was trying to say."
13. **Cardiac resynchronization therapy indications:** (1) VEF $\leq$ 35%, NYHA Class II to IV symptoms, LBBB, or QRS $\geq$ 150 ms of any morphology; (2) non-LBBB, QRS 120–150 ms, NYHA Class II to IV. Congestive heart failure (CHF) outpatient follow-up should be within 1 week.

Anesthesiology

4/27/2018 Glidoscope Intubation.

1. **Induction**: give propofol 100–150 mg → give paralytic rocuronium 36–60 mg (induction time 60–90 s) or succinylcholine 80–100 mg (30 s).
2. Feel the lash, ask to see movement or not → tilt head and neck, widely open mouth, bagging to see air in the face.
3. Bagging if CO_2 increases and to maintain SO_2.
4. Put glidoscope (C shape) in the center of the tongue and mouth, pull up → slide the tube along the C-shape glidoscope, see, and put in. Once in, inject 5 cc (half) air to secure → bagging.

4/28/2018

1. Concerns for **small bowel obstruction**: order **small bowel follow through**, order generic order for radiology, add comments: please give gastrografin via NG tube.
2. **Acute liver failure** refers to the development of severe acute liver injury with **encephalopathy and impaired synthetic function** (INR > 1.5) in a patient without cirrhosis or preexisting liver disease, disease duration <26 weeks.
3. Acute liver failure is diagnosed by all the following: **elevated aminotransferases, hepatic encephalopathy, and INR > 1.5**
4. **Diagnostic tests for acute liver failure**: PT/INR, GGT, CMP/LFT, acetaminophen level, toxicology screen, viral hepatitis, pregnancy test, arterial blood gas (ABG), autoimmune markers (ANA, anti-smooth muscle Ab, anti-liver-kidney microsomal Ab type 1, Ig levels), lactic acid, ammonia, HIV, amylase and lipase.
5. **Causes of unconjugated hyperbilirubinemia**: **overproduction** (hemolysis, Wilson disease, extravasation, shunt, hyperbilirubinemia); **reduced uptake** (portosystemic shunt, drugs, Gilbert syndrome); **conjugate defect**-acquired neonatal, maternal milk, Lucy-Driscoll syndrome, hyperthyroidism, chronic persistent hepatitis, advanced hepatitis; inherited Crigler-Najjar I&II, Gilbert syndrome.
6. **Lucey–Driscoll syndrome** is an autosomal recessive metabolic disorder affecting enzymes involved in bilirubin metabolism. It is one type of transient familial neonatal unconjugated hyperbilirubinemia.
7. **Causes of mixed conjugated and unconjugated hyperbilirubinemia**: biliary obstruction; intrahepatic cholestasis (primary biliary cirrhosis, primary sclerosing cholangitis, viral hepatitis, progressive familial intrahepatic cholestasis, intrahepatic cholestasis of pregnancy, corticosteroid use); hepatocellular injury; hepatocellular defects of canalicular excretion or sinusoidal reuptake (Dubin-Johnson, Rotor syndrome)
8. Patients with **primary sclerosing cholangitis (PSC)** usually (up to 60%–90%) also have inflammatory bowel disease, the concurrence of which increases risks for colorectal cancer. PSC occurs in 5% of inflammatory bowel disease.

5/3/2018

1. Acute dyspnea, B-type natriuretic peptide (BNP) < 100 pg/ml; congestive heart failure exacerbation unlikely (BNP not reliable in obese patients); 400 - congestive heart failure exacerbation likely; 100–400, use clinical judgment. BNP is an active hormone with a shorter half-life whereas **NT-proBNP** is not biologically active with **a longer half-life**. Pro BNP (metabolized into C-terminal BNP and N-terminal pro-BNP) is secreted by cardiomyocytes under stretch.
2. NT-pro BNP < 300 pg heart failure (HF) unlikely; age < 50, NT-pro BNP > 450-HF likely. Age 50–70, NT-pro BNP > 900 HF likely. Age > 75, NT-pro BNP > 1800 pg/ml, HF likely.
3. **Elevated BNP** is also seen in chronic kidney disease (CKD) and acute kidney injury (AKI), HTN, pulmonary diseases like chronic obstructive pulmonary dis-

ease (COPD), acute respiratory distress syndrome (ARDS), pulmonary hypertension (HTN), cardiac causes including myocardial infarction (MI), AFib, cardioversion, valvular heart disease, and myocarditis, old age, female sex, liver cirrhosis, hyperthyroidism, sepsis, chemotherapy.
4. **Conditions associated with lower-than-normal BNP**: obesity, flash pulmonary edema, and pericardial effusion.

5/6/2018

1. Shortness of breath (SOB) and tachycardia: **EKG to see whether it is AFib**. **Chest X-ray** (CXR) to see if the volume is overloaded. Lasix, Duoneb now than qid. High flow oxygen (only provides oxygen and does not help eliminate CO_2) versus BiPAP (helps get rid of CO_2 while providing oxygen). **Chest pain:** check EKG and troponin.
2. Pneumothorax, once the lung fully expands, do a CT chest to see blebs.
3. **LDH and haptoglobin** to see if hemolysis.
4. Congestive heart failure with reduced ejection fraction (CHFrEF) of 25% on Neo-Synephrine will push the patient into CHF exacerbation if, at the same time, the patient was given fluid which certainly made things worse.

Takeaway Messages

1. Ventilator medications: pain assessment and if pain, prescribe analgesic (morphine, hydromorphone, fentanyl) → decide a sedation strategy (daily interruption of sedation, sedation scale-based protocol, or no sedation) and choose sedatives: midazolam (caution use in renal failure), propofol (rapid wake-up), and dexmedetomidine (decreased sedation needs and rapid wake-up).
2. High-risk extubation management: attend to reversible risk factors, cuff leak test, pretreatment with IV steroids, and use of high flow after extubation.
3. Status epilepticus treatment: IV lorazepam 2 mg iv (may repeat another 2 mg), followed by fosphenytoin 20 mg/kg PE or Keppra and intubation, cEEG, and sedation with propofol or phenobarbital.
4. Anaphylaxis (acute dyspnea from an allergic reaction): Benadryl 50 mg IV (may add famotidine 20 mg iv), solumedrol 125 mg IV, and epinephrine 0.3 mg IM q5min for 4–5 doses.
5. Timely specialist consult and initiate goals of care discussions.

Further Readings and References

1. Patel, S.B., and J.P. Kress. 2012. Sedation and analgesia in the mechanically ventilated patient. *American Journal of Respiratory and Critical Care Medicine* 185 (5): 486–497.
2. Yang, Z., and G.L. Xiong. *Alcohol-related psychosis medication*, ed. A. Hategan. MedScape. https://emedicine.medscape.com/article/289848-medication. Accessed November 6, 2023.
3. Hopkins, C. *Hypertensive emergencies*, ed. B. Brenner. MedScape. https://emedicine.medscape.com/article/1952052-overview#a2. Accessed November 6, 2023.

4. Drislane, F.W. *Convulsive status epilepticus in adults: Management*, ed. P. Garcia, J. Edlow, and A.A. Rabinstein. Waltham, MA: UpToDate. Accessed November 10, 2023.
5. Heard, K., and R. Dart. *Acetaminophen (paracetamol) poisoning in adults: Treatment*, ed. R.G. Hendrickson. Waltham, MA: UpToDate. Accessed November 10, 2023.
6. Roy-Chowdhury, N., and J. Roy-Chowdhury. *Classification and causes of jaundice or asymptomatic hyperbilirubinemia*, ed. S. Chopra and E.B. Rand. Waltham, MA: UpToDate. Accessed November 10, 2023.

Chapter 8
The Endocrinology World

Ambulatory Endocrinology Rotation: May 7th, 2018 Through June 3rd, 2018
The endocrinology rotation is an ambulatory outpatient rotation. Per Center for Disease Control data, in the United States, 8.9% of the US population had been diagnosed with diabetes. The majority of patients in the endocrinology clinic are patients with diabetes and most of the time, diabetes management is their sole purpose for the outpatient visits. Undoubtedly, understanding the pathophysiology, treatments, and complications of diabetes is the key objective of this rotation. This chapter included the details on different categories of diabetes medications and the prescription of diabetic monitoring supplies.

Following diabetes, other common endocrinopathies include hypothyroidism and hyperthyroidism, lipid disorders, hyperparathyroidism, osteoporosis, adrenal insufficiency and Cushing disease and syndrome, hypogonadism, polycystic ovarian syndrome, premature ovarian insufficiency, pituitary gland abnormalities. While the rotation itself focused more on the treatment of specific endocrinopathies, we do need to understand the first and second lines of lab tests for the diagnosis of common endocrinological diseases: low dose cortisol suppression (24-h urine free cortisol, or 11 p.m. salivary cortisol) for Cushing's, insulin-like growth factor 1 (IGF-1) for acromegaly, plasma aldosterone renin ratio >20 for primary hyperaldosteronism, plasma-free metanephrines (after 30 min in supine position) followed by 24 h urinary fractionated metanephrines and catecholamines for pheochromocytoma.

Of note, because of the common scenarios of inpatient testing requirements, information on some of these tests was covered in other chapters, such as tests for pheochromocytoma in patients with resistant hypertension, adrenal insufficiency (morning cortisol and Cosyntropin stimulation test if morning cortisol >3–5 mg/dL but less than 10–18 mg/dL) in patients with persistent hypotension, hypercalcemia in patients on or off vitamin D and calcium supplements, autoimmune workups for type 1 diabetes in patients with latent onset type 1 diabetes, and thyroid storm and myxedema coma in patients with obvious thyroid function abnormalities.

K. Zhou, *Internal Medicine Training Notes and Survival Guide*,
https://doi.org/10.1007/978-1-0716-4039-5_8

5/7/2018

1. Cr. 1.7/1.5 for **metformin use cutpoint**; metformin should be stopped if creatinine is higher than 1.5/1.7.
2. **Hyperthyroidism ablation dose 25 mg iodine 131**; thyroid **cancer treatment** dose **100–150 mg I131**; also check thyroid stimulating hormone (TSH) and free T4 for thyroid cancer with **target TSH 1–2 after total thyroidectomy** together **with remnant ablation** for benign disease, medullary thyroid carcinoma, or anaplastic thyroid carcinoma with measurements of TSH every 4–6 weeks. Before iodine 131 ablation, optimize TSH level to ≥30 mIU/mL with **thyroid hormone withdrawal** (stop levothyroxine treatment 3–4 weeks before ablation). Exogenous administration of recombinant human **TSH (rhTSH)** or triiodothyronine can be used in the short term to prevent overt hypothyroidism during thyroid hormone withdrawal.
3. Victoza (liraglutide), and Trulicity (dulaglutide) are **glucagon-like peptide-1 (GLP-1)** agonists; Januvia (sitagliptin) is a **dipeptidyl peptidase-4 (DPP-4) inhibitor**. DPP-4 breaks down the incretins of GLP-1 and GIP (gastrointestinal hormones) which stimulate insulin release and inhibit glucagon release. Janumet = sitagliptin + metformin.
4. **Hyperparathyroidism**: check Vit D, dual X-ray absorptiometry (DEXA) scan, kidney stone, Ca++, ionized Ca++, parathyroid hormone (PTH), fracture, stones, bone density (q2y). **T score of −2.5 or less indicates osteoporosis**. **Treatment**: for medical management, prescribe moderate calcium and Vit D intake, cinacalcet if symptomatic hypercalcemia, and alendronate if osteoporosis. **Parathyroidectomy** is recommended if any one of the following: eGFR <60 mL/min/1.73 m^2, 24-h urine for calcium >250 mg/day (6.25 mmol/day) in women and >300 mg/day (7.5 mmol/day) in men, kidney stone on imaging study, vertebral fracture, osteoporosis, age < 50 years, or serum calcium >1 mg/dL above upper limit normal.
5. **Cinacalcet** (a calcimimetic) increases the sensitivity of the calcium-sensing receptor on the parathyroid gland thereby, concomitantly lowering parathyroid hormone (PTH), serum calcium, and serum phosphorus levels.
6. Normal bone density is T score ≥ −1. Osteopenia = −1 – −2.5. **Osteoporosis ≤ −2.5.**
7. **Candidates for treatment of osteoporosis in postmenopausal women**: (A) Osteoporosis or fragility fractures; (B) Osteopenia patients with a 10-year probability of **hip fracture** or combined major osteoporotic fracture of **3% or 20%** respectively [calculated using Fracture Risk Assessment Tool (FRAX)]. Treatment: alendronate, risedronate. Oral ibandronate may be used in postmenopausal osteoporosis.
8. Postmenopausal women with severe osteoporosis can be treated with anabolic agents like **teriparatide (Forteo). Severe osteoporosis = T score < −3.5 or T score ≤ −2.5 plus a fragility fracture (fracture from fall from standing height or less)**.

9. Patients with **esophageal disorders** (achalasia, scleroderma involving the esophagus, esophageal strictures, varices), **gastrointestinal (GI) intolerance to oral bisphosphonates**, **history of Roux-en-Y gastric bypass**, or an inability to follow the dosing requirement including sitting upright for 30–60 min and/or to swallow a pill, should be treated with **IV zoledronic acid or denosumab (Prolia)**.
10. **Denosumab (Prolia)** is an option for patients unresponsive to other therapies and in those with impaired renal function; however, in the absence of contraindications, it may be beneficial to treat with **teriparatide [recombinant formulation of endogenous parathyroid hormone (PTH)] first (max of 2 years) followed by denosumab forever**.
11. Thyroid gland <5 cm is normal. **Thyroid nodules ≥10 mm** need biopsy; thyroid nodules with **central vascularity** with size 5 mm or greater also need biopsy. Coarse vs. fine calcifications, **fine calcification** needs biopsy.
12. **Graves' disease takes 2 years of therapy to go back to remission**. The diagnosis of Graves' disease is based on clinical symptoms, iodine 123 (shorter half-life than I131) uptake, positive thyroid-stimulating immunoglobulin (**TSI**), and thyrotropin-binding inhibitory immunoglobulin (**TBII**).
13. **Type 2 diabetes mellitus (T2DM) regimen**: HA1c 7.5%, glimepiride 4 mg qd, metformin 1 g bid, OneTouch Delica® lancet extra Pen 33G tid, OneTouch Verio® test strips tid. Pioglitazone 30 mg qd. Tresiba flex touch 100u qd. dulaglutide (Trulicity) 1.5 mg subcu qwk.
14. Type 2 diabetes mellitus (T2DM) treatment: HA1c 6.3%, glimepiride 4 mg qd, Lantus 55u qhs, metformin 1 g bid, liraglutide (Victoza) subcu 1.8 mg qd.
15. Type 2 diabetes mellitus (T2DM) treatment: metformin 1 g bid, canagliflozin (Invokana) 300 mg qd, tresiba 130u qhs, liraglutide (Trulicity) 1.5 mg qwk, Novolog 40u with dinner.

5/8/2018

1. Type 2 diabetes mellitus (T2DM) HA1c 7% treatment: Lantus 16u qam, 18u qpm, metformin 500 mg qd. OneTouch® Delica® lancets 33G tid.
2. **Lisinopril for diabetes mellitus (DM)** should be 40 mg qd, 20 mg, or 10 mg qd as appropriate.
3. No need to put a patient on both liraglutide (Victoza) and sitagliptin (Januvia), a dipeptidyl peptidase-4 inhibitor, at the same time. **Concurrent use of GLP-1 with dipeptidyl peptidase-4 inhibitor provides no added-on benefits**.
4. Ok to combine fenofibrate (NOT other fibrates) and atorvastatin but NOT simvastatin.
5. Currently, patients with **coronary artery disease (CAD) or CAD risk equivalent** [e.g., stroke, aortic aneurysm, peripheral artery disease (PAD), diabetes mellitus (DM), metabolic syndrome] or multiple CAD risk factors conferring a risk of CVA ≥ 30%; should have an LDL target of <100 and **optimally < 70**.

5/9/2018

1. Fasting glucose not controlled; add sodium-glucose cotransporter-2 (SGLT-2) inhibitors; carvedilol (Coreg) 25 mg qd better than metoprolol succinate 100 mg qd for blood pressure control.
2. **Tresiba half-life is 28 h**, longer than Lantus. Toujeo concentrated 300 u/ml; Toujeo max
3. Gestational diabetes mellitus (DM) **glucose target is <120 mg for 2 h after meal**.
4. Electronic Libra View and Dexcom. Fine needle aspiration (FNA) atypical significance → repeat FNA in ≥ 6 weeks.
5. **AFIRMA (a molecular analysis) genetic testing of FNA if atypical cells in the thyroid gland.**
6. **Estradiol level in menopause usually is <30 pg/mL.**
7. **Insulin pump setup: basal rate** at 0.4 u/h (can set periods); **bolus** setting [sensitivity, Insulin Sensitivity Factor (ISF), correction] 50 mg/dL/u [one unit of insulin to lower a specific amount of glucose (in mg/dL)]; **insulin to carb** ratio 15 g/u. Active insulin time 4 h. Blood glucose target 12 a.m.–3 a.m. 140 mg/dL; 3 a.m.–11 p.m. 110 mg/dL; 11 p.m.–12 a.m. 140 mg/dL (blood glucose correction threshold).
8. **Pregnancy increases insulin resistance**; insulin pump for insulin dosing; Dexcom (a continuous glucose monitoring system) for glucose level monitoring.
9. Dispense as written (DAW); Synthroid (levothyroxine) is NOT generic.
10. Preferred diabetes medications (sequence of addition): **Metformin → glucagon-like peptide-1 (GLP-1) agonist → sodium-glucose cotransporter-2 (SGLT-2) → sulfonylureas.**
11. Thyroid cancer after surgery, do iodine131 reuptake → ultrasound 5 years later for follicular thyroid cancer.
12. Transgender (**male to female**) treatment: estradiol and spironolactone maintenance.
13. **Thyroid nodule tests**: TSH, FT4 in 6 m; annual US.
14. **Thyroxine complete (full) replacement** 1.6 u/kg/day.
15. **Subclinical hypothyroidism** first trimester TSH target ≤2.5; second and third trimester target ≤3.
16. **Levothyroxine half-life** is 5–7 days. It takes **4–6 weeks** to stabilize.
17. Hair loss due to fluctuating hormones (**decrease in estrogen and progesterone and increase in dihydrotestosterone**).
18. High parathyroid hormone (PTH), repeat PTH in 6 m; check Vit D; **stop hydrochlorothiazide (HCTZ)**, check **bone scan** as high PTH causes fractures and kidney stone; no need to stop Vit D in high PTH.
19. **Polycystic ovarian syndrome (PCOS)**: metformin increases pregnancy chances. **Tirosint** is gluten-free levothyroxine.
20. **Thyroid stimulating hormone (TSH)** goal 0.1–0.5 mU/L for 5–10 years in high-risk patients after thyroidectomy. TSH target is 0.1–0.5 mU/L in low-risk patients (with papillary thyroid cancer) but TSH initially should be suppressed to below 0.1 mU/L in high- and intermediate-risk thyroid cancer.

21. TSH < 0.01 check antibodies [thyroid-stimulating immunoglobulin (TSI) and thyrotropin-binding inhibitory immunoglobulin (TBII)]. **If positive → do I123 uptake scan → if a hot nodule and symptomatic, treat with thyroidectomy, radioablation, and/or methimazole. If toxic adenoma or toxic multigoiter nodules (based on TSH and thyroid ultrasound), treatment is radioiodine ablation, surgical resection, ultrasound-guided ablative procedures, or thionamide therapy.**
22. Dipeptidyl peptidase 4 (**DPP-4**) inhibitors (may need adjustment) and glucagon-like peptide-1 (**GLP-1**) agonists are safe for chronic kidney disease (CKD). Sitagliptin (Januvia) is an DPP-4 inhibitor and it needs dose adjustment for CKD.
23. **Microadenoma of pituitary workups**: TSH, free T4, T3 total, thyroid peroxidase antibodies (TPA), TSI, thyroglobulin Ab, ACTH, Am cortisol, prolactin, insulin-like growth factor-1 (IGF-1), FSH/LH, and estradiol.
24. MRI/CT adrenal protocol for **adrenal adenoma workup**: 24 h urine metanephrine/catecholamines, plasma metanephrine, morning cortisol, ACTH, salivary cortisol, urine Cr 24 h (to see the appropriateness of sample), plasma renin activity, plasma aldosterone, and urine 17-ketosteroids.

5/10/2018

1. **Humalog** acting time 15–30 min; with meals is to give insulin right away when eating.
2. HA1c 5.6%, we need to decrease Lantus even though it has been good in glucose control.
3. **Gestational diabetes mellitus (DM)**: 30–45 g carb for breakfast and lunch, 60 g or less for dinner. 2 h postprandial glucose in gestation targets <120 mg/dL; fasting glucose targets **95 or less**. If the patient fails an oral glucose tolerance test (OGTT), the patient can be started on **metformin (safe in pregnancy).**
4. Primary prevention: persons of 40–75 years old without DM with LDL of 70–189 mg/dL, estimate 10-year atherosclerotic cardiovascular disease (ASCVD) risk q4-6 y; reemphasize heart-healthy lifestyle habits and address other risk factors. **≥7.5%** risks, prescribe **moderate to high-intensity statin**. If 5%–7.5% risks of 10-year ASCVD risk, consider moderate-intensity statin.
5. Statin therapy is not recommended for individuals with NYHA class II to IV **heart failure** or who are receiving maintenance **hemodialysis** if **no other indications (peripheral artery disease, coronary artery disease, or hyperlipidemia) for statin use**.
6. **Jardiance** (empagliflozin) 25 mg qd, **Kombiglyze** (Saxagliptin/Metformin) 2.5–100 mg bid. Saxagliptin is also known as Onglyza.
7. Pregnancy diabetes screening recommends OGTT 3 h, **glucose at 1 h, 2 h, and 3 h after ingestion of 100 g glucose should be less than 180/155/140**; usually starts with OGTT with 50 g glucose and check glucose 1 h after, if abnormal (>140), perform OGTT3h.
8. Ablation for hyperthyroidism. **Stop methimazole 5 mg qd 4 days prior, ideally 7 days before ablation.**

9. **Subclinical hyperthyroidism**: if TSH < 0.01, then do radioactive iodine uptake (RAIU) 30% (<38% normal) homogenous; still diagnosed as Graves' disease (will need to check antibodies). Treatment remains controversial: **consider treatment if TSH < 0.01 and increased risk for CVD or osteopenia**.
10. **Mild ophthalmopathy** in Graves' disease: do prednisone 20 mg qd for a couple of weeks. If severe, do not prescribe steroids as it can worsen symptoms after radioactive iodine (RAI) ablation; can be treated with radiation and/or surgical decompression of orbits.

5/12/2018

1. **Cardiorenal syndrome**: Type 1 (acute)- acute heart failure (HF) results in acute kidney injury (AKI); Type II-chronic cardiac dysfunction causes progressive chronic kidney disease (CKD). Type III- abrupt and primary worsening of kidney function due to—i.e., renal ischemia or glomerulonephritis causes acute heart dysfunction. Type IV—primary CKD contributes to cardiac dysfunction. Type V (secondary)- acute or chronic systemic disease, like sepsis, or diabetes mellitus (DM) that causes both cardiac and renal dysfunction.
2. **Treatment of cardiorenal syndrome (CRS)**: (A) prescribe diuretic therapy to eliminate fluid retention even though this may cause asymptomatic mild to moderate reduction in blood pressure and renal function; (B) ok to prescribe angiotensin-converting enzyme inhibitor in CRS but should monitor for hyperkalemia and worsening kidney function; (C) ultrafiltration is reasonable for patients with refractory congestion not responding to medical therapy.

5/13/2018

1. **Heparin-induced thrombocytopenia (HIT) treatment**: argatroban and warfarin; stop argatroban when warfarin INR = 4. Anticoagulation is required for 3 months.
2. Pulmonary hypertension (HTN) from obstructive sleep apnea (OSA) can cause bradycardia. **Chronotropic response** in bradycardia is good: increased heart rate (HR) with exercise (the opposite is called chronotropic incompetence). Bradycardia will need to check head CT, Echo, stress test, and telemetry. **Corevalve in transcatheter aortic valve replacement (TAVR)** can compress the conduction system leading to **conduction blockage.**
3. Bifascicular block needs a pacemaker possibly. **Leukocytosis and/or persistent tachycardia will need blood culture to rule out endocarditis.**
4. When creatine phosphokinase also known as creatine kinase is below 5000, it is ok to stop normal saline.
5. In cardiac amyloidosis, we should **avoid digoxin (arrhythmogenic) and beta-blocker (no benefit).**
6. **Amiodarone** has to be stopped 48 h before ablation as it interferes with mapping. After cardioversion, **anticoagulation for 4 weeks**. AFib with moderate mitral stenosis should be on warfarin even if the CHA2D2VASc score is 1.
7. **Valvular atrial fibrillation** refers to **moderate or severe mitral stenosis** or a mechanical heart valve with atrial fibrillation.

8. **Echo left ventricular ejection fraction (LVEF) 35%–40%**, 40-day medical management regardless of coronary artery bypass grafting (CABG) or stenting is recommended. If no improvement after 40 days of medical treatment after myocardial infarction, will need a defibrillator.
9. If the patient is on Aldactone, we need to closely monitor K+.
10. Need fasting for 8 h or more before transesophageal echocardiogram (TEE).
11. **Coronary artery disease (CAD) with coronary artery stenosis, at least 70%, will need fractional flow reserve (FFR) and nuclear stress test to see whether it is critical ischemia**. **Intravascular ultrasound** (IVUS) may be necessary for better visualization of coronary calcification.
12. **Aldactone** is indicated in patients with diabetes mellitus (DM), low ejection fraction (EF) $\leq$ 35%, acute myocardial infarction (AMI), congestive heart failure (CHF) New York Heart Association (NYHA) stage II, or worse.
13. **If surgery is planned, no ACEi or ARB for 1–2 days given concerns for intraoperative hypotension**; beta blocker can be continued during surgery if coronary artery disease (CAD) or congestive heart failure (CHF).
14. **Takotsubo** does not require anticoagulation per se and no need for high-intensity statin if the cholesterol profile is reasonable but should be started on coronary artery disease (CAD) and/or congestive heart failure (CHF) treatment if ST-elevation myocardial infarction (STEMI). **Takotsubo syndrome has a high risk for arrhythmia**.
15. Non-ST elevation myocardial infarction (NSTEMI) with left ventricular ejection fraction (LVEF) of 40%–45%, will need **repeat echocardiogram** to see if ejection fraction (EF) recovers in 4–6 weeks.
16. **Fractional flow reserve (FFR) <0.8** indicates hemodynamically significant stenosis (70% stenosis); **abnormal wall motion →** thrombosis prone and indicates myocardial infarction.
17. **Dose-dependent benefits** with beta blocker and angiotensin-converting enzyme inhibitor (ACEi).
18. **Indications for rhythm control**: persistent symptoms despite adequate rate control; unable to attain adequate rate control to prevent tachycardia-mediated cardiomyopathy; patient preference.
19. **Causes of AFib**: thyroid issues, hypertension (HTN), CHF, obstructive sleep apnea (OSA), excess alcohol intake, cardiac surgery, pericarditis, and pulmonary embolism (PE).
20. **Wellens syndrome (STEMI equivalent)**: deeply inverted or biphasic T waves in V2-3, which is highly specific for a critical stenosis of the LAD artery. Etiologies: (1) A sudden occlusion of the LAD (angina); (2) Reperfusion of LAD (ST elevation improves and T waves biphasic or inverted identical to patients who reperfuses); (3) The coronary reperfusion is unstable and LAD can reocclude at any time, normalization of the T wave indicates pseudo-normalization. Wellens syndrome should be treated like STEMI.
21. **Low A/G ratio (albumin/globulin)** indicates ulcerative colitis (UC), burns, chronic kidney disease (CKD), cirrhosis, and multiple myeloma (MM).

22. **Combined oral contraceptives (OCP)** prevent ovulation by suppressing the release of gonadotropins. It inhibits follicular development and prevents ovulation.

5/14/2018

1. Low parathyroid hormone = low ionized calcium, but normal plasma calcium (total).
2. Cholecalciferol (D3) → 1,25-OH-Vit D (calcitriol). **Calcitriol is effective in preventing glucocorticoid-induced and post-transplant-related bone loss**.
3. Conservative management of **hyperparathyroidism-related hypercalcemia**: (A) avoid thiazides and lithium carbonate therapy, volume depletion, prolonged bed rest or inactivity and high calcium diet (>1000 mg/day); (B) encourage physical activity to minimize bone absorption; (C) encourage hydration (≥6–8 glasses of water/day) to minimize nephrolithiasis; (D) maintain calcium intake 1000 mg/day and vitamin D 400–800 mg/day; if calcitriol (1,25-dihydroxycholecalciferol) high, keep calcium intake <800 mg/day.
4. **Hyperparathyroidism history taking** focus on fractures, osteoporosis, and nephrolithiasis.
5. **Indications for surgery for hyperparathyroidism**: (A) >1 increase in serum calcium; (B) T < −2.5 at hip, lumbar spine, distal radius; (C) <60 eGFR, kidney stones, urine Calcium excretion >400 mg/day; (D) age < 50.
6. **Armour Thyroid (desiccated thyroid)** has too much T3 and less T4; need to switch to Synthroid and liothyronine first and gradually change to levothyroxine. The **half-life of T4 is 6 weeks and T3 is 2 weeks**.
7. Thyroid cancer → thyroidectomy → put on T3 to raise TSH > 50 → stop T3, **6 weeks to 1 month later after stopping T3, check for residual thyroid tissue** → give radioactive iodine.
8. After **thyroidectomy**, there is usually transient **low parathyroid hormone** (PTH), which takes a little while to recover; ok to be on **calcitriol**.
9. **Byetta** (exenatide) subcutaneous injection, bid. **Bydureon** (exenatide) subcutaneous injection once a week. GLP-1 agonist **Trulicity** (dulaglutide) is approved for diabetes while semaglutide (Ozempic) is approved for both diabetes and weight loss.
10. Angiotensin-converting enzyme inhibitor (ACEi) is recommended in diabetic patients with **hypertension (HTN) or microalbuminuria**. Urine **albumin to creatinine ratio** 30–300 = **microalbuminuria** while >300 = **macroalbuminuria**. The normal spot **urine protein to creatinine ratio** is less than 0.2 mg/mg; if >**3.5** mg/mg, it is nephrotic proteinuria
11. **Papillary thyroid cancer**: TSH should be <0.5; on Synthroid, however, his Synthroid of 250 μg daily is causing elevated FT4 2.0 (normal 0.8–1.8) and a higher dose of Synthroid causes symptoms; thus, switch to **lower dose T3 to suppress TSH** (start T3 at 10 mg and cut the dose of Synthroid).
12. **Thyroglobulin level to monitor cancer status in thyroid cancer**.
13. To see whether a patient has **thyroid cancer recurrence**: (A) prescribe synthesized TSH then radioactive iodine uptake (RAIU); (B) prescribe **liothyronine**

to raise TSH to 50 and then stop T3 to do RAIU; C. PET scan if no uptake of radioactive iodine (RAI).

14. **Metformin causes diarrhea**, need to decrease the dosage.
15. **Thyroglobulin antibody** can mask the recurrence of thyroid cancer as it binds to thyroglobulin.
16. Diabetes mellitus (DM) treatment: metformin 1 g bid, Victoza 1.2 mg qd, Basaglar 15u, Invokana 300 mg qd.

5/15/2018

1. Microalbumin/creatinine ratio random
2. **Meal-induced reactive hypoglycemia**: put a patient on acarbose and may add octreotide. It usually happens after 2–5 years after gastric bypass. **Treatment**: additionally, no glucose meal treatment. Meal-induced reactive hypoglycemia in this lady happened 15 years later after gastric bypass.
3. **Early postprandial reactive hypoglycemia** (inpatient): the patient has been having multiple frequent episodes of hypoglycemia, which usually happens right after eating, likely from **insulin secretion increase** to oral glucose stimulation which increases GLP-1 and **glucose-dependent insulinotropic polypeptide** leading to **insulin increase and glucagon suppression**. **Treatments** include medical nutrition therapy (low-carb diet), acarbose, diazoxide, calcium channel blockers, and octreotide/lanreotide may be worth trying especially given recurrent hypoglycemia for over a month while inpatient.
4. Canagliflozin (Invokana) 100 mg →300 mg qd. The use of SGLT-2 inhibitors is associated with increased **risks for amputations**: 1% had amputation which is mainly toe amputation. However, given the significant benefits, the FDA removed the black box warning of leg and foot amputations for canagliflozin in 2020.
5. In the elderly, **SGLT2 inhibitor takers may hold the medicine** if on antibiotics or at high risk for dehydration. SGLT2 has mortality benefits in congestive heart failure and can slow the decline of kidney function in chronic nondiabetic kidney disease with albuminuria ≥300 mg/day. **If eGFR < 20 mL/min/1.73 m^2, SGLT-2 inhibitors should not be initiated.**
6. In prolactin levels of 100–200, treatment is **cabergoline 0.5 mg × 2/week**. May stop treatment if prolactin normalizes for **≥2 years** and no adenoma on MRI.
7. Prolactinoma: usually complains of **headache and low testosterone** in males; **irregular periods and nipple discharge** in females.
8. **Hook effects**: prolactin level of 20–200 which is falsely low because of excessive antigen in the test. **Treatment**: dilute will eliminate the false negative.
9. **Alendronic acid** (Fosamax) 10 mg qd; risedronic acid (Actonel) 5 mg qd; denosumab (Prolia) 60 mg q6m.
10. **Repaglinide (Prandin)** lowers glucose by blocking ATP-dependent potassium channels in pancreatic beta cells, increasing insulin secretion. For light meals we can skip dosage; less risk for hypoglycemia. **Repaglinide acts like short-acting insulin**.

11. Hair loss, fatigue, weight gain → check cortisol for Cushing's: 24 h urine free cortisol, overnight 1 mg dexamethasone suppression test. Cushing disease = ACTH-producing pituitary tumor.

5/16/2018

1. 24 urine calcium for calculation of fractional excretion of calcium in urine to rule out **familial hypocalciuric hypercalcemia** (FHH).
2. **Stop methimazole 1–2 weeks** before the radioactive uptake iodine (RAUI) scan which is on 7/2, she will then have radioactive iodine (RAI) ablation on 7/19.
3. Xifaxan = rifaximin, Pepcid = famotidine; Zantac = ranitidine.
4. **Small intestine bacterial overgrowth (SIBO) syndrome**: hydrogen predominant vs. methane predominant bacterial overgrowth (treatment: neomycin 500 mg bid or rifaximin 550 mg tid for 14 days)
5. **Diabetes glucose test supplies**: glucometer, BD pen, lancet needles, OneTouch Verio® test strips.
6. **Levemir (detemir)** should be given once or twice a day.
7. **Beta hCG** shares similarities with TSH, and stimulates secretion of T3 and T4, especially at 13–15 weeks of pregnancy, suppressing TSH, thus **TSH level of 0.04 is OK** for pregnant women.
8. The HA1c target in the elderly should be **≤8.0%** (fasting and preprandial glucose between 160 and 170) in **medication-treated frail older adults** with medical and functional comorbidities and **those with a life expectancy of less than 10 years**.
9. Diabetes treatment example: Humalin RU-500 u/ml (105u subcu breakfast, 80u lunch and dinner), Invokana 300 mg, Victoza 1.8 mg qd.
10. Maximal dose: Victoza (**Liraglutide**) 1.8 mg/day; Saxenda (Liraglutide) 3 mg/week.
11. **Iron tablets and calcium pills** interfere with levothyroxine absorption; **biotin** can interfere with levothyroxine absorption too.
12. **Cushing's syndrome**: ACTH 365 high, cortisol 22.9 high, DHEA 547 high → order late-night salivary cortisol, 1 mg dexamethasone suppression test, 24 h urine free cortisol (UFC). If all tests are normal, the patient likely has physiologic hypercortisolism (stress, pain, depression, anxiety, alcoholism, eating disorder, etc.).
13. To rule out polycystic ovarian syndrome (PCOS), order **testosterone, IGF-1, ACTH, and prolactin, always 24 h Cr if 24 h UFC.**
14. **PCOS treatment**: oral contraceptive (OCP), spironolactone 50 mg bid, metformin. OCP causes mood lability, and liraglutide (Saxenda) 3 mg helps weight loss. **OCP use at age > 40 increases risks for venous thromboembolisms (VTEs) and should be stopped at age 50.**
15. **PCOS tests**: beta hCG, follicle-stimulating hormone (FSH), prolactin, TSH, free testosterone → US abdomen revealed PCOS. **Additional tests as appro-**

priate: dehydroepiandrosterone (DHEA) or 17 hydroxyprogesterone, cortisol, prolactin, TSH, and IGF-1.

16. **PCOS ovulation induction**: clomiphene (selective estrogen receptor modulator)/letrozole (aromatase inhibitor) → gonadotropin (FSH) increases → ovarian drilling—in vitro fertilization (IVF).
17. After thyroidectomy, **TSH** should go up in 8–12 weeks.
18. **Diabetes glucose testing supplies**: BD pen needles/ nano/ultrafine/32G×4 mm needles. OneTouch® Delica® lancet extra fine 33G; OneTouch Verio® test stripes 5 times a day.
19. Diabetes treatment example (HA1c 6.5%): metformin 1.5 g qd, Jardiance (empagliflozin) 25 mg qd, Toujeo 100u a.m., 50u p.m.; Humalog 46/40/48 units for breakfast/lunch/dinner, Ozempic (semaglutide) 0.5 mg sc qwk.
20. **Gestational diabetes treatment**: 30–45 g carb for each meal, <60 g for dinner; 2 h postprandial glucose target in pregnancy <120. If the patient fails an oral glucose tolerance test (OGTT), the patient may be started on metformin. Fasting glucose target <95 mg/dL; 1 h postprandial <140.
21. Clinical atherosclerotic cardiovascular disease (**ASCVD**), high-intensity statin if ≤75 yo, moderate statin if >75 yo. People 40–75 yo with DM and LDL 70–189, do moderate intensity; if **>7.5%** 10-year ASCVD, do **high** intensity.

5/17/2018

1. **Thyroiditis** takes 1 month to resolve. Methimazole has to be **stopped for 1 week** before radioactive uptake iodine (RAUI) scan.
2. Osteoporosis**, T score for post-menopause; Z score for young adults**.
3. Hyperthyroidism on methimazole: **thyroxine and TSH levels take 3 months** or longer to stabilize.
4. **Metformin** does not cause renal disease but it should be stopped if eGFR <30 or even 45.
5. If not much bolus is given, even though fasting is OK with the basal rate of 6 u/h on an insulin pump, we may still need to lower the basal rate and tell the patient to do bolus.
6. The **Z score** is scaled down by the population standard deviation. The **T score** is scaled down by the sample SD.

5/18/2018

1. Document **pager encounter** for patients from outpatient clinics.
2. **Cervical swab** tests for Chlamydia trachomatis Ag amp, N. gonorrhoeae amp, and Trichomonas vaginalis nucleic acid amplification testing (NAAT).
3. Vistaril = hydroxyzine, Zyrtec = cetirizine.
4. **Insulin pump setting example**: Basal rate 0.4 u/h, carbohydrate ratio 0:00 25, 17:00 22, insulin sensitivity 100, glucose target 110–120. 171 BG, 2 g carb, 1.3 u insulin.
5. Diabetes treatment example: Invokana (Canagliflozin) 300 mg, metformin 500 + 1000 mg, pioglitazone 25 mg, Tresiba 35u, Trulicity 1.5 mg

5/19/2018

1. **Wide QRS tachycardia**: ventricular tachycardia/fibrillation (VTach can have fusion beats, capture beats, AV dissociation); SVT with aberrancy (due to bundle branch block, WPW syndrome).

5/22/2018

1. After child delivery, cut the insulin dose in half. During pregnancy, **levothyroxine needs to be increased by 25%.**
2. **Occult premature ovarian insufficiency (POI)** is impaired ovarian responsiveness to exogenous or endogenous gonadotropin stimulation despite the presence of regular and predictable ovulatory menstrual cycles. **Overt POI** refers to the presence of irregular menses, elevated gonadotropins, and reduced fertility.
3. **Anti-müllerian hormone (AMH)** blood levels reflect the size of the remaining egg supply (**ovarian reserve**). Women with many small follicles, such as those with polycystic ovarian syndrome (PCOS) have **high AMH** whereas women with few remaining follicles and menopause have **low AMH**.
4. **Test for POI:** diagnosis with **the serum pregnancy test, TSH, prolactin, FSH, and estradiol.** After diagnosis of POI, **further testing includes** 21 hydroxylase Ab (positive in Addison disease) tests, FMR1 premutation, DEXA, and pelvic ultrasound.
5. **Treatments for POI**: estrogen-progesterone till age 50–51, IVF with donor oocytes or embryos. **Estradiol 1 mg qd and micronized progesterone 100 mg qd for 14 days on and 14 days off for POI treatments.**
6. Symptoms of **adrenal insufficiency**: weight loss, fatigue, salt craving, gastrointestinal complaints, musculoskeletal myalgia, and arthralgia. Signs: hypotension, hyperpigmentation, auricular cartilage calcification, vitiligo.
7. **Polyglandular autoimmune syndrome**. Type 1 is associated with the autoimmune regulator (AIRE) gene: **adrenal insufficiency, hypoparathyroidism, and chronic mucocutaneous candidiasis**. Type 2 is related to an unknown gene and causes **adrenal insufficiency, type 1 diabetes mellitus, and autoimmune thyroid disease**.
8. **Levemir** has research evidence for the treatment of gestational DM.
9. During the **last 8 weeks of pregnancy**, insulin requirement sharply increases, follow up with labs q4wks.
10. **Graves' eye disease** will not get better even with TSH normalization.
11. Patients with active and mild orbitopathy due to Graves' disease are candidates for thionamides, radioiodine, or surgery. For moderate to severe or sight-threatening orbitopathy, only use **thionamides or surgery**. **Selenium** helps swelling of orbitopathy in Graves' disease.
12. For patients with moderate to severe orbitopathy, initial treatment with glucocorticoids is recommended. For sight-threatening orbitopathy, use **dexamethasone 4 mg IV** and hospitalize the patient for **urgent orbital decompression**.

13. **Insulin pump**: duration of insulin action is the duration of insulin effects, usually around 6 h
14. **Creon (pancrelipase): may need to stop if weight loss, or diarrhea, then need to resume Creon once symptoms resolve.**
15. **Victoza**: 0.6 g subcu qd; **ozempic** AKA semaglutide 0.25 mg qwk for 4 weeks testing dose; **trulicity** 0.75 mg subcu qwk.
16. **PCOS** needs to ensure good periods to protect bone health till age 50: no need for TSH or FSH testing, but do testosterone check; **if testosterone is high, do spironolactone**.
17. Diabetes treatment example: Amaryl (glimepiride) 4 mg qd, Invokana (canagliflozin) 300 mg qd, metformin 1000 mg bid, Trajenta (linagliptin, a DPP-4 inhibitor) 5 mg qd.

5/24/2018

1. Nexium = esomeprazole; **high dose radioactive iodine uptake (RAIU) for ablation, stay away from children for 5 days**.
2. Follicular nodule = Hurthle cell type (undetermined significance).
3. **Neoplasm of the pituitary**: check for ACTH, cortisol, FSH, LH, estradiol, prolactin, and IGF-1.
4. **AZO go less (phenazopyridine)** is used for pain from lower urinary tract symptoms.

5/29/2018

1. Before meal glucose is good, but high postprandial glucose while on insulin pump → treat with adjusting **insulin/carb ratio (nutritional insulin dosage)**.
2. Dexcom and Medtronic care sensors require **finger stick glucose to adjust**. Omnipod is a commercial-type wearable glucometer.
3. **Cholecalciferol (vitamin D3)** has good absorption via oral.
4. Localization studies with ultrasound, technetium-99m sestamibi, CT, or MRI not for diagnosis, but along with PTH monitoring to facilitate unilateral exploration and minimally invasive surgery in those with single gland disease of primary hyperparathyroidism.
5. **Tresiba is ultralong acting** as compared to Toujeo/Lantus.
6. **Treatment of secondary hyperparathyroidism due to surgery for Crohn's disease**: Citracal® Maximum (calcium citrate with vitamin D3), Mg oxide, Vit A 25,000u qd, Vitamin D3 5000u bid, zoledronic acid (Reclast) 5 mg iv annually.
7. Fasting C peptide and glucose for differentiation between T1DM and T2DM.

5/31/2018

1. **Fructosamine test** assesses the average glucose in the previous 2 weeks.
2. **Thyroxine** half-life is 7 days. In the first trimester, low TSH is normal as beta hCG is high (**beta hCG stimulates secretion of T3 and T4**).
3. **Sensors in diabetes (DM)** glucometers: Dexcom, Meditronics, freestyle (sensors, readers, and pump).

4. Fludrocortisone corresponds with aldosterone endogenously. **Hydrocortisone 10 mg bid is used for Addison's disease, need to double the dose when sick.**
5. **Pituitary replacement**: hydrocortisone 10 mg bid, levothyroxine 125 μg qd, testosterone cypionate 0.3 ml (60 mg) q2wks-BD user locker syringe 1 ml/20 g × 1. **Growth hormone** may be necessary if <30 yo.
6. Difficulty controlling hyperthyroidism, treatment with **Synthroid 100 μg bid and Tapazole (methimazole) 10 mg qd.**
7. **80% of thyroid nodules** are **cold** nodules.
8. **Subclinical hyperthyroidism**: check thyroid-stimulating immunoglobulins (TSI) and iodine reuptake scan.
9. **Severe eye problem in Graves' disease, surgery is preferred over I131 ablation.**
10. 13 weeks of pregnancy, **TSH** 0.04, T3 total increased slightly. It's normal.
11. Zofran is not FDA-approved for use in pregnancy; **doxylamine succinate pyridoxine hydrochloride (Diclegis®)** is the only pregnancy category A drug for morning sickness during pregnancy. **Reglan** is also category A.

6/1/2018

1. Concerns for adrenal insufficiency, test **morning cortisol and ACTH (Cosyntropin) stimulation test.**
2. TSH high, a patient has sweating and palpitations → **generic T4 resistance or switch to Synthroid**.
3. Glucose in a complete metabolic panel (**CMP**) may not be reliable. If unreliable reading, do fasting glucose alone. **High C-peptide and insulin** are due to type 2 diabetes mellitus (T2DM). Order glucose monitoring, and a glucometer to check glucose if hypoglycemia.
4. **Tirosint (levothyroxine)** has no additives, no lactose or gluten, good for very sensitive patients with hypothyroidism (gluten-free).
5. Acute anemia → **HA1c** measurement may not be accurate (**moderate to severe anemia falsely increases HbA1c because of longer half-lives of red blood cells**), need to test the trend.
6. OneTouch® Delica® lancets, OneTouch® lancet extra.
7. **Synthroid**: ok to add an extra pill on Sun/Mon for the adjustment of TSH.
8. **Ectopic pregnancy, need to check transvaginal ultrasound**.
9. The T3 test is not reliable as the majority of T3 is stored inside a cell. **rT3 is usually checked in sickness euthyroid syndrome.**

6/2/2018

1. Avoid steroid and NSAIDs combination. Simultaneous use of steroids with low, medium and high NSAID doses produces odds ratios of **4 and 12.7 for gastrointestinal bleed and perforation. Dexamethasone is long-acting while prednisone is short-acting**.
2. Diagnose patient with chronic obstructive pulmonary disease (COPD) exacerbation: **increased dyspnea, sputum volume, and purulence.** If only one of the cardinal symptoms, no antibiotics, just increase bronchodilators. If moderate or

severe, check for risk factors for complicated COPD exacerbation (1 or more risk factors, >65, FEV1 < 50%, >2 exacerbations per year, cardiac disease) → do Levaquin/Augmentin. Other inpatient options: moxifloxacin, ceftriaxone, cefotaxime, cefepime, Pep/Tazo plus azithromycin. **C reactive protein ≥20–40 mg/L** can also be used as guidance for antibiotic use in COPD exacerbation.

3. Patient takes **Xanax** for 1- year, admitted for fall × 4, **check urine toxicology**.
4. There are desensitization protocols for commonly used antibiotic allergies.
5. Treatment for **bacterial meningitis**: ceftriaxone 2 g iv q12h + vancomycin 15–20 mg/kg iv q12h (if alcoholic or >50 yo or immunocompromised, add ampicillin 2 g q4h), steroid **dexamethasone 10 mg IV q6h × 4** days must be started before or with first dose antibiotics. Add acyclovir IV if unsure about herpes meningitis status.
6. The empirical initial dose of dexamethasone in brain tumor patients is an IV bolus of **10 mg Decadron followed by a maintenance dose of 4 mg given by iv q6h**. Start upon diagnosis and administer 1–2 days before brain surgery.
7. **After completion of radiation therapy, dexamethasone is tapered over 2–4 weeks and then discontinued**. Taper usually consists of an empiric reduction in a dose of 2–4 mg q1-3d by either decreasing dosing or increasing interval. After the patient is tapered to a dose of **0.75 mg/day, a morning cortisol level** should be checked to determine the steroid effect on adrenal function; if AM cortisol >10 μg/dL, the steroid can be discontinued.
8. CPAP 5 cm with auto titration.
9. **Gastrointestinal prep for colonoscopy**: electrolyte solution/PEGs (Bulk) (Colyte/Golytely) 4000 ml. May add oral bisacodyl 10 mg orally once for bowel preparation.

Takeaway Messages

1. The diagnosis of Graves' disease is based on clinical symptoms, iodine 123 (shorter half-life than I131) uptake, positive thyroid-stimulating immunoglobulin (TSI), and thyrotropin-binding inhibitory immunoglobulin (TBII).
2. Concurrent use of GLP-1 with dipeptidyl peptidase-4 inhibitor provides no added-on benefits.
3. Thyroxine complete (full) replacement 1.6 u/kg/day.
4. Toxic adenoma or toxic multigoiter nodules (based on TSH and thyroid ultrasound) treatment: radioiodine ablation, surgical resection, ultrasound-guided ablative procedures, or thionamide therapy
5. In cardiac amyloidosis, we should avoid digoxin (arrhythmogenic) and beta-blocker (no benefit).
6. Carbohydrates stimulate insulin secretion via increasing GLP-1 and glucose-dependent insulinotropic polypeptide leading to insulin increase and glucagon suppression.

Further Readings and References

1. Stuenkel, C.A., and A. Gompel. 2023. Primary ovarian insufficiency. *New England Journal of Medicine* 388 (2): 154–163.
2. Barbieri, R.L., and D.A. Ehrmann. *Diagnosis of polycystic ovary syndrome in adults*, ed. W.F. Crowley. Waltham, MA: UpToDate. Accessed November 15, 2023.
3. Barbieri, R.L., and D.A. Ehrmann. *Treatment of polycystic ovary syndrome in adults*, ed. W.F. Crowley. Waltham, MA: UpToDate. Accessed November 15, 2023.
4. Agrawal, A., M. Naranjo, N. Kanjanahattakij, et al. 2019. Cardiorenal syndrome in heart failure with preserved ejection fraction-an under-recognized clinical entity. *Heart Failure Reviews* 24 (4): 421–437.

Chapter 9
Back to General Internal Medicine Floor Rotation

June 4th, 2018 Through July 29th, 2018
At the end of my intern year, I spent another 2 months at the general internal medicine floor of two different large academic centers. The focus of the training was no longer acute coronary artery syndrome, congestive heart failure, or pneumonia, but rather other common and uncommon diseases in the field of internal medicine and disorders expanding multidisciplinary specialties.

As a general internal medicine physician, our responsibility is not only taking care of patients with common diseases but also diagnosing and treating uncommon and rare health conditions. In this chapter, topics covered included allergic bronchopulmonary aspergillosis, nephrolithiasis, triple anticoagulation, Lemierre's syndrome, hyperosmolar hyperglycemic syndrome, diabetic ketoacidosis, chronic myelogenous leukemia, blast crisis, leukostasis, surgical indications for endocarditis, toxic shock syndrome, cryoprecipitate, thalassemia, thrombocytopenia, hemolysis, hepatitis, adrenal crisis, Crohn disease, perioperative anticoagulation, cholecystitis and cholelithiasis, and anemias.

During this phase of training, interns and soon-to-be senior residents are expected to develop critical knowledge and skills in differential diagnoses, collaborate with other specialties in multispecialty care, and seek recommendations and assistance from specialists. Seeing is no longer simply believing and never say never. Understanding the uncertainties in medicine becomes very important. A patient's symptoms or presentation may have one or even multiple causes and differentiation and understanding the treatment of these different causes is key in patients' care. Meanwhile, internal medicine physicians and physicians-in-training should also recognize that general internal medicine physicians are limited by their training in procedures and surgeries. Timely requests for help from other specialties play an important role while we strive to provide the best possible care. For example, urological conditions like nephrolithiasis and hydronephrosis may require urologist interventions, and for cholecystitis, surgery team consultation is often necessary.

K. Zhou, *Internal Medicine Training Notes and Survival Guide*,
https://doi.org/10.1007/978-1-0716-4039-5_9

On top of that, even in the field of internal medicine itself, we general internal medicine physicians should recognize the limitations of us general internists. For example, in patients with blast crisis, leukostasis, and/or severe thrombocytopenias, urgent help from a hematologist and oncologist is usually necessary. Unusual or invasive infections should prompt consultations for infectious disease, and the cold and dry type of congestive heart failure likely will need assistance from a cardiologist, and the unusual ground glass changes of the lungs may require expertise from a pulmonologist with possible bronchoscopy.

6/5/2018

1. Abdominal pain not responding to Protonix and Maalox, recurrent acute on chronic pancreatitis, due to alcoholism → pancreatic enzyme replacement (**Creon**); may need to repeat **CT abdomen** to rule out complications from pancreatitis. PPI bid + sucralfate qid is good for peptic ulcer disease. Check CRP, lipase.
2. **Urology consult for kidney malignancy**: order CT abdomen/pelvis and U/S kidney prior to consult.

6/7/2018

1. Acute treatment for deep vein thrombosis (**DVT**) and pulmonary embolism (**PE**): heparin drip at 80 u/kg IV bolus, then 18 u/kg/h.
2. **ACS (STEMI, NSTEMI, UA)**: bolus 60 u/kg IV bolus (max 5000), then 12–15 u/kg/h.
3. **Gradual anticoagulation**, use nomogram by anti-Xa, in a patient treated with alteplase in the past 24 h, new mechanical valve with a high risk of bleeding.
4. **Rapid heparin nomogram by anti-Xa indications**: DVT/PE, ventricular/atrial thrombus, AFib, history of mechanical valve.
5. Initial dosing of unfractionated heparin (UFH) bolus and infusion: rapid: 80 u/kg bolus, maximal 10,000u, followed by 18 u/kg/h for PE and venous thromboembolisms (VTEs). **Gradual**: no bolus, start at 12 u/kg/h, check by 6 h after, can be used in atrial fibrillations
6. **Titration based on anti-Xa**: if <0.1, bolus 40 u/kg (20 u/kg); increase rate by 2 u/kg/h.

6/8/2018

1. **Mirabegron** is used for overactive bladder (OAB). Mirabegron is a beta-3 adrenergic receptor agonist that activates bladder beta-3 adrenergic receptors resulting in relaxation of the detrusor smooth muscle during the urine storage phase, thus increasing bladder capacity.
2. **Digoxin** inhibits Na+/K+ ATPase in myocardium → increases intracellular Na → decreases Na-Ca++ exchanger which normally transport 3Na in 1 Ca++ out → decreased heart rate (HR).
3. The combination of increased atrial arrhythmogenesis and inhibited atrioventricular (AV) conduction [e.g., **paroxysmal atrial tachycardia (PAT) with AV block**, so-called PAT with block] is pathognomonic for **digoxin toxicity**.

4. **Delirium assessment**: confusion assessment method of ICU (CAM-ICU), Richmond agitation-sedation score (RASS) while on ventilator, CAM-ICU for delirium.
5. **Confusion** (lack of coherent thinking) vs. **delirium** [decreased arousal and attention: the ascending reticular activating system (ARAS) system from mid pontine maintains wakefulness and arousal]. Decreased attention by non-dominant **parietal and frontal** lobes; insights and judgment by integrated cortical functions.
6. **Etiology for delirium**: fluid and electrolyte disturbances; infections; drug toxicity, withdrawal; metabolic disease; low perfusion; sundowning, dementia. Labs: CBC, CMP, UA/Cx, drug levels, CT head, CXR, toxicology.
7. **Consult palliative care** for frail patients, and patients with multiple comorbidities, check with family, try to discuss with family code status of do not resuscitate (DNR)/do not intubate (DNI).
8. After the decision to proceed with **percutaneous coronary intervention (PCI)**, we give unfractionated heparin 60 u/kg bolus (cardiologist to decide).
9. After PCI, post-procedural heparin is not recommended in patients with uncomplicated procedures. May need to **resume heparin drip after PCI if the patient requires coronary artery bypass grafting (CABG)**, again cardiologist to decide.
10. **Allergic bronchopulmonary aspergillosis (ABPA)** is marked by asthma and recurrent COPD exacerbations. Pathophysiology of ABPA: accumulation of mucus in the bronchial tubes, elevated levels of eosinophils, pneumonia, and bronchocentric granulomatosis. These features, along with the histological trait of asthma, are typically only observed in individuals with **asthma and cystic fibrosis (CF)**.
11. **ABPA labs** include: elevated total blood **eosinophil count** (>500 cells/μL), increased total **IgE**, precipitating **IgG Ab** (precipitins) to aspergillus, also specific IgE and IgG Ab to aspergillus on immunoassay.
12. **Stepwise evaluation for ABPA**: immediate skin test to aspergillus and/or specific IgE test; total serum IgE and peripheral eosinophil count; CT, CXR, precipitating aspergillus Abs.
13. **Treatment for ABPA**: initial dose prednisone 0.5 mg/kg qd for 14 days → every other day and taper over 3– 5 months, with or without itraconazole 200 mg tid for 3 days then bid for 16 weeks, voriconazole (loading dose 400 mg bid for two doses, followed by 200–300 mg twice daily for 16 weeks) can also be used.
14. Additional tests for ABPA include **inspiratory spirometer, mycology culture and sensitivity** with smear, and sputum culture and sensitivity with smear.

6/9/2018

1. **Hyponatremia**: true volume depletion, decreased tissue perfusions (congestive heart failure [CHF]/Cirrhosis), syndrome of inappropriate antidiuretic hormone (SIADH). Normal saline (NS) infusion makes both SIADH and decreased tissue perfusion (CHF and cirrhosis) worse. To differentiate these two, check urine Na;

less than 20 mmol/L is indicative of decreased tissue perfusion (hypovolemia like dehydration and hypervolemia like congestive heart failure both have this result), whereas a **level greater than 40 mmol/L is SIADH**.

2. **Nephrolithiasis**: calcium oxalate, calcium phosphate, uric acid, struvite (magnesium ammonium phosphate), cystine stones.
3. **Causes of** calcium oxalate **stones**: increased enteric oxalate absorption, often in the setting of malabsorption (gastric bypass, Roux-en-Y gastric bypass, short bowel syndrome). Increased intestinal fat binds diet calcium which is then unavailable to bind oxalate as usual.
4. **Struvite stones**: proteus or Klebsiella with pH >7. Treatment: **Calcium channel blocker (nifedipine) and alpha-blockers (tamsulosin)**.
5. **Work up for nephrolithiasis**: order 24 h urine profile, including appropriate serum test of renal function, uric acid, and calcium, common findings include hypercalciuria, hyperoxaluria, hyperuricosuria, hypocitraturia, and low urine volume.
6. To prevent calcium oxalate stone, **ensure adequate intake of calcium, fluid, K, and phosphate while decreasing the intake of oxalate, animal protein, sucrose, fructose, and sodium; supplement calcium and vit C.**

6/11/2018

1. **Glycopyrrolate** 0.1 mg q12h or **scopolamine** patch for excessive tracheal secretions.
2. Throat spray (**phenol**) antiseptic spray for throat pain.
3. **Fluticasone** nasal spray for nasal congestion in combination with hydroxyzine in seasonal allergies.
4. Sodium chloride spray for nasal congestion. **High CPK** can cause elevated Trop and LFT.
5. Respiratory consult for patients on ventilator or trach collar to wean off ventilator: please place the patient on **T piece** around the clock.

6/13/2018

1. Cervical swab test for **chlamydia** Ag amplification, N. **gonorrhoeae** Ag amplification, **trichomonas** vaginalis NAAT.
2. Shortness of breath (SOB) or chest pain, needs to rule out **pulmonary embolism** (PE). **Pericarditis** may be related to viral infection. **Typical PR depression and prolongation** in digoxin toxicity.
3. **Amlodipine** is good for post-PCI.

6/14/2018

1. Pancreatitis, lipase at least 3 times above the reference range. **Overnutrition with PEG** feeds can cause elevation of lipase as well. Treatment for pancreatitis is lactate ringers at 250–500 cc/h for 24 h followed by continuous IV fluid if no contraindications.
2. **Rhabdomyolysis**: 1.5 L/h bolus followed by continuous IV fluid to maintain urine 300 cc/h

3. **Post-obstructive acute kidney injury** (AKI) after correction of obstruction: 200 cc/h.
4. Typical EKG in pericarditis is **ST elevation and PR depression in most leads but reciprocal ST depression and PR elevation in lead aVR.**
5. **Elective CABG**: stop clopidogrel 5 days, ticagrelor 5 days, prasugrel 7 days prior to surgery.
6. **Cholangitis** is an abscess needing STAT/urgent endoscopic retrograde cholangiopancreatography (ERCP) after starting a broad spectrum antibiotic.

6/16/2018

1. **Pneumonia**: Sensitivity for sputum culture is only 20%–30%. Sensitivity for urine antigens is 70%–80%, and specificity is 99%.
2. Slow heart rate, ready for discharge. **Have the patient walk to make sure the patient is asymptomatic** with activities and heart rate goes up with activities.
3. **Contraindications of metoprolol**: may need to temporarily hold metoprolol if severe heart failure (HF) and/or need inotropes, decompensated HF.
4. Symptomatic sinus pauses/arrests require a pacemaker. **Asymptomatic sinus pause $\geq$ 4 s** may need a pacemaker!
5. **O_2 dissociation curve**: PO_2 60 mmHg equals 90% SO_2; PO_2 80 mmHg equals 95% SO_2.
6. **Triple oral antithrombotic therapy**, also known as triple therapy or combined antithrombotic therapy: if triple therapy is chosen, prefer (dabigatran 150 mg bid or 110 mg bid or Xarelto 15 mg bid) triple therapy for 1–6 m then aspirin is dropped, clopidogrel is continued for 6–12 m for low thrombotic and low bleeding risk. If high thrombotic risk and low bleeding risk, prefer (dabigatran 150 mg bid + Plavix) for 6–12 months; if low thrombotic and high bleeding risk, prefer dabigatran 110 mg bid + Plavix 75 mg qd for 6–12 months; if high thrombotic and high bleeding risk, prefer dabigatran 150/110 mg bid + Plavix 75 mg for 6–12 months.
7. If aspirin is used as part of the triple therapy, the dose should be 75–100 mg.
8. For patients who have completed 6–12 months of oral anticoagulation (OAC) and a P2Y12 blocker, **most continue OAC plus aspirin (ASA) 81 mg daily**. For individuals with a high risk of ischemia, some suggest OAC + Plavix.
9. AFib with cardioembolic stroke, may initiate oral anticoagulation (AC) after 24 h admission to hospital if **small stroke with minimal risk for hemorrhagic transformation**. **Withhold AC for 2 weeks if large infarct, symptomatic hemorrhagic transformation,** or poorly controlled blood pressure (BP). No need for triple therapy in stroke.
10. Give ASA 75 mg qd, Plavix 300 mg load then 75 mg for 90 days, and start both **within 24 h for ischemic stroke**.
11. Thrombolytic therapy should not be withheld for eligible patients with very early acute ischemic stroke due to **extracranial cervical artery dissection**. Give ASA 24 h after thrombolytic therapy. Give ASA for acute ischemic symptoms of both intracranial and extracranial dissection.

12. Antiplatelet for NSTEMI: the **first aspirin tablet should be chewed and contain 162–325 mg**. At discharge should be ASA 75–100 mg qd.
13. Give **P2Y12 blocker** as soon as NSTEMI diagnosis is made (defer to cardiologist given a small percentage of patients require coronary artery bypass grafting). If getting percutaneous coronary intervention (PCI), give ticagrelor.
14. **Switching from a potent P2Y12 to Plavix**: if on ticagrelor, give first Plavix dose 12 h after last ticagrelor with a 600 mg loading dose. If on prasugrel, just start Plavix 75 mg 24 h later.
15. The duration of holding a P2Y12 platelet receptor blocker before a high bleeding risk procedure is as follows: 5 days for clopidogrel; 3–5 days for ticagrelor; **7 days for prasugrel**; 7 days for ticlopidine; 1–2 days hold for novel oral anticoagulants (NOAC).

6/19/2018

1. Sinusitis symptomatic management: nasal spray- fluticasone or normal saline for stuffy nose. May add Zyrtec (Cetirizine) if allergic sinusitis.
2. **Chlorpromazine** for intractable hiccups: 25–50 mg IV, IM, po tid or qid. May also use baclofen.
3. **Meningiomas** can rise from dura at falx cerebri, tentorium cerebelli, and venous sinuses. Many patients are asymptomatic; some present with focal findings including visceral changes, loss of hearing/smell, mental status changes, extremity weakness, and obstructive hydrocephalus (benign, atypical, or malignant meningiomas).
4. **Risks for meningiomas**: prior therapeutic radiation (high grade, multiple, and recurrent). **Differential diagnoses**: Dural-based pathology mimicking meningioma including hematologic and nonhematologic malignancy, sarcoidosis, tuberculosis (TB), neurofibromatosis type 2 (NF2), schwannomas. **Diagnosis via MRI and CT with or without contrast**. **Small (<3 cm)** and **asymptomatic** meningioma only requires MRI surveillance otherwise requires surgery.
5. Gastroenterologist doc does not like **oral ferritin sulfate** before colonoscopy.
6. **Anemia increases aldosterone secretion** → increases in volume → worsening of congestive heart failure (CHF). Treatment: diuresis and transfusion
7. **Asymptomatic bradycardia**: heart rate (HR) 20–30 will need ICU admission and cardiologist consultation.
8. Dabigatran/NSAIDs should not be used together.
9. **PET/CT needs nothing per mouth (NPO)** overnight.
10. **Jugular vein suppurative thrombophlebitis** also known as **Lemierre's syndrome** or postanginal sepsis, or necrobacillosis. It's a medical emergency of peritonsillar infection involving the post compartment of the lateral pharyngeal space, complicated by suppurative thrombophlebitis of the jugular vein with Fusobacterium necrophorum, bacteremia, and metastatic abscess. The **anterior** part of this space consists of the **anterior neck muscles**; the **posterior** section **encases the carotid sheath that encloses the internal jugular vein, internal carotid artery, vagus nerve, and lymph nodes.**

11. **Jugular vein suppurative thrombophlebitis** should be suspected in patients with **antecedent pharyngitis, septic physical examination, and persistent fever** despite antibiotics. Treatments: **Zosyn, Unasyn**, or carbapenem. An **ENT physician** should be consulted for possible needs for incision and drainage.
12. Hem/Onc in general needs **tissue biopsy** results before consultation.
13. **Peak flow similar to FEV1**, peak expiratory flow variability >20% with bronchodilator is consistent with asthma. Green zone scheme: green >80% of your personal best, yellow (50%–80% of your personal best), caution airways obstructed. Red <50% of your personal best is a medical alert. If improvement is 10% with treatment, outpatient management may be appropriate.

6/22/2018

1. **Relister (methylnaltrexone)** for severe constipation in comfort care caused by large amounts of opioids.
2. Lupus and heparin-induced thrombosis (HIT) causes **arterial thrombosis**.
3. **Comfort care**: no transfers to higher levels of care, and no invasive mechanical ventilation, no CPR, no artificial hydration except for comfort care, stop dialysis if already on it.
4. **Radiation therapy causes atherosclerosis and stent restenosis**.
5. Gastrointestinal bleed, make sure to check **colonoscopy and esophagogastroduodenoscopy** history.
6. **Medications improve appetite**: mirtazapine (increase dosage after 1 m), megestrol (Megace), dronabinol (Marinol), cyproheptadine.
7. **8 stand drinks in females and 10 stand drinks** in males per day for a week will lead to minor withdrawal and 15 stand drinks in females and 19 stand drinks in males per day for a week will lead to major life-threatening withdrawal.
8. **Paraneoplastic syndrome**: Lambert-Eaton myasthenic syndrome and myasthenia gravis (MG)- treatment with plasma exchange or IVIG; encephalitis associated with Abs against neuronal cell surface antigens or synaptic proteins treatment with IV methylprednisolone, intravenous immunoglobulin (IVIG), plasma exchange; for peripheral neuropathies, and particularly those with predominant demyelinating features, plasmapheresis, IVIG, and rituximab may be effective.

6/23/2018

1. Changes in the level of **acute phase reactants** result largely from the effects of cytokines, including **IL-6, IL-1 beta, TNF-alpha, and interferon-gamma**.
2. **Erythrocyte sedimentation rate (ESR)** increases in systemic and localized inflammatory and infectious diseases, malignant neoplasms, tissue injury, and ischemia and trauma, **decreases in abnormalities of erythrocytes, extreme leukocytosis, heart failure, high serum salt of bile, hypofibrinogenemia, and cachexia**.
3. ESR normally increases with age [normal value: age in years/2 for men, (age in years + 10)/2 for women], anemia, end-stage renal disease (ESRD), and obe-

sity. In systemic lupus erythematosus (SLE), ESR is elevated, while C reactive protein (CRP) can be normal.

4. **Infection**, often bacterial, is found in **80% of patients with CRP >100 mg/L**, and 88%–94% if >500 mg/L.
5. **ESR ≥ 100** has a sensitivity of 0.36 for infection, a specificity of 97% for infection; 0.25 for sensitivity and 0.96 specificity for malignancy; 0.21 sensitivity for noninfectious inflammatory disease, and 99% specificity as a "sickness" index.
6. **Fluid maintenance** = consider normal saline or lactated ringers (weight + 40) cc/h if no contraindication.
7. Diagnostic criteria for **the hyperosmolar hyperglycemic syndrome (HHS)**: plasma glucose ≥ 600; effective serum osmolarity ≥ 320 mOsm/kg or greater; profound dehydration, up to 9 L fluid deficit; serum pH ≥ 7.3; HCO_3 ≥ 15 mEq; small ketonuria and absent to low ketonuria; **some alteration in consciousness**.
8. Diagnostic criteria in **diabetic ketoacidosis (DKA)**: blood glucose > 250 mg/dL; arterial pH < 7.3; serum bicarb < 18; AG > 10; ketonuria and/or ketonemia.
9. **Chronic myelogenous leukemia (CML)** phases: chronic phase, accelerated phase, or blast crisis. CML → acute leukemia (blast crisis) at 20% of patients a year (acute lymphocytic leukemia rather than acute myeloid leukemia) if untreated, 1% with treatment. **Treatment of CML**: potential cure with allogeneic hematopoietic cell transplantation (HCT); disease control without cure using tyrosine kinase inhibitors; or palliative therapy with cytotoxic agents.
10. Accelerated or blast phase: short-lived response to treatment. Significant relapse even after successful treatment with **imatinib, and dasatinib** and it is appropriate to consider transplantation.
11. Philadelphia translocation (Ph) with translocation t(9;22)(q34;q11) containing fusion gene (**Phi+, BCR-ABL**) is required for the diagnosis of CML.
12. **Definition of blast crisis**: ≥20% peripheral blood or bone marrow blasts; large foci or clusters of blasts on bone marrow biopsy; the presence of extramedullary blastic infiltrates (myeloid sarcoma AKA granulocytic sarcoma or chloroma). **Signs and symptoms of blast crisis include** fever, critical leukocytosis or leukostasis, fatigue, bone pain, malaise thrombocytopenia, anemia, splenomegaly
13. **Transformation** [CML transforms into AML (1/3) and ALL (2/3) in blast crisis] may be suggested if development of **signs and symptoms more typical of acute leukemia** (e.g., night sweats, weight loss, fever, bone pain, symptoms of anemia and bleeding). **Evaluation** includes CBC with differentials, CMP, unilateral bone marrow aspiration and biopsy, BCR-ABL analysis, HLA typing, and allogeneic HCT.
14. **Hyperleukocytosis** is defined as a total leukemia blood cell count greater than 50,000 or 100,000/μL. **Leukostasis** also known as symptomatic hyperleukocytosis is a medical emergency mostly seen in AML or CML as a blast crisis. It's characterized by an extremely **elevated blast cell count and decreased tissue perfusions**.

15. Cut-off points for the occurrence of symptoms of **leukostasis risks**: WBC >100 in AML, tumor lysis, and DIC are more common in ALL; WBC >400 in CLL; and CML >100 WBC. **Treatment is urgent cytoreduction** via induction chemotherapy with prophylaxis for tumor lysis syndrome.

6/24/2018

1. **Infectious endocarditis (IE)**: an early surgical approach is reserved for those with acute and refractory heart failure, perivalvular extension of infection, fungal IE, recurrent emboli, or high embolic risk (>1 cm vegetation with severe regurgitation or stenosis). Surgery is indicated for IE with heart failure or shock, evidence or risk of persistent infection, and embolic risk reduction.
2. **Acute kidney injury (AKI)**, check FENa: FENa < 1% prerenal, 1%–4% intrinsic, >4% post renal for FENa. Order indwelling Foley for all patients with concerns of obstruction.
3. **Drug overdose, call poison control**.
4. AFib etiologies (**PIRATEs**): pulmonary embolism (PE) and chronic obstructive pulmonary disease (COPD), idiopathic, rheumatic heart-mitral regurgitation, atherosclerotic, myocardial infarction (MI), coronary artery disease (CAD), endocarditis, thyroid, and sick sinus syndrome.
5. **ST depression in V1 and V2** = consider posterior ST elevation myocardial infarction (it is posterior STEMI).
6. **Type and screen** for blood transfusion only good for 3 days.
7. **Renal disease workup**: C3, C4 low in SLE; C3 also low in post-streptococcal glomerulonephritis (PSGN) while C4 usually normal. Serum protein electrophoresis (SPEP), urine protein electrophoresis (UPEP) for multiple myeloma (MM), ANA, and ANCA for autoimmune disease.
8. **Doxycycline** can be used for pneumonia with long QTc.
9. Make sure to talk to the patient to get consent before major medication changes, like initiation of anticoagulation. In modern-day clinical practice, **it is recommended to inform patients of diagnosis and treatment plans at the earliest possible time**.
10. **Toxic epidermal necrolysis (TEN):** ≥30% of the body surface. **Steven Johnson syndrome** < 10% of body surface involvement.
11. Diagnosis of **toxic shock syndrome**: fever, hypotension, diffuse erythroderma, desquamation (unless patient dies before desquamation can occur), and involvement of **at least three organ systems.**
12. **Streptococcal toxic shock syndrome (TSS)** is associated with severe pain and tenderness signifying infection at a site of local trauma in addition to the other manifestations of TSS → needs urgent debridement.
13. **Treatment for Staph and Strep TSS**: Vanco or nafcillin/oxacillin plus clindamycin.
14. **Bisphosphates** may cause irreversible acute kidney injury (AKI) due to acute tubular necrosis (**ATN**) and focal segmental glomerulosclerosis (**FSGS**).
15. **Padua score** for risk of VTE: <4 low risk; ≥4 high risk.

16. Sonosite for central line placement demos. **Flomax** causes orthostatic symptoms.

6/25/2018

1. For AFib, no need to use heparin, can go directly to **warfarin**. If DVT/PE treatment, then do heparin and warfarin at the same time and **bridge** if novel oral anticoagulation is not an option.
2. **Chest pain important differential diagnoses**: pulmonary embolism (PE) and aortic aneurysm (pleural effusion).
3. **Cerebral metastasis, structural heart disease** (fibroelastoma, valvular vegetation from IE), no need for anticoagulation if no other conditions requiring anticoagulation.
4. **Typhlitis** = neutropenic enterocolitis of the cecum.
5. **Unstable angina** is considered present in patients with ischemic symptoms suggestive of an acute coronary syndrome (ACS) without elevation in biomarkers with or without EKG changes indicative of ischemia.
6. **Angina (coronary ischemia) is considered unstable** if it is any of the following: rest angina generally lasting >20 min; new onset angina that markedly limits physical activities; increasing angina that is more frequent, lasts longer, or occurs with less exertion than previous angina.

6/30/2018

1. Gastrointestinal (GI) bleed, consider sending the patient to **ICU for complications if rapid drop in hemoglobin or blood pressure**; may need **CT angiogram GI protocol** to look for active large bleed and urgent gastrointestinal or interventional consult (embolization) depending on the location of bleeding.
2. Cardiac ischemia → stiff ventricles → **S4** → flash pulmonary edema (diastolic heart failure). Max physiological heart rate (HR) = **220-Age**.
3. **Aflutter responds well to ablation**.
4. For **larger volume paracentesis >5 L, start albumin infusion at 6–8 g per liter fluid (over 5 L) removed**.
5. Labeled red blood cell (RBC) study: Acute GI bleed loss imaging = tagged RBC scan
6. **Dakin solution**, a mixture of sodium hypochlorite (0.4%–0.5%) and boric acid (4%) diluted in water is used for contaminated wound care.

7/1/2018

1. Metabolic acidosis due to gastrointestinal diarrhea or **high output ileostomy treatment**: **NaHCO3 650 mg tid, Sandostatin, and Questran**.
2. For fever, recurrent, due to the tumor, do **naproxen 375 po tid** for 3 days. Will need to make sure to rule out infection.
3. **Short bowel syndrome**: cholestyramine/aspartame 4 g bid, add loperamide.

Resident Year 2

7/10/2018

1. **Cryoprecipitate** contains fibrinogen (factor I), factor VIII, fibronectin, factor XIII, and von Willebrand factor (VWF).
2. **Cryoprecipitate** remains an effective therapy for bleeding in patients with fibrinogen disorders, liver disease (fibrinogen < 150 or fibrinogen < 200 with massive bleeding), disseminated intravascular coagulation (DIC), or uremia after desmopressin ineffective. Cryoprecipitate may also be used for bleeding in individuals with **hemophilia A, von Willebrand disease (VWD), or factor XIII deficiency** when a purified/recombinant factor is unavailable. Cryoprecipitate is also used during pregnant patients with inherited fibrinogen disorders.

7/11/2018

1. Reticulocyte index R1 = (hematocrit/normal hematocrit) × reticulocyte %/maturation factor (45% HCT = 1, 35% = 1.5, 25% = 2). Response R1 > 2 indicates a good response from bone marrow; R1 < 2 is not a good response from bone marrow hematopoiesis.
2. **Iron deficiency anemia**: in excessive or persistent gastrointestinal (GI) blood losses, dialysis, cancer, congestive heart failure (CHF), or prior erythropoietin treatment, **IV iron (Fe-sucrose, -gluconate, -dextran) should be considered**.
3. **Celiac disease**: check for anti-TTG (**anti-tissue transglutaminase**), anti-gliadin, anti-endomysial Abs. Diagnosis requires a terminal ileum biopsy.
4. **Alpha thalassemia**: HbH (beta 4, mild form), Hb Barts (severe form, tetramer of gamma globin = gamma 4). **Beta thalassemia** (thalassemia major, minor) has **decreased HbA, normal to increased HbA2 and HbF**. Severe manifestation of thalassemia: Chipmunk facies, hepatosplenomegaly (HSM), high output heart failure, Fe overload. Diagnostic criteria for thalassemia: MCV < 70, normal Fe, **MCV/RBC < 13 (Mentzer index)**, basophilic stippling, and hgb electrophoresis. Normal hgb: **major HbA (alpha2 + beta2), minor HbA2 (alpha2 + delta2). HbF (alpha2 + gamma2).**
5. **Treatment of thalassemia**: folate, transfusion + Fe chelators (deferoxamine IV or deferasirox po)
6. **Sideroblastic anemia treatment: pyridoxine**. **Etiologies:** 5-aminolevulinate synthase gene (ALAS2) mutation, idiopathic, myelodysplastic syndrome with refractory anemia with ring sideroblasts (MDS—RARS), and reversible (alcohol, lead, isoniazid, copper deficiency) causes.
7. **Anemia of chronic disease**: microcytic or normocytic anemia (ferritin is normal or increased, hemoglobin usually typically **>8 g/dL**) with chronic illness, infection, inflammation, or cancer. **Iron deficiency anemia**: ferritin < 100 or Fe/TIBC < 20%.
8. **Pure red blood cell aplasia**: lack of erythroid precursors in bone marrow biopsy; **treatment**: thymectomy if thymoma; IVIG if parvovirus infection, immunosuppression; chemo treatment if chronic lymphocytic leukemia (CLL) or idiopathic form myelodysplastic syndrome (MDS); supportive with packed red blood cell (PRBC) transfusions.

9. **Megaloblastic macrocytic anemia**: folate, B12 deficiency, or MDS →increased LDH and indirect bilirubin. **Smear**: neutrophil hypersegmentation, macro-ovalocytes, anisocytosis, poikilocytosis.
10. **Non-megaloblastic macrocytic anemias**: liver disease, alcoholism, hypothyroidism, MDS, zidovudine.
11. **Pancytopenia**: hypocellular bone marrow (aplastic, MDS); hypercellular (MDS, leukemia, PNH, severe megaloblastic anemia); marrow replacement (myelofibrosis, tumor, granuloma); systemic disease (alcohol, sepsis, hepatosplenomegaly, toxins)
12. **Etiologies of pancytopenia**: radiation, chemo, chemicals, viruses (HHV-6, HIV, EBV, B19)
13. **Treatment of pancytopenia** (depends on etiology): allogeneic hematopoietic stem-cell transplantation (HSCT); immunosuppression [cyclosporin (CsA)/tacrolimus, anti-thymocyte globulin (ATG)]; thrombopoietin (TPO) mimetics (eltrombopag) is an option in refractory disease; supportive care: transfusions, antibiotics, granulocyte colony-stimulating factor (G-CSF), and experimental treatments.
14. **Paroxysmal nocturnal hemoglobinuria**: deficiency of glycosylphosphatidylinositol (GPI) anchors for CD55 and CD59. Causing **intravascular hemolytic anemia, and hypercoagulability**.
15. **Intravascular hemolysis**: elevated LDH, decreased haptoglobin, hemoglobinuria, hemosiderinuria, extravascular splenomegaly.
16. **Coombs test**: direct antiglobulin test (DAT). Treatment for **warm AIHA**: corticosteroid plus/minus splenectomy; IVIG, cytotoxic agents, rituximab. **Cold AIHA** treatment: avoid cold, steroids ineffective, rituximab.
17. **Drug-induced hemolytic anemia** (quinine, cyclosporin, and tacrolimus) can cause microangiopathic hemolytic anemia. **Microangiopathic hemolytic anemia**: hemolytic uremic syndrome (HUS), thrombotic thrombocytopenic purpura (TTP), disseminated intravascular coagulation (DIC), malignancy, malignant hypertension, eclampsia/HELLP (Hemolysis, Elevated Liver enzymes and Low Platelets), mechanical cardiac valves, infected vascular prosthesis).
18. For TTP, treatment with **urgent plasma exchange** to replace low ADAMTS13 and **hydrocortisone** iv may be necessary.

7/12/2018

1. Platelet (PLT) should be transfused in any patient who is bleeding with a PLT count < **50,000** (**100,000** for CNS or ocular bleeding), or in bleeding and an acquired/inherited PLT function defect regardless of PLT count. Each unit of PLT increases serum platelet **25,000–35,000**/μL.
2. **Standard dose prophylactic PLT transfusion** to prevent spontaneous bleeding in most hospitalized afebrile patients with PLT count below **10,000**/μL (with the exception of ITP which requires steroid simultaneously).

3. Other factors contributing to bleeding should also be addressed including surgical or anatomical defect, fever, infection or inflammation, coagulopathy, and acquired or inherited PLT function defect.
4. CBC: isolated decreased PLT count < 100,000; 10% have **immune thrombocytopenia (ITP) + autoimmune hemolytic anemia (AIHA) = Evans syndrome**. ITP has a large PLT in the smear. **ITP has to rule out viral etiologies** (HIV, HCV, HBV, EBV), H. pylori Ab, ANA, pregnancy APLA, TSH, parvovirus, CMV PCR, anti-PLT test not useful. **Treatment for ITP**: steroid, IVIG, splenectomy, treat with romiplostim (Nplate)/eltrombopag (Promacta) if refractory.

7/14/2018

1. **Hepatitis C assessment** includes viral genotype, liver fibrosis stage, history of prior antiviral treatment, renal functions, and medication use. Patients with **advanced fibrosis and cirrhosis** require dose modification or avoidance of certain medications. Will also require a **twice-yearly ultrasound for hepatocellular carcinoma screening and EGD**.
2. **Direct-acting antivirals** are available, highly effective, and interferon-free (in many cases, ribavirin-free) regimens are appropriate options for the majority of HCV-infected patients. HCV is treated with RNA polymerase inhibitor (RNAPi) (**sofosbuvir**), ribonucleic analog to stop RNA replication (ribavirin), and Sofosbuvir/velpatasvir (brand name Epclusa).
3. HCV subtype 1a, no cirrhosis: **sofosbuvir-velpatasvir (Epclusa)** × 12 weeks (used in cirrhosis as well), subtype 1b can also use sofosbuvir-velpatasvir. An alternative regimen includes glecaprevir/pibrentasvir for 8 weeks.
4. The **METAVIR scoring system** is a system used to assess the extent of **inflammation and fibrosis** by histopathological evaluation in a liver biopsy of patients with hepatitis C. **Activity grade**: A0 no activity; A1 mild activity; A2 moderate activity; A3 severe activity. **Fibrosis stages**: F0 no fibrosis; F1 partial fibrosis without septa; F2 portal fibrosis with few septa; F3 numerous septa without cirrhosis; F4 cirrhosis.
5. Hepatitis C from genotype 1–6 with **cirrhotic with decompensation** treatment: a daily fixed-dose combination of **sofosbuvir (400 mg)/velpatasvir (100 mg)** with weight-based **ribavirin** 600–1200 mg qd (if > 65 kg, do 1200 mg qd).
6. **Hepatitis B + D** is treated with interferon 1.5 mg/kg for 48 weeks.
7. **HBV**: LFTs, HbeAg+, **entecavir 1.5–1 mg or tenofovir**; check LFTs and US q6m for ascites, fibroscan, HBV PCR.
8. **Chronic hepatitis B**: consider liver biopsy if ALT 1–2× upper limit normal (ULN) or immune tolerated phase if age > 40. Treat if moderate to severe inflammation or fibrosis on biopsy. Treatment: entecavir/tenofovir if lamivudine-resistant, PEG-IFN (Pegylated interferon).
9. **Indications for HBV treatment**: (1) HBV DNA > **20,000** IU/mL, elevated ALT > 2× upper limit normal, no cirrhosis, regardless of HBeAg status; (2) HBV DNA ≥ **2000** IU/mL if HBeAg-negative and elevated ALT > 2× upper limit normal or evidence of advanced fibrosis; (3) compensated cirrhosis with HBV DNA > **2000** IU/mL; (4) if decompensated HBV with cirrhosis, treat with ente-

cavir right away. HBV DNA > 20,000 IU/mL, elevated ALT ≤ 2× upper limit normal, no cirrhosis, no indication for treatments.

7/15/2018

1. **Thrombotic microangiopathies** diagnosis: thrombocytopenia, usually platelet (PLT) < 20,000 + microangiopathic hemolytic anemia (MAHA) → sufficient for diagnosis. Positive schistocytes (>2–3/hpf); negative Coombs test, normal PT/PTT and fibrinogen; increased LDH (tissue ischemia and hemolysis), increased indirect bilirubin, decreased haptoglobin, and increased Cr, especially in hemolytic uremic syndrome (HUS).
2. **Treatment for hemolytic uremic syndrome (HUS) and thrombotic thrombocytopenic purpura** (TTP): decreased ADAMTS 13 activities, treatment is urgent plasma exchange ± glucocorticoids if confirmed TTP. Fresh frozen plasma (FFP) if there is a delay to plasma exchange; eculizumab in HUS and caplacizumab in TTP. **PLT transfusion is contraindicated because PLT increases microvascular thrombosis**.
3. **Heyde's syndrome** = vWF destruction by severe aortic stenosis, associated with gastrointestinal arteriovenous malformation (AVMs) and bleeding. Heyde's syndrome causes **vWF disease** which can be diagnosed with ristocetin cofactor assay. **vWF disease treatment**: dDAVP, vWF replacement; cryoprecipitate; factor VIII concentrates rich in vWF, recombinant vWF.
4. **DIC treatmen**t: support with FFP, cryoprecipitate for goal fibrinogen > 100 mg/dL, and PLTs.
5. **Hemolytic anemia**: **intrinsic**- G6PD deficiency, hemoglobinopathies including sickle cell anemia (SCA), thalassemia, membrane abnormalities like hereditary spherocytosis, paroxysmal nocturnal hemoglobinuria (PNH), spur cell anemia in liver disease. **Extrinsic**- MAHA, autoimmune, hypersplenism.
6. **Antiphospholipid syndrome (APS)** diagnosis requires ≥1 clinical and ≥1 lab test criterion. **Clinical criteria**: clinical thrombosis or complication of pregnancy (≥3 abortions < 10 weeks or >1 fetal loss after 10 weeks). **Lab criteria**: positive moderate high titer anticardiolipin, positive lupus ab, or positive beta2-GP-1 Ab on ≥2 occasions at least 12 weeks apart.
7. **Intravenous immunoglobulin (IVIG) indications**: for post-exposure prophylaxis (e.g., HAV); certain autoimmune disorders like immune thrombocytopenic purpura (ITP), Guillain-Barré syndrome (GBS), myasthenia gravis (MG) (MG),? chronic inflammatory demyelinating polyneuropathy (CIDP), common variable immunodeficiency (CVID), and chronic lymphocytic leukemia (CLL).
8. **Transfusion reactions**: acute hemolytic, delayed hemolytic, febrile nonhemolytic, allergic, transfusion-associated circulatory overload (TACO), and transfusion-related acute lung injury (TRALI).

7/17/2018

1. **Metabolic acidosis**: anion gap (AG) or non-AG; if pH < 7.1 or bicarb < 10, start bicarb drip; otherwise normal saline (NS) bolus and NS at 120 cc/h; may use BiPAP 14/6, with backup respiratory rate of 14, 50% FiO_2 if trouble breathing.
2. **Type 1 diabetes mellitus (T1DM)** is usually due to autoimmune destruction of beta cells. Testing for **islet cells Abs** (ICA, against cytoplasmic proteins in the beta cell) or other islet autoantibodies: Ab to **glutamic acid decarboxylase (GAD) 65**, insulin autoantibodies (**IAA**), protein tyrosine phosphatase antibodies, insulinoma associated protein 2 (IA-2) and IA-2 beta, and zinc transfer ZnT8.
3. **Latent autoimmune diabetes in adults (LADA)**: usually has positive islet cell antibody (ICA) or GAD65; LADA adults do not require insulin at diagnosis but progress to insulin dependence after several months to years.
4. Patients with T2DM can develop diabetic ketoacidosis (DKA) in **severe infection or other illnesses**. Sodium-glucose cotransporter-2 (**SGLT2**) inhibitors can cause **euglycemic DKA**.
5. **Maturity onset diabetes of the young (MODY)** is a clinically heterogeneous disorder characterized by noninsulin-dependent diabetes diagnosis at a young age (<25) with autosomal dominant transmission and lack of antibodies. **Heterogeneous genetic mutations in MODY**: hepatocyte nuclear factor -4alpha (HNF4A), glucokinase gene (GCK gene), hepatocyte nuclear factor -1 alpha (HNF1A), insulin promoter factor 1 (IPF1), hepatocyte nuclear factor-1 beta (HNF1B), neurogenic differentiation factor −1.
6. **Diabetes mellitus (DM) from other etiologies:** cystic fibrosis (CF), hereditary hemochromatosis, chronic pancreatitis, fibrocalculous pancreatic diabetes, Cushing, acromegaly, pheochromocytoma, glucagonomas, somatostatinomas, and hyperthyroidism.

7/20/2018

1. Ischemic stroke outside thrombolytic window (4.5–6 h), not candidate for endovascular intervention such as mechanical thrombectomy. **Treatment**: IV normal saline (NS) at 80 cc/h, allow for permissive hypertension (HTN) for initial 24, not treating HTN unless sBP > 220 or dBP > 120. Give aspirin 81 mg daily, check HA1c, lipid panel, ESR, CRP, and serial serum glucose, tele, 2D echo, MRI and MRA head and neck, neuro check q1h. **A neurologist recommended additional treatment**: low dose heparin drip without bolus for first 24 h given fluctuating symptoms and apparent proximal R MCA stenosis (update: this case should be discussed for mechanical thrombectomy).
2. Symptoms and signs of **myxedema coma**: altered mental status, depressed respiratory rate, hypothermia, hypotension, bradycardia, hyponatremia, and hypoglycemia. **Treatment**: load 5–8 ug/kg (300–600) **T4 IV**, then 50–100 ug IV qd T4; **triiodothyronine** 5–20 μg intravenously, followed by 2.5–10 μg every eight hours; **hydrocortisone** 100 mg iv q8h.
3. **Adrenal crisis** should be considered in cancer patients taking ipilimumab (CTLA4), nivolumab or other immunotherapy medications as these agents cause adrenalitis. Alternatively, medications such as **antiepileptics, barbiturates, and**

antifungals can also interfere with steroid metabolism and cause acute adrenal insufficiency.

4. **Adrenal crisis diagnosis** requires at least 2 of the following symptoms: hypotension, nausea and vomiting (N/V), fatigue, low Na, hypoglycemia, hyperkalemia; improves with IV steroids. May require **Cosyntropin stimulation test** with 250 ug ACTH stimulation (if the morning cortisol level **5–15 ug/dL**) and initiate glucocorticoid replacement if the increase in cortisol <9 ug/dl or absolute cortisol level <10 ug/dL. **Treatment**: hydrocortisone 50–100 mg IV q6-8h IV. Before the ACTH stimulation test, use dexamethasone 2–4 mg q6h IV + fludrocortisone 50 ug daily if steroids are absolutely needed.
5. **Ten endocrine emergencies**: myxedema coma (300–600 T4 loading followed by 50–100 μg T4 qd + hydrocortisone and T3), thyroid storm (IV propranolol, IV methimazole or PTU, hydrocortisone, Lugo's solution, cholestyramine), adrenal crisis (Waterhouse-Friderichsen syndrome), congenital adrenal hyperplasia (treatment with oral hydrocortisone for glucocorticoid replacement), pheochromocytoma (treatment with doxazosin or prazosin), diabetic ketoacidosis (DKA), hyperglycemic hyperosmolar syndrome (HHS), pituitary apoplexy, hypercalcemic crisis, and acute hypocalcemia.

7/21/2018

1. **Crohn disease**: 80% small bowel involvement, 50% ileocolitis, 20% limited to colon, 1/3 perianal disease. **Clinical manifestations**: crampy abdominal Pain; diarrhea (excessive fluid secretion and impaired fluid absorption), bile salt malabsorption, steatorrhea, small intestine bacterial overgrowth (SIBO), overlapping irritable bowel syndrome, bleeding, fistulas, phlegmon/abscess, perianal disease, malabsorption, and **rectal sparing**. Bile acid is normally absorbed in the ileum.
2. **Extraintestinal manifestations of Crohn's disease**: arthritis or arthropathy; eye involvement like uveitis, iritis, and episcleritis; skin disorders (erythema nodosum, pyoderma gangrenosum); primary sclerosing cholangitis; secondary amyloidosis; venous thromboembolism (VTE); renal stones; bone losses and osteoporosis; pulmonary involvement.
3. **Diagnosis of Crohn's disease**: pANCA, ASCA (anti saccharomyces cerevisiae antibodies).
4. The **typical course in Crohn's disease**: intermittent exacerbations of symptoms followed by periods of remission.
5. **Surgical indications for Crohn's disease**: bowel perforation (surgical emergency); intra-abdominal retroperitoneal or abdominal wall abscess refractory to nonoperative management; gastrointestinal (GI) bleed refractory; fibrotic stricture causing obstruction; refractory fistula.
6. **Treatment for Crohn's disease**: 5-aminosalicylates, like sulfasalazine, mesalamine; glucocorticoid, like prednisone, budesonide; immunomodulators, like azathioprine, 6-mercaptopurine, methotrexate; biologic therapies, like infliximab, adalimumab.

7. **Crohn disease activity indices**: Crohn disease activity index (CDAI) and the Harvey Bradshaw Index. **Severity of Crohn's disease**: clinical remission, mild, moderate to severe, severe fulminant (step-up therapy vs. top-down therapy)
8. **Ileum and or proximal colon involvement treatment**: budesonide is first line for low-risk patients with mildly active Crohn's disease of the ileum and proximal colon. Budesonide 9 mg qd for 4 weeks followed by taper by 3 mg for a total of 8–12 weeks. Alternatively, prednisone 40 mg qd for 1 week followed by taper 5–10 mg per week to discontinue over 1–2 months.
9. **Diffuse colitis or left colonic involvement treatment**: prednisone 40 mg qd for 1 week followed by taper over 1–2 months. Alternative sulfasalazine 3–6 g qd for 16 weeks.
10. **Management of asymptomatic diagnosed incidentally** (shallow small aphthous ulcers: oral aphthous ulcerations, can be treated with topical triamcinolone), a repeat ileocolonoscopy is performed in 6–12 months in addition to clinical monitoring.
11. **Other therapies for mild Crohn's disease**: loperamide, cholestyramine, colestipol, colesevelam, probiotics, and diet.
12. **High-risk, moderate to severe Crohn's disease treatment**: fluids IV and electrolyte replacement, IV broad-spectrum antibiotics, nutritional assessment, gastrointestinal (GI) consultation, and surgery.
13. **Partial small bowel (SB) obstruction in Crohn's disease with no evidence of long strictures (>10 cm) treatment**: IV hydration, may add IV glucocorticoids, intermittent nasogastric wall suction, and parenteral nutrition
14. **Localized peritonitis in Crohn's disease treatment**: bowel rest and antibiotics for 2–4 weeks.
15. **Patients with intra-abdominal abscess treatment**: antibiotics with drainage.
16. **Top-down approach for Crohn's disease**: a biologic agent, like tumor necrosis factor (TNF) inhibitor, together with an immunomodulatory like azathioprine (AZA), methotrexate (MTX), 6-6-mercaptopurine (6-MP) for induction therapy.
17. **Nonresponders to standard induction therapy**: anti-integrin natalizumab (Tysabri) or anti-IL-12/23 Ab ustekinumab (Stelara) and vedolizumab (Entyvio) for both induction and maintenance.
18. **HCO_3** in the basic metabolic panel (BMP) is high, will need to check venous or arterial blood gas (VBG or ABG).

7/24/2018

1. **Drug allergy**, skin peeling, treatment: stop antibiotic (ABX), start Solu-Medrol 40 mg IV stat, famotidine 20 mg bid × 3 days, Medrol dose pack, can give Benadryl iv or oral and hydroxyzine if necessary.

7/25/2018

1. **Non-ST elevation myocardial infarction (NSTEMI)**: old adults should receive cardiac catheterization; call cardiologist; do heparin drip. Plavix loading per cardiologist. Timely communications with attending at all times.

2. Altered mental status (AMS) at the same time with NSTEMI, needs CT/MRI brain to rule out **stroke, seizure, and possible other infections**.
3. D5-1/2NS + $NaHCO_3$ 8.4% at 125 cc/h, add 2 amp for each liter.

7/26/2018 Perioperative Anticoagulation

1. Estimate thromboembolic risk, estimate bleeding risk, determine the timing of anticoagulant interruption, and determine whether to use bridging anticoagulation.
2. **Indications for IVC filter**: if cessation of anticoagulation is required for 24 h or longer such as acute bleeding in acute venous thromboembolisms (VTEs), surgery using general or neuraxial anesthesia within 3–4 weeks of an acute VTE.
3. Settings in which **the anticoagulant (including warfarin with INR < 3) can be continued**: dental procedures, superficial abscess drain, cutaneous procedures (like thoracentesis and paracentesis), selected cardiac procedures (cardiac implantable devices, endovascular procedures, and catheter ablation). However, always check with the person who does the procedure.
4. **Warfarin discontinuation**: if INR > 1.5, administer po vit K 1–2 mg (IV vit K 10 mg may be necessary if INR > 5); proceed with surgery if INR ≤ 1.5, restart warfarin 12–24 h after surgery in the evening of the day of surgery or the day after surgery (heparin bridging).
5. **Dabigatran discontinuation**: 2 days hold before surgery, may hold up to 3–4 days before surgery if GFR 30–50. Restart dabigatran 2–3 days after high bleeding risk procedures, if needed, administer a lower dabigatran 110 mg qd, or DVT ppx LMWH for the initial 2–3 days after surgery. **Novel oral anticoagulants (NOACs)** like rivaroxaban, apixaban, edoxaban, do the same as dabigatran.
6. **Bridging indications**: embolic stroke or systemic embolic event within the previous 3 months, venous thromboembolisms (VTEs) in the previous 3 months, mechanical mitral valve; AFib with CHAD2S2VASc score 5–6 or stroke or systemic embolism within the previous 12 weeks; recent coronary stenting within the previous 12 weeks; previous thromboembolism during interruption of chronic anticoagulation.
7. **Timing of bridging**: initiate heparin bridging 3 days before a planned procedure (i.e., 2 days after stopping warfarin when INR is below therapeutic range), discontinue LMWH 24 h or unfractionated heparin 4–5 h before a procedure. For high-bleeding-risk procedures, restart the therapeutic dose of unfractionated heparin or LMWH 2–3 days after hemostasis. For low bleeding risk procedures in which bridging is used (eg, laparoscopic hernia repair), restart therapeutic LMWH or unfractionated heparin 24 h after the procedure.
8. **Neuraxial anesthesia** is contraindicated in anticoagulated individuals due to the risk of potentially bleeding before surgery. Wait at least 10–12 h after the last dose of LMWH or at least 24 h after therapeutic LMWH before neuraxial anesthesia.
9. In general, **diagnostic endoscopic procedures are low risk** whereas therapeutic procedures are high risk.

10. Warfarin can be reversed by **prothrombin complex concentrate** (PCC), FFP, vit K. Dabigatran can be reversed by **idarucizumab** (Praxbind). Eliquis and Xarelto can be reversed by K centra or **andexanet alfa** (Andexxa).

7/28/2018 Cholecystitis and cholelithiasis

1. **Biliary pain (colic)** = episodes of right upper quadrant (RUQ) pain or epigastric abdominal pain from gallstones, lasting 30 min to 3 h. **Treatment**: cholecystectomy, usually laparoscopic if symptomatic.
2. **Cholecystectomy (CCY) indications in asymptomatic patients with gallstones**: gallbladder (GB) calcification, GB polyps > 10 mm, native Americans, stone > 3 cm, or bariatric surgery or cardiac transplant candidates. NSAIDs diclofenac 50 mg intramuscular ⇒ consider opiates for pain.
3. **Complications of gallstones**: cholecystitis, choledocholithiasis (common bile duct stone, may lead to cholangitis and gallstone pancreatitis), cholecystoenteric fistula, gallstone ileus (small bowel obstruction at ileum due to stone through fistula), gallbladder cancer. **Mirizzi syndrome—common hepatic duct compression** by cystic duct or infundibulum stone—jaundice, biliary obstruction.
4. **Acalculous cholecystitis**: gallbladder stasis and ischemia → inflammatory response, mainly in critically ill hospitalized patients such as postop of major surgery, total parenteral nutrition, sepsis, trauma, burns, opiate use, immunosuppression, infection of CMV, Cryptococcus, campylobacter, or typhoid fever.
5. **Laboratory evaluation**: increased WBC +/− mild increase in bilirubin, ALP, AST/ALT, and amylase. **Diagnosis** of cholecystitis, right upper quadrant ultrasound (RUQ U/S), high sensitivity and specificity for stones. **Gallbladder wall thickness > 4 mm**, pericholecystic fluid, and a sonographic Murphy sign. HIDA has a 10%–20% false positive rate (cystic duct obstructed from chronic cholecystitis, lengthy fasting liver disease).
6. **Treatment for cholecystitis**: NPO, IV fluid, nasogastric tube if intractable vomiting, analgesia, CCY. **Alternatives**: endoscopic ultrasound (EUS)-guided transmural or endoscopic retrograde cholangiopancreatography (ERCP)-guided transcystic duct drainage or **percutaneous cholecystostomy** (if without ascites or coagulopathy), usually if a patient is not a surgical candidate. Intraoperative cholangiogram or ERCP to rule out choledocholithiasis in **patients with jaundice, cholangitis, or stone in the bile duct (BD) under ultrasound**.
7. **Choledocholithiasis**: right upper quadrant pain **cholestatic pattern** elevation of liver enzymes (increase in ALP ⋙ AST/ALT elevation); may have acute cholangitis, total bilirubin > 4 mg/dL, common bile duct stone or dilation. RUQ ultrasound common bile duct (CBD) stone seen in 50% of cases, inferred from **dilated CBD > 6 mm**. ERCP is the preferred diagnosis modality when suspicion is high. Cholangiogram (**percutaneous drainage**, intraoperative gallstone removal) when ERCP is unavailable or unsuccessful. EUS/MRCP may be ordered to exclude bile duct stones when suspicion is low. **Treatment**: ERCP, CCY in 6 weeks unless contraindicated. **Complications**: cholangitis, cholecystitis, pancreatitis, and strictures.

8. **Cholangitis**: bile duct stones (malignant biliary/pancreatic) or benign stricture, infection/flu-like (Opisthorchis viverrini and Clonorchis sinensis). **Charcot's triad** (biliary obstruction with upper abdominal pain, fever, and jaundice) and **Reynolds pentad** (Charcot's triad plus confusion and hypotension). **Diagnosis**: RUQ ultrasound, increased WBC, bilirubin, ALP, amylase, positive blood culture, ERCP, percutaneous transhepatic cholangiogram if ERCP is unsuccessful. **Treatment**: conservative antibiotics with biliary drainage on an elective basis, 20% require urgent biliary decompression via ERCP (papillotomy, stone extraction, and/or stent placement). If **sphincterotomy** cannot be performed (larger stones), **a biliary stent or nasobiliary catheter** can be done otherwise **percutaneous transhepatic biliary drainage** or surgery.
9. **Hyoscyamine** indications: as a gut antispasmodic and anti-tremor agent for muscle cramps in bowels or bladder; symptoms of IBS, colitis, and other digestive problems; pain caused by kidney stones or gallstones, and muscle problems (tremors and rigidity) related to Parkinson disease.

7/31/2018

1. **Ferritin levels** >100 ng/mL are rarely seen in iron deficiency anemia, even with associated inflammation. Elevated methylmalonic acid is specific for B12 deficiency. Iron deficiency versus celiac disease.
2. Differential diagnoses (DDx) for **hypoproliferative normocytic anemia**: anemia of chronic disease (ACD), aplastic, pure red blood cell (RBC) aplasia, and chronic kidney disease (CKD).
3. **Spherocytosis** DDx: autoimmune hemolytic anemia and spherocytosis. Normal red cell distribution width (RDW) is seen in thalassemia.
4. **Hypoproliferative microcytic anemias** DDx: FLATs (Fe/iron deficiency, Lead poisoning, Anemia of chronic disease, Thalassemia, Sideroblastic anemia). **Hypoproliferative macrocytic anemia** DDx: B12/folate, myelodysplastic syndrome (MDS), hypothyroidism, liver disease, alcohol, drugs. **Hypoproliferative normocytic anemia** DDx: renal failure, aplastic anemia, pure RBC aplasia, thyroid disease, MDS, and multiple myeloma (MM).
5. **Erythropoietin** indication: end-stage renal disease (ESRD) with Hgb < 10 with a target hemoglobin of 10–11.5 g/dL. ESRD patients with **transferrin saturation ≤ 30 and ferritin < 500** require iron supplementation, preferably IV.
6. **Lichen planus** is characterized by multiple discrete intensely pruritic, polygonal-shaped violaceous papules/plaques involving the flexure surfaces of extremities (commonly wrist), buccal mucosa, or external genitalia.
7. Uncomplicated **bacterial rhinosinusitis** in an individual without antibiotic exposure in the past 6 weeks' treatment: amoxicillin, doxycycline, TMP-SMX; others like Augmentin, moxifloxacin, levofloxacin may also be used.
8. Most common bacterial bronchitis is caused by **mycoplasma and Chlamydophila** pneumonia; wheezing is common in both viral and bacterial bronchitis.
9. In otherwise healthy patients presenting with radicular complaints, no red flags, and no evidence of major neurologic abnormalities, imaging is not necessary **unless symptoms persist beyond 6 weeks**.

Takeaway Messages

1. Confusion (lack of coherent thinking) vs. delirium (decreased arousal and attention).
2. Allergic bronchopulmonary aspergillosis (ABPA) is marked by asthma and recurrent COPD exacerbations from accumulation of mucus in the bronchial tubes, elevated levels of eosinophils, pneumonia, and bronchocentric granulomatosis.
3. Urine sodium less than 20 mmol/L is indicative of decreased tissue perfusion whereas a level greater than 40 mmol/L is SIADH.
4. Infection, often bacterial, is found in 80% of patients with CRP > 100 mg/L, and 88%–94% if >500 mg/L. ESR $\geq$ 100 has a sensitivity of 0.36 for infection, and a specificity of 97% for infection.
5. Blast crisis refers to $\geq$20% peripheral blood or bone marrow blasts. Leukostasis has elevated blast cell count and decreased tissue perfusions.
6. For larger volume paracentesis >5 L, start albumin infusion at 6–8 g per liter fluid (over 5 L) removed.
7. Cryoprecipitate remains an effective therapy for bleeding in patients with fibrinogen disorders, liver disease (fibrinogen < 150 or fibrinogen < 200 with massive bleeding), disseminated intravascular coagulation (DIC), or uremia after desmopressin ineffective.
9. Antiphospholipid syndrome diagnosis requires positive moderate high titer anticardiolipin, positive lupus ab, or positive beta2-GP-1 Ab on $\geq$2 occasions at least 12 weeks apart.

Vacation time
July 30th, 2018 through August 26th, 2018.

Further Readings and References

1. Akuthota, P., and P.F. Weller. *Treatment of allergic bronchopulmonary aspergillosis*, ed. C.A. Kauffman and P.J. Barnes. Waltham, MA: UpToDate. Accessed December 8, 2023.
2. Akuthota, P., and P.F. Weller. *Clinical manifestations and diagnosis of allergic bronchopulmonary aspergillosis*, ed. C.A. Kauffman and P.J. Barnes. Waltham, MA: UpToDate. Accessed December 8, 2023.
3. Senapati, J., K. Sasaki, G.C. Issa, et al. 2023. Management of chronic myeloid leukemia in 2023— common ground and common sense. *Blood Cancer Journal* 13 (1): 58.
4. Pyrsopoulos, N.T. *Hepatitis B treatment and management*, ed. B.S. Anand. MedScape. https://emedicine.medscape.com/article/177632-treatment#d1. Accessed December 8, 2023.
5. Bhattacharya, D., A. Aronsohn, J. Price, et al. 2023. Hepatitis C Guidance 2023 update: AASLD-IDSA recommendations for testing, managing, and treating Hepatitis C virus infection. *Clinical Infectious Diseases*: ciad319.
6. Douketis, J.D., and G.Y.H. Lip. *Perioperative management of patients receiving anticoagulants*, ed. Leung LLK. Waltham, MA: UpToDate. Accessed December 8, 2023.
7. Peppercorn, M.A., and S.V. Kane. *Clinical manifestations, diagnosis, and prognosis of Crohn disease in adults*, ed. J.A. Hashash. Waltham, MA: UpToDate. Accessed December 8,.
8. Hashash, J.A., and M. Regueiro. *Medical management of moderate to severe Crohn disease in adults*, ed. S.V. Kane. Waltham, MA: UpToDate. Accessed December 8, 2023.

Chapter 10
The ICU Observer, Nocturnist with Closed ICU, and Palliative Care Medicine

August 27th, 2018 Through September 23rd, 2018
At the beginning of my second year of residency, I had a half-month rotation at the medical intensive care unit shadowing fellowship-trained intensivists in a different hospital. Although I was promoted to a senior resident, my job responsibility was really as an observer for this rotation despite daily responsibilities of data gathering, patient assessment, and clinical decision-making. Nonetheless, during this rotation, I had the opportunity to revisit the topics of sedation medications for ventilation, management of acute respiratory distress syndrome, pressor support in septic shock, thrombolytic therapy for massive and submassive pulmonary embolism, hepatorenal syndrome, angioedema, cerebral salt wasting, hepatorenal syndrome and cirrhosis complications.

After the relatively smooth sailing through the medical intensive care unit, I returned to the largest hospital in south Buffalo as a senior resident admitter working nights for a month. The job duty as a senior resident night time admitter who also provided cross-coverage for inpatients inside the hospital during nights changed significantly from my experiences as an intern. Grasping the knowledge and skills for taking care of usual medical emergencies/urgencies on top of small trivial issues for patient care like pain medications, diabetes care, and sleeping medications on the general medicine floor is the key to a successful night rotation. Meanwhile, as a nocturnist admitter, appropriate workup, diagnosis, and management of patients with acute medical conditions were the daily routine that also defined the quality of my patient care as a nocturnist.

As a senior resident nocturnist, the learning experiences were no longer about congestive heart failure and pneumonia and COPD management, although taking care of these patients remains a major part of the job. Differential diagnoses of common symptoms and workup for atypical presentations became more important during this month's rotation. Patients with chest pain, abdominal pain, dyspnea, altered mentation, and cavitary lung lesions were common clinical scenarios for life as a nocturnist. Topics covered in this section were more miscellaneous and included

K. Zhou, *Internal Medicine Training Notes and Survival Guide*,
https://doi.org/10.1007/978-1-0716-4039-5_10

HIV, malaria, headache, skin lesions [urticaria, bullous pemphigoid, toxic epidermal necrolysis (TEN), and Stevens-Johnson syndrome (SJS)], thalassemia and sickle cell anemia, and extrapyramidal symptom management.

The later portion of this chapter included notes for palliative care and ambulatory medicine rotations which were my clinical rotations after the night flow. The rotation of palliative care medicine was to drill a concept that quality of life, many of the times, is more valuable than the length of life. As a doctor, we strive to provide patients with the best possible care. Yet, at times, we will have to provide patients and their families the information about the quality versus quantity of life with medical care. Besides goals of care discussions with family, improving the quality of care also depends on controlling patients' symptoms. It is worth noting that palliative care does not preclude aggressive care or treatment. The topics covered in this section included lithium toxicity management, anticoagulation strategies for valve replacements, thyroid assessments after radioactive iodine, schizophrenia prognostic factors, pneumococcal and shingles vaccination, and syphilis diagnosis and treatment.

1 Special Procedures and the ICU Observer

August 27, 2018 Through September 23, 2018

9/4/2018

1. **Acute pulmonary embolism (PE)** = symptoms immediately after the initial event; subacute PE = days or weeks after the initial event; chronic PE = slowly developing symptoms of PE over many years, i.e. chronic thromboembolic pulmonary hypertension (TEPH).
2. **Size: massive**/high-risk PE, **submassive** or **intermediate**-risk PE, low-risk PE.
3. **Anatomic location:** saddle, lobar, segmental, subsegmental PE.
4. **Hemodynamically unstable PE** is defined as sBP < 90 or drop in sBP > 40 cm Hg from baseline for >15 min.
5. Prognostic models for low vs high-risk PE: **pulmonary embolism severity index (PESI)** (≥85); simplified PESI (≥1).
6. Diagnosis of PE: **CT angiogram**; if contraindicated due to kidney function, order **V/Q scan**. For massive and submassive PE, also recommend **echo** (right ventricular enlargement/hypokinesia, regional wall motion abnormalities that spare the right ventricular apex (**McConnell's sign** or Visualization of a clot).
7. **Treatment of PE**: respiratory support; IV fluid (limited); vasopressors (Levophed, or dobutamine plus Levophed). **Wells score** for anticoagulation (AC), if contraindicated for AC, do **inferior vena cava (IVC)** filter.
8. For patients with **high-risk PE and possibly intermediate-risk PE** with large clot burden, severe right ventricle (RV) enlargement or dysfunction, high O_2 requirement, and or tachycardiac, need to consult invasive cardiologist or interventional radiologist for **thrombolysis or mechanical embolectomy**.

9. Hemodynamically unstable PE treatment: **thrombolytic therapy**; if contraindicated, do **catheter-directed thrombus removal with or without thrombolysis. Thrombolysis contraindications**: high risk of bleeding, patients-in-shock who will die before thrombolysis can take effect and in those with unsuccessful thrombolysis, prior intracranial bleeding or stroke history in the previous 3 months, tumor of brain, aortic dissection.
10. **Special populations anticoagulation** (AC): malignancy—preferring the use of low molecular weight heparin (LMWH); pregnancy-unfractionated heparin; heparin-induced thrombocytopenia (HIT) -argatroban and direct oral anticoagulation (DOAC)
11. **Thrombolytic agents**: tPA (alteplase), streptokinase, recombinant urokinase.
12. Anticoagulation therapy is typically discontinued during **thrombolytic therapy** (clear diagnosis of PE/DVT, potential contraindication reviewed, delivery via a peripheral intravenous line, initiate/continue other supportive therapy, discontinue heparin). tPA 100 mg over 2 h.
13. **Massive proximal** lower extremity (LE) or **iliofemoral thrombosis associated with severe symptomatic swelling or limb-threatening ischemia** for less than **14 days** is the only widely accepted indication for thrombolytic therapy for lower extremity deep vein thrombosis (DVT), provided that the patient has good functional status and low risk of bleeding.
14. **Screening for inherited thrombophilia** should include Factor V Leiden mutation, prothrombin gene mutation, antithrombin (AT), protein C/S, prothrombin G20210, antiphospholipid antibody.
15. Venous thromboembolism (VTE) prophylaxis (ppx) **in pregnant women with thrombophilia**: anticoagulation with intermediate dose or therapeutic dose LMWH.
16. **Heparin-induced thrombocytopenia (HIT)**: argatroban 1–2 mg/kg per min continuous drip. If a patient develops HIT while on warfarin, d/c warfarin and reverse it with vit K. Warfarin restart only if stably anticoagulated with alternative AC and platelet (PLT) >150,000. If **argatroban** treatment for HIT, argatroban can be stopped if INR >4, but repeat INR in 4–6 h after stopping argatroban.

9/5/2018

1. Acute onset muscle pain with passive muscle stretching may indicate **acute compartment syndrome**; this is a surgical emergency.
2. **Wolff-Parkinson-White (WPW)** treatment is cardiac ablation.
3. Low erythropoietin = consider **polycythemia vera** (PV); if high erythropoietin = consider secondary causes.
4. **Candida endophthalmitis** with vitreous involvement is typically treated with amphotericin B, intravitreal antifungal injection, and vitrectomy. An **urgent ophthalmologist** consultation is needed.
5. **Eccentric, punctate, and reticular** but not popcorn calcifications of lung nodules are suspicious for **malignancy**.
6. The use of erythromycin in breastfeeding women has been linked to the development of **infantile hypertrophic pyloric stenosis**.

7. **Azithromycin** is used in **cat scratch disease** (Bartonella henselae, a gram-negative rod, regional lymphadenitis).
8. **Pneumocystis pneumonia** (PCP): increased LDH, reticular infiltrates, induced sputum or BAL PCR), treatment: **TMP-SMX; add prednisone** if Aa gradient >35 and/or $PaO_2 < 70$ mmHg.
9. **Acute ischemic colitis** = consider acute abdominal pain followed by bloody diarrhea, and significantly high lactic acid. Central venous pressure target 8–12 mm H_2O.
10. **Infectious endocarditis** ⇒ mycotic aneurysm (aneurysms from infection of the arterial wall).
11. Treatment with **antithyroid medication or radioactive iodine** is indicated if TSH <0.1, age >65, CAD, or osteopenia in **subclinical hyperthyroidism**.
12. **Shaken baby syndrome**: look for retinal hemorrhage, and will need a CT head.
13. **Hypertrophic cardiomyopathy** treatment: **beta blocker, verapamil, or disopyramide; if low blood pressure, give phenylephrine and volume infusion while beta-agonists are contraindicated**. HIV needs statin; caspofungin for severe candida and aspergillus.
14. **Parathyroidectomy indications**: symptomatic hypercalcemia; complications like osteoporosis, nephrolithiasis, CKD; severe HTN, age <50
15. In mitral regurgitation (MR), a left ventricular ejection fraction (LVEF) of 55% may indicate left ventricular systolic dysfunction. Symptomatic and **asymptomatic severe mitral regurgitation** with valve hemodynamics [central jet MR >40% left atrium or holosystolic eccentric jet MR, vena contracta width (VC) >0.7 cm, mitral regurgitant volume (Rvol) >60 mL, regurgitant fraction (RF) >50%, effective regurgitant orifice (ERO) >0.40 cm^2] may need valvular surgery. **Aortic stenosis (AS)** needs aortic valve replacement if LVEF <50%, dobutamine stress echo $V_{max} > 4$ m/s, aortic valve area < 1 cm^2, or $\Delta P_{mean} \geq 40$ mmHg.
16. **Sinus bradycardia** is common in inferior wall myocardial infarction (MI).
17. **Persistent hypotension** after atropine for bradycardia should receive normal saline (NS).
18. Repeated episodes of vomiting, chest pain, and fever in an alcoholic raise concern for **esophageal perforation with acute mediastinitis**.
19. **Rocky Mountain Spotted Fever (RMSF)**: rash on the 3rd to 5th day, treat early fulminant cases, can develop changes in mental status, focal neurological deficits, seizures, multiorgan failure, leading to death. **Treatment**: Doxycycline for 7 days minimum and at least 3 days after being afebrile.
20. AIDS patient with headache (HA), visual changes, **papilledema, and cranial nerve palsies** = consider **cryptococcal meningoencephalitis**. Extremely elevated cerebrospinal fluid (CSF) pressure and molluscum contagiosum. Treatment: induction therapy with **amphotericin B and flucytosine** for >2 weeks → consolidation with **high dose oral fluconazole** for 8 weeks → maintenance with **low dose fluconazole** for ≥1 year.
21. **Weakness of 1-sided body** raises concerns for acute stroke, call code stroke → tPA in 3–4.5 h, check for bleeding risk.

22. **Ceftriaxone can displace albumin-bound bilirubin in neonates**; thus, cefotaxime is used. ≤28 days neonate, use ampicillin + gentamicin or cefotaxime. >28 days infant, ceftriaxone/cefotaxime ± vancomycin.
23. The test for the **urethral diverticulum** is pelvic MRI or transvaginal US. **Symptoms of urethral diverticulum** include frequent urinary tract infections, dyspareunia, urinary incontinence (UI), or malignancy. Treatment is urethral **diverticulectomy excision and reconstruction** but may involve complications of urethrovaginal fistula, urinary incontinence, and rarely urethral stricture.
24. **Gestational diabetes mellitus (DM)** screening at 24–28 weeks with 1 h 50 g oral glucose tolerance test (OGTT); if ≥140, do 3 h 100 g OGTT (180, 155, 140, 95).
25. **Torsade de pointes (Tdp) treatment is magnesium IV.**
26. Renal transplant: **hypertension** likely due to renal artery stenosis if within the first 6 months after renal transplant. In this condition, **angiotensin-converting enzyme inhibitor (ACEi) is contraindicated** because of renin-angiotensin-aldosterone system (RAAS) activation.
27. **Tuberculosis (TB)** in pregnant treatment: isoniazid (INH), rifampin (RIF), ethambutol (EMB) for 2 months, then INH and RIF for 7 months. No use of pyrazinamide. Infants and children with TB meningitis, miliary TB, and TB osteomyelitis should receive anti-TB therapy for 12 months.
28. **Disseminated herpes** is characterized by the appearance of lesions outside of the primary or immediately adjacent dermatomes. Disseminated infection requires **standard precautions plus airborne and contact precautions**.
29. **Acute rhinosinusitis** is most commonly due to viral pathogens and usually resolves within 10 days. Patients with symptoms greater than 10 days, severe symptoms, or deterioration after several days of improvement often have **bacterial rhinosinusitis**. **Treatment**: 7–10 days of Augmentin.
30. **Biliary colic** test is abdominal ultrasound (US). **Dyspepsia** in patients of >55 yo or with alarm symptoms (vomiting, bleeding or anemia, abdominal mass or unintended weight loss, and dysphagia) need EGD. <55 years old if H. pylori prevalence <10%, can do PPI trial. If the prevalence of H. pylori is >10%, test for H. pylori.
31. **Pneumoperitoneum** is a surgical emergency: in preparation for expedited surgical intervention, start treatment with IV fluid, broad-spectrum antibiotics (ABX), and IV proton pump inhibitor (PPI) if concerns for peptic ulcer perforation.
32. **Genetic testing** is indicated in high-risk family history: 2 first degree relatives with breast cancer, one ≤50, 3 first or second with breast cancer, first or second relative with both breast and ovarian cancer, first degree relative with bilateral breast cancer, male breast cancer, Ashkenazi Jews.
33. **High-risk nodules** require direct VATS or bronchoscopy excision.
34. Treatment for **toxic thyroid nodules** is radioactive iodine ablation and surgery.
35. The most common microorganism from **corneal foreign body culture** is staphylococcus; if contact lenses, risks of pseudomonas are high.

36. **Akathisia** treatment: propranolol or lorazepam.
37. **Lobular carcinoma in situ (LCIS)** needs an excisional biopsy to rule out invasive breast cancer ductal carcinoma in situ (DCIS).
38. For **multiple sclerosis** (MS), IV steroids should be first given because oral steroid is associated with optic neuritis. **If refractory, do plasmapheresis.** Prevention of exacerbation using interferon (**IFN**) or **glatiramer acetate**: both are mainstay treatments for relapsing-remitting multiple sclerosis.

9/6/2018

1. Amoxicillin administration in infectious mononucleosis from Epstein-Barr virus (EBV) causes a generalized **maculopapular rash**.
2. Topical oxymetazoline (**Afrin**) and **Rhino rocket** are used for nosebleeds.
3. **Plasmapheresis and intravenous immunoglobulin (IVIG)** are the mainstay treatments for severe and progressive Guillain-Barré syndrome (GBS).
4. **Peripheral arterial disease (PAD)** treatment: statin, aspirin (ASA), Plavix, blood pressure control, screening and treatment of DM.
5. **Hemolytic crisis** in G6PD deficiency: **splenic sequestration** is seen in young children. **Aplastic crisis** is seen in the transient failure of erythropoiesis.
6. **Anomalous origin of the coronary artery** is a common cause of sudden cardiac death in young adults. Symptoms include exertional chest pain, syncope, and sudden cardiac death. **Treatment** may include restriction in strenuous exercise, beta blocker, and surgery.
7. **Pancreatitis predictor** for persistent organ failure and pancreatic necrosis: **HCT > 44% and increased B**UN.
8. **Benzo withdrawal**: confusion, restlessness, psychosis, and autonomic instability (increased heart rate, blood pressure and temperature).
9. **Incidentaloma of the adrenal gland** workup: electrolytes, dexamethasone suppression test, 24-h urine-free, and plasma-free metanephrines (creatinine, total catecholamines, vanillylmandelic acid, and metanephrines) or plasma free metanephrine and urine 17-ketosteroid.
10. **Obsessive-compulsive disorder** treatment is cognitive behavioral therapy (CBT). The most common CBT is **exposure and response prevention via confronting the subject** or event or thoughts that make you anxious & provoke obsessions.
11. **Phencyclidine (PCP) intoxication** leads to severe agitation and violent behavior. Should be **treated STAT with benzos**. Urine drug screening (UTox) is needed but not required.
12. For all possible depression patients, the first step is always screening the patient for **suicidal ideation**.
13. In refeeding chronic alcoholics, particularly if respiratory alkalosis is present, phosphate will shift into cells causing a decrease in **phosphate**.
14. **Celiac disease** is associated with **dermatitis herpetiformis**; **Crohn's disease** is associated with **perianal skin tags** and **pyoderma gangrenosum**. **HCV** is associated with **lichen planus, porphyria cutanea tarda, and cryoglobulinemia** causing leukocytoclastic vasculitis.

15. **Acrochordons** = skin tags, obesity, insulin resistance. HIV/Parkinson's disease is associated with severe seborrheic dermatitis.
16. **Serum uric acid level is low** in syndrome of inappropriate antidiuretic hormone (**SIADH**).

9/7/2018

1. 74 yo F status post (s/p) bifemoral bypass with pH 7.11 from **metabolic acidosis**. Treatment: **Bicarb** 100 mEq (3 amps) in D5W 1000 mL at 150 cc/h; **BiPAP** I = 12, E = 6, FiO_2 40%, backup rate 20 to keep $SO_2 > 92\%$.
2. **Liver failure, alcoholic hepatitis**: AST/ALT > 2, decreased PLT, consider steroid if MDE > 32, MELD >18, or presence of encephalopathy. Methylprednisolone decreases death but increases infection.
3. **Magnetic resonance cholangiopancreatography (MRCP)** is indicated if biliary dilatation without biliary stones on other imaging studies.
4. **Hypotension pathophysiology in liver failure**: severe portal hypotension (HTN) and bacterial translocation (initially in lymph nodes) → severe splenic arterial vasodilation → increased cardiac output (CO) and plasma volume insufficient to normalize effective arterial blood flow → sodium retaining and ascites → further activation of the vasoconstrictive system, leading to impairment of CO.
5. Differential diagnoses of **renal failure in cirrhosis/liver failure**: hepatorenal, acute tubular necrosis (ATN), **presence of renal tubular epithelial cells favors ATN**, Fena <1% favors hepatorenal. Other causes include hypovolemia, parenchymal disease, and the use of certain drugs.
6. **Hepatorenal syndrome** treatment: if critically ill, do Levophed + albumin 1 g/kg to increase mean arterial pressure (MAP) 10 mmHg. If not critically ill, do **octreotide** 100–200 tid subcutaneously + **midodrine** max 15 mg pot id + 1 g/kg **albumin** followed by 20–60 g albumin.
7. **Angioedema requiring intubation, interventions before extubation**: cuff leak test, famotidine 20 mg iv q12h + Benadryl 50 mg iv q6h, Decadron 4 mg iv q6h, avoid angiotensin-converting enzyme inhibitor (ACEi).
8. **Intracranial bleed with brain metastatic mass**, treatments: Keppra 1500 mg iv bid; Decadron 4 mg iv q8h. **Vasogenic edema in brain tumor**, treatments: 10 mg Decadron loading dose, followed by 4 mg 4 times daily or 8 mg bid. However, smaller doses (4–8 mg qd) are adequate and less toxic. A total maintenance dose of **16 mg per day** is typically reserved for patients with **significant edema and deficits**.
9. **Wean off sedation**: change to Precedex from versed; pressure support ventilation (PSV) for 1 h then extubate, may check VBG before and after extubation, may transition to high flow first.
10. **Diabetic ketoacidosis (DKA)** fluid speed: NS at 200 cc/h if young; bolus 2 L if LVEF ok. When K 4–5, add KCl 20 mEq to each liter IVF.
11. **Seizure treatment**: carbamazepine 300 mg bid; Lexapro (escitalopram) 5 mg qd.

12. pH = 7.19 in alcoholic liver failure treatment, do BiPAP at the same time, $NaHCO_3$ 8.4% 100 mEq in D5W 2 amp, and BiPAP 12/6, backup rate 12.

9/8/2018

1. **C. diff infection (CDI)** treatment: oral vancomycin 125 mg qid or fidaxomicin 200 mg bid (expensive, treatment may not be covered by insurance) is recommended for 10 days in both severe and non-severe CDI. In patients with fulminant disease or severe complicated CDI with shock, hypotension, ileus, or megacolon, **vancomycin 500 mg qid is recommended together with parental metronidazole**. Patients with ileus can be treated with vancomycin via retention enema.
2. For **recurrent C. diff**, if oral Vanco is used initially, use the following: use fidaxomicin; use a prolonged tapered and pulsed vancomycin regimen that is administered over 6–12 weeks; repeat Vancomycin 125 mg qid for 10 days. Patients may also be managed with 10 days of vancomycin followed by 20 days of rifaximin or a fecal transplant.
3. **C. diff toxin negative but PCR positive is considered as carrier status which may need treatment if symptomatic**.

9/9/2018

1. **Cerebral salt wasting (CSW)**, similar to a combination of syndrome of inappropriate antidiuretic hormone, in a patient with subarachnoid hemorrhage (SIADH + SAH) differs from SIADH in the fact that **CSW is hypovolemic and SIADH is euvolemic**.
2. **SIADH + SAH**, the patient may be treated with **mineralocorticoids**, such as fludrocortisone and normal saline.
3. **Hyponatremia patients with SAH** should be treated with **hypertonic saline** to both preserve cerebral perfusion and prevent complications from hyponatremia-induced brain swelling. One proposed regimen is an infusion of hypertonic saline at **20 cc/h** with subsequent dosing dependent on the measurement of sodium. One time of maximal dose of **100 cc** NS3% raises Na 1.5 mEq.
4. **SIADH**: severe symptoms to prevent cerebral edema: 100 cc 3% NS bolus with 10 min interval to raise Na 4–6 mEq in the first 3–4 h. If urine osmolarity >500, may give Lasix 20 mg po bid can expedite increase in serum Na.
5. **SIADH** (<120): mild to moderate symptoms, use 3% NS to raise 4 mEq (in reality, we tend to prefer no higher than 0.5 mEq raise per hour) in 4 h; then fluid restriction to 800 cc/day; oral salt 1–3 g tid; oral urea 15–30 g/day → furosemide 20 mg bid po (excretion of free water → increase in serum Na).
6. The presence of a **reset osmostat** should be suspected in any patient with apparent SIADH who has mild hyponatremia 125–135, no treatment is necessary.
7. **SIADH characteristics**: hyponatremia, hypoosmolality in serum, **urine osmolarity >100 and greater than serum osmolarity, urine Na typically >40, low uric acid in plasma**.
8. **Causes of SIADH**: CNS disease; malignancy with ectopic ADH; drugs (chlorpropamide, carbamazepine, cyclophosphamide...); surgical procedure; pulmonary disease, especially pneumonia; hyper/hypopituitary.

9. In **severe hyponatremia** (<105), the goal of initial therapy is to raise Na 4–6 mEq/L in a 24 period, maximal 8 mEq/L.
10. Risk factors for **osmotic demyelination syndrome**: Na < 105, concurrent hypokalemia, chronic excessive alcohol intake, acute or chronic hepatic disease, and malnourishment.
11. **Acute hyponatremia** is Na decrease in 48 h. Severe hyponatremia symptoms include seizures, obtundation, coma, and respiratory arrest.
12. If urine Na > 40 and urine Osmo >100, consider checking **morning cortisol and ACTH stimulation test and TSH**.
13. **Tolvaptan** should not be used in most patients with cirrhosis (it is somewhat dangerous to prescribe Tolvaptan and thus it is recommended to leave this medication to nephrologists and cardiologists).

9/10/2018

1. Major **complications of cirrhosis**: variceal bleeding, ascites, spontaneous bacterial peritonitis (SBP), hepatic encephalopathy, hepatocellular carcinoma, hepatorenal syndromes, hepatopulmonary syndrome (decompensated cirrhosis).
2. The diagnosis of **hepatopulmonary shunt** is empirical in a patient who has evidence of liver disease, impaired oxygenation, and intrapulmonary shunt when other etiologies have been sufficiently excluded. Diagnostic criteria may include **portal hypertension plus A-aO_2 gradient ≥ 15 mm** (>20 mmHg if over 64 years of age) while breathing room air.

9/13/2018

1. **Hyperkalemia treatment**: do 4 Neb treatment, 1 neb is 2.5 mg albuterol; give calcium gluconate 2 g to stabilize the heart; order D50 25–50 g followed by iv regular insulin 8–10 units, plus Lokelma or Kayexalate. Additionally, bicarb bolus and drip can also be given.
2. **Cardiopulmonary resuscitation** (CPR) on septic shock? need to clarify the code status in the meantime.
3. **Half-life of amiodarone** is 30 days if acute use.
4. **Pressor support**: first line Levophed, then vasopressin and epinephrine as second line vasopressors.
5. **IV hydrocortisone** 50 mg iv q6h if pressors can't get blood pressure up.
6. **Pressors**: Levophed 500 mg bag, vasopressin 20u in NS at 12 ml/h (0.4 u/min); epi 32 mg IV 64 mg/ml to maintain MAP >65. **Sedation**: fentanyl citrate 50 μg to >100 μg IV q1h for critical-care pain observation tool (CPOT) ≥3
7. **VFib**: needs Echo, ischemic workup, and EP studies. Amio 300 mg rapid bolus, repeat 150 mg prn → amio drip (cardiologist consult to decide).

9/16/2018

1. **Neupogen** = filgrastim. Used in myelosuppressive chemotherapy with non-myeloid malignancies, AML following induction, consolidative chemo, or bone marrow transplant.

2. **Opdivo (nivolumab)** is a fully human IgG4 monoclonal Ab that selectively inhibits programmed cell death-1 activity by binding to the PD-1 receptor to block the ligands PDL1 and PDL2 from binding.
3. **Revlimid (lenalidomide)** causes **DVT, and bone marrow suppression** (neutropenia and thrombocytopenia). Revlimid is a treatment for MM, MDS, CLL.

9/20/2018

1. **Acute respiratory distress syndrome (ARDS)** diagnosis is based on PO_2/FiO_2 ratio, acute bilateral pulmonary infiltrate, and respiratory distress not from cardiac causes. **Settings of the ventilator** in a patient with ARDS: 70%/16PEEP/RR34/250 tidal volume, mv 8.5, pPEAK 38, pH 7.33/56.1CO_2/145O_2/28.7HCO_3, 99%. Changed to settings 60%/14PEEP/RR34/250tidal volume, pH 7.32/51.2CO_2/95.7O_2/30.3HCO_3, 97%.
2. **3 factors that decrease ARDS mortality**: low tidal volume ventilation, prone positioning, and the use of Nimbex (cisatracurium).
3. **pPeak** = pPlateau + respiratory resistance. If pPeak differs greatly from pPlateau, it means high resistance from the respiratory tract, and may respond to **steroids and duoneb**. If there is no difference in pPeak, no benefit from steroids and duonebs.
4. **Low tidal volume ventilation**: (A) predicted by body weight. M: 50 + 0.91 (height in cm—152.4); F: 45.5 + 0.91 (height in cm—152.4). (B) plateau pressure goal (inspiratory hold) pPlateau <30 cmH_2O. (C) check inspiratory plateau pressure with 0.5 s inspiratory pause q4h and after each change in PEEP or tidal volume. **If pPlateau > 30 cm H_2O**, decrease the tidal volume in 1 mL/kg to 5 or 4 cc/kg if needed. If pPlateau <25 cmH_2O and tidal volume < 6 cc/kg, increase by 1 cc/kg or to 6 cc/kg. If **breath stacking (auto-PEEP) or severe dyspnea, can increase tidal volume** to 7 or 8 cc/kg predicted ideal body weight (PIBW) if pPlateau <30 cmH_2O.
5. **Goal O_2**: PaO_2 55–80 mmHg or SpO_2 88%–95% (PEEP/FiO_2 5/0.3, 10–14/0.7, 14/0.8, 10/0.6)
6. The **setup of minute ventilation**: set initial RR to approximate baseline minute ventilation (not >35 breaths per minute), and adjust Vt and RR according to minute ventilation.
7. **RR X tidal volume = minute ventilation** which is approximately 5–6 L/min in healthy individuals at rest, but increases among patients who are mechanically ventilated.
8. **ARDS sedation**: propofol and fentanyl 2500 μg titrate, start at 50 μg/h and 50 μg bolus, maximal 200 μg/h. Nimbex (cisatracurium) load 0.2 mg/kg/dose (29 mg/dose) then 200 mg/100 mL titrate.
9. **Vasopressors**: Levophed, vasopressin, and epinephrine are the only three pressors with mortality benefits. Beware of autoPEEP and permissive hypercapnia with 7.25 may be Ok in ARDS. **Flolan (epoprostenol)** was also used at 1.5 mg inhalation at 6 cc/h. **Flolan is a prostacyclin that increases levels of intracellular cyclic adenosine monophosphate leading to vasodilation in the lungs**.

10. **Ventilator adjustment example**: ABG at *9/19/2018 13:28*: 7.25/58.8CO_2/25/84%

At *14:20* ventilator setting 100%/PEEP8/RR18/450tidal volume. I:E = 1:1.7. Patient breaths at 32. ABG at *15:12* pH 7.31/56.1/49.2/27.1/78%. Increase PEEP to 18 ⇒ ABG at *18:37* pH 7.29/62.2/64.5/29/89%. Ventilator *19:19* setting 100%/PEEP18/RR32/248 tidal volume, ABG at *19:27* pH 7.25/72.4/59/30.7/80.4%. Ventilator setting at *20:24* was 100%/22/32/250, PEEP increased to 20 ⇒ ABG at *21:43* pH 7.24/77.5/155/31.7/99%. Ventilator at *22:23* setting 100%/18/RR32/250 ⇒ FiO_2 90% and PEEP 18.

ABG at *9/20/2018 at 2:10 a.m.*, pH 7.3/61/217/29.2/100%, PEEP decreased from 18- > 16. ABG *5:53 a.m.* pH 7.33/56.1/145/28.7/99% ⇒ 70%/16PEEP/34RR/250 tidal volume (8 a.m.?). ABG at *9:54 a.m.* pH 7.32/61.2/95.7/30.3/97% ⇒ 60%/16/34/250 (*10,35 a.m.*). *13:56* ABG 7.32/62.1/65.8/31.3/91%. *15:18* 60%/14/34/250 ⇒ 17:44 ABG 7.36/53.9/105/29.7/98%. *19:00* ABG 60%/14/34/250 ⇒ *21:49* 7.38/51.8/125/30/99%. ABG 23:00 50%/14/34/250 ⇒ *9/21/2020 1:59 a.m.* 7.37/53.7/83.6/30.4/97%. *2:55 a.m.* ABG 60%/14/34/250, *5:56 a.m.* 7.38/53.5/103/31.1/98%.

9/21/2018

1. **Pulmonary edema** (bilateral infiltrate on CXR, no leg edema, BNP <400, no wheezing, chest pain), need to think of acute respiratory distress syndrome (ARDS).
2. A scrotal **pyocele (urological emergency)** can be distinguished from a **hydrocele** by the presence of debris, septations, or loculations in **scrotal ultrasound**. A 78-year-old male with paraplegia was brought to the hospital for encephalopathy. He was previously discharged from the emergency room for epididymitis with Bactrim. He was treated with Rocephin and doxycycline this time after admission. However, his fever continued. **Repeat scrotal ultrasound revealed hydrocele with septations and debris**. Urologist was consulted and the patient was diagnosed with pyocele and brought to the operation room right away for incision and drainage with resolution of fever thereafter.
3. **Retroperitoneum free air (surgical emergency)**: air on both sides of the bowel, lack of gastric air-fluid level, and/or visible falciform ligament. Worsening abdominal pain after EGD, repeat KUB 2 days later, the patient was found to have a 1.3 cm **gastric ulcer perforation**.
4. **Initiation of suboxone treatment** in a patient with acute femur fracture sp. intramedullary nailing: Prescription for Naloxone 0.4 mg intranasal as needed for opioid overdose, acetaminophen 1000 mg 3 times daily, oxycodone 5–10 mg every 4–6 h as needed for acute pain. Because of his acute pain with femur fracture, recommend a low dose suboxone initiation protocol: 0.5 mg daily—day 1; 0.5 mg twice daily—day 2; 1 mg twice daily—day 3; 2 mg twice daily—day 4; 4 mg twice daily—day 5; 4 mg three times daily—day 6; 4 mg four times daily—day 7 (stop other opioids (oxycodone) at this time. But may need to continue short-term for him because of his acute pain). Avoid alcohol, marijuana, benzodiazepines, and any intoxication.

2 Second Taste of Being a Nocturnist

September 24th, 2018 Through October 21st, 2018

9/29/2018

1. **Vit B12 supplement for severe B12 deficiency**: im B12 1000 mg one to three times a week or daily for 7 days, followed by 1000 mg im for 3 weeks, then monthly forever.
2. **Candida esophagitis**: fluconazole 400 mg po load, then 200–400 mg po daily for 2 weeks.
3. Use broad-spectrum antibiotics in the setting of severe disease if WBC increases, abdominal pain → ceftriaxone and Flagyl. If further concerns, do vancomycin and Zosyn.
4. **Isolated elevation of ALP** can be seen in infiltrative liver disease if gamma-glutamyl transpeptidase (GGT) elevation which includes **malignancy, granulomatous disease, infectious, and certain medications**. Other causes of ALP elevation can be seen in bone disease and TSH abnormalities.
5. **Acne treatment**: topical retinoids and benzoyl peroxide → consider the addition of topical antibiotics (erythromycin or clindamycin) → consider oral antibiotics → consider oral isotretinoin.

10/6/2018

1. **Metabolic acidosis**: Bicarb drip if severe ($pH < 7.1$ or bicarb <10 in BMP) and BiPAP if respiratory distress. BiPAP may also be used to compensate for metabolic acidosis.
2. **Differentials of dyspnea**: pulmonary embolism (PE), congestive heart failure (CHF), pneumonia (PNA), obstructive sleep apnea (OSA), obesity hypoventilation syndrome → consider CPAP, non-rebreather.
3. A patient with **chest pain** was later diagnosed with pulmonary embolism (PE). A patient with **abdominal pain** and lactic acidosis = consider bowel ischemia.
4. Status post (S/p) percutaneous coronary intervention (PCI), abdominal pain, cold legs or feet → Treatment: NPO, cefepime, and Flagyl → NS at 100 cc/h for lactic acidosis → stat general surgery consult for **acute abdomen** and vascular consult for **critical limb ischemia**.
5. **Switching between P2Y12 inhibitors requires a loading dose**. If temporarily held, just start without loading.
6. Acute kidney injury (AKI) or acute tubular necrosis: if BiCarb <21, may start bicarb drip until bicarb normalizes, 75 mEq. **Bicarbonate drip** is appropriate in AKI with severe metabolic acidemia (i.e., pH, $\leq$7.20; bicarbonate, $\leq$20 mmol/L; partial pressure of carbon dioxide, $\leq$45 mm Hg). **Mild metabolic acidosis** in AKI should be only treated with normal saline drip.
7. **Order CT chest** if drop in O_2 and chest X-ray can't tell the exact cause. Check procalcitonin, erythrocyte sedimentation rate, and C reactive protein to assess the chances of infection.

8. **Be liberal about consulting specialists**. If something is not right/patient not getting better, better to get other people involved.
9. Be broad about antibiotics if not sure of the source of infection.
10. **Crackles**: order diuretics. **Wheezing**: order DuoNeb and steroids.
11. **IgG deficiency, start atovaquone if high dose steroid use**.
12. **HIV patient with significant headache** management: lumbar puncture (LP) with fluid analyses, send fluid for JC virus, cryptococcus, HSV1 and HSV2, VZV, HSV6, CMV.

10/7/2018

1. **Mild gallstone pancreatitis** should undergo cholecystectomy within 7 days of clinical improvement, usually in the same hospitalization. Delayed cholecystectomy should be considered for severe gallstone pancreatitis which is characterized by the **persistent failure of one or more organ systems** (e.g., hypotension not responding to fluid resuscitation)
2. **Ursodeoxycholic acid** is a 2nd line option for symptomatic cholelithiasis who don't desire cholecystectomy.
3. AFib not controlled with Cardizem drip, give **amiodarone** 150 mg load.
4. Cancer patients may need to discuss goals of care.
5. **Postprandial syncope** due to a drop in blood pressure after a meal, common in patients with underlying conditions like diabetes and Parkinson's disease. Possibly due to **increased blood supply diversion to the GI tract**.
6. **Bowel ischemia**, has to call surgery consult stat!
7. **Coronary artery bypass grafting (CABG)** preop workup: vein mapping, echo, carotid Doppler, and pulmonary function test.

10/8/2018 Malaria

1. Area with **chloroquine-resistant P. falciparum**, common in sub-Saharan Africa and south and southeast Asia, start prophylaxis with **atovaquone-proguanil** (may cause liver function abnormalities), **doxycycline** (causes GI disturbance), **or mefloquine** (agent of choice in pregnancy) weekly dosing.
2. Areas with **chloroquine-sensitive P. falciparum**, start prophylaxis with **chloroquine**, or **hydroxychloroquine**, need to start 1–2 weeks in advance before travel.
3. Areas without P. falciparum (parts of South Africa, Mexico, and Korea), start prophylaxis with **primaquine** (may cause G6PD hemolysis), and weekly dosing.

10/16/2018

1. Heart failure, respiratory failure, lactic acidosis, low blood pressure, may need ICU care, BiPAP, and pressors. Be vigilant for patients in need of ICU care, call ICU provider for suggestions and recommendations.

10/17/2018

1. Preferred medications for **rhythm control** (maintaining sinus rhythm) in AFib: no structural heart disease-**flecainide** and propafenone; **left ventricular hypertrophy -dronedarone** and amiodarone; coronary artery disease -sotalol and

dronedarone; **heart failure**-amiodarone and dofetilide; **recurrent AFib**- symptoms refractory to antiarrhythmic drugs-**radiofrequency catheter ablation**.

2. 1st line treatment for cluster headache (HA) is **100% oxygen inhalation**, if partial or no response, give **intranasal sumatriptan** contralateral to HA. **Verapamil** is the agent of choice to prevent cluster HA.
3. **Persistent chest pain** in cocaine abusers needs **CT angiogram** to rule out acute dissection of the ascending aorta.
4. **Rheumatoid arthritis (RA)** is a clinical diagnosis; rheumatic factor (RF) can be negative in 20% of patients; **erosive joint disease requires methotrexate**. If refractory, order purified protein derivative (PPD) test then give tumor necrosis factor (TNF) inhibitors (etanercept and infliximab). **Anti-cyclic citrullinated peptides (anti-CCP)** have a high sensitivity for RA.
5. **HIV in pregnancy treatment-** the preferred backbone treatment options: abacavir and lamivudine (ABC/3TC), emtricitabine/tenofovir alafenamide (FTC/TAF) or emtricitabine/tenofovir disoproxil fumarate (FTC/TDF). **Efavirenz** should not be started; if already on it, should not be stopped. Postnatal infants should be treated with zidovudine for ≥6weeks. Three drug combinations in highly active antiretroviral therapy (HAART) = 2 NRTIs with 1 NNRTI or PI.
6. The diagnosis of **respiratory syncytial virus (RSV)** is primarily clinical (treatment is palivizumab), lab screening RSV Ag in nasal/pulmonary secretions. RSV infection requires **contact isolation. Palivizumab** is recommended for infants at high risk for RSV due to conditions such as prematurity or other medical problems including heart or lung diseases.
7. **Primary biliary cholangitis**, formerly known as primary biliary cirrhosis (PBC) is a chronic progressive liver disease in middle-aged women: **progressive cholestasis** (without extrahepatic biliary obstruction) and **liver failure**, can have **hyperlipidemia** (HLD) and **xanthomas**. 95% of patients with PBC have **positive antimitochondrial antibodies** whereas 70% of patients with PBC have **positive ANA**. Treatment: **ursodeoxycholic acid** and **liver transplantation**; steroid is not useful. **Primary sclerosing cholangitis (up to 90%) is closely associated with inflammatory bowel disease** and has typical imaging findings of multifocal, short, annular strictures of bile ducts.
8. **HCV Ab +** requires further investigation: HCV RVA quantity and type to persistent infection, cleared infection vs. false positive test?
9. **Somatic symptom disorder** has ≥1 systemic symptom versus illness anxiety disorder (no actual symptoms).
10. **Rhinocerebral mucormycosis** (Rhizopus organisms) is seen in diabetes and other immunosuppressive conditions. **Treatment**: surgery debridement and IV liposomal amphotericin B.
11. **Bacterial vaginosis**: diagnosed with cervical discharge swab with wet mount to look for clue cells (epithelial cells); bacterial vaginosis is a risk factor for pelvic inflammatory disease, sexually transmitted infections, and other obstetric disorders. Treatment: **metronidazole oral or topical or clindamycin**. Prenatal treatment for symptom relief. Treatment has no impact on pregnancy complications.

12. **Porphyria cutanea tarda**, due to deficiency of uroporphyrinogen decarboxylase (UROD) in the liver, is strongly associated with HCV infection.
13. **Abdominal ultrasound** is the best diagnostic test for a suspected subphrenic or other abdominal abscess.
14. **Raynaud's phenomenon** treatment: nifedipine or amlodipine. If there is no response, check ANA, RF, C4, C3, CBC, and CMP.
15. **Pregnant women with acute urinary tract infection** treatment: cefalexin, nitrofurantoin (should not be used in pyelonephritis), or Augmentin 3–7 days.
16. **Mycosis fungoides/Sezary syndrome** is a type of cutaneous T-cell lymphoma.
17. **Clinical features of melanoma** (ABCDE): asymmetry, border irregularity, color variation, diameter >6 mm, evolving size, shape, color.
18. **Nelson syndrome** is characterized by pituitary enlargement, hyperpigmentation, and visual field defects following bilateral adrenalectomy. Signs and symptoms include headache, weakness, fatigue, and **hyperpigmentation**.
19. **Alopecia-areata** can commonly recur in patients, even after successful treatment and normal hair growth.
20. **Ecthyma gangrenosum** does not require surgical debridement. **Ecthyma gangrenosum** treatment: two antipseudomonal antibiotics.
21. **Clostridium myonecrosis** (also known as gas gangrene) does require surgical debridement.
22. End-stage renal disease (ESRD) patients with transferrin saturation **≤ 30% and ferritin < 500 mg/mL** require preferred IV supplementation of iron.
23. Exposure to tuberculosis (TB) should receive screening of **TB with tuberculin skin testing or IFN-r release assay. If negative, repeat in 8–10 weeks.**
24. Patients with **≥3 polyps, large (1–2 cm) adenomas, villous adenomas, or 5–10 adenomas** with high-grade dysplasia should have repeat colonoscopy in 3 years. Repeat colonoscopy in 1 year if >10 adenomas. Patients with very large polyps **(>2 cm)** or **carcinoma in situ** should have a second look colonoscopy in 2–6 months to verify complete excision. Small <10 mm hyperplastic polyps (n<20), do colonoscopy in 10 years. 1–2 small (<10 mm) tubular adenomas, repeat colonoscopy in 5–10 years.

10/18/2018

1. **Ischemic stroke treatment**: tPA or TNK (tenecteplase) in 4.5 h. Then, no antiplatelet or anticoagulation therapy for at least 24 h until a repeat CT head is done to confirm no delayed hemorrhage.
2. **Amaurosis fugax** is a sudden and transient mononuclear blindness = consider carotid artery atherosclerotic disease.
3. **Hot flashes treatment in menopause**: menopause hormone therapy, or selective serotonin reuptake inhibitor (SSRI), or serotonin and norepinephrine reuptake inhibitor (SNRI) like venlafaxine.
4. **Naloxone** to reverse opioid overdose. **Naltrexone** is an option for maintenance treatment to prevent relapse in opioid use disorder (OUD). **Buprenorphine** is a partial agonist which can worsen withdrawal symptoms in long-term opioid users.

5. **Endometritis** is caused by ascending infection from the cervix and vaginal vault by **Chlamydia** or **Gonorrhea** and others, commonly seen in sexually transmitted infections, chronic pelvic inflammatory disease, and postpartum infections. **Endometritis treatment**: clindamycin and gentamicin. **Pelvic inflammatory disease (PID)**: cefoxitin and doxycycline (should be avoided in breastfeeding)
6. **Urticaria treatment**: first or second generation H1 blocker; increase to 2–4 times standard dose of H1 blocker → add H2 blocker → add hydroxychloroquine, tacrolimus, omalizumab.
7. **Endometriosis** presents with pelvic pain, dyschezia (pain with bowel movements), rectovaginal nodularity, ovarian mass ⇒ consider infertility, and chronic pelvic pain.
8. **Meningococcal (Neisseria meningitidis) prophylaxis** in close contacts (>8 h, <3 feet, direct exposure to respiratory secretions in 7 days before symptom onset of the patient) regardless of vaccination status: rifampin 600 mg bid for 2 days, Cipro 500 mg single dose, or ceftriaxone 250 mg iv single dose in 24 h after exposure. In adults, except for tuberculosis meningitis, **only Neisseria meningitis requires droplet isolation in the first 24 h of antimicrobial therapy with mask and face protection for intubation**.
9. Post coronary artery bypass grafting (CABG), the patient appears drowsy, lethargic, and difficult to arouse, check for **opioid sedation and overdose**.
10. **Sleep terror**: non-rapid eye movement (NREM) sleep arousal disorder, treatment with benzodiazepines (BZDs). **Nightmares**: rapid eye movement (REM) sleep with clear dream recall and complete awakening.
11. **Cavitary apical lung lesion** is common at higher CD4 counts, but patients with advanced HIV can have lobar, pleural, or disseminated disease as well. **TB pleural effusion** is typically **lymphocytic and exudative with high adenosine deaminase (ADA)** levels. The smear is often negative for acid-fast bacilli, and diagnosis requires a **pleural biopsy** with a histopathological demonstration of pleural granulomas.
12. **Workups for cavitary lung lesions**: check serum Aspergillus, serum cryptococcal Ag, QuantiFERON gold, urine Histoplasma Ag, urine Blastomyces Ag, urine Strep and Legionella Ags, sputum culture PJP; and biopsy vs bronchoalveolar lavage.

10/19/2018

1. **Hepatitis C virus (HCV)** infection is confirmed with HCV PCR RNA. **HCV Ab test** is not reliable as it takes up to 12 weeks or longer to become positive in acute HCV.
2. 56 yo M with fatigue (fever, malaise, myalgia), bilateral knee and ankle pain, left side chest pain, cardiomegaly, small pleural effusion, and multiple systemic involvement. Diagnostic test: **ANA and anti-histone Ab positive**. Final diagnosis: **drug-induced lupus.** The **culprit**: procainamide, hydralazine, minocycline, etanercept and infliximab.

3. **Hepatorenal syndrome treatment**: a combination of octreotide and midodrine or Levophed alone can be used while cautioning the use of intravenous fluids. **Albumin** should also be continued for 2–3 days.
4. **Keratitis**: photophobia, blurred or impaired vision, and a foreign body sensation with difficulty opening the affected eye. Treatment: **urgent referral to an ophthalmologist**. Keratitis common in contact lenses, can be due to Pseudomonas infection with contact lens.
5. **Bacterial conjunctivitis** treatment: erythromycin ointment, polymyxin-trimethoprim drops, or azithromycin drops. Use fluoroquinolone drops if contact lens use. **Viral conjunctivitis** treatment: warm/cold compression; plus, or minus antihistamine/decongestant drops. **Allergic conjunctivitis** treatment: topical antihistamines.
6. **Common causes of papilledema**: mass lesion, cerebral edema, increased cerebrospinal fluid (CSF) production, decreased CSF outflow (venous thrombosis), and pseudotumor cerebri (idiopathic intracranial hypertension).
7. Hypertension diagnosis → **evaluation of urine protein excretion** (protein–to-creatinine ratio normally should be **<200 mg/g**). If >500–1000 mg/g, give ARB/ACEi, add diuretics → calcium channel blocker (CCB). Normal urine albumin/creatinine ratio should be <30 mg/g. Urine albumin/creatinine ratio **30–300 mg/g** in random urine sample = **microalbuminuria**.
8. **Fat malabsorption and steatorrhea** → Diagnosis of chronic pancreatitis (MRCP or CT) vs. celiac disease (no abdominal pain).
9. **Pneumothorax** diagnosis can be based on bedside ultrasound or other imaging studies.
10. **Renal ultrasound** should be performed in children <2 years old after symptoms resolve or fail to respond to appropriate antibiotics in urinary tract infection (UTI). **Voiding cystourethrogram** is performed in neonates with first-time febrile UTI or children <2 years old with recurrent infection or abnormal renal ultrasound.
11. **IV steroids are indicated in infectious mononucleosis with severe complications** (airway obstruction, overwhelming infection, aplastic anemia, thrombocytopenia).
12. Risk factors of colorectal cancer: alcohol > smoking.
13. **Traveler's diarrhea**: bacteria E. coli is more common than rotavirus (vomiting and fever). **Enterotoxigenic Escherichia coli (ETEC)** has no vomiting or fever. **Giardia** causes symptoms over 1 week after exposure and has a foul smell. **Vibrio parahaemolyticus** causes fever and bloody diarrhea.
14. Patients with severe pancreatitis, signs of sepsis, or evidence of deterioration ≥72 h after presentation should undergo **CT abdomen with contrast** to evaluate for potential complications (**pancreatic pseudocyst, pancreatic necrosis, pancreatic fistula, infected/walled-off pancreatic necrosis**) or evidence of infection.
15. Diagnosis of **acute pancreatitis** requires 2/3 criteria: abdominal pain, elevated amylase or lipase (3 times upper limit normal), and imaging findings.

16. Construction/dressing apraxia is caused by the lesion(s) in the **non-dominant parietal lobe**. Wernicke aphasia is caused by the lesion(s) in the **dominant temporal lobe**. Acalculia, finger agnosia, agraphia, and right-left confusion are caused by lesion(s) in the **dominant parietal lobe (Gerstmann syndrome).**

10/20/2018

1. **Extensive cutaneous bullous lesion** differential diagnoses: erythema multiforme vs. toxic epidermal necrolysis, Steven-Jonson syndrome, autoimmune disease, or paraneoplastic bullous disease, or mycoplasma.
2. **Toxic epidermal necrolysis (TEN)/ Stevens-Johnson syndrome (SJS)**: a. referral to intensive therapy/burn unit; b. prompt withdrawal of culprit drugs (allopurinol, antiepileptic drugs, lamotrigine, sulfonamides, mycoplasma pneumonia infection); c. supportive care, same as major burns and wound care, fluid and electrolyte management, nutritional support, temperature management, pain control, and monitoring for or treatment of superinfections. Mortality rate 10%–30% (25%)
3. **Adjunctive therapies for TEN/SJS** include systemic corticosteroids, IVIG, cyclosporine, plasmapheresis, and TNF Abs.
4. **Impetigo**: nonbullous impetigo, bullous impetigo, ecthyma (patient is not that sick). It is characterized by erythematous plaques with a yellow crust due to S. aureus (80%) or S. pyogenes (10%) infections.
5. **Ecthyma gangrenosum** is associated with Pseudomonas bacteremia.
6. In **bullous impetigo**, pustules and blisters form at the initial site of infection that trigger widespread blistering and sloughing of the skin and multiple mucous membranes.
7. **Bullous pemphigoid**: diagnosis with biopsy and serum tests for autoantibodies to the hemidesmosomal **bullous pemphigoid antigens 180 and 230**; treatment with **clobetasol topical ointment**, **doxycycline**, prednisone, and **nicotinamide**.
8. **SJS/TEN** are severe allergic reactions triggered by medication that trigger widespread blistering and sloughing of the skin and multiple mucous membranes.
9. **Staphylococcal scalded skin syndrome**: total body reddening of the skin and blistering and sloughing of the skin resembling a hot water burn or scalding of the skin, mucous membrane not involved.

10/21/2018

1. **Normal blood pressure (BP)**: <120/<80 mm Hg; **elevated BP** 120–129/<80 mm Hg. **Stage 1 hypertension**: sBP 130–139 or dBP 80–89 mm Hg, and **stage 2 hypertension**: sBP $\geq$ 140 or dBP $\geq$ 90 mm Hg. In patients with coronary artery disease, diabetes, hyperlipidemia, smokers, and CKD and an estimated 10-year ASCVD risk of $\geq$10%, **goal BP is < 130/80**. In persons with no history of CVD and with an estimated 10-year ASCVD risk <10%, **goal BP is < 140/90**. Chlorthalidone (12.5–25 mg) is the preferred diuretic for hypertension treatment.

2. **Initial treatment for hypertension**: African-American, use thiazide or calcium channel blocker (CCB); others, use thiazide, CCB, angiotensin-converting enzyme inhibitor (ACEi), or angiotensin II receptor blocker (ARB).
3. **Urine immunoassay** is urine toxicology. Chromatography is more accurate but expensive.
4. **Antibiotic prophylaxis** can be considered in young female patients who have had at least 2 urinary tract infections (UTIs) in 6 months or 3 UTIs in a year.
5. **Exercise-induced bronchoconstriction** can occur with or without pre-existing asthma. Diagnosis is made through bronchoprovocation testing.
6. **P450 system inducers**: **BCG PQRS** (Barbiturates, Carbamazepine, Griseofulvin, Phenytoin, Quinidine, Rifampin, St. John's Wort). **P450 system inhibitors**: **PICK EGS** (Protease inhibitor, INH, Cimetidine, Ketoconazole, Erythromycin, Grapefruit juice, Sulfonamides). Oral contraceptive pill (OCP) failure can be caused by the use of phenytoin.
7. In pulmonary embolism (PE), the patient has a **small amount of hemoptysis is normal**. Anticoagulation should be continued if the patient is otherwise stable.
8. **Drusen spots**: macular degeneration (cellular debris). Central retinal artery occlusion (CRAO): **cherry red macula.**
9. For older patients with memory and concentration issues, we should **assess mood and affect to screen for major depression**. High risk for Alzheimer's dementia (AD).
10. **Newborn jaundice**: Unconjugated hyperbilirubinemia (from high cell turnover), **phototherapy** should be continued until bilirubin declines to below threshold levels. **Exchange transfusion** should be considered if bilirubin is at toxic levels (>20–25 mg/dL)
11. Chest pressure with walking uphill, do **exercise stress test** to rule out coronary artery disease.
12. **Acute rheumatic fever (JONES)**, Sydenham chorea (emotional lability, distal handwriting), mitral stenosis. **Sydenham chorea develops** 1–8 months after initial Streptococcus infection. **Carditis and arthritis** develop in 3 weeks. **Sydenham chorea patients should receive long-acting im penicillin until adulthood for second prevention**. Corticosteroids can reduce the duration of symptoms but are reserved for severe cases.
13. **Huntington's disease** is an autosomal dominant (AD) disease; psychiatric symptoms, chorea, and **dementia typically manifest at age 30–50**.
14. **Rotavirus** in children can cause fever; **norovirus** causes prominent vomiting, usually in institutional settings, and causes epidemic gastroenteritis in adults and children.
15. **Campylobacter**: acute onset of cramping abdominal pain and inflammatory diarrhea (mucus and blood). Diagnosis via stool culture.
16. **Listeria** is usually associated with deli meats and soft cheese.

10/21/2018 2

1. **Molluscum contagiosum** is caused by a poxvirus, not itchy. **Chickenpox (variola)** causes an itchy rash. **Lichen planus**: intense, discrete pruritic,

polygonal-shaped violaceous papules or plaques involving the flexural surfaces of extremities (wrists), buccal mucosa, or external genitalia. Dx via biopsy.

2. **Unilateral headache** (HA) presenting with associated Horner syndrome should consider **carotid artery dissection** until proven otherwise.
3. **Physiologic jaundice** manifests 24 h after birth. Neonatal jaundice in the first 24 h is always pathologic, immune or non-immune hemolysis; G6PD is the most common cause of nonhemolytic neonatal jaundice.
4. **HbC** (glutamic acid to lysine mutation); **HbS** (glutamic acid to valine mutation, sickle hemoglobin), autosomal recessive (AR), either **HbSS** (the most common and most severe form of sickle cell disease) or **HbSC** (a milder form of sickle cell disease) is required for disease expression. **Sickle/β0-thalassemia (HbSβ0)**: complete loss of beta-globin chain = severe form of sickle cell disease. **Sickle/β+-thalassemia (HbSβ+)**: underproduction of beta-globin chain = mild to moderate sickle cell disease. **HbAS** (sickle cell trait, usually asymptomatic). **HbSβ0** thalassemia has higher hemoglobin levels and risks for acute chest syndrome compared to **HbSS**.
5. **Hemophilia A** (Factor VIII deficiency) and **B** (Factor IX deficiency) are inherited X-linked recessive patterns.
6. **Alpha thalassemia**: **No alpha globin** = $\gamma 4$ (**Hb Barts**) = hemoglobin made of four gamma chains. 4 alle, very little alpha globin, $\beta 4$ (**HbH**) = hemoglobin mainly made of four beta chains as only one α-globin gene is functional.
7. **Beta thalassemia minor** = beta chain underproduced, **HbA2**. Beta thalassemia major, marrow expansion, parvovirus B19 induced aplastic crisis. **HbS-beta** thalassemia heterozygote: mild to moderate sickle cell disease, depending on beta globin production. **HbF = $\alpha 2\gamma 2$.**
8. **Rabies prophylaxis**: pre exposure prophylaxis (ppx): rabies vaccine on days 0, 7, 21, and 28. Post-exposure, previously unvaccinated: rabies vaccine on days 0, 3, 7, 14, and rabies immunoglobulin on day 0. Post-exposure, previously vaccinated: rabies vaccine on days 0 and 3.
9. In patients with deep vein thrombosis (DVT) as a result of a **reversible or time-limited risk factor** (e.g, surgery, pregnancy, OCP use, or trauma), anticoagulation should be continued for a minimum of **3** months, no more than **6** months.
10. **Chronic bacterial prostatitis** typically presents with >3 months of urinary tract infection (**UTI**), **pain in the genitourinary** (GU) region, or pain with ejaculation, urine leukocytes, and bacteriuria typically present, especially after prostate massage. Treatment: **6 weeks of fluoroquinolone or TMP-SMX**. Fever, chills, and constitutional symptoms together with **prostate edema and tenderness upon digital rectal exam** differentiate prostatitis from lower UTI.
11. Bilateral symmetrical facial involvement, carpopedal spasm on occlusion of blood supply after parathyroidectomy = relative hypoparathyroidism also known as (AKA) **hungry bone syndrome**.
12. Hemifacial involvement, a preceding history of upper respiratory infection, and facial asymmetry = **Bell's palsy**.
13. **Lupus treatment**: **prednisone + hydroxychloroquine** for arthritis, aortitis, and cutaneous symptoms in systemic lupus erythematosus (SLE).

Prednisone + cyclophosphamide for serious manifestations like lupus nephritis, central nervous system (CNS) involvement, and vasculitis. **Methotrexate** for significant organ involvement with incomplete response to prednisone.

14. **Monoclonal antibodies, including natalizumab, rituximab, efalizumab, and eculizumab** are associated with the development of **progressive multifocal leukoencephalopathy**.
15. **Antipsychotic extrapyramidal effects** and their treatments: **acute dystonia**—benztropine/diphenhydramine; **akathisia**—propranolol, benzodiazepines (BZDs) like lorazepam; **Parkinsonism**—benztropine or amantadine; **tardive dyskinesia**—no definitive treatment, but clonazepam may help.
16. Cough after common cold (upper respiratory infection) 10 days ago; cough 5 day-3 weeks = consider **acute bronchitis**, no treatment necessary. **H. influenza B**: thumbprint sign X-ray indicating epiglottitis.
17. **Congenital 21 hydroxylase** deficiency has elevated hydroxyprogesterone; treatment: hydrocortisone.
18. **Multiple sexual partners** are associated with the highest increase in risk for pelvic inflammatory disease (PID).
19. **Huntington's disease**: memory is preserved until the late stage, but executive functioning, attention, and judgment dysfunction happen early on.
20. **Staccato cough**—chlamydia; **whooping cough**—pertussis; **barking cough**—parainfluenza (croup), steeple sign.

10/21/2018 3

1. In **reactive arthritis**, we need to repeat **urine culture for chlamydia**.
2. **NSAIDs** can reduce pain and erythema and minimize damage to the epidermis after **excessive sun exposure**.
3. First line treatment for toxic megacolon is medical management with **glucocorticoids and antibiotics (ABX)**. 5ASA compounds like sulfasalazine and opioids should be avoided in patients with toxic megacolon. Causes of toxic megacolon include inflammatory bowel disease, infection, and ischemia. Of note, **cytomegalovirus** is the leading cause of toxic megacolon in HIV and AIDS patients
4. **Renal failure is an indication to manage diabetes mellitus (DM) with insulin**; it's recommended to be cautious or even stop metformin and sulfonylureas in chronic kidney disease (CKD).
5. **Hypertensive emergency** in pulmonary hypertension (HTN): use **nitroglycerin** or **nitroprusside**.
6. **Exchange transfusion**: the removal of bilirubin and Ab with replacement of RBC is indicated for neonates with severe (>20–25 ug/dL) hyperbilirubinemia, worsening hyperbilirubinemia on phototherapy, or signs of bilirubin induced neurologic dysfunction.
7. **FT4** is unreliable in pregnancy; **total T3** is used when suppressed TSH and normal T4.
8. **Poison ivy contact dermatitis** is usually a pruritic linear lesion; when severe, papules can evolve into vesicles with serous fluid.

9. **Gestational diabetes**: can discontinue hyperglycemic therapy after delivery; however, a 2 h oral glucose tolerance test (OGTT) is needed 6–12 weeks postpartum.
10. **Localized herpes zoster** should be given oral antiviral, ideally, initiated within 72 h: acyclovir 200 mg 5×/day or valacyclovir 1 g bid for 10 days for the initial episode; acyclovir 400 mg bid for 5 days or valacyclovir 500 mg bid for 3 days if recurrent. **Prophylaxis**: 400 mg bid acyclovir or 500 mg–1 g daily valacyclovir. There is no benefit in using steroids.
11. **Linagliptin** is a dipeptidyl peptidase-4 (DPP4) inhibitor; sulfonylureas like glimepiride and meglitinides (an ATP-dependent K+ (KATP) channel agonist on pancreatic beta cells) cause weight gain and hypoglycemia. Meglitinides include nateglinide and repaglinide.
12. **Premature labor managements**: 34-week 0/7-to-36-week 6/7: ± betamethasone, penicillin if GBS+ or unknown; 32-week 0/7 to 33 week 6/7: ± betamethasone, tocolytics, penicillin if positive or unknown GBS; < 32 weeks: betamethasone, tocolytics, MgO_2, penicillin if GBS + or unknown.
13. Behavioral therapy is the preferred initial treatment for preschool children (3–5 years) and drug therapy is the first line for ≥6 yo with attention-deficit/hyperactivity disorder (ADHD).

3 Palliative Care and Ambulatory Medicine

October 22nd, 2018 Through December 16th, 2018

10/22/2018

1. After adjusting for age, **FEV1** remains the single most important factor in determining the prognosis of COPD.
2. The initial treatment of squamous cell carcinoma of the glottis confined to vocal cord T1N0M0 is **radiation therapy, lasor excision, or partial vocal cordectomy**.
3. INR for mechanical aortic valve with high-risk features (e.g., AFib, LVEF ≤30%, prior VTE, presence of hypercoagulable state) and the mechanical mitral valve is **2.5–3.5**.
4. **Aspirin** 75–100 mg/day **in addition to warfarin** is recommended in all patients with mechanical valves if low bleeding risks.
5. For **transaortic valve replacement**, **aspirin** 75–100 **mg** is recommended for life long after surgery, plus the addition of Plavix 75 mg daily or warfarin with target INR 2.5 for 3–6 months if low risk of bleeding. For surgical **bioprosthetic mitral** and **aortic valve** replacement, **aspirin** 75–100 **mg daily lifelong** plus **warfarin target INR 2.5** (range 2–3) is recommended for the first 3–6 months after surgery.
6. A lower INR target of **1.5–2.0** is recommended for patients with an **On-X bileaflet mechanical aortic valve** and no additional thromboembolism risks

7. **Total T3 and FT4** are used to assess thyroid function soon after radioactive iodine (RAI) ablation. TSH remains suppressed for weeks or even months following RAI treatment and does not reliably reflect thyroid function status.
8. **Good prognostic factors in schizophrenia**: later onset, female, acute onset with precipitant, no family history, short duration of symptoms.
9. Dengue: **hemorrhage and decreased platelet** (PLT). Plasmodium falciparum malaria: **anemia**
10. All patients with asymptomatic **LVEF ≤ 40%** should be treated with **ACEi**, or **ARB** to delay onset of symptomatic heart failure and improve long-term cardiac mortality and morbidity using 5 mg and up and then add beta blocker.
11. Newborns whose mothers did not receive indicated **Group B Streptococcus (GBS) prophylaxis must be observed for 48 h**. A CBC with differentiation and blood culture are indicated if the infant is preterm or exposed to premature rupture of membranes (PROM). **Antibiotic prophylaxis** is recommended during preterm labor and delivery in a pregnant woman with unknown GBS status, or if maternal fever during labor, or with rupture of membranes greater than 18 h.
12. **Neuroblastoma**: originates from immature nerve cells in the adrenal medulla and paraspinal or periaortic regions, 90% patients are <5 years old, has abdominal distension, and a firm irregular mass that can cross the midline. **Wilms tumor** also known as nephroblastoma is a rare type of kidney cancer in children; it has smooth margins on ultrasound and is unilateral. Neuroblastoma can cause **hypertension** and **opsoclonus-myoclonus** (dancing eye and dancing feet) syndrome.
13. The initial exam for renal imaging of renal cell carcinoma (RCC) is CT.
14. **Seborrheic keratosis** (stuck on appearance), no treatment is necessary.
15. Elderly patients should check **TSH** for apathetic thyrotoxicosis (lethargy, confusion, weight loss, heart failure, and depression)
16. Lyme disease is transmitted by **Ixodes** tick after 36–48 h of attachment. **Erythema migrans** take >**3 days** to develop.
17. Patients with a history of renal disease, diabetes, hypertension (HTN), or prior preeclampsia (particularly preterm preeclampsia with severe features) are at high risk for **preeclampsia recurrence**. In high-risk patients, **aspirin is used for preeclampsia prevention and is started at 12 weeks of gestation**.
18. Lithium **>4 mmol/L** (normal kidney function) in serum needs dialysis; may also need dialysis if lithium **>2.5 mmol/L** with renal insufficiency or contraindication for aggressive fluid hydration. **Hidradenitis suppurativa** (acne inversa) treatments: topical clindamycin → oral doxycycline → TNF inhibitors. **HELLP** (hemolysis, elevated liver enzymes, and low platelets) is a variant of preeclampsia, treated with **magnesium sulfate**.
19. Target of HA1c 7%–8%. **Beta-blockers** are indicated in prior myocardial infarction (MI), left ventricular dysfunction, and coronary artery disease (CAD).
20. **Q waves** and **T wave** inversion may suggest a prior MI.
21. **A sleep study** is needed for the diagnosis of **narcolepsy** (excessive daytime sleepiness), and **cataplexy** (a brief sudden loss of muscle tone). **Narcolepsy** is treated with **modafinil** and **sodium oxybate**. **Cataplexy** is treated with selective serotonin reuptake inhibitors (**SSRIs**), serotonin and norepinephrine reuptake inhibitors (**SNRIs**), tricyclic antidepressants (TCAs), and sodium oxybate.

22. **Chronic adrenal insufficiency** = hyponatremia, hyperkalemia, and hyperchloremic acidosis.
23. Physicians must consider the possibility of misuse, abuse, and diversion when **confronted with new patients requiring stimulants**.
24. **Cardiac tamponade** causes an increase in the right atrium (RA) and right ventricle (RV) pressures along with characteristic equalization of RA, right ventricular end-diastolic pressure (RVED), and pulmonary capillary wedge pressure (PCWP).
25. **Cutaneous cryptococcus** is diagnosed by lesion biopsy. Treatment: **fluconazole** 400 mg qd for 6–12 months.
26. Pregnancy-related skin changes: **pemphigoid gestationis**.
27. **Pseudohypoparathyroidism (PHP)** pathophysiology: target organ resistance or unresponsiveness to parathyroid hormone (PTH); labs: low Ca++, high P, high PTH, normal 25-OH vit D. **Albright hereditary osteodystrophy** is the phenotype of pseudohypoparathyroidism type 1A with manifestations of facial and skeletal deformities with short stature, round face and short fourth finger.
28. **Pseudopseudohypoparathyroidism (PPHP)** is an inherited condition without an increase in phosphorus or decrease in calcium due to mild PTH resistance. PPHP is similar to Albright hereditary osteodystrophy but with normal PTH and serum phosphorus and calcium.
29. **Withdrawal from family is a sign of depression**.
30. **Zyprexa** is not approved for dementia-related psychosis but use may be justified in care-interfering **agitations**.

10/23/2018

1. Hypertension (HTN) in patients with **gout**: use **angiotensin II receptor blocker (ARB)** as it has a uricosuric effect. Thiazides, loop diuretics, and aspirin should be avoided.
2. Exogenous hyperthyroidism, **thyroglobulin** is low as there is no inflammation or destruction of the native thyroid gland, helping distinguish this problem from thyroiditis.
3. **Reconstruction of the cleft lip** is performed at 3 m of age: 10 lbs, 10 weeks, 10 g Hgb. Cleft palate surgery should be performed between 6 and 12 months of age.
4. Clinical presentation of substernal chest pain or discomfort, relief with nitroglycerin, EKG ST depression in leads III, aVF, V5-V6 is consistent with **acute coronary syndrome** (ACS)-NSTEMI, should be managed with dual antiplatelet therapy (DAPT, if approval by cardiologist given possible need for coronary artery bypass grafting), statin, beta blocker, and anticoagulation with heparin.
5. Emergency cardiac catheterization and revascularization within **90 min from first medical contact** is for ST-elevation myocardial infarction (**STEMI**).
6. **Pneumococcal conjugate vaccine (PCV15 or PCV20)** for all adults 65 years or older as well as adults 19 through 64 years old who have certain chronic medical conditions or other risk factors. Per the CDC, "If PCV15 is used, a dose of PPSV23 should be given one year later. The minimum interval is 8 weeks

after PCV 15 for PPSV 23 and can be considered in an immunocompromising condition (immunocompromised- alcoholism, chronic heart disease, not hypertension, chronic liver or kidney or lung disease, cigarette smoking, diabetes), cochlear implant, or cerebrospinal fluid leak. If PCV20 is used, no PPSV23 is necessary." "If PPSV 23 or PCV 13 administration history, give 1 dose of PCV20 at least 1 year after PCV13; give 1 dose of PCV15 or PCV20 at least 1 year after the most recent PPSV23."

7. **Seborrheic dermatitis** is commonly seen in HIV and Parkinson's disease (PD).
8. **Small intestine bacterial overgrowth (SIBO)** is a malabsorption syndrome due to anatomical or motility (diabetes mellitus, systemic sclerosis) disorders. **The jejunal biopsy** is the diagnostic test for SIBO.
9. **Cough variant asthma** presents with a chronic nonproductive cough that is typically worse during the night and triggered by exercise, forced expiration, and allergen exposure.
10. **Cremasteric reflex** corresponds with the **L1-L2 level of the spinal cord**. Normal ambulation and motor strength indicate **diabetic neuropathy** rather than L1 and L2 spinal cord injury.
11. **Primary and secondary and early latent (<12 m) syphilis** treatment: benzathine penicillin G 2.4 million IV single dose. **Latent > 12 m**, unknown duration, gummatous or cardiovascular (CV) syphilis, Treatment: **benzathine penicillin G 2.4 million IM weekly for 3 weeks. Neurosyphilis** treatment: aqueous penicillin G 3–4 million IV q4h for 10–14 days. **Congenital syphilis** treatment: aqueous penicillin G 50,000 u/kg/dose q8-10 h for 10 days.
12. The **diagnosis of syphilis** requires positive results for both of the two-step tests: **a nontreponemal test** (Venereal Disease Research Laboratory [VDRL] or rapid plasma reagin [RPR] test) and a **treponemal test** (the T. pallidum passive particle agglutination [TP-PA] assay, fluorescent treponemal antibody absorption [FTA-ABS]). Patients with a **history of previous treatment do not need treatment even if treponemal test positive unless sexual history indicates a reexposure** (warrants a repeat nontreponemal test 2–4 weeks to evaluate for early infection).
13. **Status epilepticus** treatments: midazolam, lorazepam, diazepam → consider fosphenytoin, phenytoin, valproic acid → consider continuous EEG, phenobarbital, propofol, midazolam.
14. **Pediatric inguinal hernia should be repaired ASAP**.
15. **Renovascular hypertension** (HTN): no angiogram is necessary, do abdominal duplex Doppler ultrasound.
16. **Oral contraceptive pill (OCP)** contraindications: migraine headache (combined OCP increases risks for stroke) with aura; stage 2 hypertension (HTN); ≥35 yo with ≥15 cigarettes/day. For these patients, give progestin only.
17. **Blastomycosis** causes various skin lesions with heaped-up borders (non-papular ulcerative lesions). Disseminated histoplasmosis may be associated with nodular, papular or plaque-like skin lesions, also systemic signs, usually critically ill.

18. **Sporotrichosis**: painless papule ulcerates and drains a nonpurulent odorless fluid, along the proximal lymphatic chain.

10/24/2018

1. Fever, cough, and chest pain, probable sinus infection in an immunocompromised = consider invasive fungal infection like **Aspergillus**. Treatment: fluconazole is Not effective. Use **voriconazole 6 mg/kg IV bid** for day 1 followed by 4 mg/kg qd for ≥7 days. Can add caspofungin.
2. **Giardia** infection treatment: 5-day course of Flagyl.
3. Pain crisis in sickle cell disease = sickle cell crisis. Patients with **sickle cell crisis** should only use **progestin-containing (progesterone, levonorgestrel)** intrauterine device (IUD). **Copper** IUD is associated with **heavy menstruation** and **dysmenorrhea**.
4. Cholesterol screening is universally recommended for individuals ages 9–11 and 17–21. Screening should be performed at age > 2 if risk factors (family hx of premature cardiovascular disease (CVD) or diabetes mellitus, dyslipidemia, obesity).
5. **An old patient with obesity** and memory problems likely has **obstructive sleep apnea** (OSA). **Diuretics** (HCTZ, chlorthalidone, furosemide) can cause **pancreatitis**.
6. Patients with **panic attacks** have recurrent, unexpected anxiety attacks with multiple somatic symptoms.
7. Verapamil, quinidine, and amiodarone can potentially potentiate **digoxin toxicity**.

10/25/2018

1. Patients with **central venous thrombosis** usually develop a gradually worsening **headache** due to elevated intracranial pressure and may have focal **neurological deficits** or **seizures** due to cerebral venous congestion. Although focal cerebral hemorrhage may be present on injury, **anticoagulation with heparin or LMWH** is considered safe and standard care.
2. **Preeclampsia** with severe features requires stabilization with blood pressure control using **hydralazine, labetalol,** and **magnesium sulfate** for seizure prophylaxis. At >**34 weeks**, **delivery is initiated after maternal stabilization** is established.
3. **Alcoholics** with depression can be treated with depression medication using selective serotonin reuptake inhibitors **(SSRIs).**
4. **Nonallergic rhinitis** typically presents after age 20 with nasal blockage, rhinorrhea, and postnasal drip. Treatment: topical intranasal steroids like **fluticasone, intranasal antihistamines azelastine**.
5. **Non-hepatic encephalopathy** is often due to infection, GI bleed, metabolic abnormalities, or sedatives.
6. **Juvenile myoclonic epilepsy** EEG shows bilateral polyspikes and slow discharges during the interval period; treatment: valproic acid for 7 months.

7. **Tuberculosis (TB) in pregnancy** should be treated with 3 drugs: isoniazid (INH), rifampin (RIF), and ethambutol for 2 months followed by INH and RIF for 7 months.
8. **Osteomyelitis** should be suspected in patients with fever, focal bone pain, and elevated inflammatory markers. In **sickle cell disease with osteomyelitis**, should cover **staphylococcus and salmonella** with **ceftriaxone** and **clindamycin**.
9. **Postoperative atelectasis** is common 2–5 days following thoracoabdominal surgery. Presents with hypoxemia or respiratory difficulty may be treated with CPAP → BiPAP, chest physical therapy, and suctioning.
10. **Infectious mononucleosis** has post-cervical lymphadenopathy and severe fatigue while strep throat does not.
11. **Microangiopathic anemia** differentials: disseminated intravascular coagulation (DIC); thrombotic thrombocytopenic purpura (TTP)/hemolytic uremic syndrome (HUS); systemic lupus erythematosus (SLE); hemolysis, elevated liver enzymes, low platelet count (HELLP).
12. First line treatment for **anorexia nervosa** involves **psychotherapy** and **nutritional rehabilitation**, medication treatment may include **olanzapine**. Bulimia nervosa treatment: **SSRI**.
13. **Benzodiazepines** should be **avoided in older patients** due to tolerance, excessive sedation, cognitive impairment, falls, and dependence.
14. Active cardiac conditions that require further evaluation and treatment before noncardiac surgery: **unstable coronary syndrome, decompensated congestive heart failure, significant arrhythmia, and severe valvular disease**.
15. **Tardive dyskinesia** on Haldol. If discontinuation is not feasible, switch to 2nd generation like **Seroquel** or add **clozapine**.
16. All children <2 years with urinary tract infection (UTI) should undergo renal ultrasound and bladder ultrasound. if abnormal or recurrent UTI, should go **voiding cystourethrogram (VCUG)**.
17. Treatment of neonatal infections due to C. trachomatis (i.e., **conjunctivitis**, **pneumonia**) requires **systemic macrolides**. **IV ampicillin and gentamicin are for neonatal sepsis**.
18. **Viral conjunctivitis (watery mucoid), is no longer contagious once discharge resolves**. **Erythromycin** ointment to prevent **gonococcal** conjunctivitis.
19. **Naltrexone is a 1st line treatment** for moderate to severe alcohol use disorder.
20. **Psychogenic nonepileptic seizure** also known as pseudoseizure has normal video EEG.
21. **Polyhydramnios, an amniotic fluid index** ≥ 24 may be due to maternal diabetes mellitus (DM), congenital anencephaly, or duodenal atresia.

10/26/2018

1. **Haldol** is safe and effective for severe mania or bipolar in pregnancy. Other treatments include **lithium** and 2nd generation atypical antipsychotics (**valproate and carbamazepine**) should be avoided. **Electroconvulsive therapy**

(ECT) should be reserved for treatment-resistant cases or those at imminent risk to themselves or their fetus.

2. **Bell's palsy** treatment: corticosteroid and supportive care for eyes (prednisone 60 mg for 7 days). **Ramsay Hunt syndrome** (the triad of ipsilateral facial paralysis, ear pain, and vesicles in the auditory canal or on the auricle) treatment: **valacyclovir 1 g tid for 7–10 days and prednisone 1 g/kg for 5 days**.
3. **Tinea capitis** treatment: oral terbinafine or griseofulvin.
4. **Dysmenorrhea** treatment: NSAIDs for 2–4 months oral contraceptive pills (OCP). Identifying **depression in Parkinson's disease (PD)** is difficult, an empiric trial of selective serotonin reuptake inhibitors (SSRIs) could be helpful if concerns.
5. **Strep throat** treatment: penicillin oral 10 days to prevent rheumatic fever.
6. **Intravenous drug abusers** (IVDAs) have a high risk for infective pulmonary embolism (PE), infective endocarditis, mycotic aneurysm, echo is needed.
7. A **case-control study** is the most appropriate study design to investigate an outbreak of acute infectious disease.
8. In HCV infection, the patient should **avoid alcohol and also get a vaccination against HBV and HAV**.
9. **Female with breast mass**: if <30, do U/S only; if ≥30, do mammogram and ultrasound.
10. **Mitral valve prolapse** in Marfan syndrome → rupture of chordae tendineae in Ehlers-Danlos syndrome.
11. **Gag reflex** is frequently impaired in botulism, and may result in aspiration if the airway is not protected.
12. Use amiodarone, **decrease warfarin dose by 25%–50%** to compensate.
13. **Epiglottitis** thumbprint sign = consider **H. influenza** B. **Steeple sign** = consider **parainfluenza virus** (croup).
14. Treatment of croup = consider **racemic epi and dexamethasone 0.6 mg/kg**, barking cough.
15. Pancreatic cyst diagnosis: **endoscopic ultrasound.**
16. Patients with unknown GBS status should receive **penicillin prophylaxis** if pregnancy is preterm (<37 weeks) or if develop an intrapartum fever or have a rupture of membrane >18 h.
17. Concerns of intimate violence, **open-ended questions**. How are you feeling about your relationship with your husband?
18. **Doxycycline** is contraindicated if age < 8 yo.
19. About **60%** of **head** and **neck cancers** are locally advanced at the time of diagnosis and are **inoperable**. **Chemoradiation** is the treatment.
20. **Necrotizing fasciitis** treatment: surgical exploration, antibiotics (Zosyn/meropenem, Vanco, and clindamycin in combination), hemodynamic support.
21. **Hemophilia** is an X-linked recessive disease. **Tuberous sclerosis** needs EEG monitoring, and often death from epilepsy.

11/9/2018

1. **Hospice orders**: care management referral (hospice team will be notified), spiritual care referral (pastor will be notified), morphine oral (Roxanol solution) 5 mg prn, atropine 1% optic 1 drop prn, hyoscyamine sublingual prn or scopolamine patch for secretions, Ativan 1 mg subcu q4h (can be oral).

11/19/2018

1. **Chronic bacterial prostatitis** treatment: 6 weeks of Cipro/Levaquin or Bactrim.
2. **Allergic rhinitis** treatment: desloratadine or cetirizine, naphazoline-pheniramine eye drop, and fluticasone nasal spray.
3. F17.210 for cigarette nicotine dependence. Breo elipta = fluticasone vilanterol 100–25, similar to Advair. Ellipta = umeclidinium/vilanterol.
4. **Lichen sclerosus** treatment: Clobetasol emollient base cream. **Lichen planus** may be associated with hepatitis C.
5. **Dyspepsia** if age < 60 years old: check for H. pylori and then start proton pump inhibitor (PPI) for **4–8 weeks**.
6. **Headache** (HA) differential diagnoses: cluster, tension-type, migraines, or rhinosinusitis.

11/21/2018

1. Senior female needs **surgery medical clearance** as outpatient: order EKG, echo, chest X-ray (CXR), cardiologist consult if major cardiac disease history.
2. Uncontrolled **hypertension** (HTN), unable to make sure the patient is taking his medications, have the patient coming back in 1 week to bring all his/her medications to the clinic and check.
3. **Diabetes** supplies: one touch test strip 1 box, 5 refills; lancet in vitro 2–3/day × 100, 5 refills; diabetes monitor device and alcohol swabs.
4. Old adults, do a **mini mental exam** and complete advanced directives as a primary care physician.
5. If a patient declines to take **chlorthalidone**, offer **hydrochlorothiazide** (HCTZ).

11/27/2018

1. **Prograf = tacrolimus, Epivir = lamivudine**, for hepatic transplant. **Calcium channel blockers** are the preferred blood pressure medication in **transplant patients** because they can alleviate cyclosporine-induced nephrotoxicity, control hypertension, and prevent post-transplantation acute tubular necrosis.
2. Saxenda = liraglutide (Victoza); Byetta = exenatide.

11/28/2018

1. When fasting glucose is at goal, but HA1c remains at 10%, we will need to add **premeal insulin or GLP-1 agonist** or add 1 additional injection of long-acting insulin. **GLP1 agonists and SGLT2 inhibitors decrease post meal glucose**.
2. **Inpatient diabetes mellitus** (DM) care: most often universally order basal long-acting insulin like Lantus and sliding scale insulin, may also order pre meal nutritional insulin.

3. **Lofexidine** has similar efficacy as **clonidine** in helping **opioid withdrawal**; Suboxone (buprenorphine and naloxone) is recommended to be changed to **Subutex (buprenorphine) in pregnancy**. Buprenorphine is Ok to use in pregnancy and breastfeeding.
4. **Altered mental status (AMS)** in the outpatient setting: finger stick glucose, SO_2, send the patient to ER via emergency medical service (EMS), vitals. For home health aid, a primary care physician will need to fill out a form.

11/29/2018

1. **Medicare wellness exam**: need to do the mini mental exam (MME) and advanced directives; nebulizer; CPAP requires sleep study. The Medicare wellness exam requires primary care physicians to address all the issues: **vaccination, cancer screening, and all chronic conditions**.

11/30/2018

1. Invokana = canagliflozin, Jardiance = empagliflozin, Steglatro = ertugliflozin.
2. Dipeptidyl peptidase 4 (DPP4) inhibitors: Onglyza = saxagliptin; Januvia = sitagliptin.
3. **Otitis externa** treatment: Ciprodex suspension and Levaquin 500 mg daily for 5–7 days. **Benign prostate hyperplasia** (BPH) treatment: Flomax (tamsulosin), alfuzosin 10 mg qd. **Alfuzosin** is an alpha1-adrenergic receptor blocker.
4. Anoro ellipta = umeclidinium vilanterol. Trelegy ellipta = fluticasone umeclidinium vilanterol.
5. **Diabetes insulin and supply prescriptions**: BD insulin syringes, ultra-fine III bid e11.9, 100, refill 5. Pen needles, 1/16″ 31G × 8 mm. Lantus solo star 100 u/mL, 1 box refill 5, e11.9. One-touch test strips.
6. Methadone and teriflunomide (for multiple sclerosis) simultaneous use needs close monitoring. **Teriflunomide** increases methadone concentrations. Teriflunomide is an immunomodulatory drug inhibiting pyrimidine de novo synthesis and is used for **multiple sclerosis**.

12/5/2018

1. Levsin = hyoscyamine 0.175 mg q6h for **irritable bowel syndrome (IBS)**.
2. Libre glucose monitor and reader is a continuous glucose monitoring system.
3. Depo-Provera im = **medroxyprogesterone** q3m im
4. **Desipramine** for dysmenorrhea 100 mg qd; **mirabegron** beta 3 activations ⇒ muscle relaxation for overactive bladder (OAB).
5. Pap smear 21–65 q3y (for **age 30–65,** can also do HPV test with or without Pap smear q5y), no need for pap smear or HPV testing if total hysterectomy with cervix removal.
6. **Shingles vaccination** is recommended in healthy adults ≥ 50 yo with two doses of Shingrix, separated by 2–6 months (or in immunocompromised >19 yo with two doses of Shingrix separated by 1–2 months). *Zostavax* is no longer on the market in the US. Patients who received Zostavax still should get Shingrix.

7. **Bone scan** every other year if female age **≥ 65 or male ≥ 70**. Low-dose CT lung cancer screen is recommended in patients with **20 pack-year** or more smoking history and current smokers or quit less than 15 years and age **50–80** q1y.

12/7/2018

1. **Synthesized opioid**: fentanyl, methadone. Buprenorphine will not show up in urine immunoassay.
2. **Heroin** is often mixed with fentanyl. 6-monoacetyl morphine (6-MAM) is a unique metabolite of heroin.
3. **Morphine** and **hydrocodone** both can be metabolized to hydromorphone.
4. Provigil = modafinil; gas chromatography includes immunoassay.

12/9/2018

1. Surgery: hold the morning dose of Lovenox on the day of surgery, and resume the day after surgery.
2. Family history **of breast cancer increases risk for pancreatic adenocarcinoma**, needs to check BRCA1 & 2.
3. SGLTis like Farxiga (**dapagliflozin**) are associated with acute **pancreatitis**.
4. **Multiple myeloma** tests: bone marrow biopsy is the golden standard, together with urine and serum immunofixation (IFE), kappa and lambda light chain, urine and serum electrophoresis.
5. **EBV** IgM and IgG increase risks for **nasopharyngeal cancer** and **Burkitt's lymphoma**.
6. **Antiphospholipid syndrome** tests: beta2 glycoprotein Ab IgM and IgG, anti-lupus antibody, anti-cardiolipin antibody.
7. **Parkinson's disease (PD)** treatment: Sinemet (levodopa + carbidopa). Nuplazid (**Pimavanserin**) is used for Parkinson's disease psychosis.
8. **Pseudogout** treatment: NSAIDs or prednisone until flare resolution then taper >7–10 days.

12/15/2018

1. **Entresto** = sacubitril/valsartan, is an angiotensin receptor-neprilysin inhibitor, has to stop Lisinopril for 48 h before starting Entresto.
2. **Revlimid** = lenalidomide, used for myelodysplastic syndrome (MDS), multiple myeloma (MM), and mantle cell lymphoma (MCL). Will need to **hold lenalidomide if infection, absolute neutrophil count (ANC) < 500, or platelet < 50**. Lenalidomide causes hematologic toxicity and infection, hepatotoxicity, angioedema, and anaphylaxis, as well as secondary malignancies like myeloid leukemia, and skin cancers. **Lenalidomide** also has been linked to **deep vein thrombosis**, pulmonary embolism, acute myocardial infarction, and **cerebrovascular accidents**.
3. **Eliquis** dose adjustment only for atrial fibrillation: ≥80 yo, wt ≤ 60 kg, egfr ≤40 or Cr > 1.5. If fulfill ≥2 criteria, prescribe/decrease to 2.5 mg bid.

4. Switch from Lantus to Toujeo, 100 units Lantus = 125 units Toujeo; 100 units Toujeo = 80 units Lantus. Basaglar = Lantus. Switching from basal insulin to once-daily Toujeo, approximately **10%–18% more** insulin Toujeo is needed.
5. **Edema whole body (anasarca), do Lasix drip at 5 cc/h, 200 ml in total**.

Takeaway Messages

1. High-risk pulmonary embolism (PE) and possibly intermediate-risk PE with large clot burden, severe right ventricle (RV) enlargement or dysfunction, high O_2 requirement, and or severe tachycardia may benefit from thrombolysis or mechanical embolectomy.
2. Massive proximal lower extremity (LE) or iliofemoral thrombosis associated with severe symptomatic swelling or limb-threatening ischemia will likely need thrombolytic therapy.
3. Urethral diverticulum diagnosis requires MRI and treatment with diverticulectomy excision and reconstruction.
4. Emergency conditions requiring surgery or an ophthalmologist: acute compartment syndrome, Candida endophthalmitis, keratitis, retroperitoneum free air, bowel ischemia.
5. Pressor support: 1st line Levophed, then vasopressin and epinephrine as 2nd line vasopressors.
6. Mild gallstone pancreatitis should undergo cholecystectomy within 7 days of clinical improvement, usually in the same hospitalization.
7. Bullous pemphigoid: diagnosis with biopsy and serum tests for autoantibodies to the hemidesmosomal bullous pemphigoid antigens 180–230; treatment with clobetasol topical ointment, doxycycline, prednisone, and nicotinamide.

Further Readings and References

1. Palmer, B.F. *Cerebral salt wasting*, ed. R.H. Sterns. Waltham, MA: UpToDate. Accessed January 30, 2024.
2. Stern, R.H. *Pathophysiology and etiology of the syndrome of inappropriate antidiuretic hormone secretion (SIADH)*, ed. M. Emmett. Waltham, MA: UpToDate. Accessed January 30, 2024.
3. Stern, R.H. *Treatment of hyponatremia: Syndrome of inappropriate antidiuretic hormone secretion (SIADH) and reset osmostat*, ed. M. Emmett. Waltham: UpToDate. Accessed January 30, 2024.
4. Whelton, P.K., R.M. Carey, W.S. Aronow, et al. 2017. ACC/AHA/AAPA/ABC/ACPM/AGS/APhA/ASH/ASPC/NMA/PCNA Guideline for the prevention, detection, evaluation, and management of high blood pressure in adults: A report of the American College of Cardiology/American Heart Association Task Force on Clinical Practice Guidelines. *Journal of the American College of Cardiology* 2018 (71): e127–e248.
5. Writing Committee Members, C.M. Otto, R.A. Nishimura, et al. 2021. 2020 ACC/AHA guideline for the management of patients with valvular heart disease: A report of the American College of Cardiology/American Heart Association Joint Committee on Clinical Practice Guidelines. *Journal of Thoracic and Cardiovascular Surgery* 162 (2): e183–e353.

Chapter 11
Sports Medicine, Rheumatology, Admitter, Followed by General Medicine Floor

December 17th, 2018 Through April 7th, 2019

At the beginning of the second year of residency training, internal medicine residents face the decisions for their life after residency training: entering the job market versus fellowship training. Besides preparing to work as a primary care physician or hospitalist, internal medicine residents can apply for a vast category of fellowships. While the actual fellowship application submission typically is due in mid-July of the PGY2 year, preparation for fellowship application starts one or more years before that. The chances of successful fellowship matching (fellowship match day: early December of the PGY3 year) is largely determined by the readiness of the resident applicant and the competitiveness of the specific fellowship program.

When I looked back at my journey in residency training, I enjoyed my days for my one-month training at the sports medicine clinic and the one-month training at the rheumatology clinic. Because of my physical therapy education background, I was originally thinking of pain management or sports medicine fellowships. Even though later on, my interests changed to hematology and oncology, and eventually I landed as a full-time hospitalist, the training for sports medicine and rheumatology enhanced my understanding of the management of chronic musculoskeletal pain which emphasizes exercise, judicious use of opioid medications, joint injections, and the use of biologic agents.

As for sports medicine training, concussion and pain management including steroid injections were the major components of my clinical experiences. Understanding the human anatomy and movements together with the vestibular system serves as the foundation, and the procedures of joint injection per se require practice and additional training in ultrasound-guided procedures. As for rheumatology, objectives for the rotation included diagnosis and treatments for common rheumatological diseases, understanding the inflammatory pathway including tumor necrosis factor and interleukins, and the use of various biological agents. During these two rotations, I had the chance to take care of both professional athletes and regular patients with musculoskeletal pain disorders.

K. Zhou, *Internal Medicine Training Notes and Survival Guide*,
https://doi.org/10.1007/978-1-0716-4039-5_11

Although this chapter encompassed notes taken during the four rotations (4 weeks for each) of sports medicine, rheumatology, admitter, and general medicine floor, the notes mainly focused on sports medicine and rheumatology with additional topics of preoperative medicine, Langerhans cell histiocytosis, and polycystic ovarian syndrome.

1 Sports Medicine

12/16/2018

1. **Concussion diagnosis**: a traumatic brain injury from kinetic energy to the head causing an immediate and transient dysfunction of the brain with vestibular, balance, and vision impairment and cognitive thinking, functional capability, and mood symptoms.
2. **Physical exam focuses** when concussion concerns: vestibular-ocular reflex look between fingers, convergence (<10 cm), smooth tracking, tandem gait (heel to toe open and closed eye walk), back of neck palpation, orthostatic vital signs.
3. Additional symptoms of concussion: headache (HA), dizziness, trouble sleeping.
4. **Treadmill test** for heart symptoms and concussion symptoms: cognitive intolerance versus exercise intolerance or both. **Treatment**: aerobic exercises at the specific level that causes symptoms.
5. **Treatments for concussion:** physical activity and aerobic exercise treatment should be initiated as early interventions; cervicovestibular rehabilitation should be recommended for patients with neck pain, headaches, dizziness, and/or balance problems (especially if lasting longer than 10 days).
6. If there is symptom exacerbation during cognitive activity or screening, difficulties with reading, concentration or memory, or other aspects of learning, a **Return to Learn (Return to Sport)** strategy should be implemented at the time of diagnosis and during the recovery process. **Light physical activities** and prescribed **sub-symptom threshold aerobic exercise** treatment in a safe and supervised environment should be encouraged. Persistent symptoms over **2–4 weeks** require further evaluation and referral.
7. **Proximal fifth metatarsal fracture**: also known as Jones fracture; it is one type of stress fracture (healing 3 months; treatment is non-weight bearing 6–8 weeks). **An avulsion fracture** is also known as (AKA) pseudo-Jones fracture.
8. **Injection medications for osteoarthritis of the knee**: dexamethasone 4 cc + lidocaine 1 cc + Synvisc One (hylan G-F 20) to the knee. **Synvisc** is a type of hyaluronic acid injection.
9. **Radial neck fracture treatment**: sling for 2–3 weeks, then range of motion (ROM) exercises as tolerated.

10. **Platelet-rich plasma (PRP)** injection for muscle, tendon, and joint problems, usually only once; dosage is 8 cc.
11. **Preparation of PRP**: Anticoagulant Citrate Dextrose Solution A (ACD-A) 8 cc (anticoagulant) + 60 cc venous blood ⇒ centrifuge PRP injection. No NSAIDs for a week, short arc terminal knee extension exercise in 1 week, biking after 24 h.

12/19/2018

1. **Flexor carpi ulnaris (FCU) tendonitis** is diagnosed via MRI. **Triangular fibrocartilage complex (TFCC)**—major stabilization of the ulnar carpus and distal radioulnar joint, absorbs 20% axial load across the wrist, made of ulnotriquetral ligament, meniscal homolog, articular disc, dorsal radioulnar ligament, volar radioulnar ligament, ulnolunate ligament, and ulnar collateral ligament. Patients with TICC injury may need arthroscopic surgery.
2. **Trochanteric bursitis**: lateral hip pain with radiation to the anterior thigh. Treatment: steroid injection.
3. **Patellofemoral pain** after steroid shot and worsening with physical therapy exercise, needs MRI to look for infection.
4. **Diabetes mellitus**: be cautious about joint infections in joint injections.

12/20/2018

1. **Migraine, depression, and anxiety** cause prolonged recovery from concussion. Magnesium tablets may help concussion recovery. **Concussion treatment**: vestibular rehab + magnesium tablets + massage.
2. Lidocaine epinephrine for local subcutaneous anesthesia. **Joint injections**: Marcaine + lidocaine + dexamethasone
3. **Injection while withdrawal technique**. Lidocaine to induce subcutaneous wheal, then 45-degree needle insertion, and then inject while withdrawal.
4. **Pain after injection treatment**: ice, NSAIDs, Motrin.
5. **Rotator cuff tendonitis** treatment: subacromial bursa injection with 5 cc lidocaine + 1 cc dexamethasone OR 5 cc bupivacaine + 1 cc dexamethasone.
6. **Ankle sprain** in brace: 80% better, then get rid of brace. Tylenol 625 mg 2 tablets, bid for 7 days of shoulder pain. No heavy exercises, stretch ⇒ strength ⇒ range of motion (ROM).

1/2/2019

1. For concussion treatment: if the patient wears lenses and glasses, keep them on during the exam. Vision therapy, do different lenses, then vision practices.
2. **Return to play 5-day protocol**, concussion at sports, check at scene, no play if symptoms, rest, athletic trainer (AT) check at scene → nurse check next day.
3. Joint injection: **shoulder joint injection**: 22-gauge spinal needle (10 cc), give 6 cc lidocaine + 1 cc dexamethasone/Kenalog. **Hip joint injection**: 22-gauge spinal needle, give 9 cc or 6 cc lidocaine + 1 cc dexamethasone (or 2 cc steroid + 3 cc ropivacaine). **Knee joint injection**: 22-gauge spinal needle, give 5 cc

lidocaine + 1 cc dexamethasone/Kenalog. **Iliopsoas injection**: 22-gauge needle, 2 cc Kenalog (40 mg/cc) + 3 cc ropivacaine 0.5% in a 5 cc syringe.

1/7/2019

1. **Knee at 90-degree flexion** for lateral injections.
2. Psych disorder attention deficit hyperactivity disorder (ADHD) versus **concussion**: do treadmill test, if positive, do **suboptimal exercise (90% HR for stress test) training.**
3. **Patelloneovascularization** → tendonitis → plasma-rich platelet (PRP). Trochanteric bursitis is due to imbalanced muscle of the hip.
4. **Box fracture**: healing with a splint for 6–8 weeks, recheck in 2 weeks; angulated degrees for splinting (45 degrees fifth, 30 degrees fourth, 15 degrees second, 0-degree index finger)
5. **Non-displaced radial head fracture treatment**: sling for 2 weeks, then active range of motion (AROM) as tolerated. After 2 months, start resistive range of motion (ROM) exercises if no pain.
6. **Migraine/headache treatments**: Excedrin = aspirin/paracetamol/caffeine. Fioricet = acetaminophen/butalbital/caffeine. Doxepin is a TCA.
7. After a head injury, need to check the ophthalmoscope for **optic swelling** (see trauma protocol for cervical spine clearance).

1/8/2019

1. **Knee injection**: 3 cc lidocaine + 3 cc bupivacaine + 10 mg dexamethasone at lateral side of knee.
2. Shoulder pain for a long time in a young suspicious male, check MRI of the shoulder.
3. Wrestler presents with joint effusion and pain at the elbow after 1 week (injury): consider **MRI to see whether growth plate fracture**.
4. Stress fracture at tibia (pain at tibia in a runner): consider MRI (the best method to diagnose stress fracture) ⇒ consider **resting in a pneumatic cast for 6 weeks**.
5. **Shoulder injection**: 2 cc lidocaine + 2 cc bupivacaine + 4 mg dexamethasone, 22G needle injection at shoulder.
6. **Shoulder injection**: insert the needle beneath the acromion, the tip of the needle toward the coracoid process.

1/9/2019

1. **For radial head fracture**, check supination and pronation which comes back first, may heal in 4–6 weeks if no major passive range of motion limitations.
2. **Shoulder injection**: 6 cc lidocaine + 10 cc dexamethasone using 22G needle at shoulder.
3. **18G** to draw lidocaine/steroid, then use **22G** needle for injection.
4. 1.5 cc lidocaine + 0.5 mg dexamethasone, 25G needle for **Morton neuroma**. If it is Morton neuroma of the finger, use 27G. In joint injection, we usually use a 22G needle.

1/10/2019

1. Knee injection, needle parallel to the transducer with ultrasound guidance.
2. **Second metatarsal fracture** treatment: CAM boot for 6 weeks or surgical shoe.
3. **Stress view** for fibular fracture, separation greater than **4 mm** at tibia from calcaneus medially or fibular separation >**1 cm** with stress view ⇒ consider surgery, it's not going to heal.
4. 40 mg Kenalog + 4 cc lidocaine/bupivacaine for lateral knee injection.
5. Young male with hip osteoarthritis and pain → **do MRI to rule out avascular necrosis**.

1/11/2019

1. Requip = ropinirole; Gilenya = fingolimod for MS.
2. **Acute gout attack**: colchicine 0.6 mg qd for 4 weeks with allopurinol started after acute gout attack, overlap 1 month; colchicine can be used for 6 months.

1/13/2019

1. CellCept = mycophenolate; Cytoxan (cyclophosphamide) or Rituxan (rituximab) for lupus maintenance therapy, also serve as steroid avoidance therapy; long-term use of these medications can cause **leukemia and lymphoma**.
2. Acute kidney injury (AKI) on chronic kidney disease (CKD), kidney function keeps getting worse and K+ elevation, give Bicarb 150 mEq/D5W 1 L at 150 cc/h; 150 mEq = 3 amps, albumin 25% 50 cc IV bid.
3. **Lupus nephritis**, getting worse, do solumedrol 1 g qd × 3 then continue prednisone 1 mg/kg/day in divided doses. Watch for **sigmoid perforations**, need to add Protonix for GI prophylaxis given steroids + mycophenolate mofetil 500 mg bid use in lupus.

1/14/2019

1. CKD V treatment: if chronic compensated metabolic acidosis, use NS + 2 amps $NaHCO_3$ at 60 cc/h, and then $NaHCO_3$ 650 mg tid po.

2 Rheumatology Rotation, Admitter, Followed by General Medicine Floor

1/15/2019

1. Simponi Aria = Golimumab, a monoclonal Ab to tumor necrosis factor (TNF) alpha. Remicade = infliximab, a monoclonal Ab to TNF.
2. Enbrel = etanercept, TNF inhibitor. **Orencia = abatacept** is a soluble fusion protein that consists of the extracellular domain of human cytotoxic T-lymphocytes associated antigen 4 (**CTLA-4**) linked to the modified Fc (hinge CH2 & CH3 domains) portion of human immunoglobulin G1 (IgG1).

3. Humira = adalimumab, a recombinant human IgG monoclonal Ab against TNF alpha.
4. Xeljanz = tofacitinib, an anti-JAK targeting a specific cellular process in RNA.
5. Methotrexate 2.5 mg, 3 tablets AM, 3 tablets PM, qwk. **Methotrexate overlaps with Medrol (methylprednisolone) over 2 weeks** (8 mg qd for 1 week, and 4 week for 1 week) for rheumatoid arthritis.
6. **Diagnosis of rheumatoid arthritis (RA)**: X-ray of hands and fingers, QuantiFERON, rheumatic factor (RF), anti-cyclic citrullinated peptide (CCP), antinuclear antibody (ANA), extractable nuclear antigen (ENA) panel (anti-RNP, anti-smith, anti-SS-A, anti-SS-B, anti SCL-70, anti Jo-1), dsDNA, hepatitis profile, trial steroid, No NSAIDs while on steroids.
7. **Cosentyx (Secukinumab)** is a human IgG1k monoclonal Ab that binds to the protein interleukin 17A to inhibit its interaction with its receptors, used for **psoriasis, ankylosing spondylosis (AS), psoriatic arthritis**.
8. Cimzia = certolizumab pegol, a monoclonal Ab to TNF-alpha.
9. As on Enbrel with multiple infections: switch to Humira, add Celebrex 200 mg qd, Flexeril 10 mg tid prn.
10. Actemra = tocilizumab, a **monoclonal Ab against IL-6R**.
11. **Not to take biological agents when sick/febrile or on antibiotics (ABX)**.
12. A rheumatoid arthritis patient has responded well to Medrol (methylprednisolone) for weeks, can bridge the patient with methotrexate (MTX) 2.5 mg 6 tablets per day with Medrol **overlapping 2 weeks**.
13. Cosentyx (Secukinumab) 300 mg subcu q4wks, to 200 mg q2wks.
14. **ENA** = extractable nuclear antigen; extractable nuclear antigen (ENA) panel includes anti-Ro, anti-La, anti-Sm, anti-RNP, anti-Jo-1, anti-Scl 70, anti-centromere

1/16/2019

1. **Granuloma lymphadenopathy** indicating sarcoidal lymphadenitis, urine Ag for histoplasmosis negative, but lymph node biopsy grew **Histoplasma capsulatum. Treatment**: itraconazole 200 mg bid for 1 year, hold statin for liver toxicity, monitor CBC, CMP, and CPK.
2. **Polymyalgia rheumatica** is common in patients with ulcerative colitis and may indicate multiple myeloma. Polymyalgia rheumatica treatment includes **prednisone 15 mg for 2 months, 10 mg for 2 months, then cut down by 1 mg every month and taper**. May continue low-dose prednisone for a year or longer.
3. For ulcerative colitis, if joints are involved, give **sulfasalazine**. If only the intestines are involved, give **mesalamine**.

1/17/2019

1. 70 yo male with **ulcerative colitis**, 10/16/2017 started on adalimumab; on 1/31/2018, he was diagnosed with multiple myeloma (MM) while on azathioprine and mesalamine.
2. **Fibromyalgia**: if inflammatory pain, give prednisone 10 mg daily for 2 weeks, then 5 mg daily for 2 weeks.

3. **Phenazopyridine** (Pyridium) can relieve pain and dysuria in urinary tract infection (UTI) and symptoms of bladder cancer.
4. **Fibromyalgia**, will need to rule out (r/o) ankylosing spondylitis (AS), rheumatoid arthritis (RA), and lupus: order rheumatic factor (RF), anti-cyclic citrullinated peptide (CCP), ESR, ENA, ANA, ds-DNA, CRP, C3&C4, HLA-B27; imaging hands and feet.
5. No NSAIDs while on steroids.

1/20/2019

1. **Tumor necrosis factor (TNF) alpha inhibitors**: TNF receptor blockage refers to TNF alpha inhibitors binding to transmembrane TNF which causes apoptosis, cytotoxicity, diminished cell influx or reduction in cytokines, and chemokines (inflammatory mediators).
2. The terminal deoxynucleotidyl transferase dUTP nick end labeling (**TUNEL**) technique has been used to detect apoptotic cells with TNF alpha inhibitor or placebo.
3. Infliximab promotes apoptosis in **activated T lymphocytes** (TUNEL-positive CD3 cells) but not in resting T lymphocytes.
4. **Soluble TNF-alpha** acts on many hematopoietic and nonhematopoietic cell types through two main receptors: **TNF receptor I and receptor II**. Transmembrane TNF binds only to TNF receptor II, coupling to intracytoplasmic domains (**TNF receptor-associated factors**) that activate other gene transcription factors such as **NF-kB** (causing inflammation) and **activator protein 1** inducing the synthesis of a range of proinflammatory cytokines and chemokines (responsible for differentiation, proliferation, and apoptosis).
5. Promotion of inflammation by TNF alpha via stimulating **IL-1, IL-6,** regulation of Th1 and TNF alpha via inducing **IL-2 and IL-8**. TNF alpha is capable of amplifying the TH1 type response triggered by IL-12 and IL-18 activation of CD4 T cells and promoting increased **IFN-gamma** production. **IFN-gamma** activates innate and adaptive immunity against viral, some bacterial, and protozoan infections. IFN-gamma activates macrophages and induces major histocompatibility complex class II molecule expression.
6. **Infliximab, adalimumab, and etanercept** are all TNF alpha inhibitors based on human IgG1 Fc, which have the capability of complement fixation and binding to Fc receptors.
7. **Infliximab**, 3 mg/kg/IV infusion, given at weeks 0, 2, 6, and then q8wk, can be combined with methotrexate (MTX)
8. Etanercept, 50 mg subcu once a week; 25 mg subcu, twice a week.
9. Adalimumab, 40 mg subcu, q14d, may increase to 40 mg qwk if not on methotrexate.
10. Certolizumab, 400 mg subcu wk. 0, 2, 4 followed by 200 mg subcu q2wk.
11. Golimumab 50 mg subcu qmonth with methotrexate.
12. **Azathioprine** takes 8–12 weeks to work, and causes bone marrow (BM) suppression, especially in chronic kidney disease (CKD), need to check thiopurine methyltransferase (TPMT) before initiating therapy. **TPMT genotype and**

TPMT enzyme activity (phenotype) testing are both required in all patients who are evaluated for treatment with azathioprine (**AZA**) or 6-mercaptopurine (**6-MP**). Dysfunctional TPMT causes severe drug-induced bone marrow toxicity when these agents are used.

1/22/2019

1. **Enbrel and other TNF alpha inhibitors need to be stopped 2 weeks before knee replacement and restarted 2 weeks after surgery (after wound closure).**
2. Xeljanz (tofacitinib) has to be used concomitantly with methotrexate (MTX) for **psoriatic arthritis**. Xeljanz can be used with or without methotrexate for **rheumatoid arthritis** (RA).
3. **RA**: methotrexate and Plaquenil, and if not effective, switch to TNF inhibitors, and if not effective, switch to Janus kinase 1 (JAK1) inhibitor (Xeljanz), and if not effective, switch to IL-6 inhibitor (Actemra), and if not effective, switch to rituximab.
4. **Psoriasis**: methotrexate, if not effective, use TNF alpha inhibitor; if not effective, use IL-17 inhibitor Cosentyx (Secukinumab).
5. **Ankylosing spondylitis** (AS): TNF alpha inhibitor, and if not effective, switch to IL-17 inhibitor Cosentyx.

1/23/2019

1. **Chondrocalcinosis** treatment: colchicine 0.6 mg qd for 3–6 months. Chondrocalcinosis refers to the calcium-containing deposits in cartilage on joint X-rays. It is usually caused by calcium pyrophosphate crystals in **pseudogout**.
2. **Cimzia (certolizumab pegol)** is a tumor necrosis factor (TNF) alpha inhibitor.
3. **Rheumatoid arthritis (RA)**, once started on Enbrel (etanercept), can continue or stop methotrexate (MTX).
4. Cosentyx (Secukinumab) 2 doses per week for 5 weeks, and then 2 doses per week every month for psoriatic arthritis and skin rash.
5. Order **QuantiFERON GOLD** before initiating TNF alpha inhibitors.

1/24/2019

1. Tumor necrosis factor (TNF) alpha inhibitor medications should be **in room air for over 1 h before injection**.
2. **Plaquenil (hydroxychloroquine)** is less potent than methotrexate (MTX); it is used in young, pregnant, or no joint involvement cases of rheumatoid arthritis (RA) and lupus.
3. **Discoid lupus**: on Plaquenil 400 mg qd and prednisone 5 mg qd; no response, can add methotrexate (MTX) 4 tablets per week.
4. **RA**: start methotrexate and then initiate prednisone taper.
5. **Allopurinol** in chronic kidney disease (CKD) should be ≤100 mg qd. **Uloric** (Febuxostat) does not require renal adjustment and thus can be used in CKD, usually starting with 40 mg qd, but still requires dose adjustment if CrCl <30 mL/min.

6. **Gout flare-up** treatment: colchicine 0.6 mg qd for ≤6 months, add allopurinol when asymptomatic, **uric acid goal < 6**.
7. Prednisone tapering dose for gout: 10 mg tablet 6 tablets qd for 2 days, 4 tablets for 2 days, 3 for 2 days, 2 for 2 days, and 1 for a day.
8. Compared to Plaquenil, methotrexate has stronger effects.

1/31/2019

1. ST elevation myocardial infarction (STEMI): start NS at 80 cc/h 8 h prior and 8 h after angiogram. Needs to call code STEMI.
2. **Left ventricular (LV) failure**: decrease afterload can help increase stroke volume and cardiac output (CO), decrease myocardial O2 demand. If chest pain or uncontrolled hypertension, can use **IV nitroglycerin (NTG) or nitroprusside** (risk of coronary steal), add short-acting angiotensin converting enzyme inhibitor (ACEi). If congestive heart failure with shock despite diuretics and decreased afterload, may start **dopamine, dobutamine, or milrinone**.
3. Dizziness after acute coronary syndrome on heparin drip, will have to rule out **retroperitoneal bleed**, can order CT head and abdomen/pelvis (dry CT).
4. **Drug-eluting stents are safe for MRI, even immediately after stent implantation.**
5. After the coronary artery angiogram study, the patient is a candidate for coronary artery bypass grafting (CABG), **heparin should be held for 4 h after angiogram then restarted**.
6. After the coronary artery angiogram study, the patient was recommended for CABG, **we assume severely decreased left ventricular ejection fraction (LVEF)** unless stated otherwise by a cardiologist.
7. For **relapsed or refractory multiple myeloma (MM),** monoclonal antibodies (daratumumab, isatuximab), protease inhibitors (bortezomib, carfilzomib, ixazomib), alkylating agents (melphalan, cyclophosphamide), bendamustine, CAR-T cell therapy and steroids may be used. Velcade = bortezomib.
8. Initial regimens for **MM treatment** include 3–6 cycles of DVRd (daratumumab, bortezomib, lenalidomide, low-dose dexamethasone) followed by hematopoietic cell transplantation (HCT) if high risk; VRd (bortezomib, lenalidomide, low-dose dexamethasone), DRd (daratumumab, lenalidomide, low-dose dexamethasone). Followed by maintenance therapy with **lenalidomide and bortezomib** (if DRVd) or lenalidomide and daratumumab (if DRd) or single agent with lenalidomide. **Hematopoietic cell transplantation if appropriate should be after induction therapy with the aforementioned regimens.**
9. Patients with MM have high risks of developing **acute myeloid leukemia (AML) and myelodysplastic syndrome (MDS)**.

2/6/2019

1. **Symptoms of uremia**: fatigue, anorexia, pruritus, altered mental status (AMS), shortness of breath (SOB), pruritic pain, and loss of ambition.
2. **Pericardial friction rub** indicates uremic pericarditis and will need dialysis treatment. **Classic indication for dialysis** includes: pulmonary edema which is

resistant to diuretics, refractory hyperkalemia, refractory metabolic acidosis, uremic complications (pericarditis, encephalopathy, bleeding); dialyzable intoxications (e.g., lithium, toxic alcohol, and salicylates)

3. **Continuous renal replacement therapy (CRRT)** is mainly used in hemodynamically unstable patients.
4. **Dialysis disequilibrium syndrome**: urea decrease causes osmotic changes leading to a shift of water in the brain, thus seizure. **Treatment**: dialysis in 3 days at a slow rate, limit urea clearance of urea and increase dialysate sodium level.
5. **AV fistula needs 6–8 weeks** after AV fistula (connects an artery and vein directly) surgery to be used. **AV graft** (connects the artery and vein via a tube and graft) can be used in **2 weeks**. Benefits of AV fistula as compared to AV graft: less likely to become infected, less likely to clot, and is longer lasting. The life span for an **AV fistula is 10 years while only 2 years for an AV graft**.
6. If dialysis is started on diabetic patients, the mean life expectancy is >2 years (usually between 5 and 10 years) unless transplantation (**survival rate of 71% in T2DM and 94% in T1DM at 3 years**). Common causes of death are acute myocardial infarction (AMI) and sepsis. **The mean life expectancy on dialysis is 4.5 years for patients aged 60–64**.
7. When to start **CRRT**: can't tolerate hemodialysis (HD), acute, not responding to HD, and unstable patients.
8. **Pericardial effusion in renal dialysis** patients, especially if seen with chest wall veins and upper extremity vein enlargement, needs STAT echo to rule out **cardiac tamponade. Call cardiologist consultant for stat pericardiocentesis**.

2/23/2019

1. For high bleeding risk, anticoagulation (AC) should be discontinued if surgical bleeding risk is high. **Cardiac implantable devices or catheter ablation for atrial fibrillation** have a low risk of bleeding and should continue warfarin or defer to the cardiologist who performed the procedure.
2. **Syndrome of inappropriate antidiuretic hormone (SIADH)** has low BUN and plasma uric acid.
3. Procalcitonin if >0.25, community-acquired pneumonia (CAP) is likely. For infection, procalcitonin level daily may be appropriate for determination of antibiotic duration, and consider discontinuing antibiotics (ABX) if levels are <0.5 or decrease by 80% from peak procal >4 ng/uL and the patient has stabilized. **Procalcitonin is not reliable for bloodstream infections.**
4. Stanford classification of aortic dissection: **Type A dissection**—ascending aorta and may progress to involve the aortic arch and thoracoabdominal aorta. **Type B dissection**—descending aorta (thoracic) or thoracoabdominal aorta distal to left subclavian artery without involvement of the ascending aorta. Palpate carotid, subclavian, and femoral pulses, obtain BP in bilateral arms.
5. Type A aortic dissection is a medical emergency and needs vascular surgery consult stat; Type B can be managed medically unless end-organ ischemia, progression, or rupture.
6. **Acute medical treatment for aortic dissection** if unstable: surgery consult STAT; 2 large bore IVs; monitor HR and BP continuously, control HR and

BP. Target goal heart rate (HR) < 60 bpm and systolic blood pressure (sBP) between 100 and 120 mmHg, administer **esmolol 250–500 mg/kg loading, then 25–50 mg/kg/min titrate or give labetalol or verapamil/Cardizem**. Once heart rate < 60, give vasodilators, if sBP > 120, give **nitroprusside 0.25–0.5 mg/kg or nicardipine**. Give iv opioids for pain, place Foley for strict I&Os.

2/24/2019

1. **Lupus anticoagulants** are autoantibodies against negatively charged phospholipids or complexes of phospholipids with either beta-2-glycoprotein 1 or clotting factors such as prothrombin. Lupus anticoagulants can be first screened using **aPTT-lupus anticoagulant (LA)**, also checked with **dilute Russell Viper Venom test (dRVVT)** and **Kaolin clotting time** (KCT). All these tests are phospholipid-responsive clotting tests.
2. **dRVVT** activates factor X while bypassing FVII and contact system or plasma kallikrein–kinin system and antihemophilic factors of the intrinsic pathway. Thus, dRVVT test is not affected by contact factor abnormalities, deficiency or antibodies. **Mixing study is useful to exclude factor II, V, and X deficiencies**.
3. **Contact system**, also named as **plasma Kallikrein-kinin system**, consists of three serine proteinases: coagulation factor XII and XI, plasma prekallikrein, and the nonenzymatic cofactor high molecular weight kininogen.
4. **Antiphospholipid Abs** are Ab against phosphorus fat components of the cell membranes, lanterin blood proteins (bind with phospholipids), and the complexes when phospholipids and proteins bind.
5. Common antiphospholipid Abs are **lupus Ab and cardiolipin Ab**; others include anti-beta2 glycoprotein-1 (anti-beta2 GP1) and anti-thrombin.
6. **Anticardiolipin IgG** is highly related to complications (like thrombo-occlusive events and death after focal cerebral ischemia) whereas high **anticardiolipin IgM** is associated with autoimmune hemolytic anemia.
7. PTT-LA is a modified aPTT with dilute phospholipids. It is very sensitive but not specific to LA. PTT-LA can be prolonged in patients on anticoagulation. If not on anticoagulation and PTT ≤50 s, need to repeat a PTT with a routine agent.
8. Both of the following tests should be ordered for lupus anticoagulant profiling because LAs are heterogenous with variations in titer, avidity, and isotype. (1) PTT-LA if positive, do **hexagonal phase confirmation**; (2) dRVVT screen, if positive, do **dRVVT confirmation**, if again positive, do **dRVVT1:1 mix study**.
9. The combination of aPTT that does not correct after 1:1 mix and positive Hexagonal Phase Phospholipid (HPP) confirmations consistent with a lupus anticoagulant. **Direct antithrombin inhibitors and factor VIII inhibitors** can cause a false positive and should be ruled out if positive lupus anticoagulants.

3/2/2019 Preoperative Cardiac Assessment for Noncardiac Surgery

1. Calculate the estimated perioperative risk of major adverse cardiac events (MACEs) based on combined clinical and surgical risks: low risk (<1%) or elevated risk (>1 = 1%). If elevated risk (moderate or greater risks), check **baseline functional status** (≥4METs functional capacity may indicate medically opti-

mized for surgery). **4METs = climbing ≥ 1 flight (12 stairs) of stairs without stopping**. If <4 METs or unknown → will test further to help maximize the patient's condition, such as a Cardiolite stress study and echocardiogram.
2. **Revised Cardiac Risk Index (RCRI)** also known as the Lee Index or the American College of Surgeons National Surgical Quality Improvement Program Risk Prediction is usually used to establish the patient's risk.
3. Preoperative medical evaluation of the healthy adult patient: (1) **Hgb measurement** if ≥65 and young patients with risk for lots of blood loss; (2) **Measurement of Cr** in ≥50 undergoing intermediate or high-risk surgery; (3) **Risk of renal injury** in young patients.
4. **Dry nose, and nose bleed**, can be treated with oxymetazoline 0.05% spray + NS 0.65% (ocean nasal spray).
5. Patient sick, trop 0.06, need to **trend troponin** to rule out acute coronary syndrome while understanding troponin elevation is also a severity index factor.

3/3/2019

1. Constant and uncontrolled nausea and vomiting, treatment: may **apply nasogastric (NG) tube** (especially if confirmed bowel obstruction or ileus) and **order CT abdomen/pelvis** to rule out bowel obstruction, ileus and place the **patient on nothing per mouth** to prevent aspiration.
2. **Altered mental status (AMS)** requires the exclusion of encephalitis, meningitis, stroke, and seizures.
3. **Leukemia** needs to look at monocytes and basophils. If high monocytes, the patient may have myelomonocytic leukemia.
4. **Hematuria** (may require urologist consultation and continuous bladder irrigation with Foley insertion), hematochezia, bruising, need to check PT/INR.

3/9/2019

1. For **aspiration pneumonia**, usually begins with just pneumonitis, and may be observed off antibiotics. Procalcitonin can also be used; however, low procalcitonin can happen in the early stages of aspiration pneumonia. Therefore, may also simply be treated with antibiotics for 7 days if suspicions of pneumonia increase.
2. **Cavernous hemangioma**, no need for treatment and no anticoagulation; if myocardial infarction (MI), go directly to angiogram. However, research evidence indicates no increase in bleeding risks or focal neurological deficit with antithrombotic therapy and antiplatelet therapy in patients with cavernous malformation.

3/12/2019

1. Alogliptin is a dipeptidyl peptidase-4 (DPP-4) inhibitor; Dyazide = hydrochlorothiazide and triamterene
2. d-**lactic acidosis** in short bowel syndrome (can also be seen in patients with ingestion of a large amount of propylene glycol and patients with diabetic keto-

acidosis) will not correct with fluid hydration. Typical serum lactic acid test is not sensitive for D-lactic acidosis; diagnosis requires high suspicion and clinical history with lab showing anion gap is lower than expected for the decrease in bicarbonate (HCO_3-)

3. **Causes of d-lactic acidosis**: short bowel syndrome, ingestion of a large amount of propylene glycol, diabetic ketoacidosis. **Diagnosis**: unexplained high anion gap metabolic acidosis or hyperchloremic metabolic acidosis. **Treatment**: Sodium bicarbonate. Oral **antimicrobial** agents (such as metronidazole, neomycin, or vancomycin) can be used in short bowel syndrome.
4. **Type A lactic acidosis is caused by systemic hypoperfusion; Type B lactic acidosis is due to toxin-induced impairment of cellular metabolism and localized ischemia.**
5. In general, those taking prednisone dosage equivalents **of at least 20 mg/day for 1 month or longer with another cause of immunocompromise should receive P. jirovecii pneumonia** prophylaxis.

3/16/2019

1. **Tamiflu prescription**: if eGFR >60, prescribe 75 mg bid, no renal adjustment necessary; if eGFR 30–60, prescribe 30 mg bid; if eGFR 30–10, prescribe 30 mg qd. If ESRD is not on HD, do not use.
2. Non-valvular AFib: Eliquis dosing 5 mg bid unless 2 of the following: **≥80 yo, <60 kg, Cr > 1.5. If yes, do 2.5 mg bid**
3. New chronic obstructive pulmonary disease (COPD) diagnosis with COPD exacerbation: discharge on Stiolto Respimat (olodaterol/tiotropium) plus albuterol inhaler.
4. **Multiple sclerosis (MS) pulmonary function test** (PFT): respiratory muscle strength check with MIP (maximum inspiratory pressure) and MEP (maximum expiratory pressure).
5. **Normal D-dimer** upper limit: 50 yo = 500, 60 yo = 600, 70 yo = 700.
6. Zio cardiac patch for remote cardiac rhythm monitoring.
7. **Gastrointestinal (GI) symptoms** on exertion may indicate inferior wall myocardial infarction; circumflex artery provides blood supply to the inferior artery in 10%–15% of patients.
8. Amiodarone use, if still irregular rhythm, may simply stop it.
9. If left ventricular ejection fraction (LVEF) is normal, there is no need for Coreg (carvedilol). Get an echocardiogram and if LVEF ok, may discontinue Coreg and add Cardizem for blood pressure (BP) control.
10. Chest pain with tachycardia = if **stress test + , consider calling cardiologist consultant** for cardiac catheterization; Zio patch for AFib and flutter monitoring or rule out.

3/20/2019

1. Maximum urine dilution 50–100 Osm.

2. **HA1c to serum fasting glucose transformation**: 30 mg Glu each percentile above 4 on the base of 60 mg/mL for HA1c estimate. 6 = 2 × 30 + 60 = 120; 7 = 3 × 30 + 60 = 150.
3. Combivent = ipratropium bromide and albuterol sulfate. Stiolto Respimat = olodaterol—tiotropium combination, 2 puff qd.
4. **Lymphoma workup**: SPEP, UPEP, LDH, HBV/HCV, serum beta2-microglobulin.
5. **Trospium** is a muscarinic antagonist for OAB.
6. **Quetiapine** and many other antipsychotics can cause increased mortality.
7. **Digoxin** loading 0.5 g, then 8 h later 0.25 g, then 8 h later 0.25 g, then 0.125 g qd.
8. Benign prostate hyperplasia (BPH) or urinary retention, add finasteride and tamsulosin after discontinuing terazosin.

3/22/2019

1. **Congestive heart failure (CHF)**, upon discharge, recommends weighing daily, if gained ≥ 3lbs, double the dose of Lasix.
2. Fall, if **loss of consciousness**, then structural and functional heart diseases including aortic stenosis, VFib, and sick sinus syndrome will have to be ruled out.
3. **Strep A (Streptococcus pyogenes)** causes necrotizing fasciitis, septic shock, and Strep throat. CT and MRI to look for necrosis and **tissue gas** are the best tests to look at **necrotizing fasciitis.**
4. **Fetty syndrome** = rheumatoid arthritis (RA), neutropenia, and splenomegaly, leading to increased susceptibility to bacterial infections.
5. **Ipratropium** (blockade of muscarinic cholinergic receptors causing smooth muscle relaxation and bronchodilation) is not good for expectoration, **albuterol** (beta-2 adrenergic receptors to relax the bronchial smooth muscle) can loosen sputum.
6. Tobramycin is a better eye drop.
7. **Low left ventricular ejection fraction (LVEF), do not use Cardizem or verapamil.**

3/25/2019

1. **Bell's palsy treatment**: treatment with prednisone 60 mg po qd × 7 days, ideally within 3 days of symptom onset, definitely within 7 days of symptom onset. For patients with severe facial palsy (House-Brackmann grade IV or higher), order adjunctive valacyclovir 1000 mg 3 times daily for 1 week. Close follow-up for **MRI brain if incomplete recovery after 3–4 months**.
2. **Stercoral colitis** is inflammation of the colon from chronic severe constipation. If sepsis, treat with antibiotics. Monitor for bowel perforation and peritonitis which require surgery for bowel resection.
3. **Free water flush** in chronic vent patients can cause aspiration with PEG but does help with hypernatremia.
4. Unknown benefits for beta-blocker if left ventricular ejection fraction (LVEF) is normal.

5. Flomax 0.4 mg qd, finasteride 5 mg qd for BPH; **Pyridium** 100 mg tid for dysuria.
6. Patiromer (Veltassa), sodium polystyrene sulfonate (Kayexalate), and sodium zirconium cyclosilicate (Lokelma) are all used for hyperkalemia.
7. **Cilostazol is contraindicated in congestive heart failure (CHF).**
8. **Peripheral arterial disease (PAD)**: Plavix + aspirin is used for 6 m after stent placement. The **Angiojet thrombectomy system** needs heparin during and before the procedure for severe critical limb ischemia (vascular surgery consult).

3/26/2019

1. **After ureteral stent placement**, may need 3-day Zosyn (can also use Cipro) treatment; 1 dose before procedure.
2. **After pacemaker placement**: cefazolin/Keflex for 5 days; 1 dose prior to the procedure. No water over the surgical site for 1 week; no large amplitude movement of the shoulder, ok to use walker, and bandage for 5 days after pacemaker placement.
3. If the left ventricular ejection fraction (LVEF) is low, Cardizem will have to be replaced with a beta-blocker.
4. **Right ventricular failure** with normal LVEF: no benefit for beta-blocker; need to **increase heart rate** if cardiac index low (normal cardiac index 2.5–4.2 L/min/m^2). Can increase pacemaker rate, add Bumex, cardiovert if atrial fibrillation. If cardiorenal, can also give **dopamine**.
5. **Anticholinergic** can decrease secretion, not good for expectoration.
6. Moxifloxacin causes QTc elongation. **Acapella and incentive spirometry** are good for the prevention of aspiration pneumonia and after surgery.
7. Sucking lemon for dry mouth; adding calcitriol for low Vit D and hypocalcemia in chronic kidney disease (CKD). **Do not use calcitriol if phosphorus is above normal or calcium $\geq$ 9.5**. Use **cinacalcet** in hemodialysis patients.
8. **Adrenal insufficiency** outpatient treatment: hydrocortisone 10 mg qam + 5 mg qpm (can go up to 25 mg total daily dose).
9. **Bactrim** blocks Cr excretion by 10% and also increases serum potassium, but has no effect on chronic kidney disease (CKD).
10. COPD discharge: Combivent (ipratropium + albuterol) for 1-week qid + albuterol prn
11. **Scopolamine** patch for excessive secretion.
12. C. diff + bacteremia = 7 days daptomycin + 7 additional days po vancomycin after completion of daptomycin.
13. Need to adjust allopurinol and gabapentin for CKD. Hydroxyzine for agitation 25 mg q6h prn.
14. **Kidney injury etiologies**: acute tubular necrosis (ATN), dehydration, cardiorenal, drug toxicity and others.
15. If the O2 requirement is too high, $\geq$7 lpm, may not be a good candidate for bronchoscopy or endoscopy. This may require **intubation** to get **bronchoscopy and endoscopy** if deemed appropriate.

16. Heparin and Lovenox can cause hyperkalemia via the aldosterone pathway. Metoprolol can cause increased potassium in 0.5% of the patients without acute renal failure.

4/3/2019

1. Simvastatin (40 mg) and diltiazem interaction results in **rhabdomyolysis and hepatitis**.
2. Simvastatin max dose 20 mg when used together with amlodipine due to risk for rhabdomyolysis.
3. **Albumin/globulin ratio** (normal 0.8–2): the major proteins in serum are albumin and globulin. Globulin includes alpha1, alpha2 globulin, beta, and gamma globulin. Albumin accounts for 50% of total serum proteins. **Total globulins** can be increased in certain chronic inflammatory diseases (tuberculosis and syphilis), multiple myeloma, collagen diseases, and rheumatoid arthritis (RA). Decreased levels of globulin in hepatic dysfunction, renal disease, and cancer. **Gamma gap** = total protein − serum albumin.
4. **Minoxidil** 5 mg qd causes pericardial effusion, T wave changes in EKG, edema, and sodium retention.
5. **Hard to control blood pressure in end-stage renal disease (ESRD)**: Coreg 25 mg bid, clonidine 0.2 mg tid, isosorbide dinitrate 20 mg tid, nifedipine 90 mg tid, hydralazine 100 mg tid, and terazosin 2 mg increased to 6 mg bid.
6. Calcium low in ESRD: calcitriol 0.5 mg qd + calcium carbonate 1350 mg bid.
7. **Acyclovir causes crystallization induced crystals**; its infusion requires hydration with normal saline. Uremic encephalopathy requires urgent dialysis.
8. On aspirin, still developed stroke 1 year later, add Plavix or even Brilinta. Altered mental status (AMS) may require ICU admission or transfer.
9. **Trihexyphenidyl** (anticholinergic) is used for symptomatic treatment of tremors, spasms, and stiffness in Parkinson's disease. It is also used to treat **extrapyramidal side effects** during antipsychotic treatments. **Adverse events**: drowsiness, vertigo, dizziness. It's an anti-muscarinic.
10. **Contrast dye allergy protocols for CT with contrast**: Oral prednisone 50 mg at 13, 7, and 1 h prior to contrast administration plus 50 mg diphenhydramine 1 h prior. Urgent: Hydrocortisone 200 mg IV 5 h and 1 h before contrast administration and 50 mg IV diphenhydramine 1 h before contrast administration.
11. Before or after percutaneous coronary intervention (PCI): Imdur 30 mg for chest pain, Nitro-Bid Ointment, nitroglycerin drip for hypertension and chest pain in coronary artery disease (CAD).
12. **Dangerous renal diuretic drip**: furosemide 100 mg in D5 at 10 cc/h. Can also use Bumex drip in **anasarca**. Will need to monitor BMP q12h.
13. Hemoptysis may require Ear Nose Throat (ENT) doctor consultation to look at the throat. Prednisone 60 mg daily can be used to treat asthma.
14. Hydralazine 100 mg tid can cause **drug-induced lupus**.
15. Chronic obstructive pulmonary disease (COPD) and asthma, outpatient treatment regimen: Spiriva, betamethasone, Advair (fluticasone/salmeterol)

16. **Coreg has alpha-blocker effects** and drops blood pressure more than metoprolol; **urine RBC (hematuria)** requires cystoscopy either as inpatient or outpatient to rule out malignancy of the bladder and potentially also CT scan to look for renal cell carcinoma (urologist referral needed).
17. **Memory loss differential diagnoses** (DDx): stroke, transient ischemic attack (TIA), drug side effects, transient global amnesia, and seizures.

Langerhans Cell Histiocytosis (LCH): Most Common in Children 1–3 yo.

1. Langerhans cell histiocytosis with one organ system involvement like **bone** happens in ½ patients. The majority of patients have raised soft tender masses or lytic punched out the appearance of bone lesions. **Skin** involvement happens in 40% patients with **lung** in 10% patients.
2. Patients with lung involvement may be asymptomatic or develop spontaneous pneumothorax or with nonproductive cough, dyspnea, and chest pain, together with possible constitutional symptoms. Diagnosis via CT high resolution which shows **cysts and nodules** and via biopsy of an osteolytic bone or skin lesion showing **histiocytes on biopsy** with or without infiltration of extraskeletal lesions.
3. If the central nervous system is involved, **diabetes insipidus and symptoms of neurodegenerative changes of ataxia, and cognitive dysfunction** are common.
4. Differential diagnosis of LCH include other **histolytic and dendritic cell disease**, metastatic malignancies, and **hemophagocytic lymphohistiocytosis** (HLH) and **macrophage activation syndrome**.
5. **Macrophage activation syndrome** is mostly seen in juvenile idiopathic arthritis (JIA), but also happens in systemic lupus erythematosus (SLE) and Kawasaki disease. It is systemic hyperinflammation leading to a **cytokine storm** causing hemophagocytosis and multi-organ failure, associated with **autoimmunity**, infection, and malignancy.
6. **Hemophagocytic lymphohistiocytosis (HLH)** is a disorder of immune dysregulation that leads to ***excessive macrophage activity***, often with life-threatening consequences, caused by ***infections, malignancies, rheumatologic conditions, and genetic defects***.
7. Treatment for LCH: single organ LCH- **prednisone, the combination of prednisone + vinblastine**, curettage of bone lesions; multi-system LCH (hematopoietic organs, liver, spleen)—clinical trial, induction chemo with vinblastine plus prednisone or cytarabine.

4/4/2019

1. Addison disease, adrenal insufficiency: cortisol at 8 a.m., cortisol <3–5 is diagnostic (if borderline or unsure, do ACTH stimulation); >5 is normal. ACTH stimulation 250 mg → if cortisol >18, it is normal and adrenal insufficiency is ruled out.
2. **Follicular stimulating hormone (FSH)** normal value in postmenopausal is >30. **Morning testosterone** normal value should be >300 in male.

3. **Polycystic ovarian syndrome (PCOS)** + hyperandrogenism **treatment** (Rx): combined oral contraceptive (OCP) is the first-line treatment; progesterone is not good for hyperandrogenism. For patients with hyperandrogenic symptoms after 6 months of contraceptive symptoms, **spironolactone** 50–100 mg twice daily can be added.
4. Chronic obstructive pulmonary disease (COPD) newly diagnosed discharge medications: Symbicort (Budesonide / Formoterol) bid, tiotropium.
5. **Diagnosis of PCOS**: menstrual irregularity; polycysts in ovary; labs showing hyperandrogenism (**DHEA, testosterone, serum 17-hydroxyprogesterone**). If met 2/3 = diagnosis. DHEA = Dehydroepiandrosterone.
6. Peripherally inserted central catheter (PICC) line and dialysis line contraindication: vein mapping for preparation of dialysis. Avoid PICC in the dominant hand.
7. After transcatheter aortic valve replacement (TAVR): do **Plavix and Coumadin for 3 months, then drop Plavix in AFib**.
8. When hgb drops in a patient's status post transcatheter valve replacement, left ventricular assist devices, or surgical valve replacement, will have to rule out **prosthesis-related hemolysis**. Check hemolysis labs, get echo, and possibly CT angiogram. Treatments for prosthesis-induced hemolysis include supplementation with **folic acid, iron, and pentoxifylline on top of device-specific treatments from specialists**.
9. Right heart failure: right heart catheterization if not much pressure in the right heart → stop diuresis. If wedge pressure is high, start diuresis
10. If the patient has a PICC line, think of infection.
11. **Thyroid cancer (papillary), thyroid nodule** treatment: 24 mg lenvatinib, lymph node dissection at cancer center, and 2–3 radioactive iodine ablation treatment.
12. Ativan for EToH withdrawal: may consider 2 mg qid for 48 h, tid for 24 h, and qd for 24 h. May also use Librium 25–50 mg q6-8h.

Takeaway Messages

1. Concussion is a traumatic brain injury with vestibular, balance, vision, and cognitive and functional symptoms. Physical activity and aerobic exercise treatment are early interventions together cervicovestibular rehabilitation if neck pain, headaches, dizziness, and/or balance problems. Return to Learn/Sport includes a series of graded subsymptomatic threshold exercises.
2. Promotion of inflammation by TNF alpha via stimulating IL-1 and IL-6, regulation of Th1 and TNF alpha via inducing IL-2 and IL-8.
3. Enbrel and other TNF alpha inhibitors need to be stopped 2 weeks before knee replacement and restarted 2 weeks after surgery (after wound closure).
4. Multiple myeloma (MM) treatments include different combinations of DVRd (daratumumab, bortezomib, lenalidomide, low-dose dexamethasone) with or without hematopoietic cell transplantation. MM has risks for developing acute myeloid leukemia (AML) and myelodysplastic syndrome (MDS).
5. For Bell's palsy (treatment: prednisone 60 mg daily and valacyclovir 1000 mg tid for a week), if incomplete recovery after 3–4 months, need MRI brain.

6. Diagnosis of PCOS: menstrual irregularity; polycysts in ovary; labs showing hyperandrogenism (DHEA, testosterone, serum 17-hydroxyprogesterone). If met 2/3 = diagnosis. Treatment of PCOS is an oral combined contraceptive; for patients with persistent hyperandrogenic symptoms after 6 months of contraceptive symptoms, spironolactone 50–100 mg twice daily can be added.

Further Readings and References

1. Decq, P., D. Brauge, A. Calmat, et al. 2021. Diagnosis clinical criteria of sport related concussion: Toward an operational criteria definition in France. *Neurochirurgie* 67 (3): 222–230.
2. Patricios, J.S., K.J. Schneider, J. Dvorak, et al. 2023. Consensus statement on concussion in sport: the sixth International Conference on Concussion in Sport-Amsterdam, October 2022. *British Journal of Sports Medicine* 57 (11): 695–711.
3. Silva, L.C., L.C. Ortigosa, and G. Benard. 2010. Anti-TNF-α agents in the treatment of immune-mediated inflammatory diseases: mechanisms of action and pitfalls. *Immunotherapy* 2 (6): 817–833.
4. Zhou, K., D. Mehedint, and H. Khadim. 2019. Prolonged activated partial thromboplastin time due to plasma prekallikrein deficiency: A case study and literature review on its clinical significance. *Blood Coagulation Fibrinolysis* 30 (6): 300–303.
5. McClain, K.L., and G. Goyal. *Clinical manifestations, pathologic features, and diagnosis of Langerhans cell histiocytosis*, ed. P. Newburger. Waltham, MA: UpToDate. Accessed December 12, 2023.
6. McClain, K.L., and G. Goyal. *Treatment of non-pulmonary Langerhans cell histiocytosis*, ed. P. Newburger. Waltham, MA: UpToDate. Accessed December 12, 2023.

Chapter 12
Senior Resident at ICU and Back Being a Nocturnist

April 8th Through May 5th, 2019 and June 2nd Through June 30th, 2019
The oncology clinic: May 6th, 2019 through June 2nd, 2019 (notes for the oncology clinic were reorganized in later chapters).

My last three rotations in the 2nd year of residency training included one-month rotation each for the medical intensive care unit (ICU), oncology clinic (at a large NCI-designated cancer center), and night flow. At that time of the residency training, action plans for life after residency already began and were in full speed ahead. While taking care of patients in the ICU and admitting patients as a nocturnist were my major job responsibilities, I also spent a one-month elective rotation at the large cancer center (notes were adapted at later sections of the book) for my hematology/oncology fellowship application which eventually did not work out.

Lessons from my fellowship application experiences included the following: (1) Networking with fellows, faculty members, and program directors can offer valuable insights and potentially open doors for future opportunities. (2) Strong research experience and publications in the relevant field can bolster our fellowship application and demonstrate our commitment to advancing the field. (3) Demonstrating strong clinical skills, professionalism, and dedication to patient care can make a positive impression on program directors and faculty members. The preparation for fellowship application starts with day 1 of or even way before residency training.

For residents aspiring to secure fellowship positions, seeking advice and guidance from forerunners or mentors in fellowship training in their desired specialty is essential as they can provide valuable insights and recommendations to help residents navigate the fellowship application process successfully. One common recommendation is to undertake an away-elective rotation at hospitals or institutions known for their excellence in the resident's targeted specialty. Away electives offer residents the opportunity to gain exposure to different clinical environments, work alongside renowned experts in the field, and showcase their skills and dedication. It allows residents to assess the culture and learning environment of potential fellowship programs firsthand. It also provides them with the chance to establish

K. Zhou, *Internal Medicine Training Notes and Survival Guide*,
https://doi.org/10.1007/978-1-0716-4039-5_12

connections with faculty members, fellows, and residents at other institutions, which can be advantageous during the fellowship application and interview process.

Besides fellowship applications, the conclusion of the second year of residency training is also a crucial juncture for the preparation of independent practices of internal medicine residents. By the end of the second year, resident physicians should have acquired all the foundational knowledge and skills of internal medicine. Rotation as a senior resident in the ICU provided me another chance to review the knowledge in ventilator management, sedation medications, different pressors, and the care for various medical emergencies and polish my skills in taking care of sick patients. While the majority of the required knowledge was mentioned in previous chapters or was touched upon in later chapters, this chapter did encompass topics in thyroid storm, microangiopathic hemolytic anemia, and multiple sclerosis. The subchapter for back being a nocturnist only touched on arrhythmias as the majority of the survival pearls were discussed in previous chapters.

1 ICU as a Senior Resident

4/8/2019

1. **Thyroid storm** clinical signs: hyperpyrexia with T > 103 F, goiter, cardiovascular (CV) dysfunction (HR > 120), altered mentation, and tachycardia including atrial fibrillation (Afib). **Risk factors** include cessation of antithyroid medication for hyperthyroidism, recent thyroid or non thyroid surgery, and recent exposure to iodine-containing contrast. Additionally, labs are consistent with hyperthyroidism. The aforementioned information aids the empirical diagnosis of thyroid storm.
2. **Treatment for thyroid storm**: beta blocker, thionamide, an iodine solution to block the release of thyroid hormone; glucocorticoids to reduce T4 to T3 conversion, promote vasomotor stability, and treat relative adrenal insufficiency; bile acid sequestrants to decrease enterohepatic recycling of thyroid hormone.
3. **Propylthiouracil** (PTU) 200 mg q4h or **methimazole** 20 mg q4–6h; can add **sucralfate** to aid gastrointestinal (GI) clearance of thyroxine.
4. **Thyroid storm treatment example**: Cholestyramine (Questran) light 4 g q6h, hydrocortisone (Solu-Cortef) 100 mg iv q8h, propranolol 60 mg po q6h, Propylthiouracil (PTU) 200 mg q4h (preferred over methimazole 20 mg q4h), Lugol's solution (potassium iodine) 5 drops po q6h via Wolff–Chaikoff effects; continue treatment until shows clinical improvement.
5. **Atrial fibrillation with uncontrolled blood pressure**: IV Cardizem drip and IV metoprolol if rate consistently >120 bpm but not episodic. Repeat metoprolol as needed; discontinue amiodarone. When a patient can take po, convert medications to PO. If blood pressure (BP) is soft and heart rate (HR) is consistently above 120, after the replacement of electrolytes, may use 1–2 doses of IV digoxin.

4/9/2019

1. **AKI** treatment: LR 150 cc/h, or $NaHCO_3$ 8.4% in D5W at 100 cc/h.

4/10/2019

1. **Secondary hypertension workup**: renin, aldosterone, 24-h urine fractionated metanephrine fractionated, plasma free metanephrines. **Treatments** while the secondary workup is in process: hydrochlorothiazide (HCTZ) 12.5 mg, nifedipine 60 mg, Lisinopril 20 mg

4/14/2019

1. In pulmonary hypertension, goal oxygen saturation is **90% SO_2**. In metabolic acidosis with a high anion gap, will need to look at the **osmolar gap** for intoxications. Gastrointestinal (GI) bleed, look at HCO_2 of the basic metabolic panel for intoxications.
2. Short procedure, ok to do sedation with **propofol with versed 2 mg iv prn** under mechanical ventilation.

4/17/2019 Thrombotic Microangiopathy (TMA)

1. The primary TMA syndromes include thrombotic thrombocytopenic purpura (**TTP**, can be hereditary or acquired), Shiga toxin-mediated- hemolytic uremic syndrome (**HUS**), **drug-induced TMA syndrome**, **complement-mediated TMA** (hereditary or acquired).
2. Additionally, rare hereditary disorders of **Vit B12 metabolism**, factors involved in hemostasis pregnancy associated syndromes (e.g., **severe preeclampsia/ HELLP), severe HTN, systemic infections and malignancies, autoimmune diseases such as SLE** and complications of **hematopoietic stem cell or solid organ transplantation** can also present with **microangiopathic hemolytic anemia (MAHA) and thrombocytopenia**.
3. A history of cancer warrants **bone marrow biopsy with special stains** for cancer cells to rule out systemic metastatic cancer-associated TMA.
4. **MAHA**: helmet cells (schistocytes) and other fragmented red cells, microspherocytes. **TTP**: deficiency of ADAMTS13 activity, can be hereditary (Upshaw-Schulman syndrome) or acquired as a result of inhibition of ADAMTS13 activity by an autoantibody. In TTP, abnormalities of the **central nervous system (CNS), heart, pancreas, thyroid, adrenal glands, intestinal mucosa,** and other tissues may occur, but the lungs are usually spared. **Upshaw-Schulman syndrome (USS)** is a congenital bleeding disorder with repeated episodes of thrombocytopenia and MAHA that respond to infusions of fresh frozen plasma.
5. **Shiga toxin-mediated hemolytic-uremic syndrome** (O157:H7 and O104:H4): Shiga toxin causes damage to kidney epithelial cells (podocytes and tubular cells), kidney mesangial cells, and vascular endothelial cells.
6. **Complement-mediated TMA**: hereditary deficiency of complement factor H and 1 (can be acquired), membrane cofactor protein (MCP, CD46), or heredi-

tary abnormality of protein that accelerates the activation of this pathway (e.g., CFB, C3).

7. **Drug-induced TMA**: immune-mediated (quinine, gemcitabine, oxaliplatin, and quetiapine); dose-dependent, toxicity-mediated due to direct cellular damage (A) chemotherapeutic agents like gemcitabine and mitomycin; (B) immunosuppressive agents like cyclosporine and tacrolimus; (C) VEGF inhibitors bevacizumab; (D) opioids like morphine and cocaine).
8. **Metabolism-mediated TMA**: hereditary mutations in MMACHC gene (methylmalonic aciduria and homocystinuria C), cobalamin deficiency (coagulation-mediated TMA: mutations in genes encoding thrombomodulin), plasminogen, and diacylglycerol kinase epsilon.
9. **Systemic disorders** associated with MAHA and thrombocytopenia: **HELLP** (hemolysis, elevated liver enzymes, low platelet count), **severe hypertension** (HTN), **systemic infections** like bacterial endocarditis, HIV, CMV, Rocky Mountain spotted fever, RBC parasites like malaria and babesia, and systemic aspergillosis, **systemic malignancies, systemic rheumatic diseases** like systemic lupus erythematosus (SLE), systemic sclerosis (SSc) and antiphospholipid syndrome (APS), **hematopoietic stem cell transplant and organ transplantation, DIC, severe B12 deficiency**.
10. Diagnostic approach: verify MAHA and thrombocytopenia → exclude systemic disorders → identify which type of **primary TMA, PLASMIC score, TTP (treatment with plasma exchange and eculizumab), complement-mediated TMA (treatment with eculizumab, prevent and treat acute kidney injury).**
11. Suspected TTP: start plasma exchange (Plasmapheresis). **Plasmapheresis adverse events**: central **venous catheter-associated hemorrhage, infections, or thrombi**, and plasma-associated transfusion reactions.
12. Suspected complement-mediated TMA: use **eculizumab** if rapid kidney function decline.
13. If anaphylactic reaction to plasma, **a factor VIII concentrate that contains a high concentration of ADAMTS 13 (<10% activity)** can be used together with plasma removal.
14. TTP can be acquired, due to an auto-antibody inhibitor, or hereditary due to mutations in ADAMTS13.
15. TTP should be suspected in a patient present with **MAHA, hemoglobin < 10, and severe thrombocytopenia, PLT < 30,000, with or without symptoms of organ involvement and without an apparent etiology**.
16. **Diagnostic testing in TTP**: CBC, review of blood smear, CMP, LDH, bilirubin, haptoglobin, coagulation testing (PT, aPTT, fibrinogen, D-dimer, negative direct antiglobulin/Coombs test), **ADAMTS13 activity and inhibitor** testing, MRI of brain, and stool for Shiga toxin and bacteria.
17. The diagnosis of acquired TTP is confirmed by **severe ADAMTS13 activity deficiency (e.g, <10% of normal) and the presence of an ADAMTS 13 inhibitor (autoantibody)** in the appropriate clinical setting.

18. **Paroxysmal nocturnal hemoglobinuria (PNH):** lack of decay-accelerating factor (DAF) CD55 and CD59; **venous thrombosis including thrombosis at unusual sites such as portal vein** which may ultimately occur in up to 40% of individuals with PNH.
19. Most TTP is acquired and caused by autoantibody inhibition of ADAMTS13 activity. Hereditary TTP caused by ADAMTS13 gene mutation is uncommon. **Hereditary TTP is present during childhood and pregnancy**. **Treatment**: plasma exchange.
20. Treatment for drug-induced TMA: drug discontinuation and supportive care for DITMA; If confidence of DITMA is high, **plasma exchange or anti-complement therapy** (only for rapid kidney worsening) is not necessary.
21. **Treatment for acquired TTP**: response (normalization of PLT), remission (30 days after stopping plasma exchange), exacerbation versus relapses.
22. **Plasma exchange** is recommended for all patients with a presumptive diagnosis of TTP. **Steroids and rituximab** in addition to plasma exchange may be given to all patients with a presumptive TTP. May give **anti-vWF antibody caplacizumab**, especially if severe disease (caplacizumab and **IV solumedrol 1 g qd for 3 days** → switch if improving to prednisone 1 mg/kg/day oral or solumedrol 125 mg bid for 3 days).
23. Thrombocytopenia is not protective against thrombosis. **Venous thromboembolism (VTE) prophylaxis may be needed in certain patients and treatment of thrombosis (venous or arterial)** should not be withheld if indicated.
24. Treatment for acquired TTP: **steroids, caplacizumab, FFP, or plasmapheresis.**
25. After acute phase TTP: monitor for clinical signs of relapse; monitor ADAMTS13 activity (should improve from <10%)
26. A finding of **drug-dependent Ab together with absence of severe ADAMTS13 deficiency** is supportive of DITMA.

4/21/2019

1. **Abdominal distension** → bowel obstruction → check lactic acid and order nasogastric (NG) tube.
2. **Pneumothorax <3 cm usually does not need a chest tube**. It can be treated with high to medium-flow oxygen.

4/24/2019

1. **Subdural hematoma** evacuation (Borehole): labetalol 10 mg iv q15 min to maintain systolic blood pressure (sBP) < 160 mmHg. Keppra 500 mg bid po; Protonix 40 mg iv bid.
2. Concerns for hepatocellular carcinoma (HCC), MRI of the liver is diagnostic. Treatment: sorafenib + nivolumab.
3. **Pulmonary embolism EKG** presentation: S1Q3T3. **McConnell sign**: only the RV apex wall contracts while the rest of the right ventricular wall does not contract on echocardiogram; this can be seen with pulmonary embolism and may require **thrombolysis vs thrombectomy**.

4. **Sedation medications** in the intensive care unit: **avoid midazolam (Versed) in kidney deficiency, avoid dexmedetomidine (Precedex) in liver dysfunction, and avoid ketamine in either liver or kidney dysfunctions.**
5. Elevated **procalcitonin** can also be seen in **noninfectious conditions** like surgery, trauma, cardiogenic shock, multiorgan dysfunction, pancreatitis (severe), severe systemic inflammatory response syndrome (SIRS), and prolonged resuscitation. These conditions most often do not require antibiotics if there are no clinical signs or symptoms of infection.
6. **Acute respiratory distress syndrome (ARDS)**: no clinical evidence of an elevated left atrial pressure, pulmonary capillary wedge pressure $\leq$ 18. However, 20% of patients with ARDS have concomitant left ventricular dysfunction.

4/25/2019

1. **$PCO_2 < 30$ in subdural hematoma** may cause seizures. For intracranial hemorrhage (ICH) hemorrhage, we may need to **increase respiratory rate (RR)** transiently to **decrease edema**.
2. **Aortic murmur** radiates to the neck; **mitral regurgitation** murmur radiates to the left axilla. **Pulmonic murmur** is localized with no radiation.
3. tPA for stroke → hemorrhagic conversion. If **NIHSS > 20, the risk for hemorrhage is ≥17%**; hemorrhage (50% mortality) → check stat PT/PTT, PLT, fibrinogen, Type, and Cross, give **cryoprecipitate and platelet (PLT)** if confirmed with CT.

4/26/2019

1. **Metabolic alkalosis** from over diuresis; treatment: may give temporarily acetazolamide 250 mg bid.
2. **Ischemic stroke**: tPA → need MRI in 12 h and CT in 12 h to look for hemorrhagic conversion. If yes, do reversal, and consult neurology and neurosurgery.

4/28/2019

1. MRI compatible with chronic microvascular white matter change, episodes of left hemiparesis with facial drop in light of abnormal findings suspicious for **possible demyelinating disease**. Management includes order lumbar puncture (LP) with CSF analysis to look for markers of demyelinating disease such as **oligoclonal bands, IgG index, and IgG synthesis rate** (these are markers for inflammation of the central nervous system). Can give a trial of IV solumedrol 1 g per day for 3 days to facilitate quicker recovery if multiple sclerosis.

4/29/2019

1. Angiography → Transjugular intrahepatic portosystemic shunt (TIPS). Chest pain, may need to rule out **dissection.**
2. Pleural fluid can help diagnosis of malignancy; pleural biopsy can also help with the diagnosis of tuberculosis. If pleural fluid is **transudate** (like from congestive heart failure or liver failure), **diuretics** like Lasix may be helpful.
3. Random urine protein–to-creatinine ratio should be **<200 mg/g.**

4. Diagnosis of **hepatorenal**: presentation of acute kidney injury in patients with decompensated liver failure without other explanation for worsening kidney function besides liver failure. Treatments include **albumin, midodrine, and octreotide**.
5. Pneumothorax treatment: if unstable, call an interventional radiologist or surgeon STAT for a chest tube. If small, may resolve with supplementary oxygen treatment.

2 Back Being a Nocturnist

6/13/2019

1. Dyspnea in a patient status post abdominal aortic aneurysm (AAA) stent → SO_2 keeps dropping → consider **intubation**
2. In rapid response or urgent conditions, may need to **check troponin, lactic acid, arterial or venous blood gas, d-dimer, and EKG on top of routine labs**.
3. Sotalol initiation: needs to **do 6 doses in hospital, check EKG 2 h after each dose for QTc**, then discharge home on 80 mg bid.
4. The European Respiratory Society (ERS) and the American Thoracic Society (ATS) recommend **mucolytic (N-acetylcysteine)**, **long-acting muscarinic antagonist inhalers**, **phosphodiesterase-4 inhibitor (roflumilast)** and **macrolide therapy [Azithromycin (250 mg/d or 500 mg 3 times per week) or erythromycin (500 mg 2 times per day]**, as well as a conditional recommendation against fluoroquinolone therapy for prevention of chronic obstructive lung disease (COPD) exacerbations.

6/14/2019

1. Conversion from Toujeo to Lantus, the same dose; but a higher daily Toujeo may be needed.
2. **Torsade de pointes** risk in patients on sotalol is 2%.
3. Per epidemiology, **20% of patients with COPD** are non-smokers.
4. Nonspecific ST-T wave changes with significant troponin elevation may be diagnosed as NSTEMI; it may not be a good idea to give Brilinta/Plavix as it can be a **multivessel disease**.
5. A **wide QRS complex** (LBBB, RBBB, WPW, and nonspecific intraventricular conduction) on an EKG may give the appearance that the QT interval is prolonged. However, a wider QRS complex represents **depolarization** in these conditions; whereas long QT syndrome is a disorder of repolarization (**J point**) in wide QRS complex cases. J point refers to the end of depolarization (QRS) and the start of repolarization (ST portion). **JTc = QTc – QRS duration**.
6. Sotalol is better for the lung than metoprolol than Coreg in reactive airway disease.

7. **Wolf-Parkinson-White** (WPW) syndrome: delta wave indicates that the accessory pathway conducts faster than the atrioventricular (AV) node, thus resulting in **pre-excitation**. Characteristics: **short PR interval, delta wave with wide QRS**.
8. **WPW**: bundle of kent can communicate between: (1) **Left atrium and left ventricle**—Type A pre-excitation pattern reacting in a positive R wave and delta wave in V1. Tall R wave and inverted T waves in **V1 through V3** mimic right ventricular hypertrophy; aVL has a negative delta wave mimicking q wave. (2) **Right atrium and right ventricle**—Type B preexcitation and results in a negative delta in V1; tall R and inverted T waves in **V2 through V6** mimicking left ventricular hypertrophy (LVH); pseudo-infarct in III and AVF.
9. **Atrioventricular (AV) reentry tachycardia (AVRT)** in WPW when the accessory pathway has a refractory period longer than the AV node.
10. AVRT is a type of SVT, often triggered by a premature atrial contraction (PAC). A reentry circuit forms using the AV node (AVN) and the accessory pathway. The impulse from atrium → AVN → His Purkinje system results in a **narrow QRS (narrow complex tachycardia AVRT = orthodromic conduction)**. Then the impulse travels up the accessory pathway in a retrograde manner, creating a reentry circuit into the AVN. **Rate 200–300 often with T wave inversion and ST wave depression = orthodromic conduction**. **Wide complex tachycardia AVRT**: in 5% WPW, the impulses pass down the accessory pathway in an antegrade fashion. The impulses arise in the ventricular myocardium; however, they propagate less rapidly than if conducted via the His-Purkinje system, resulting in a wide QRS, then moving retrogradely via AVN creating a circus movement = antidromic.
11. Differential diagnoses (DDx) for **wide irregular tachycardia**: WPW with AFib; polymorphic VTach; AFIb with interventricular delay; Aflutter with WPW.
12. WPW treatment (Rx): no adenosine, amiodarone, digoxin, or Cardizem, but **only with procainamide or ibutilide; cardioversion is the best option for treatment.**

6/20/2019

1. Tikosyn (dofetilide) 250 mg bid, 2 h EKG after dosing, reduced LVEF; **left ventricular assistive device may be used for bridging to transplantation**.
2. **Types of atrial fibrillation**: paroxysmal <7 days; persistent >7 days; long standing persistent >12 m; permanent is continuous AFib after cardiac ablation.

6/28/2019

1. History (Hx) of paroxysmal atrial fibrillation (PAF), status post maze/Afib ablation procedure with mitral valve (MV) repair → developed Aflutter → transesophageal echocardiogram (TEE). Treatment options include antiarrhythmic therapy with Multaq (dronedarone 400 mg bid), sotalol, and Tikosyn (dofetilide) versus ablation. We agreed to proceed with antiarrhythmic therapy with dronedarone. If she has a recurrence of atypical Aflutter, will consider ablation. She is now status post TEE with DCCV and restoration of sinus rhythm with

good rate control. **Need to be on anticoagulation 1 night before and 2 months after cardioversion with Eliquis at minimum**.

2. Screening for **coronary artery disease** before starting Class Ic (flecainide and propafenone) antiarrhythmics.
3. Rarely uses Tikosyn (dofetilide) for paroxysmal AFib and infrequently uses dronedarone for persistent AFib due to reduced efficacy compared with amiodarone.
4. For **vagally** mediated AFib (characterized by AFib with atrioventricular block, asystolic periods, sinus bradycardia and an increase in heart rate variability), use **disopyramide**. If not tolerated, use flecainide or amiodarone.
5. For **adrenergically** mediated AFib (e.g., during exercise or other activity), use **beta blockers** as 1st line followed by sotalol and amiodarone.
6. In patients **without structural heart disease** (may have hypertension) and no left ventricular hypertrophy, use **flecainide or propafenone**.
7. **Structural heart disease**, prefer to use **sotalol, amiodarone, or dofetilide** (all are 1st line therapies)
8. **For coronary artery disease (CAD) without heart failure, use sotalol, dronedarone**, dofetilide, or amino (all are 1st line therapies). Ic is contraindicated in CAD.
9. Heart failure: **amiodarone and dofetilide** are used in AFib with concomitant congestive heart failure with reduced ejection fraction (CHFrEF) < 35%.
10. Patients with significant **left ventricular hyperplasia (LVH) with wall thickness >1.4 cm** due to HTN, hypertrophic cardiomyopathy, or aortic stenosis, have underlying subendocardial ischemia and electrophysiologic abnormalities, **dronedarone** can be used. **Sotalol, flecainide, and propafenone may cause significant arrhythmia in LVH.**
11. Drug resistant AFib: rate control or surgery (**Maze operation**) **or catheter ablation** such as pulmonary vein ablation preferred.
12. Inpatient initiation with **continuous telemetry of high-risk drugs such as dofetilide and sotalol** is done in 3 days.
13. Type Ic drugs, **QRS widening should not be permitted to exceed 150% of baseline QRS duration**. May use exercise testing.
14. For Type Ia and III except amiodarone anti-arrhythmics, the **corrected QT interval in sinus rhythm should be no longer than 520 ms**.
15. The presence of chronic kidney disease (CKD) warrants dose reductions or cessation of **sotalol and dofetilide**. In liver dysfunction, adjust the amiodarone dosage.
16. Patients with severe heart failure (NYHA III or IV CHF or those who have been hospitalized with heart failure in the previous 4 weeks) or those with left ventricular ejection fraction (LVEF) < 35% **should not receive dronedarone**.
17. For AFib >48 h or duration unknown, a **minimum 3 consecutive weeks of anticoagulation** (AC) before cardioversion for symptomatic patients in whom there is a strong preference to not delay cardioversion or in whom there is a concern about bleeding with prolonged oral AC, do TEE and therapeutic anticoagulation throughout peri-cardioversion period. After cardioversion, the

patient will need oral **AC for 4 weeks; and 6–48 h before cardioversion**, start anticoagulation if CHA2DSc-VASc ≥1.

18. AFib with rapid ventricular rate (RVR): beta-blocker → digoxin if congestive heart failure (CHF) or systolic dysfunction; may also use calcium channel blocker (CCB) diltiazem if no systolic CHF. Amiodarone can be used for short term.
19. After cardioversion for patients with AFib but no structural heart disease, use flecainide or propafenone to maintain sinus rhythm after cardioversion. If **structural heart disease, use amiodarone, sotalol or dofetilide.**

Takeaway Messages

1. Thyroid storm treatment example: Cholestyramine (Questran) light 4 g q6h, hydrocortisone (Solu-Cortef) 100 mg iv q8h, propranolol 60 mg po q6h, Propylthiouracil (PTU) 200 mg q4h (preferred over methimazole 20 mg q4h), Lugol's solution (potassium iodine) 5 drops po q6h via Wolff–Chaikoff effect.
2. Plasmapheresis adverse events: central venous catheter-associated hemorrhage, infections, or thrombi, and plasma-associated transfusion reactions.
3. Differentials for MAHA: TTP, HUS, PNH, DIC, HELLP, systemic metastatic cancer-associated TMA, systemic infections, drug-induced/complement-mediated/metabolism-mediated TMA.
4. Treatment for acquired TTP: steroids (hydrocortisone 100 mg iv q8h or solumedrol 1 g daily × 3 days or Prednisone 1 mg/kg daily), caplacizumab, FFP or plasmapheresis.
5. Avoid midazolam (Versed) in kidney deficiency, avoid dexmedetomidine (Precedex) in liver dysfunction, and avoid ketamine in either liver or kidney dysfunctions.
6. In rapid response or urgent conditions, may need to check troponin, lactic acid, arterial or venous blood gas, d-dimer, and EKG on top of routine labs.

Further Readings and References

1. George, J.N., and C.M. Nester. *Diagnostic approach to suspected TTP, HUS, or other thrombotic microangiopathy (TMA)*, ed. M. Crowther. Waltham, MA: UpToDate. Accessed January 24, 2024.
2. Ers, Wedzicha J.A., Miravitlles M. Co-Chair, J.R. Hurst, et al. 2017. Management of COPD exacerbations: A European Respiratory Society/American Thoracic Society guideline. *European Respiratory Journal* 49 (3): 1600791.
3. Buttner, R., and E. Burns. 2022. Pre-excitation syndromes. In *Life in the Fast Lane*. https://litfl.com/pre-excitation-syndromes-ecg-library/. Accessed January 24, 2024.

4. Buttner, R. 2022. Atrioventricular re-entry tachycardia (AVRT). In *Life in the Fast Lane*. https://litfl.com/atrioventricular-re-entry-tachycardia-avrt/?_thumbnail_id=189428. Accessed January 24, 2024.
5. Kumar, K. *Antiarrhythmic drugs to maintain sinus rhythm in patients with atrial fibrillation: Recommendations*, ed. P.J. Zimetbaum and B.P. Knight. Waltham, MA: UpToDate. Accessed January 24, 2024.

Chapter 13
The Last Year of Residency Training

July 1st, 2019 Through June 30th, 2020

The three-year-long residency training prepares an internal medicine resident to be successful in his/her future career as an internist. The career path after residency graduation consists of primary care service and hospital medicine on top of subspecialty fellowship training. The last year of internal medicine residency is the last chance before graduation for a doctor-in-training to get supervision and guidance from experienced physicians before becoming an independent practicing attending physician. The learning experiences at this time were more like the summary of knowledge and skills learned during residency training. The 3rd year residency training targeted at honing and refining skills and knowledge in patient care for the job as a primary care physician, hospitalist, or soon-to-be fellow in subspecialty training.

The last year of residency training can be likened to the final touches on a painting on a blank canvas. Just as an artist adds depth, detail, and refinement to their canvas to bring their vision to life, the last year of residency is a time for physicians-in-training to add the finishing touches to their medical training before transitioning to independent practice. Throughout residency training, we gradually layer on experiences, learning from each patient encounter, procedure, and clinical decision. These layers represent the accumulation of knowledge, skills, and clinical experiences over time. By the last year of residency, the canvas is nearly complete, with the outlines of a well-rounded physician beginning to take shape. Like a skilled artist putting the final strokes on their masterpiece, residents use this final year to refine their skills, polish their clinical judgment, and perfect their bedside manner.

Ultimately, the goal of the last year of residency is to produce a work of art—a competent, compassionate, and capable physician ready to embark on their professional journey. Like a finished painting that reflects the artist's dedication and skills, a resident physician completing their training emerges as a fully-formed clinician, equipped with the knowledge, experience, and confidence to provide excellent patient care and make meaningful contributions to the field of medicine. When I

K. Zhou, *Internal Medicine Training Notes and Survival Guide*,
https://doi.org/10.1007/978-1-0716-4039-5_13

ponder the traits of the excellent role model physicians that I have encountered or heard about, I find that they are usually highly motivated, engaged, committed, empathic, compassionate, and enthusiastic about patient care. Additionally, they are also humble, flexible, and have a sense of humor.

Topics covered in this section included Parkinson's disease, seizures, multiple sclerosis, neuromyelitis optica, ischemic stroke, ASPECTS score, immune thrombocytopenic purpura (ITP), acute GI bleed workup and management, serotonin syndrome, neuroleptic malignant syndrome, retina abnormalities. This section also included notes during an infectious disease rotation which included topics of infectious diseases in renal transplants, rapidly growing mycobacterium, vaccination for urgent splenectomy, SPICE-producing bacteria, and G+ rods. Additionally, I also had a rotation at the palliative care department at a National Cancer Institute-designated cancer center. Notes of palliative care medicine covered topics of malignant bowel obstruction, blast syndrome, and differentiation syndrome, carcinomatous meningitis.

7/3/2019

1. **Allergic rhinitis** treatment: Flonase and Claritin (or cetirizine).
2. **Otitis externa**: Ciprodex (Ciprofloxacin/Dexamethasone), or neomycin-polymyxin ear drops. May need to add oral Levaquin in some patients.

7/4/2019

1. Oral **sodium-glucose co-transporter-2** (SGLT-2) inhibitors: Farxiga (dapagliflozin) Steglatro (ertugliflozin), Invokana (canagliflozin), Jardiance (empagliflozin)
2. **Dipeptidyl peptidase 4** (DPP4) inhibitors: Trajenta (linagliptin), Januvia (sitagliptin), Onlyza (saxagliptin))
3. **Sulfonylureas**: glipizide, glimepiride, glyburide.
4. **GLP-1 agonist**: Victoza (liraglutide), Trulicity (dulaglutide), Bydureon (exenatide), Ozempic (semaglutide).

8/4/2019

1. **Prophylactic acyclovir** is recommended for Velcade (bortezomib), a 26S proteasome inhibitor, for multiple myeloma (MM).
2. **Colovesical fistula** should be treated with surgery consult and Foley catheter. **Fournier's gangrene** = necrotizing fasciitis of the genital and peritoneum.
3. **Trach removal** depends on trach secretion, swallowing, and O_2 requirement. Respiratory therapists and pulmonologists are usually handling this. Decrease the size of the trach and then ENT consult for decannulation.
4. The most common causes of **acute scrotal pain** are acute **epididymitis** and **testicular torsion**. Testicular ultrasound can help with diagnosis.
5. **Empiric antibiotics for epididymitis**: ceftriaxone 500 mg im once plus doxycycline 100 mg bid for 10 days (alternative is azithromycin 1 g once, not fluoroquinolones if gonorrhea as **gonorrhea resistance to fluoroquinolones is common**). If low risk for sexually transmitted disease, can be treated with

Levaquin 500 mg daily for 10 days or ofloxacin 300 mg bid for 10 days or DS Bactrim for 10 days.

8/20/2019

1. Status post (Sp) abdominal aortic aneurysm (AAA) rupture repair transfer to intensive care unit (ICU) medication treatments: cefazolin 1 g q8h for 2 doses right after surgery; heparin 5000 q8h, Dilaudid, Zofran, NS at 150 cc/h, nothing per mouth (NPO) or except ice chips, nasogastric tube (NG) tube to wall suction, no feed or oral med unless essential.
2. **Massive transfusion (6 units of PRBC or more)** of blood products like red blood cells (RBC), plasma for clotting factors, and platelet (PLT) should be given **1:1:1** ratio, especially for trauma patients.
3. In adults, each 10–12u of transfused RBC is associated with a 50% drop in platelet count; thus, significant thrombocytopenia can be seen after 10–20u of RBC with platelet <50,000. For replacement in this setting, 6u of whole blood derived platelet (a pooled unit of platelets) or one apheresis platelet concentrate should be given, **1u increases serum platelet by 20,000–40,000/μl.**

9/2/2019

1. **Orlistat (Xenical), phentermine/topiramate (Qsymia), naltrexone/bupropion**, and nowadays **GLP-1 agonists** for weight loss, long term use. **Lisdexamfetamine** (Vyvanse) is used for attention deficit hyperactivity disorder (ADHD) and binge eating disorder.
2. **Bariatric surgeries**: Roux-en-Y gastric bypass, sleeve gastrectomy, adjustable gastric bands. After surgery, patients are encouraged to consume at least 60–80 g of protein daily.
3. **Routine supplement after bariatric surgery**: Vit A 5000–10,000 u qd; Vit B1 12–50 mg daily, Vit B9 (folate) 400–800 mg qd; B12 sublingual 500 μg daily or parental 1000 μg qmonth; D3 3000IU qd, VitE 15 mg qd, vit K 90–120 mg, calcium 500–600 mg tid; iron 18 mg qd, 40–60 mg qd for absorption concerns; zinc and copper 100%–200% recommended dietary allowance (RDA).
4. **Weight maintenance strategies after weight loss**: high level of physical activity 60 min qd; low-fat, low-calorie diet; self-monitoring weight; constant eating pattern across the week.
5. **Brief counseling** has been shown to reduce unhealthy alcohol use for up to 4 years.
6. **Pharmacology therapy for sobriety maintenance**: disulfiram, naltrexone, acamprosate, topiramate, and gabapentin.
7. For patients with three or more revised cardiac risk index factors, we need to **initiate perioperative beta blockers.**

9/5/2019

1. **Noninvasive imaging ultrasound** to rule out abdominal aortic aneurysm: especially important in known atherosclerotic diseases, including peripheral arterial disease (PAD), coronary artery disease (CAD), cerebral vascular accident

(CVA), and abdominal bruit. A rise in serum creatinine after initiation of ACEi or ARB, or at the onset of hypertension at a young age could represent **fibromuscular dysplasia**.

2. **Primary aldosteronism**: unilateral aldosterone-producing adenomas; bilateral idiopathic hyperaldosteronism (IHA: bilateral adrenal hyperplasia).
3. **Diagnosis of primary aldosteronism**: check plasma aldosterone concentration (PAC >10 dg/mL) and plasma renin activity (PRA < 1 mg/mL) or plasma renin concentration (PRC) ⇒ diagnosis confirmed. **Aldosterone suppression testing**: orally administered NaCl and measurement of urine aldosterone excretion or with IV NaCl loading and measurement of PAC. Confirmation testing not necessary for: spontaneous hypokalemia, undetectable PRC or PRA, or PAC ≥20 ng/mL
4. **Mineralocorticoid receptor antagonists** spironolactone and eplerenone can interfere with the results of primary aldosteronism labs, but not ACEi and ARB.
5. **Secondary hyperaldosteronism**: diuretic therapy, renovascular or malignant hypertension (HTN), Cushing syndrome, certain forms of congenital adrenal hyperplasia, Liddle syndrome, and rare renin-secreting tumors, non-aldosteronism-mineralocorticoid excess.
6. **Adrenal CT** is needed to determine the subtype (adenoma versus hyperplasia) and exclude adrenal carcinoma.
7. ≥35 years old, would recommend **adrenal vein sampling** to confirm unilateral disease if the patient would like to pursue surgical management of their primary aldosteronism.
8. Indications for **renovascular hypertension**: progressive decline in renal function; recurrent episodes of flash pulmonary edema; uncontrolled hypertension. **Diagnosis**: duplex Doppler US, CTA, MRA. The gold standard is **renal arteriography**.

9/30/2019

1. **Baclofen** can cause withdrawal if discontinued suddenly.
2. **Daptomycin use** should check CPK weekly.
3. **Keppra check does not need to be in the therapeutic range as the range is broad and can be different for different patients/diseases**.
4. **Bloody diarrhea** with antibiotics may indicate **hemolytic uremic syndrome (HUS) with microangiopathic hemolytic anemia, thrombocytopenia, and acute kidney injury**. Antibiotics increase risks for full-blown **HUS from Shiga toxin–producing Escherichia coli (STEC)** leading to death; thus, no antibiotic if diarrhea by E coli.
5. Dialysis patients with endometrial bleeding can be treated with **megestrol 5 mg q8h**.
6. Bleeding vagina is common in ESRD on hemodialysis (HD), Treatment: **megestrol 40 mg qd.**
7. **Siponimod** (**Mayzent**) is a sphingosine-1-phosphate receptor modulator. Used in multiple sclerosis (MS) and can cause **headaches** (HA). Copaxone = **glat-**

iramer acetate is an immunomodulator used in MS; glatiramer acetate decreases the frequency of relapses, but not the progression of disability.

Neurology Service

10/1/2019 Neuromyelitis Optica Spectrum Disorders (NMOSD)

1. NMOSD also known as **neuromyelitis optica** (NMO) is an inflammatory disorder of the central nervous system (CNS) characterized by severe immune-mediated demyelination and axonal damage predominantly targeting optic nerves and the spinal cord. **Necrosis and cavitation** involve both gray and white matter.
2. **Neuromyelitis optica** (NMO) has a disease-specific serum **NMO-IgG Ab binds to aquaporin 4 (AQP4)**. NMO is mediated by the humoral immune system.
3. **Hallmark features** of NMO include **bilateral or rapidly optic neuritis** leading to severe visual loss together with **transverse myelitis** (limb weakness, sensory loss, and bladder dysfunction). Other suggestive symptoms include intractable nausea, vomiting, hiccups, excessive daytime somnolence or narcolepsy, reversible posterior leukoencephalopathy syndrome, neuroendocrine disorders, and (in children) seizures.
4. **Treatment of neuromyelitis optica**: solumedrol 1 g qd × 5 day → plasmapheresis → eculizumab.

10/6/2019

1. **Parkinson's disease (PD)**: change frequency and dosage of sinemet (Carbidopa/Levodopa) from dosing at 7, 12, 5 to dosing at 7, 11, 3, 7 for better symptom control. Comtan = entacapone, Tasmar = tolcapone, and both are catechol-O-methyltransferase (COMT) inhibitors. Rasagiline = monoamine oxidase-B (MAO-B) inhibitor.
2. **Apomorphine** is a fast-acting subcutaneous dopamine agonist for rapid relief of symptoms caused by sudden wearing off of a Parkinson's medication; **droxidopa** for orthostatic hypotension in PD.
3. Current dopamine agonists used for Parkinson's disease (PD) and restless leg syndrome (RLS) include **pramipexole, ropinirole, and rotigotine (Neupro)**; injectable **apomorphine** is also a dopamine agonist.
4. No seizure for 2 years, may stop seizure meds.
5. MRI susceptibility-weighted imaging **(SWI) is used for bleeding**. Diffusion-weighted imaging (DWI) is used for **acute anemia (stroke) in 4wks**. MRI Flair = T2 − (ventricle + sulci).
6. MRI with/without contrast brain, MRA with and without contrast neck, MRA without contrast brain for **brain vascular disorders**.

10/7/2019

1. Psychogenic nonepileptic spells/events (PNES).
2. **Thunderclap headache (HA)** is characteristic of reversible cerebral vasoconstriction syndrome (**RCVS**). Diagnosis: MRI or CT angiography. Treatment:

verapamil and nimodipine. Predisposing factors: triptans, cocaine, and cannabinoids.

3. Dystonic tremor, cerebellar tremor, essential tremor, parkinsonian tremor, rubral tremor.
4. **Rubral tremor**: focal injury to cerebellar outflow pathways and is characterized by a coarse tremor that is present at rest but most severe during action. Prominent proximal components.
5. **Convulsive status epilepticus** is defined as persistent tonic-clonic activity with impaired mental status lasting longer than 5 min or recurrent seizures without recovery between seizures. **Treatment**: IM midazolam, IV lorazepam, IV diazepam → phenytoin and valproic acid.
6. **Anti-NMDA receptor encephalitis**: fever, headache, feeling tired, psychosis, hallucinations, and delusions. It is associated with ovarian cancer. **Diagnosis**: serum antibody positive.
7. **Paraneoplastic syndrome** with anti-Hu, anti-LGI1, anti-CV2/collapsin response mediator protein (CRMP)5 and other serum markers can be seen in autoimmune encephalitis (generalized cortical hyperexcitability and subclinical seizures).
8. Metoprolol, propranolol, timolol, Divalproex, and topiramate are used for migraine with a frequency of **≥5 days per month**.
9. **Chronic migraine** is defined as headache ≥15 days/month, with at least 8 days meeting full criteria for migraine or responding to migraine specific medications.
10. Child-bearing potential women, **levetiracetam and lamotrigine** are the most appropriate treatments for seizure → consider discontinuing oral contraceptive (OCP), start **folic acid**, and taper off valproic acid. **Juvenile myoclonic epilepsy requires long-term treatment**.
11. **POEMS syndrome (polyneuropathy, organomegaly, endocrinopathy, monoclonal gammopathy, and skin changes)**.
12. The classic presentation of chronic inflammatory demyelinating polyradiculoneuropathy (**CIDP**) is **generalized areflexia and progressive or relapsing symmetric sensory and motor neuropathy**. Acute inflammatory demyelinating polyradiculoneuropathy (AIDP) = Guillain-Barré syndrome (GBS).
13. **Obsessive-compulsive disorder (OCD), Tourette syndrome**: first line agents used to treat Tourette syndrome when the associated tics interfere with education, daily function, or work are **clonidine, guanfacine, topiramate, and tetrabenazine**.
14. **Convulsive syncope** is a seizure-type syncope typically associated with tunnel vision, palpitations, short duration of loss of consciousness (<1 min), movements, and shaking, and immediate and complete neurologic recovery right after waking up. **Convulsive syncope = tonic and myoclonic phenomena during syncope without epileptic EEG activity**. Treatment is similar to other types of syncope based on etiology and seizure medications have no role in its treatment.
15. **Myoclonic seizures**: brief <1 min, limb jerking, all limbs.

16. In multiple sclerosis (MS) with liver disease, **glatiramer acetate is preferred to interferon (IFN) and fingolimod.**
17. **Granulomatosis with polyangiitis** (Wegner, C-ANCA, anti-proteinase 3) causes mononeuropathy multiplex.
18. Diagnostic angiography is not routinely indicated to confirm the degree of stenosis before carotid revascularization. **After CT head and neck angiography, it may be necessary to order carotid Doppler.**
19. **Failing two anti-epileptic drugs (AEDs), this patient should be referred to an epilepsy center for video EEG, and may be a candidate for epilepsy surgery**.
20. All the **synucleinopathy** is caused by abnormal accumulation of aggregates of **alpha-synuclein protein** in neurons, nerve fibers, or glial cells. There **are three main types of synucleinopathy**: Parkinson's disease (PD), dementia with Lewy bodies (DLB), and multiple system atrophy (MSA). They all have a much higher rate of **rapid eye movement (REM) sleep behavior disorder.**

10/8/2019

1. Commonly used treatments for **essential tremor (ET)**: propranolol 40 mg bid to 320 qd, primidone (Mysoline) 50–75 qd. **Next line of treatment**: gabapentin, topiramate, nimodipine, or combining propranolol with primidone.
1. **Tremor differential diagnoses**: essential, cerebellar, Parkinson's, dystonia, rubral (one type of cerebellar tremor with large amplitude during activities). **Three major types of tremors**: (1) cerebellar tremor (large amplitude), Parkinson's disease (small resting tremor), (2) medication-induced tremors, and (3) essential tremor (happens with movements).
2. 62 yo F was diagnosed with multiple sclerosis (MS) in 1992, was taking daily copaxone (glatiramer acetate) till 2013, was put on Mayzent (siponimod, a sphingosine-1-phosphate R modulator), then developed seizure 3 weeks later ⇒ consider stop Mayzent, start Keppra 500 mg bid, may taper off Keppra in a few weeks.
3. Discharge instructions for **patients with seizure**: no driving, operating machinery, unprotected heights, swimming alone, contact sports, or other potentially hazardous activity till cleared by neurology in the future, and no missing medication or sleep.
4. For **relapsing-remitting MS**, use im INF-alpha, subcu INF 1alpha/1beta, subcu glatiramer acetate, IV natalizumab, IV ocrelizumab, or po teriflunomide (Aubagio) /siponimod (Mayzent) /fingolimod (Gilenya).
5. **Primary progressive MS** treatment: ocrelizumab (Xolair). Secondary progressive MS Treatment: siponimod, or cladribine (Mavenclad).
6. **Attacks/exacerbations of MS** are defined as episodes of focal neurologic disturbances lasting >24 h with a preceding period of clinical stability of at least 30 days and without an alternate explanation such as infection or fever.
7. **Concerned about MS exacerbation:** consider MRI brain and spine to look for new lesions.

8. **Treatment (Rx) of MS exacerbation**: solumedrol 500–1000 mg qd (1 g for 5 days) with or without prednisone taper. **Plasma exchange** may be beneficial for acute central nervous system (CNS) inflammatory demyelinating disease that does not respond to glucocorticoid steroids.
9. **Uhthoff phenomenon**: a small increase in body temperature worsens MS symptoms.
10. **Syncope differential** diagnoses (DDx): transient ischemic attack (TIA), seizure, ventricular fibrillation (VFib), orthostatic; check TSH, B12, and T4.

10/9/2019

1. 35-year-old lawyer presented with headache and dizziness: **MRI with contrast** to rule out focal pathology; **MRA head** without contrast to rule out stenosis or aneurysm. **MRA neck** to rule out stenosis or dissection.
2. Epilepsy with breakthrough seizure: alcohol withdrawal seizures; management: MRI brain to rule out acute pathology, possible EEG. **Seizure medications are generally not recommended in alcohol withdrawal seizures.**

10/10/2019

1. Dilantin also known as **phenytoin** is a P450 **inducer**; Depakote also known **as valproic acid** is a P450 **inhibitor**.
2. Passing out differentials: syncope, transient ischemic attack (TIA), seizure, Vasovagal, vasomotor.
3. **M1 lesion** → define it with CTA or MRA. In stroke patients, if symptoms onset <24 h, it is an indication for thrombectomy.
4. Group home resident with developmental delay presented with syncopal event-induced seizure: not on antiepileptic drug (AED), do EEG → abnormal EEG → start **Trileptal (Oxcarbazepine) 150 mg bid.**
5. **Altered mental status (AMS) differentials:** metabolic vs. toxic encephalopathy vs. disease progression from traumatic brain injury (TBI) vs. seizure vs. stroke. Workups: EEG abnormal → consider increasing Keppra, MRI flair and diffusion, EEG, may need lumbar puncture, review medical records to rule out medication side effects.
6. **Status epilepticus**: home medications include Depakote 750 mg tid, lacosamide (Vimpat) 200 mg bid, and Dilantin 200 mg bid. STAT Treatment: Ativan 2 mg, **Depakote (Sodium valproate)** 1 g IV stat → continuous EEG shows periodic lateralized epileptiform discharge (PLED) → increase Depakote to 500 mg tid, continue lacosamide 200 mg bid, Dilantin (Phenytoin) 200 mg bid. After STAT load **fosphenytoin 500 mg** IV × 1, still, frequent PLED, treatment: **Keppra 1 g IV** stat followed by 500 mg iv bid, continue Depakote 500 tid, change phenytoin 200 mg bid to fosphenytoin 200 mg iv q12h, continue Vimpat 200 mg iv bid, give **fosphenytoin 1 g IV stat →** still frequent left temporal spikes → increase Keppra to 1 g bid IV, keep fosphenytoin 200 mg q12h iv, Vimpat 200 iv bid → Depakote later was discontinued, give additional fosphenytoin 500 mg × 1 IV.

7. A 71-year-old female with **anxiety disorder** presented to the ER for "numbness to her tongue (tongue biting and bleeding) that started about 1.5 h prior to arrival when she woke up. Patient states she also was not able to move her arms or legs well and they ached." She does seem to have some **histrionic** tendencies. The neurologist commented, "Given her behavioral health history I would recommend **divalproex (Sodium valproate)** rather than levetiracetam." The patient was thus discharged on divalproex (24-h) 500 mg tablet daily.

10/11/2019

1. **Paraproteinemia neuropathy** can present with symptomatic distal sensory neuropathy or as sensorimotor multifocal motor or cranial neuropathies.
2. **Idiopathic intracranial hypertension (CSF opening pressure ≥ 25 mm H_2O)**: headache, vision changes, intracranial
3. **Amitriptyline** can be used for the prevention of chronic tension-type headaches (HA).
4. All patients on **chronic antiepileptic drugs** (AEDs) with phenytoin, carbamazepine, phenobarbital, or valproic acid should undergo **an initial DEXA scan after 5 years of therapy**. If osteoporosis, **change AED to Lamictal or Keppra**.
5. **Primary stabbing pain**: transient localized stabs, no organic disease, common in **migrainers**, usually lasting seconds.
6. **Hemicrania continua**: continuous, occasional stabbing pain with ipsilateral autonomic features.

10/12/2019

1. Only a few antiepileptic drugs (AEDs) including **lamotrigine, levetiracetam, topiramate, valproic acid, and zonisamide** are considered broad-spectrum agents and can be used to treat both generalized and partial epilepsy syndromes. Other narrow-spectrum AEDs including carbamazepine, gabapentin, oxcarbazepine (Trileptal), phenobarbital, phenytoin, and pregabalin have the potential to exacerbate seizures in generalized epilepsy.
2. **Oxcarbazepine** causes hyponatremia; **phenytoin** causes dizziness, ataxia, tremors, peripheral neuropathy, cerebellar atrophy, and agranulocytosis.
3. **Kidney stones and cognitive impairment can be exacerbated by topiramate**.
4. **Valproic acid** can cause tremors, cognitive dysfunction including Parkinsonism-associated dementia in older persons, and thrombocytopenia.
5. **Keppra** can worsen depression, topiramate can cause or worsen psychosis, and Lamictal is good for women.
6. The combination of parkinsonism, cerebellar ataxia, dysautonomia, and early postural instability characterizes multisystem atrophy = **Parkinson's plus syndrome**.
7. Patients **with ischemic stroke and large vessel occlusion** have low recanalization with tPA (tPA still should be given if candidate) → need CT angiography to determine endovascular therapy candidacy.
8. For stable patients with small strokes, prior full anticoagulation is typically **resumed 24 h after hospitalization** to reduce hemorrhagic transformation

which happens more often in **larger infarcts (>1/3 brain) and with cardioembolic cause**.

9. **Intracranial hypotension headache**: orthostatic headache, MRI with contrast can show diffuse **nonnodular patchy meningeal enhancement** (diagnostic). Cerebellar tonsillar descent and insignificant bilateral subdural fluid collection are common in intracranial hypotension from CSF leaks; treatment is with an epidural blood patch, especially if a recent history of lumbar puncture → CT myelography.
10. **MRI brain** is needed for red flag headaches: **anticoagulation use, ≥50 yo, or progressive headache (HA) pattern**.
11. **Indomethacin** is the treatment for chronic paroxysmal hemicranias; **Lamictal** is the treatment for short-lasting unilateral neuralgiform headache attacks with conjunctival injection and tearing (**SUNCT**).
12. Signs and symptoms (S&S) of **transverse myelitis**: pain, motor and sensory loss, bowel and bladder dysfunction. Treatments for transverse myelitis: first line treatment is high dose steroid, **1 g solumedrol qd × 5 ⇒ plasma exchange**.
13. **Cognitive dysfunction** in multiple sclerosis (MS) needs cognitive rehab, not memantine, donepezil, or methylphenidate.
14. **Keppra, carbamazepine, and Lamictal are choices for seizure treatments in pregnancy**.

10/13/2019

1. **Valproic acid** toxicity causes side effects from mild drowsiness to coma or fatal cerebral edema → monitor vitals (respiratory depression, hypotension, tachycardia, hyperthermia), metabolic (hyperammonemia, metabolic acidosis, hyperosmolarity, hypernatremia, hypocalcemia), gastrointestinal (vomiting, diarrhea, and hepatitis), additional neurologic (miosis, agitation, tremors, myoclonus) symptoms.
2. **Focal seizure** treatment: Lamictal and/or Keppra. **Myoclonic seizures** treatment: Keppra and/or valproate.
3. Treatments for **generalized convulsive status epilepticus**: Ativan, Versed, meanwhile loading fosphenytoin 20 mg/kg or valproate 30 mg/kg, or Keppra 40–60 mg/kg max 4500 mg IV ⇒ continuous infusion of Versed, propofol or phenobarbital.
4. **Ketogenic dietary therapy** is a valid treatment option for patients who have failed at least 2 antiepileptic drugs (AEDs): the classic long-chain ketogenic diet; the median chain triglyceride (TG) diet; the modified Atkins diet; the low glycemic index diet.
5. For the treatment of **nonconvulsive status epilepticus (NCSE)**: lorazepam 0.1 mg/kg (max 4 mg at a time) combined with one of the following: fosphenytoin at 20 mg/kg, valproate 40 mg/kg, Keppra 2500 mg IV over 15 min, or lacosamide 400 mg over 15 min.

10/14/2019

1. **Basilar artery occlusion**, we can do stenting and ballooning, but most importantly, endovascular thrombectomy within 24 h of symptom onset reduces dis-

ability and mortality, particularly in patients with moderate-to-severe symptoms. However, thrombectomy in basilar artery occlusions is associated with procedural complications and more cerebral hemorrhages.
2. **Criteria for thrombectomy**: occlusion of the internal carotid artery (ICA) or M1 lesion of the middle cerebral artery, NIHSS ≥10, mismatch volume, and NIHSS ≥7.
3. **6%–13%** chance of hemorrhagic transformation after tPA; **3%** mortality after tPA.
4. **Symptomatic, midline shift, >0.5 ml bleeding in SAH**: neurosurgery may take the patient for evacuation.
5. **Exclusion criteria for tPA**: significant head trauma or prior stroke in the previous 3 m, subarachnoid hemorrhage (SAH), intracranial hemorrhage (ICH), arteriovenous malformations (AVM), aneurysm, internal bleed, platelet (PLT) < 100,000, INR > 1.7 or PT > 15, or anticoagulation (A/C) use.

10/15/2019

1. **Seizure** ≥ 2 episodes equals **epilepsy**. After first unprovoked seizure, 1/3 will have recurrent seizures in 5 years. Increased chance of recurrent seizure in epileptiform abnormalities on EEG, structural changes in brain MRI, remote symptomatic causes, abnormal neurological exam, and a first seizure during sleep.
2. **Types of seizure**: focal seizure with retained awareness (impaired awareness), generalized seizure (absence seizure also known as petit mal, clonic seizure, myoclonic seizure, tonic seizure, and atonic seizure)
3. **Differential diagnoses (DDx) for altered mental status (AMS):** infection including encephalitis and meningitis, seizure, stroke, metabolic (B12, TSH, ammonia), and drug side effects
4. **Diffusion-weighted imaging (DWI)** bright and apparent diffusion coefficient (ADC) black = consider **ischemia, seizure, and vasogenic**. MRI-based diffusion-weighted imaging (DWI)–fluid-attenuated inversion recovery (FLAIR) mismatch is defined as an ischemic lesion visible on DWI without parenchymal hyperintensity on FLAIR sequence indicating infarct **less than 4.5 h**.

10/23/2019

1. **Cecal bascule** is a large bowel obstruction folding of the cecum anteriorly over the ascending colon. It is one of the three types of cecal volvulus; the other two being **axial ileocolic volvulus** (a twisting or torsion of a portion of the cecum and a portion of the terminal ileum) and a **clockwise axial twisting** or torsion of the cecum along the long axis.
2. Cecal bascule can be complicated by **necrosis or organ dysfunction** before the diagnosis is made, particularly if the ileocecal valve is competent, preventing retrograde decompression of the cecum into the ileum.
3. **Air fluid level** = consider **bowel obstruction**.
4. Continue **Zemplar (paricalcitol)** 10 mg IV during dialysis prn for secondary **hyperparathyroidism** and **erythropoietin (EPO)** 4000 u IV during dialysis for anemia from chronic kidney disease.

5. Treatments for chronic kidney disease (CKD) on hemodialysis (HD): **lanthanum, paricalcitol, calcium, Vit D, epoetin**.
6. **Medication-induced pancreatitis** includes immunologic reactions (i.e, 6-mercaptopurine, aminosalicylates, sulfonamides), direct toxic effects (diuretics, sulfonamides), accumulation of toxic metabolites (i.e., valproic acid, didanosine, pentamidine, tetracycline), ischemia (i.e., diuretics, azathioprine), intravascular thrombosis (e.g., estrogen), and increased viscosity of pancreatic juice (diuretics and steroids)
7. **Diarrhea treatment**: diphenoxylate-atropine (Lomotil) slows GI motility, loperamide.
8. **Oxacillin side effects**: C. diff-associated diarrhea, liver function test (LFTs) abnormalities, acute interstitial nephritis, and acute tubular disease.
9. **Treatment for immune thrombocytopenic purpura** (ITP): **steroid** for 4 weeks → **IVIG** for 2–3 days; second line includes splenectomy, rituximab, ltrombopag (Promacta). Refractory ITP: romiplostim (**Nplate**), eltrombopag (**Promacta**), and autologous hematopoietic stem cell transplantation (HSCT).
10. **Side effects of eltrombopag (Promacta)**: rebound thrombocytopenia, increased LFTs, and venous thromboembolisms (VTEs).
11. Among patients with PTH persistently > **150–300 pg/mL** despite treatment of hyperphosphatemia and Vit D deficiency, will need to add **calcitriol** or **active Vit D analog** (paricalcitol and doxercalciferol). **Calcitriol** 0.25 mg tid, do not use **calcitriol** if serum phosphate is above the normal range or if the corrected serum total calcium concentration is above **9.5 mg/dL**.
12. Use **cinacalcet** if calcium ≥ 9.5 or P > 5.5 after treatment using lanthanum or sevelamer.

10/25/2019

1. Gastrointestinal (GI) bleed in a 47 yo with bright red blood per rectum (BRBPR): planning esophagogastroduodenoscopy (EGD) and colonoscopy, **2–4 L GoLYTELY (Polyethylene glycol) prep (can add one dose oral bisacodyl 10 mg),** results in negative bleed → CT angiogram abdomen/pelvis GI bleeding protocol → acute GI bleed loss imaging (**RBC tag scan**) → repeat colonoscopy (pan-diverticular disease and blood throughout colon, mostly sigmoid colon) → if further bleed, **CT angiogram GI bleed protocol** (acute bleed, large bleed) followed **by mesenteric angiogram for embolization**. Surgery: if further bleeding, repeat bleeding scan then partial resection vs. subtotal colectomy with colostomy.
2. GI bleed in an 87 yo bleeding through ostomy site: **EGD and enteroscopy → outpatient capsule endoscopy**. If bleeding acutely → acute GI bleeding scan after CT angiogram GI bleeding protocol.
3. Diagnostic studies of GI bleed: nasogastric tube, EGD, colonoscopy, push enteroscopy, anoscopy, capsule endoscopy, tagged RBC scan (>**0.04 cc/min**), CT angiogram (arteriography) (≥**0.5 cc/min**).
4. **Enteroscopy**: single balloon, double balloon, or spiral.

10/27/2019

1. **Liver failure workup, nonalcoholic steatohepatitis (NASH)** workup: autoimmune screen (anti-mitochondrial Ab, anti-smooth muscle Ab, ANA, antiphospholipid syndrome), alpha-1 antitrypsin level and phenotype, serum ceruloplasmin, fasting iron studies, hepatic vein Doppler and 2D echo (abdominal US to rule out portal vein thrombosis), US duplex abdomen/pelvis limited, and alpha-fetoprotein (AFP).
2. **Alcoholic hepatitis**: consider steroids if Maddrey's Discriminant Function (MDF) score ≥ **32**. Treatment: **methylprednisolone 32 mg qd iv or prednisolone 40 mg qd oral for 4 weeks with 4–6 weeks taper**. **Contraindicated** in active gastrointestinal bleeding (GIB), pancreatitis, untreated HBV, and uncontrolled infections. **Pentoxifylline** can be considered as an alternative to steroids if prednisolone cannot be used.
3. **Medications that can't be crushed** to fit percutaneous endoscopic gastrostomy (PEG): Cardizem CR (switch to short-acting), pantoprazole (switch to lansoprazole or esomeprazole), tamsulosin (switch to doxazosin).
4. Large volume paracentesis: order IV **albumin 6–8 g of albumin/L** of fluid removed when above **5 L of ascites** removal.
5. Primary prophylaxis with a **nonselective beta blocker (NSBB) or endoscopic band ligation** should be initiated upon detection of high-risk varies (i.e, small varices) with red signs, medium or large varices irrespective of Child-Pugh classification or small varices in Child-Pugh C patients.
6. In patients with progressive hypotension with **sBP < 90**, or in patients who develop an acute intercurrent condition such as **bleeding, sepsis, spontaneous bacterial peritonitis (SBP), or acute kidney injury (AKI)**, NSBB should be discontinued. After recovery, NSBB can be resumed. **If failed NSBB or intolerant to NSBB, do transjugular intrahepatic portosystemic shunt (TIPS)**.
7. **Libman-Sacks endocarditis**, also known as **verrucous marantic** or **nonbacterial thrombotic endocarditis**, is the most characteristic manifestation of the autoimmune disease systemic lupus erythematosus (SLE). Most commonly affects the mitral and aortic valves, but all four cardiac valves can be affected and so does the endocardial surfaces. **Malignancy and hypercoagulable state** are also associated with verrucous endocarditis, usually in patients with positive antiphospholipid Ab with impaired antithrombotic mechanisms. No specific treatment is indicated in these conditions.
8. Persons with Libman-Sacks endocarditis are usually asymptomatic. When symptomatic, usually presents with **cardiac failure, cerebrovascular embolism, and systemic thromboembolism**. **Secondary infective endocarditis** can also happen.
9. G+ rods: **bacillus, clostridium, Corynebacterium, Listeria, and Gardnerella**.
10. **Serotonin syndrome**: a combination of autonomic hyperactivity, hemodynamic changes, and neuromuscular (NM) derangements. **Treatment**: discontinuation of all serotoninergic agents, and supportive care to normalize vital

signs. **Sedation with benzodiazepines (BZDs), may give serotonin antagonists, like cyproheptadine.**

11. **Diagnosis of serotonin syndrome** requires a serotoninergic agent administration within the preceding 5 weeks together with one of the following symptoms: **muscle rigidity, temperature ≥ 38, ocular clonus or inducible clonus, ocular clonus plus agitation or diaphoresis, inducible clonus plus agitation or diaphoresis, spontaneous clonus, tremor plus hyperreflexia, and hypertonia.**
12. **Neuroleptic malignant syndrome (NMS)** of extrapyramidal side effects includes muscle **rigidity** and **rhabdomyolysis** (increase in WBC, Cr, and LFTs and metabolic acidosis). Unlike serotonin syndrome, NMS is rarely associated with **hyperreflexia and myoclonus**.
13. Serotonin syndrome usually presents within 24 h of exposure; altered mental status (AMS) with agitation and delirium; may have seizures and rhabdomyolysis.
14. **Common meds related to serotonin syndrome**: MAOIs, SSRIs, TCAs, SNRIs, and bupropion.
15. **Pneumococcal endocarditis, meningitis, and pneumonia triad from pneumococcal infection = Austrian syndrome.**
16. In severe infection, may use double coverage, usually Vanco and cefotaxime for patients with known or suspected pneumococcal infections until susceptibility results, **mortality of pneumococcal endocarditis is 15%–20%.**
17. Pneumococcal endocarditis is often a fulminant disease and causes severe valve damage and embolic complications. **Valve replacement** may be necessary. Pneumococcus can cause suppurative infections anywhere, **purulent endocarditis, septic arthritis, osteomyelitis, and abscesses in the abdomen**.
18. Abruptly stopping or rapidly tapering antidepressants often causes **discontinuation symptoms** including agitation, anxiety, chills, diaphoresis, dizziness, dysphoria, fatigue, headache, insomnia, irritability, myalgia, paraesthesias, rhinorrhea, and tremor. **Correct tapering regimen**: SNRI taper and TCA taper in 2–4 weeks, and MAOI taper in ≥4 weeks.
19. It's not common to experience bupropion withdrawal symptoms, but those who do may become **agitated and irritable**.

10/29/2019

1. **Skin rash and endocarditis**, may consult an allergist for antibiotic allergy and prescribe prednisone 30 mg bid for 3 days.
2. Check O_2 in ambulation and rest before discharge if the patient is on oxygen in hospital.
3. History of heart failure (HF), AFib, rhythm control use Tikosyn; **initiation of Tikosyn (dofetilide)**: start Tikosyn 500 mg bid, EKG 2 h after each dose, keep K > 4 and Mg > 2; if no spontaneous conversion to normal sinus rhythm (NSR), plan to do direct current cardioversion (DCCV) before discharge.
4. Percutaneous endoscopic gastrostomy (**PEG**) feeds, give **thyroxine**, need to hold feeds 1 h prior and 1 h after thyroxine administration

5. **Opioid tapering inside hospital**: clonidine 0.1 mg qid, Trileptal (oxcarbazepine) 150 mg qid, methadone 2.5 mg (bid to qid depends), Wellbutrin 150 mg qd, Lexapro 10 mg bid, Buspar 5 mg qd.

11/3/2019

1. 49 yo F shortness of breath, drinker, Hgb 4, acute kidney injury (AKI) with creatinine 7.87. Anemia workup. In reviewing the patient's smear, we see very prominent rouleaux, schistocytes, and tear drop cells, suggesting possible myelocytic changes. **Differential diagnoses**: bone marrow stress, multiple myeloma (MM); rule out thrombotic thrombocytopenic purpura (TTP) or paroxysmal nocturnal hemoglobinuria cause (PNH). Labs: **LDH, UPEP, SPEP, kappa and lambda light chains, HBV, HCV, serum immunofixation, IgA, IgG, IgM, cold agglutinins, serum immunofixation essay (IFE) diagnostics, cryoglobulin, ADAMTS13, beta2-microglobulin**.
2. **AKI workup** for the above patient: urinalysis (UA), urine Na, K, Cl, C3, C4, and C50, ANA, ANCA, antiglomerular basement membrane antibodies, protein/creatinine ratio.

11/10/2019

1. **Keppra** can cause agitation in dementia patients, 48 h monitoring is needed
2. **Respiratory bronchiolitis**-associated interstitial lung disease (RBILD) is a smoking-related interstitial pneumonia and is one of the idiopathic interstitial pneumonia. Other major **idiopathic interstitial pneumonia** includes idiopathic pulmonary fibrosis (IPF), nonspecific interstitial pneumonia (NSIP), desquamative interstitial pneumonia (DIP, another smoking-related ILP), acute interstitial pneumonia, and cryptogenic organizing pneumonia (COP).
3. Respiratory bronchiolitis **key features**: the presence of **tan-pigmented macrophages**. Respiratory bronchiolitis **pathology**: **respiratory bronchiolitis** (RB) changes as the sole findings with history of smoking and clinical evidence of ILD. Seen in patients aged 30–50 s with subacute symptoms of dyspnea, wheezes, cough, and or sputum production. **Diagnostic tests**: alpha-1 antitrypsin (AAT), pulmonary function testing (PFT), imaging (diffuse, fine reticular or nodular opacities with preserved lung volumes, diffuse or patchy ground glass opacities, bronchoscopy or surgical lung biopsy).
4. Treatment for RBILD: smoking cessation, supportive therapy including O_2, pulmonary rehab, vaccination of flu and pneumonia. **If there is a lack of response, give prednisone 0.5 mg/kg up to 30 mg per day for 1 month following 20 mg daily for 2 months**.
5. **Daptomycin** is not good for pneumonia
6. Long-term daptomycin needs weekly CPK; for long-term ceftriaxone, do weekly CBC and CMP.

12/16/2019: Life-Threatening EKG Findings

1. **Hyperkalemia** EKG: a flattened P wave; a prolonged PR interval; borderline widened QRS complex and more pathognomic pointed, **narrow, and tented tall T waves**.
2. **Digitalis** toxicity: **junctional tachycardia** with **variable conduction delays** in AFib.
3. Clinically significant manifestations of digitalis poisoning can be treated with **digoxin-specific Ab (Fab) fragments**: **life-threatening arrhythmia (VTach, VFib, asystole, complete heart block, Mobitz Type II block, symptomatic bradycardia), evidence of end-organ dysfunction (renal failure, altered mental status), and/or hyperkalemia.**
4. **Torsades de pointes**: sinus rhythm with long QT, followed by wide complex tachycardia = Tdp.
5. **Wellens' sign/syndrome = marked biphasic T waves with deep T wave inversions seen in precordial leads, namely V2 and V3 (may also be in leads V1, V4, V5, and V6)** ⇒ high suspicion for a very proximal LAD lesion. Wellens' syndrome = ST-elevation myocardial infarction (**STEMI**).

12/17/2019

1. **Jewell-Lange-Nielson syndrome** (JLNS) is a long QT syndrome (LQTS) with severe bilateral sensorineural **hearing loss**. Signs and symptoms: congenital deafness, syncope, seizures, palpitations, sudden cardiac death. Treatment: **defibrillator in addition to a beta-blocker**. LQTS + skeletal abnormalities (short stature and scoliosis) = Long QT syndrome 7 (**Andersen syndrome**).
2. Diagnosis of **long QT syndrome**: suspected long QT syndrome should undergo pharmacologic provocation with epinephrine or isoproterenol in patients with borderline presentation.
3. **Treatment of congenital long QT syndrome**: (1) Beta-blocker: nadolol 50 mg qd > propranolol > metoprolol > atenolol; (2) Surgical option: implantation of cardioverter-defibrillator, and pacers.
4. Treatment for acquired LQTS: **$MgSO_4$**, isoproterenol, lidocaine, phenytoin, $NaHCO_3$ for quinidine-related arrhythmia; temporary pacing (atrial of ventricular).
5. **Sydenham chorea also known as rheumatic chorea** is characterized by chorea, emotional lability, and hypotonia. Other manifestations of **rheumatic fever** include carditis and valvulitis, migratory polyarteritis, subcutaneous nodules, and erythema marginatum.

1/7/2020 Retina Abnormalities

1. **Hypertensive retinopathy**: retinal hemorrhages, exudates and cotton wool spots.
2. **Ischemic optic neuropathy**: afferent pupillary defects and pallid disc swelling of the right optic nerve.
3. **Retinal whitening and cherry red spot** and amaurosis fugax (fleeting visual loss/blindness): acute central retinal artery occlusion.
4. **Hollenhorst plaques** are cholesterol emboli (occlusion of the carotid arteries common). They are bright white spots on the retina.

5. **Superficial hemorrhages** seen in central retinal vein occlusion (CRVO).
6. **Cotton wool spots** represent a micro infarct of the retina caused by small vessel occlusions; can be seen in **CMV infection** in HIV infection.
7. **Flame and blot hemorrhages** scattered throughout the retina and boat-shaped preretinal hemorrhage in macule = consider **acute leukemia**.
8. **Roth spots**: white-centered hemorrhage in the macular region. The white center is coagulated fibrin and/or microinfarcts. **Differential diagnoses**: bacteremia endocarditis, leukemia, severe anemia, HIV-related retinopathy.
9. **Scattered intraretinal hemorrhage** = non-proliferative diabetic retinopathy or neovascularization. **Exudate and hemorrhage in the macula** = consider diabetic macular edema.

1/12/2020

1. Chronic ill patients, **frequent pressure relief** to prevent pressure ulcers.
2. Ask why medication is being used; discharge barriers, and physical findings.
3. Ask about antibiotic indications, length, and need for IV line.
4. Old anterior infarct, **no identifiable R wave in V1 and V2.**
5. Old inferior myocardial infarct, **a Q wave in lead II, III, aVF**.
6. **Guttate psoriasis**: development of inflammatory plaques on the skin, erythrodermic, related to strep infection or Pityrosporum (Malassezia) folliculitis infection. **Treatment**: phototherapy, topical steroids, Vit D analogs (calcitriol, calcipotriene)
7. **LAFB EKG**: a Q wave in lead I; rS in lead II, III, aVF, LAD, QRS duration normal or slightly prolonged.

Infectious Disease Rotation

1/13/2020

1. Ceftriaxone 2 g qd for most infections; **2 g q12h for meningitis, and endocarditis (may require ampicillin synergy).**
2. **Fournier's gangrene** is a necrotizing fasciitis; it requires STAT surgical debridement.
3. Patients on highly active antiretroviral therapy (HARRT), check **HIV RNA every half a year**.
4. Documentation, two symptoms per system.
5. Rapidly growing mycobacterium: **abscessus, fortuitum, chelonae**.
6. Diagnosis of necrotizing soft tissue infections: **crepitus**, skin discoloration or **necrosis**, thin foul-smelling wound discharge, rapid progression of clinical manifestations; **severe pain** (gas in CT).
7. **M. abscessus**: single lesion, causes lung infection in patients with lung disease. **M. fortuitum**: multiple lesions, causes skin, soft tissue, wound, and catheter infection through direct inoculation. **M. chelonae** causes infection in immunosuppressed patients, including hematogenously disseminated disease and also causes wound infection and keratitis.
8. **M. abscessus and M. fortuitum cause lymphadenitis**.

9. A 60-year-old male with a history of renal transplant and prostate cancer for which he received penile implant was found to have an abscess in implant. Culture showed **acid fast stain +** and eventually grew Mycobacterium fortuitum.
10. Treatment for mycobacterium abscessus/fortuitum/chelonae**: amikacin, tigecycline, imipenem, cefoxitin, or doxycycline**.
11. Common slowly growing NTM (non-tuberculosis mycobacterium) include **Mycobacterium avium complex (MAC), M. kansasi, M. haemophilum, M. marinum**.

1/14/2020

1. **Renal transplant treatment**: cyclosporine 175 mg bid, daily trough 150–200; prednisone 5 mg qd. Hx of CMV, give Valcyte (valganciclovir) 450 mg bid.
2. **Mycobacterium fortuitum** treatment: **tigecycline + Cipro**, monitor QTc
3. Graft loss, renal transplant, treatment: tacrolimus 1 g bid, mycophenolate stopped, prednisone 10 mg bid, **PJP prophylaxis, still needs to check CMV PCR, BK PCR**.
4. G+ rods: Mycobacterium, Nocardia (steroid injection at SIJ). Treatment: Bactrim, imipenem, amikacin. **Actinomyces, Listeria, Clostridium, Bacillus, and Corynebacterium** are all gram-positive rods.
5. **Linezolid** causes peripheral **neuropathy, seizures,** and **serotonin syndrome**.
6. Beta-D-Glucan assay, can aid the diagnosis of invasive fungal infection (aspergillus and PJP). But can be falsely positive in **hemodialysis** with cellulose membranes, **IVIG**, **albumin**, **gauze packing** of serosal surfaces, IV **amoxicillin–clavulanic acid**, and **infections** with certain **bacteria** that contain cellular beta glucans like **pseudomonas**.

1/15/2020

1. **Renal transplant immunosuppression**: cyclosporine 175 mg bid (daily trough 150–200), prednisone 5 mg qd.
2. **Vaginal discharge** check labs for trichomonas, gonorrhea, chlamydia, influenza A&B, tick-borne or other zoonotic infection.
3. **Osteomyelitis**, monitor for weekly ESR and CRP. Outpatient treatment: Keflex and Bactrim DS for **4 weeks**.
4. Hip **septic arthritis**: IV ceftriaxone for **6 weeks** (strep).
5. **Empyema** treatment: Augmentin for **4 weeks**.
6. **Renal transplant**: **pentamidine** for PCP, **valganciclovir** (Valcyte) for CMV, **acyclovir** for herpes, **Diflucan** 100 mg qd for fungi prophylaxis.
7. Routine **follow-up labs for renal transplants**: serum CMP, trough tacrolimus, cyclosporine, everolimus, or sirolimus, urinalysis (UA), urine protein-to-creatinine ratio, HA1c, lipid profile, PTH, 25-hydroxyvitamin D, BK virus, and CMV check.
8. Immunosuppression in renal transplant (solid organ transplant): **induction therapy** typically consists of biologic antibodies of Rabbit antithymocyte globulin (thymoglobulin), basiliximab (Simulect) and high dose glucocorticoids; **maintenance regimens** include glucocorticoids, calcineurin inhibitors (tacroli-

mus, cyclosporine), antimetabolic agents (mycophenolate, azathioprine), mammalian target of rapamycin (mTOR) inhibitors (sirolimus, everolimus) or costimulatory blockade agents (belatacept).

9. **Calcineurin inhibitors (CNI)** cause kidney injury **hypertension and neurotoxicity**, permanent fibrosis in the kidney. Check trough level. **CNI level increases with the use of calcium channel blockers (CCB) or antifungal agents**; CNI level decreases with the use of anticonvulsants.
10. Side effects (SEs): **CNI causes hirsutism, gingival hyperplasia with cyclosporine, and alopecia with tacrolimus. Mycophenolate causes GI disturbances and diarrhea**.
11. **Opportunistic infection in transplant**: CMV, BK (polyomavirus), Nocardia, Listeria, Aspergillus, PCP, HCV, HBV, VZV, EBV, mycobacterium, TB.
12. **Malignancies in renal transplant**: skin cancer, lip cancer, **post-transplant lymphoproliferative disorder (PTLD)**, Kaposi sarcoma, and renal carcinoma.
13. **BK virus infection**: asymptomatic viruria, viremia, renal tubular damage, and nephropathy. Treatment: reduce immune suppression.
14. **Post-transplantation prophylaxis for 3-6-12 months**: TMP-SMX for PCP (sulfa allergy, use pentamidine), Listeria, and Toxoplasma; Diflucan 100 mg qd; valganciclovir/ganciclovir for CMV; acyclovir for patients who are not receiving CMV prophylaxis.
15. For **mild to moderate hypercalcemia** from hyperparathyroidism, use **cinacalcet**. If serum calcium >12, do parathyroidectomy.
16. **Hyperuricemia** and gout in transplant treatment options: intra-articular steroid injection → po steroid → colchicine and NSAIDs. Allopurinol → febuxostat, or possibly probenecid can be used to lower uric acid after acute symptom resolution.
17. **CKD secondary hyperparathyroidism**: if PTH persistently above 150–200 pg/ml despite treatment for hyperphosphatemia, low phosphate intake, and Vit D supplement, give calcitriol 0.25 mg tid. Do not use calcitriol if P is above normal or calcium ≥ 9.5. Use cinacalcet in hemodialysis patients.
18. Strep pyogenes, septic shock, AKI, fever, necrotizing fasciitis, 33 yo female. Necrotizing soft tissue infection: discontinue the vancomycin and piperacillin-tazobactam; initiate **penicillin** infusion; initiate **clindamycin** for toxin mediation; initiate **metronidazole** for empiric anaerobic coverage; send screening HIV, syphilis, urine gonorrhea, and chlamydia.

1/16/2020

1. 66 yo ESRD due to polycystic kidney disease (PCKD) sp. kidney transplant on immunosuppression (belatacept), mycophenolate, and prednisone came in for community-acquired pneumonia (CAP). Treatment recommendation: stop Vanco/Zosyn, check **mycoplasma** and **chlamydia**, **beta D glucan**, add atovaquone 750 mg, renal adjust, continue azithromycin 500 mg qd, add prednisone 40 mg po, check **Histo Ag**, **fungus**, **Blasto Ag**, **PJP sputum**, **CMV DNA**, **flu**, **hepatitis**, **RSV**.

2. Cerebrospinal fluid (CSF) exam additional labs: HSV1&2 DNA, VZV DNA, CMV DNA, EBV DNA, toxoplasmosis.
3. **Complicated urinary tract infection (UTI)**, use Cipro for 10 days or beta-lactam for 14 days.
4. **Broth vs. agar plate**, bacterial growth difference: broth is a liquid form while plate is a solid form culture. Agar is for bacterial isolation and preservation while broth is for growth and cultivation for the production of bacterium.
5. HIV treatment example: a combination of **Prezcobix** (darunavir & cobicistat) + **Tivicay** [dolutegravir (integrase)].
6. **Nafcillin**: increases serum transaminase.
7. **EVD** = external ventricular drainage. If given dapsone, check G6PD.
8. **Osteomyelitis** with MRSA treatment in a patient with intramedullary nail: 3 months Doxy + rifampin. May need long term suppressive therapy.
9. **Urgent splenectomy** requires vaccination in 14 days: PCV20 alone or PCV15 plus PPSV23 (PCV13 → 8 weeks later, PPSV23); Hib; MenACWY; MenB-4 or MenB-FHbp; seasonal influenza virus vaccination for the prevention of **pneumonia, H influenza infection, meningitis, and influenza**. Revaccinate PPSV 23 and MenACWY q5y.
10. Functional asplenia: **penicillin V or amoxicillin** till age 5 for ≥1-year-old children; if also immunocompromised, give antibiotic ppx till at least age 18 or for life if immunocompromised for life.
11. Adults undergoing splenectomy will need **daily antibiotic prophylaxis** for ≥1 year after splenectomy using penicillin V or amoxicillin.
12. High risk in asplenic patients for the following infections: **animal bite (Capnocytophaga including C. canimorsus); babesiosis, malaria**.
13. Antibiotics for procedures involving paranasal sinuses or respiratory tract (endoscopic sinus surgery, bronchoscopy), do antibiotic prophylaxis (amoxicillin 2 g orally, 30–60 min before procedure); antibiotic prophylaxis in clean procedures is not supported by research evidence.
14. **Detection of fungal Ags**: blood & bronchoalveolar lavage (BAL) fluid, test galactomannan, or beta-D-glucan.

1/17/2020

1. **Aspergillosis**: invasive aspergillosis (risk factors: chronic granulomatous disease, neutropenia); chronic pulmonary aspergillosis (risk factors: structure lung disease, emphysema, intact immune system); aspergilloma; allergic bronchopulmonary aspergillosis (ABPA).
2. **Actinomyces**: filamentous G+ rods, anaerobes, not acid-fast (Nocardia is acid fast), slowly growing, colonizing the upper respiratory gastrointestinal (GI) and female genital tracts, sulfur granules.
3. **G+ rods: bacillus (anthrax), clostridium, Corynebacterium, listeria, Gardnerella.**
4. **Nocardiosis**: bronchopulmonary (cavitary lesion in immunocompromised, can disseminate to CNS); cutaneous or lymphocutaneous lesions leading to mycetoma. Treatment: Bactrim.

1/20/2020

1. **Overflow bacterium** (MRSA, Strep. pyogenes) in urine, need blood cx, less likely urinary tract infection (UTI).
2. **Sick septic shock**, do empirical clindamycin for toxin suppression and other antibiotics (ABX), like penicillin (Group A strep bacteremia).
3. Tuberculosis (TB), multiple myeloma (MM), malignancy, and sarcoidosis can all cause **hypercalcemia**.
4. Hardware with an abscess at the elbow, treat with Keflex for **6 weeks**.
5. **Fulminant septic shock**: *Staph*, *Streptococcus* pyogenes, *Rocky Mountain* spotted fever (RMSF), *Vibrio*, *West Nile*, *Clostridium perfringens*.
6. **Pneumocystis jiroveci Pneumonia (PJP) Ag** in sputum, galactomannan, beta-D-glucan, LDH tests are used in concerns for PJP infection. **ASO titer is only used for Strep infection in pediatric patients**.
7. **SPICE produces AmpC beta-lactamase** (cephalosporinases): Serratia, Pseudomonas, indolent proteus Citrobacter, Enterobacter. Serratia infection in joints, prescribe Cipro, Bactrim po or IV ertapenem/cefepime.
8. **Epidural abscess** with bacteriuria of S. pyogenes, use **nafcillin better than cefazolin** for CNS coverage. Needs neurosurgery consult stat consult!
9. **Indications for funguria** treatment: identification of **fungal casts in urine** cytology specimens stained with periodic acid-Schiff or silver stains is diagnostic of **kidney involvement**; **persistent candiduria**, esp. in **diabetes**, with CT or US showing **hydronephrosis**, **fungus ball** or **perinephric abscesses** associated with ascending infection; otherwise, if asymptomatic, no treatment. Treatment, if necessary, do fluconazole 200–400 mg qd for 14 days.
10. **Daptomycin** needs weekly CK. **MRSA endocarditis** is treated with daptomycin and cefazolin for 6 weeks.
11. Right leg and arm weakness → MRI head and spine → **cervical discitis**. Need antibiotics with good CNS coverage.
12. **PCP pneumonia** treatment: atovaquone 75 mg bid for 21 days; alternatives include trimethoprim–dapsone, and clindamycin-primaquine. **Preferred is Bactrim, pentamidine**. Dapsone and primaquine need to check G6PD.
13. If **PO2 < 70 mmHg on RA and or an A-a gradient of ≥ 35 mmHg**, start steroids in patients with PCP infection. **Steroid regimen**: prednisone 40 mg bid for 5 days, 40 mg qd for 5 days, followed by 20 mg qd for 11 days.

1/21/2020

1. **G+ bacteremia** needs IV antibiotics for 14 days. **G- bacteremia** can be treated with po for 7 days.
2. Staph, and Streptococcus mutans/viridans need echocardiogram checks.
3. **Streptococcus constellatus** is part of the normal flora in the oral cavity, urogenital region, and intestinal tract. However, it can frequently cause infection in other parts of the body with purulent infection, like the liver.
4. **Osteoarthritis** follow-up, do ESR, CRP in 8 weeks. If increased, do suppression therapy.

5. **Tigecycline** needs to monitor LFT and INR; **fluconazole** increases QTc.
6. **Dalbavancin** can be used for 2 doses for G+ bacteremia, MRSA, and MSSA, 1 week apart.
7. In **MRSA** non-responsive to Vanco, can do **ceftaroline + daptomycin** (synergism).
8. **Endophthalmitis** etiologies: fungus, candida, staph, Klebsiella, aspergillus, toxoplasma, onchocera/Taenium, histo, blasto.
9. **Listeria** CSF studies show results consistent with nonspecific bacterial meningitis. **Lyme disease**: **ELISA/IFA → western blot IgM and Ig G**, CSF **lymphocytic** pleocytosis.
10. Rash, fever = consider **vasculitis**. pANCA + from the use of hydralazine.
11. Decreased C3, C4 seen in **infective endocarditis, systemic lupus erythematosus (SLE), hydralazine vasculitis, and hepatitis**.
12. **Fulminant sepsis** with multi-organ involvement etiologies: **Staph, Strep, RMSF, Vibrio, West Nile, Clostridium toxin**.

1/22/2020

1. **Prepatellar septic bursitis**, drainage grew MRSA, treatment: vancomycin for 3–5 days, then Bactrim for 2–3 weeks.
2. **Hold Remeron while on Linezolid**, and restart once Linezolid is completed. **For gangrene finger** sp. amputation, do linezolid for a total of 7 days.
3. **Hydronephrosis: need to rule out obstructive nephropathy, please consult Urology!**
4. **Discitis** and **osteomyelitis** with difficulties ambulating, treatment: cefepime 2 g q8h + Flagyl po after biopsy. Duration is usually 6 weeks.
5. **MRSA abscess aspiration** for abscess of right leg status post tibial intramedullary nail and open reduction internal fixation (ORIF) of right ankle (July, 2019); fell 5 days ago. Low trough for Vanco despite q8h dosing. Change to daptomycin, weekly ESR, CRP, CMP, CK.
6. **Prior MRSA infection of knee hardware** treatment: Vanco IV for 6 weeks then doxy suppression for 7 months, completed in 3/2019. Presented with wound dehiscence → If biopsy culture positive, needs 6 weeks IV then po doxycycline suppression for 12 m. If negative, go directly to po doxy or Bactrim suppression.
7. **MenACWY-D (Menactra):** recommended for ≤55 years not previously vaccinated and who have **persistent complement deficiencies (including eculizumab use), functional or anatomic asplenia**, or who have HIV infection, 2 doses, 2 months apart.
8. **MRSA bacteremia** and endogenous MRSA endophthalmitis (Vanco eye drop) treatment: Vanco for 4 weeks, once clearance of bacteremia is confirmed, will need her **hemodialysis (HD) catheter** changed. No need for empirical antifungal treatment.
9. **ESRD with tunneled dialysis** catheter and diabetic foot ulcer (DFU) came in with fever, blood culture positive for G- bacilli. Treatment: aztreonam. Later, culture was positive for pseudomonas. **Management**: remove HD catheter once

repeat blood culture negative (3/26–3/28). if negative till Saturday (3/28)—place a new tunneled dialysis catheter. Then, also place midline for continuous **aztreonam for 14 days** from the first negative blood culture.

10. Flomax causes **postural hypotension**. Recurrent UTI with hydronephrosis → treatment with Foley and urology consult. **Transplant patient, if urine retention in the old kidney → nephrostomy tube is needed.**
11. **Actinomyces** should be treated with penicillin G or ceftriaxone for **2–6 months**. It causes slow infection and colonizing bacteria in the mouth and urinary tract, GI tract.
12. **Dalbavancin** 1500 mg per week for 2 weeks for MRSA.
13. **AUC vs. MIC** = area under the curve vs. minimum inhibitory concentration.

1/23/2020

1. **Fluconazole** causes QTc elongation.
2. **Cryptococcus meningitis** treatment: amphotericin B 3–4 g/kg qd + flucytosine 100 mg/kg/day in 4 doses daily for ≥2 weeks → repeat lumbar puncture (LP) → fluconazole 800 mg bid for 8 weeks.
3. **Neostigmine** po 15 mg tid for **myasthenia gravis** (MG); 5 mg IV for reversal of neuromuscular (NM) **blockade after surgery**; 0.25 mg subcutaneously for **postop urinary retention**; 2 mg IV over 3–5 min for **Ogilvie syndrome**.
4. Rapid right-sided weakness on top of MRSA bacteremia: MRI brain with contrast, MRI C/T/L, EMG/NCS, **sensorimotor polyneuropathy with severe degree of axonal cell loss** → diagnosis: **critical illness polyneuropathy**.
5. **Intravesicular** temperature is **1° higher** than regular temperature!
6. **HIV infection additional lab tests**: check Toxoplasma gondii IgG, Hep A IgG, Hep B surface Ab, acid-fast (AF) stain blood for Mycobacterium avium complex (MAC).
7. 57-year-old African American female with **fever and intractable vomiting** → candida fungemia from infected central line. Treatment: **micafungin 100 mg (150 mg in refractory disease) qd iv × 2 weeks**. The patient was told to notify the MD immediately if any visual changes, and repeat the dilated exam in 2 weeks with ophthalmology.
8. **Serological workup for kidney disease**: acute kidney injury (AKI) with high anion gap metabolic acidosis (HAGMA) - 7.23 bicarb 10, order bicarbonate 2–3 amp at 150 cc/h. glomerulonephritis (RBC cast), then serology (C3, C4, ANCA, anti-GBM).
9. **Recurrent UTI** → nitrofurantoin suppression for 3 m. For acute complicated UTI, do beta-lactam for 10–14 days, fluoroquinolone (FQ) for 5–7 days, or Bactrim for 7–10 days.
10. **Low QRS voltage** → pericardial effusion, fever, chest pain, back pain, and generalized body achiness = consider **pericardial effusion infection with MRSA**. **Cardiology consult** for possible need of pericardiocentesis and/or pericardial window.

1/29/2020

1. AFib with RVR, HR 170 s, sBP 100, LVEF 20% → cardiology and **EP consult**, metoprolol, may use digoxin or amiodarone.
2. **Permacath has to be removed by an interventional radiologist or nephrologist**.
3. **Fecal elastase** is used in the diagnosis of chronic pancreatitis.
4. Gallstone pancreatitis has to get cholecystectomy before discharge.
5. Check **digoxin** level, and pay attention to social issues.
6. **Mepolizumab** and **reslizumab** are monoclonal Abs against IL-5 which can reduce hospitalization of uncontrolled eosinophilic asthma. **Omalizumab** for symptoms not controlled with inhaled steroids, perennial allergic allergies, and **IgE** between 30 and 700 u/mL.

2/2/2020

1. **Digoxin is good for resting heart rate** but not during movement.
2. GERD mild → H2 blocker once a day → 4 weeks later, H2 blocker bid → 2 weeks later, PPI once daily for 4–8 weeks. **If asymptomatic for 8 weeks**, can taper and discontinue.
3. Diabetic ketoacidosis (DKA) can have **normal pH**.
4. Right heart failure (RHF), pain at chest, nitrate is of no benefit, will need **morphine**.

2/3/2020

1. Gastroenterologist consult for dysphagia and achalasia. **Aspiration concerns →** get speech for modified diet and do CT chest.
2. AFib on **amiodarone** maintenance dose **200 mg qd**; VFib maintenance dose **400 mg qd**.

3/2/2020

1. **Olanzapine** 2.5 mg bid for nausea and hiccups. Low-dose **baclofen** can also be used for hiccups.
2. **Octreotide + Reglan + dexamethasone** for malignant bowel obstruction.
3. **Hypoactive delirium**: unusual drowsiness, lethargy, and inactivity, diagnosis via the 4 As test (Arousal, Attention, Abbreviated Mental Test—4, and Acute change) for **attention and awareness**. Management of hypoactive delirium: explanation to the patient and family of the symptoms and diagnosis, treatment of reversible causes, **cognitive stimulation, reorientation, early mobility, improved hearing and vision, sleep-wake cycle preservation, and hydration**.
4. **Hyperactive delirium**: disturbance in awareness and attention, characterized by predominantly restlessness and agitation.
5. **Liver mass pain**: may give non-steroidal anti-inflammatory drugs (NSAIDs) and Decadron.

3/2/2020–3/5/2020

Palliative Care at Cancer Center

1. **Octreotide 300 mg IV tid + reglan 5 mg iv q6h + dexamethasone 4 mg bid** for malignant bowel obstruction.
2. Use **olanzapine** for hiccups, nausea, and vomiting.
3. "If you get sicker, what the plan will be". **Emphasis on social and family issues.**
4. Total parenteral nutrition (TPN) for small bowel obstruction in cancer patients; if not improving or re-obstruction, will need **venting percutaneous endoscopic gastrostomy (PEG) tube**, 3 months of life left.
5. **Senna** may work better than docusate/senna combination.
6. Nausea and constipation orders: Zofran 8 mg tid iv, Compazine 10 mg iv, miralax 17 g qd, senna 2 tablet bid, lactulose 20 g tid, magnesium citrate 300 mg po qd prn.
7. **Long-acting opioids**: oxycontin, transdermal fentanyl, and MS morphine. **Methadone and buprenorphine** are the true actual long-acting opioids.
8. **Cytoreduction** with HIPEC (hyperthermic intraperitoneal chemotherapy) after neoadjuvant FOLFOX for **intraperitoneal carcinomatosis**.
9. **Malignant bowel obstruction**: if re-obstruction, she would require **venting G tube and +/− TPN**. Poor prognosis needs discussion of hospice and DNR/DNI.
10. Hospice referral if life expectancy is less than 6 months. With hospice care, the **hospice nurse will visit the patient twice a week** or so, a couple of hours each time.
11. **Chondrosarcoma** in a 29 yo treatment: pazopanib (multiple kinase inhibitor) 400 mg → 600 mg → 800 mg qd. **Radiation** for **spine metastasis** if spinal cord injury from metastasis → pembrolizumab.
12. **Myxoid high-grade sarcoma** treatment processes: en bloc resection of sigmoid mesocolon, bilateral distal ureterectomies/cystectomy, ileal conduit urinary diversion → recurrence 3 years later → 2 cycles of gemcitabine → recurrence, thus 50 Gy preoperative radiation → wide resection of recurrent tumor → gemcitabine → trabectedin → doxorubicin × 4 cycles → eribulin (microtubule inhibitor) → pembrolizumab.
13. **Social history**: family support (marital status/relationship, children, siblings/parents, friends); occupation/education; military history/PTSD, smoking/alcohol/illicit drug abuse. Function before admission. Spiritual support.
14. How do you cope with anxiety?
15. Nausea goes away with opioids in 3 days with **Cannabidiol (CBD) + 10 mg Marinol (Dronabinol, insurance coverage).**
16. Steroids can be used for end of life: **Decadron** at a dosage of 8 mg a day can help with fatigue, pain, trouble breathing, nausea, vomiting, and poor appetite.
17. **Hospice**: oral antibiotics and stool softeners can be used.
18. 1 mg IV Dilaudid (Hydromorphone) = 12 mg po morphine; 1 mg methadone po = 10 mg po morphine.

19. **Patient-controlled analgesia (PCA) pump**: basal rate 0.5 mg/h, bolus rate 0.4 mg, lockout frequency to 10 min, maximal dosage 3 mg/h = basal rate + bolus rate × 1 h/lockout frequency

3/11/2020

1. **Hemodialysis** (HD) may be necessary if BUN >100, biopsy planned. Before biopsy, give **DDAVP** (desmopressin) to end-stage renal disease patients.
2. In **post-streptococcal glomerulonephritis (PSGN**), steroids may not provide benefits; use steroids for other ANCA + glomerulonephritis (GN).
3. As long as the patient is producing urine, the patient can continue to take **ACEi and water pills** even if the patient is on hemodialysis (HD).
4. Acute kidney injury (AKI), if **serum bicarbonate is low**, may use Bicarb drip or add oral bicarbonate till hemodialysis (HD) or improvement of serum bicarbonate to normal.

3/21/2020

1. Systemic antibiotics are not recommended for the prevention of surgical site infection in elective colon surgery. In patients with intra-abdominal infections who had undergone an **adequate source-control procedure**, the outcomes after fixed-duration antibiotic therapy (**approximately 4 days**) were similar to those after a longer course of antibiotics (approximately 8 days) that extended until after the resolution of physiological abnormalities.
2. **Adrenal crisis**: hydrocortisone 50 mg IV q6h → stable then transition to 50 mg IV bid → 50 mg bid → 25 mg bid. Will change to 50 mg hydrocortisone twice daily × 5 days (or shorter if blood pressure reasonable) followed by **25 mg of p.o hydrocortisone** divided into two doses upon discharge with follow-up as an outpatient and to reestablish home dose.

3/22/2020

1. Diabetic patients in the hospital getting steroids, may use **NPH once daily** in the morning to control **steroid-induced hyperglycemia**.
2. Normally hospitalized patients with not well-controlled diabetes, can give 1/2 **home dose Lantus and 1/2 premeal lispro tid**.

3/26/2020

1. **Hypercalcemia** from B cell lymphoma, status post rituximab + ibrutinib, found to have 1,25-di-Vit D elevation. **Treatment**: prednisone 50 mg qd for 5 days, taper to 10 mg then 7.5 mg daily. Labs include beta-2 microglobulin, LDH, TSH, 1,25$(OH)_2$VitD.

4/10/2020

1. **Seroquel** for patient agitation during nights.
2. Tachy-Brady (Tachycardia-bradycardia) syndrome, may need a **pacemaker**. When **supraventricular tachycardia (SVT)** is nonresponsive to adenosine, will

need to make sure it is not ventricular tachycardia (VTach). Once VTach is ruled out, can use diltiazem.

3. **Coronary artery disease (CAD) status post coronary artery bypass grafting (CABG) provides a protective function for the heart for 5 years, but not during the first 1–6 months**.
4. Heparin drip, if given Lovenox (Enoxaparin) in the morning, no bolus for heparin drip use on the same day.
5. **Chest pain**, decreased CO_2 in ABG, D-dimer 3400, do CT angiogram which revealed **pulmonary embolism** (PE).
6. Repeat everything as new, post-obstruction diuresis needs to make sure **input matches output**.
7. **Acetazolamide** (**Diamox)** may be used briefly for metabolic alkalosis, acute mountain sickness/high-altitude cerebral edema, and elevated intraocular pressure associated with acute angle-closure glaucoma (adjunct).
8. **Mirtazapine** 15 mg qd for depression and decreased oral intake; 1 month later, increase to 30 mg daily.

4/19/2020

1. On meropenem, from urinary sepsis ⇒ consider CT abdomen/pelvis to rule out hydronephrosis and stones; if any, consult urology to fix the urinary tract with stenting ⇒ continues to have increased WBC → repeat CT. Echocardiogram to look for endocarditis; at the same time, consult **urology** to use **transrectal ultrasound** to look at the prostate.
2. On fluid, not eating, may need **tube feeding** if not improving after 24 h.
3. **Tumor encasement of the superior mesenteric artery (SMA)**, possible thrombosis in CT, needs discussion with radiologist, MRI may be needed.
4. Understand why the patient is here, fix it, and prevent the situation from happening again.
5. Longer than **3 weeks of need for nasogastric tube feeding** is an indication of percutaneous endoscopic gastrostomy (PEG). **PEG in old dementia and stage IV malignancy increases mortality and morbidity** and thus is not recommended.
6. **Chronic kidney disease (CKD) Stage IV-V**: needs nephrology consultation.

4/20/2020

1. A patient found to have increased **peripheral blasts up to 33% (oncologic consult stat)** with WBC 27 K. **Treatment**: hydroxyurea and allopurinol 300 mg qd, check FLT3 (FMS-like receptor tyrosine kinase 3) gene. CD 135 is the receptor for FLT3 ligand. FLT3 gene negative → pathology diagnosis for **bone marrow aspiration** ⇒ acute myeloid leukemia (AML), **treatment**: azacytidine (Vidaza, methylation of DNA) 75 mg/m^2 SQ × 7 days plus venetoclax (cytotoxic for BCL2) daily → developed headache and pain → CT brain for bleed negative, bloodstream infection of Nocardia ⇒ **bone marrow restaging consistent with variable cellular marrow with trilineage dyspoiesis** (10% cellularity, raging 0%–60%), 8% blasts consistent with relapsed leukemia—IDH 2 positive (isoci-

trate dehydrogenase 1 & 2). Start **IDH2 inhibitor Enasidenib** for relapsed or refractory AML with mutant IDH2 ⇒ developed differentiation syndrome.

2. **Differentiation syndrome**: fever, dyspnea, acute respiratory distress, pulmonary infiltrates, pleural or pericardial effusions, rapid weight gain or peripheral edema, lymphadenopathy, bone pain, hepatic, renal or multi-organ dysfunction (3 or more of the aforementioned features).
3. Differentiation syndrome is a type of **cytokine release syndrome** from the large and rapid release of cytokines (immune substances) from leukemia cells after cancer treatments.
4. **Causes** of differentiation syndrome: treatment of acute promyelocytic leukemia (APL) with all-trans-retinoic acid (ATRA) and/or arsenic oxide; treatment of AML with IDH inhibitors (IDH2 inhibitor **enasidenib**; IDH1 inhibitor **ivosidenib**); treatment of AML with FLT3 mutant inhibitor **gilteritinib**.
5. **Differential diagnoses** of differentiation syndrome: sepsis, infection, thromboembolic, alveolar hemorrhage, allergy, and acute kidney injury (AKI).
6. **Treatment** of differentiation syndrome: **Decadron 10 mg bid** → q6h for greater than 3 days till defervescence symptom resolution, antibiotics, supportive care (fluid, renal replacement therapy); treat coagulopathy with **cryoprecipitate, fresh frozen plasma, and fibrinogen**.

4/27/2020

1. **Digoxin loading of 1 g in 24 h (iv and oral have almost the same bioavailability)**: 250 μg→ 6 h later 250 μg → 6 h later 250 μg → 6 h later 250 μg → next day 125 μg daily. Check digoxin level before discharge. Need to **decrease digoxin dosage to half or less** in patients with **chronic kidney disease or combination with amiodarone.** Will need to monitor the **digoxin trough** level, which should be <1.2.
2. **AFib**, uncontrolled HR 170 s, LVEF <25% on **metoprolol** 200 mg bid, can add **digoxin or amiodarone**. Diltiazem should not be used in patients with decreased ejection fraction.
3. **Seizure**: Keppra 250 mg bid, carbamazepine 100–100-50 mg, breakthrough seizure, add Vimpat 100 mg iv bid

4/28/2020

1. **Diuresis till no JVD**, IV diuresis, looking for body weight and getting the ideal body weight (BW) to know the need for diuresis dosage, ideally twice daily (BID) dosing. This patient has an LVEF <20%.
2. Death, contact the funeral home, arrange for the morgue, and contact relatives (these are nursing staff responsibilities).
3. **Uncontrolled sinus tachycardia:** look for myocardial infarction (MI), infection including endocarditis, pulmonary embolism, and other causes.

5/1/2020

1. **Arrhythmia**: abnormal impulse function: (A) automaticity (enhanced pacer); (B) early after depolarization; (C) delayed after depolarization. Reentrant: (A) antidromic- wide QRS; (B) orthodromic—narrow QRS. (LBBB and RBBB)
2. Right bundle branch block (**RBBB**) has a higher risk of atrioventricular nodal reentrant tachycardia (**AVNRT**).
3. Regular sinus tachycardia: AVNRT, atrial flutter (atrial depolarization, 2–1, 3–1, check p wave/atrial depolarization), atrial tachycardia.
4. With adenosine, AVRT/AVNRT breaks back to normal. **Heart rate (HR) 110–120 s often indicates atrial tachycardia; if HR > 200 s, it often indicates atrial flutter**.
5. Vimpat 50 mg bid, increase to 100 mg + 50 mg after 1 week; keep carbamazepine 100 mg tid, Keppra (250 mg qam, 500 mg qhs). After 3 days, cut carbamazepine to 50 mg qd.
6. **P wave morphology**: normally upward in lead I and II, biphasic or inverted in V1, inverted in aVR.

5/2/2020

1. **Digoxin toxicity**: PR interval prolongation, scooped or slurred ST wave, **T wave inversion (digoxin trough should be less than 1.2).** Digoxin toxicity risk increases in chronic kidney disease.
2. Digoxin, dosage decrease to qod once trough is 1.24 (ideally <1.2), continue metoprolol, add spironolactone.
3. **A typical central line should be used for < 7 days**. A non-tunneled CVC is usually used for 2–3 weeks.
4. Depakote 500 mg bid → increase to 1 g bid 1 week later. Check Depakote level 2 weeks later.
5. Kidney stone, order CT/US kidney.
6. **If AAA sp repair, check Doppler renal artery for AKI**.
7. **Metolazone** causes disturbances in Mg and K.
8. Longer than 3 weeks nasogastric tube feeding, do percutaneous endoscopic gastrostomy (PEG). Nasogastric tube feeding is a short-term fix.

5/3/2020

1. Stone, treatment with **tamsulosin,** and add intravenous fluid if inpatient to flush the stone out.
2. **Levaquin** needs to be dosed **750 mg qod** if renal dysfunction.
3. Family friend → conflicts of interests, transfer the patient to a different team
4. **Ureteral stones → urology consult especially if concerns for infected kidney stone**, do stent if renal function is not getting better. Hydroureter or hydronephrosis requires urology consults.

Neurology

5/4/2020

1. Keppra 1 g load, then 500 mg bid.

2. **Intracranial hemorrhage** on antiplatelet therapy (APT), no need for **platelet** (PLT) **transfusion** unless neurosurgery or PLT < 50–100 depending on neurosurgeon or neurologist recommendations.
3. **Contraindications for tPA**: intracranial neoplasm, arteriovenous malformation (AVM), or aneurysm.
4. Coronary artery bypass grafting (CABG) → stroke days later after CABG → ICA stenosis → perform carotid bypass of ICA. Of note, **carotid bypass** is usually performed only if revascularization via **endarterectomy** and primary patch closure or **stenting** cannot be performed. **Stenting for symptomatic carotid stenosis may be associated with a higher risk of periprocedural stroke or death than endarterectomy**.
5. Left large cerebellar infarct thus increased risk for **hemorrhagic transformation**; thus, no anticoagulation (A/C).
6. **Seizure**: postictal confusion period, has no memory. **The commercial driver requires 10 years with no seizure to get a license**. Some states require a report to the Department of Motor Vehicle (DMV) for seizure.

5/6/2020

1. **Right parietal lobe**: contralateral **neglect**, constructional apraxia, denial of the defect.
2. **Left parietal lobe**: Gerstmann's syndrome (dysgraphia, dyscalculia, L-R disorientation, finger agnosia).
3. **Gliomas and meningiomas** are the most common intracranial tumors in adults.
4. **Astrocytoma**, homogenous in CT/MRI, seizure after resection of astrocytoma.
5. **3 types of tremors**: (1) cerebellar tremor (large amplitude), Parkinson's disease (small resting tremor), (2) medication-induced tremors, and (3) essential tremor (happens with movements).

5/7/2020

1. **Seizure + hallucination =** consider **autoimmune encephalitis**. Treatment: if confirmed, IVIG 25 g qd × 5 days (20 g IVIG alternates with 30 g IVIG, 0.4 g/kg) → IV solumedrol × 5 days.
2. **Bilateral motor weakness** only = consider metabolic problems (hypokalemia), check deep tendon reflex (DTR) to rule out Guillain-Barré syndrome (GBS).
3. Patients with **acute intermittent porphyria** usually present with **paralysis** + **hallucinations** or **seizures** + **abdominal pain** and not eating.
4. **The pontine gaze center, medial longitudinal fasciculus** (MLF), can affect both sides of the brain at pontine lesions (**internuclear ophthalmoplegia**).
5. **Carcinomatous meningitis** also known as leptomeningeal metastases from solid tumors, commonly seen in **melanoma**, **breast**, **lung**, and GI cancer. The most common presenting signs and symptoms were **headache** (39%), **nausea** and **vomiting** (25%), leg weakness (21%), **cerebellar dysfunction** (17%), altered mental status (16%), diplopia (14%), and facial weakness (13%)

6. **Seizure**: Depakote 500 mg bid → 500 mg tid. Depakote and Keppra used together can increase delirium, drowsiness, confusion, and difficulty concentrating.
7. CT head showing general vascular disease, can be treated with **aspirin** and **statin**.

5/8/2020

1. Stroke imaging: **DWI** shows a high-intensity signal of stroke within 3–30 min and lasts 6 h–4 weeks; **DWI-Flair mismatch** indicates stroke time < 4.5 h and is a candidate for tPA. Development of **hyperintense** signal on FLAIR is a sign of **vasogenic edema** which typically happens after 4.5 h since the onset of stroke. CT perfusion and MRI **DWI with FLAIR** (rapid tests for stroke of unknown duration) for endovascular procedures (mechanical thrombectomy vs tPA or both) 6–24 h after stroke.
2. Suspected **embolic stroke characteristics**: location over the **peripheral** cortex, **multiple** locations, **cryptogenic**. Will need a loop recorder or event monitor to rule out cardiac arrhythmia.
3. Hyperdensity of artery (**dense artery sign**) on non-contrast CT = consider **ischemic stroke**, indicates embolic or atherosclerotic occlusion of an artery, usually middle cerebral artery (MCA), posterior cerebral artery (PCA), vertebral artery, or basilar artery. **CTA spot sign** is a sign of intracerebral hemorrhage.
4. **ASPECTS score** (total 10) is used for MCA stroke: caudate, lentiform nucleus (pallidum + putamen), internal capsule, M1-3, M4-6, insular cortex. Striatum = caudate + lentiform nucleus. Every region's involvement is counted as **-1**. ASPECTS score of **≤7** indicates a **poor prognosis in 3 months** and high risks for hemorrhage and more likely to benefit from thrombolysis. ASPECTS score **≤ 4** indicates a high risk for symptomatic **hemorrhage and mortality**.
5. **SWI** bleeding is black. **T1** weighted MRI **enhances fat** and is good for looking at **mass**, and tumor (high-intensity signals = white)
6. **Active thrombosis with malignancy** on aspirin and Eliquis. Treatment: switch to aspirin & Lovenox plus minus Plavix or Brilinta (ticagrelor).
7. **Small ischemic stroke** may or may not need to hold anticoagulation (A/C) for 24 h. If ba large stroke, hold A/C for 48 h to 2 weeks for concerns of hemorrhagic conversion.
8. Dual antiplatelet therapy (DAPT) in large vessel atherosclerotic stenosis. In acute stroke **large vessel occlusion**, will need to assess the eligibility for **mechanical thrombectomy**.
9. **Transient ischemic attack**: start aspirin 162–325 mg daily alone if **ABCD2** score < 4; if ≥4, give dual antiplatelet therapy with aspirin and Plavix for 21 days. If **thrombocytopenia**, maybe monotherapy with aspirin is more appropriate.

5/12/2020

1. **New seizure** from brain metastasis. Treatment: **Keppra** 1 g load followed by 500 mg bid po.

2. **Amantadine** side effects include **psychosis**, and central nervous system (CNS) **depression**, and if it happens, it has to be **weaned off**.
3. Low blood pressure (BP) can give **global hypotension** causing altered mental status (AMS).
4. Combination or overlapping of tyrosine kinase inhibitors (**TKIs**) with **immunotherapy** or shortly after carries a high risk for **pneumonitis**.
5. (A) **High-grade glioma**: hypointense mass on T1 that enhances after contrast infusion. **Glioblastoma multiforme (GBM)** has rim enhancement with central necrosis and cystic changes.

   (B) **Primary CNS lymphoma**: lesions are hypointense or isointense on T2 weighted MRI and tend to enhance homogenously after contrast. Typical locations of lesions include white matter, basal ganglia, and corpus callosum.

   (C) **Low-grade glioma**: T2 FLAIR hyperintense expansive lesion.

   (D) **Brain metastasis**: rounded, well-circumscribed masses that enhance after contrast; >0.5–1 cm will have **vasoedema**.

   (E) **Meningiomas**: extra-axial, dura-based mass that is isotense or hypotense to gray matter on T2 and isotense or hypertense on T2.
6. **Glioma** classification: astrocytoma, oligoastrocytoma, oligodendroglioma, glioblastoma.
7. **Dizziness**: neuro-TIA, seizure; peripheral vs. central vertigo; vestibulopathy.

5/29/2020

1. **High-risk chest pain**: typical features including high-risk factors, worse with exertion, better with rest, and relief with nitroglycerin. In high-risk chest pain, even with no troponin leak, treat as unstable angina with **heparin drip if no major contraindications ⇒ cardiology** consult.
2. CT abdomen/pelvis revealed **moderate stenosis of celiac artery** → vascular consult → CTA → angiogram.
3. Follow other specialty recommendations.
4. The patient's **health** is more important than **economic costs**.

5/31/2020

1. **Sinus node dysfunction or sick sinus syndrome (SSS)**: typically, symptomatic with fatigue, lightheadedness, palpitations, presyncope, and or syncope. EKG: sinus bradycardia, sinus pauses, arrest, sinoatrial exit block, and alternating bradycardia with atrial tachycardia. Diagnosis and treatment: ambulatory **EKG** monitoring and **pacemaker**.
2. **Aortic stenosis management**: avoid aggressive diuresis, keep euvolemic rather than hypervolemic, control hypertension, and maintain sinus rhythm.
3. **Bradycardia**: hold atrioventricular node blocker, stop Cardizem and metoprolol if any.
4. **AFib**: no P wave, irregular rhythm, tele.
5. Pay attention to tele readings, read them thoroughly.
6. On chronic steroids while needing to check morning cortisol level: **check morning cortisol 24–48 h** after stopping Decadron or steroids.

7. **Altered mental status (AMS) etiologies**: seizure, metabolic encephalopathy, sepsis, infarcts
8. **VTach/VFib case (stat cardiology consult)**: treat with amiodarone → developed long QTc → stop amio, start lidocaine IV and mexiletine 100 mg tid → 200 mg tid mexiletine and stop lidocaine → Automatic Implantable Cardioverter Defibrillator (AICD) revealed further episodes of VTach → order sotalol 80 mg bid (EKG 2 h after each dose); monitor inside hospital for 48 h → VTach again → EP study and ablation.
9. **Non-sustained VTach**: greater or equal to 3 beats of VTach ≥100 bpm, but less than **30 s**.

6/1/2020

1. **SVT vs. VTach**: SVT with aberrancy (aberrant conduction due to WPW or LBBB/RBBB). RS complex → R to S interval > 100 ms → AV dissociation: these are morphology criteria for **VT presentation** in V1-V2 and V6.
2. EKG tutorial, **5 boxes is 1 s**. Types of SA nodal dysfunctions: (A) **sinus pause or arrest** (<2×PP); (B) **SA nodal exit block** (first, second, and third degree). **Variants of SA nodal dysfunction**: (A) sinus arrhythmia (variation of PP interval > .12 s, common with digoxin or morphine); (B) wandering atrial pacemaker.
3. **Atrial and AV nodal (SV) arrhythmias**: (A) escape atrial beats; (B) atrial tachycardia; (C) atrial tachycardia with AV block; (D) wandering atrial pacemaker; (E) multifocal atrial tachycardia; (F) PAC; (G) AVNRT.

1/28/2021

1. Indications for removal of nasogastric (NG) suction tube: passing gas, bowel movement, clamp for 24 h before removal; **no more than 300 cc suction per 8 h shift**.
2. If no improvement, a timely specialist consultation is vital.
3. Make sure to mention the **severity or gravity of the disease** to the patient's family with the patient's permission if the patient is his/her own decision maker.
4. **Furosemide 10 mg/ml 200 mg in 50 ml NS at 70 cc/h plus metolazone 5 mg daily** for anasarca.
5. Indications for **removal of chest tube**: drainage threshold of **200 mL** or less per day, no more air leaking/escaping through the tube. **Clamp 6 h** before removing the chest tube with chest **X-ray before and after clamping** as well as daily chest X-ray to monitor chest condition.

Takeaway Messages

1. Massive transfusion: red blood cell (RBC), plasma, and platelet (PLT) should be given a 1:1:1 ratio.
2. Orlistat (Xenical), phentermine/topiramate (Qsymia), naltrexone/bupropion, and nowadays GLP-1 agonists for weight loss, long-term use.
3. Serum Keppra check does not need to be in the therapeutic range.
4. Bloody diarrhea with antibiotics may indicate hemolytic uremic syndrome (HUS) with microangiopathic hemolytic anemia, thrombocytopenia, and acute

kidney injury. Antibiotics increase risks for full-blown HUS from Shiga toxin–producing Escherichia coli (STEC) leading to death.

5. MRI brain is needed for red flag headaches: anticoagulation use, ≥50 yo, progressive headache (HA) pattern.
6. DWI-FLAIR mismatch indicates infarct less than 4.5 h.
7. Digitalis toxicity: junctional tachycardia with variable conduction delays in AFib.
8. Indications for removal of a nasogastric (NG) suction tube include no more than 300 cc suction per 8 h shift. Indications for removal of the chest tube include a drainage threshold of 200 mL or less per day and no more air leaking/escaping through the tube.

Further Readings and References

1. Lefort, A., J.L. Mainardi, C. Selton-Suty, et al. 2000. Streptococcus pneumoniae endocarditis in adults. A multicenter study in France in the era of penicillin resistance (1991–1998). The Pneumococcal Endocarditis Study Group. *Medicine (Baltimore)* 79 (5): 327–337.
2. Hosker, C., and D. Ward. 2017. Hypoactive delirium. *British Medical Journal* 357: j2047.
3. Müller, M.D., P. Lyrer, M.M. Brown, and L.H. Bonati. 2020. Carotid artery stenting versus endarterectomy for treatment of carotid artery stenosis. *Cochrane Database Systematic Reviews* 2020 (2): CD000515.
4. Oliveira-Filho, J., and O.B. Samuels. *Mechanical thrombectomy for acute ischemic stroke*, ed. J. Biller and A.A. Rabinstein. Waltham, MA: UpToDate. Accessed January 31, 2024.

Part II
Ambulatory Medicine

My ambulatory medicine rotation during internal medicine residency training was a pivotal experience that exposed me to the unique challenges and rewards of providing primary care service in an outpatient setting, especially in underserved populations. Throughout the rotation, I had the opportunity to immerse myself in the practice of ambulatory medicine, caring for patients with a diverse range of medical conditions and health needs, and socioeconomic backgrounds. One of the most rewarding aspects of my ambulatory medicine rotation was the opportunity to develop long-term relationships with patients and families.

Internal medicine residency training in ambulatory medicine prepares physicians to excel as primary care providers, outpatient clinicians, and future leaders in healthcare delivery. Goals of ambulatory medicine in residency training included: (1) gain expertise in managing chronic medical conditions commonly seen in the outpatient setting; (2) develop competencies in preventive healthcare practices, including health screenings, immunizations, lifestyle modifications, and risk factor reduction; (3) collaborate with interdisciplinary healthcare teams, including nurses, nurse practitioners, physician assistants, pharmacists, dietitians, social workers, and other allied health professionals, to deliver comprehensive care to patients; (4) develop strong communication skills to engage patients in shared decision-making, educate them about their health conditions, and empower them to actively participate in their care.

Additionally, ambulatory medicine training incorporated principles of quality improvement and population health management to enhance the delivery of healthcare services and improve patient outcomes. I learned to identify gaps in care, implement evidence-based interventions, and measure outcomes to drive continuous improvement in clinical practice. Prevention is a major component of ambulatory medicine; I conducted routine screenings, administered vaccinations, and provided counseling on topics such as smoking cessation, diet and exercise, and cancer screening. I learned that patients are the major deciders of their health and by empowering patients to take ownership of their health and adopt healthy behaviors, patients themselves can mitigate disease burden and improve quality of life.

Overall, my ambulatory medicine rotation was a transformative experience that deepened my appreciation for the art and science of primary care. Through patient-centered care, preventive medicine, diagnostic challenges, interdisciplinary collaboration, and lifelong learning, I gained invaluable insights and skills that have shaped my practice as a compassionate and competent physician in the outpatient setting and beyond.

Notes of this section were based on the American College of Physicians (ACP) Online, UpToDate, and MedScape websites, supplemented and revised per journal articles and guidelines. Topics in this section included addiction medicine, anemia, adolescent medicine, alcoholism, anxiety, depression, dementia, chronic kidney disease, gout, dizziness, statin use, GERD, headache, obesity, immunization, hypertension, common eye problems, HIV, chronic musculoskeletal pain, asthma, thyroid issues, upper respiratory disease, pneumonia, and osteoporosis.

Chapter 14
Behavioral Health

Addiction: Illicit Drugs

1. **Marijuana** use impairs neurocognitive function. Marijuana can cause cannabinoid hyperemesis syndrome and on rare occasions, high-grade heart block.
2. Diagnosis of a **substance use disorder** is based on the presence of ≥2 of 11 criteria which can be categorized into impaired control, social impairment, risky use, and pharmacological dependence.
3. **MDMA (ecstasy)** and **amphetamines** are phenethylamines mediating the actions of dopamine, norepinephrine, and/or serotonin. **Adderall** = amphetamine and dextroamphetamine.
4. **Adderall** can cause insomnia and hypertensive urgency; treatment of hypertensive urgency is not to add more and more quetiapine and blood pressure medications but to decrease or even stop Adderall. **Vyvanse** = lisdexamfetamine. **Vyvanse** and **Adderall** and other stimulants may cause **peripheral vasculopathy** and **Raynaud's phenomenon** from the peripheral release of catecholamines.
5. Risk for **opioid overdose**: recent abstinence, detoxification, incarceration. **Treatment for opioid overdose**: naloxone 0.4 mg or 0.8 mg subcu or iv, may repeat every 2–3 min. In some patients, **naloxone** continuous drip and usually overnight hospital observation is necessary.
6. **Opioid withdrawal**: treatment with partial opioid agonists (i.e., buprenorphine) and clonidine are available to primary care providers. "All practitioners with a current DEA registration that includes Schedule III authority may now prescribe buprenorphine for **Opioid Use Disorder** if permitted by the local state law."
7. Buprenorphine can **precipitate opioid withdrawal**: buprenorphine is not good for pain control in acute conditions. Patients on a full opioid agonist regularly should be in mild opioid withdrawal (stop all full opioid agonist analgesics) before restarting buprenorphine therapy.

K. Zhou, *Internal Medicine Training Notes and Survival Guide*,
https://doi.org/10.1007/978-1-0716-4039-5_14

8. **Buprenorphine**: 2 mg and 8 mg pills and the typical dose is 8–24 mg/day as a combination with **naloxone** in a film strip formulation (Suboxone) or a sublingual tablet formulation (**Zubsolv**).
9. **Initiation of suboxone treatment** in a patient with acute femur fracture sp. intramedullary nailing: Prescription for Naloxone 0.4 mg intranasal as needed for opioid overdose, acetaminophen 1000 mg 3 times daily, oxycodone 5–10 mg every 4–6 h as needed for acute pain. Because of his acute pain with femur fracture, recommend a low dose suboxone initiation protocol: 0.5 mg daily- day 1; 0.5 mg twice daily- day 2; 1 mg twice daily- day 3; 2 mg twice daily- day 4; 4 mg twice daily- day 5; 4 mg 3 times daily- day 6; 4 mg 4 times daily - day 7 [stop other opioids (oxycodone) at this time. But may need to continue short-term for him because of his acute pain]. Avoid alcohol, marijuana, benzodiazepines, and any intoxication.
10. Agents with alpha and beta blockade such as **labetalol** or **carvedilol** (not metoprolol) are effective at **reducing blood pressure without potentiating vasoconstriction**, and thus they are possibly safe to use in patients with **cocaine abuse**.
11. **Cocaine abuse treatment**: diazepam 10 mg q3-5 min, nitroglycerin, nitroprusside 0.3–.5 mg/kg/min (maximal dose 10 mg/kg/min), phentolamine (usually reserved as the last resort for hypertension) 1–2.5 mg q 5–15 min, or give valium 5 mg q3–5 min or lorazepam 1 mg IV q5-10 min.
12. Most patients with cocaine-induced myocardial infarction (MI) have underlying coronary artery disease (CAD). As such, coronary angiography is recommended in these patients.
13. Antidepressants **dopamine agonists/antagonists and anticonvulsants** may not be effective in stimulant abusers.
14. Phencyclidine (PCP) and ketamine cause **dissociative symptoms**. Lysergic acid diethylamide (LSD) causes **flashbacks**. Ecstasy or MDMA causes amphetamine-like effects including hypertension, hyperthermia, rhabdomyolysis, and arrhythmias.
15. Six components of **motivational interviewing** (Feedback, Responsibility, Advice, Menu Options, Empathy, and Self-Efficacy, FRAMES): Feedback of personal risks, emphasis on personal Responsibility for change, clear Advice for change, offering a Menu of options, therapeutic Empathy as part of the intervention, and enhance Self-efficacy.
16. The patient who takes methadone is overdosed, then revived with naloxone ⇒ consider **admitting to observation because of concerns of recurrent overdose effects** when naloxone wears off.

Alcoholism

1. **Patients with alcohol use disorder often develop fasting ketosis and alcoholic ketoacidosis. Clinical Institute Withdrawal Assessment (CIWA)** protocol.

2. **Alcoholism** diagnostic criteria: impaired control over drinking, preoccupation with the drug alcohol, use of alcohol despite adverse consequences, and distortion of thinking, most notably denial.
3. **Alcohol withdrawal**: do lorazepam 1 mg im, po, or iv, can increase to 2 mg or diazepam 5–10 mg po as needed. If in active withdrawal, will need admission for scheduled and prn benzodiazepines.
4. A **drink** is defined as 12 oz. of beer, 5 oz. of wine (table wine, a standard glass), or 1.5 oz. of distilled spirits (a shot glass), each containing about 0.5 fl oz. or 12 g of alcohol. **1 pint = 16 oz.**
5. **Limits of healthy** drinks: daily 2 drinks for males and 1 drink for females; 4 per occasion for males (3 for females).
6. **Brief counseling** has been shown to reduce unhealthy alcohol use for up to **4 years**.
7. There is **no maximum dosage** of benzodiazepines for the treatment of alcohol withdrawal, reports of >2000 mg of diazepam over 48 h for severe withdrawal. Treatments of benzodiazepines for typically 3 days are sufficient, but may need a week or longer.
8. Medications for alcohol use disorder or **alcoholism**: disulfiram (causes unpleasant feeling with drinking) 250–500 mg qd, naltrexone (reduces heavy drinking and promotes abstinence) 500–1000 ng qd, acamprosate (reduces heavy drinking and maintains abstinence) 666 mg tid. Off label use medications include topiramate (may reduce heavy drinking while treat comorbid migraine headaches or obesity/binge eating disorder) 100–250 mg bid, gabapentin (relieves symptoms while treating neuropathy, restless legs syndrome, insomnia, or anxiety) 300–600 tid, baclofen 30–80 mg qd, and ondansetron 4–8 mg bid.
9. **Unhealthy alcohol use** screening is recommended for all adults ≥18 years old: if positive, counsel on the healthy limits of drinking. **Unhealthy alcohol use** = 4 drinks/day or 14 drinks/week for healthy men aged 21–64 years; or 3 drinks/day or 7 drinks/week for women of any age and men 65 years or older.
10. The **CAGE** is used to screen for alcoholism, not unhealthy alcohol use. **Alcohol-related disorders**: alcohol abuse, alcohol dependence, alcohol use disorder.
11. **Setting clear goals** is key for effective counseling in alcoholism.
12. **Blood alcohol level (BAL) 0.08%**: 0.08 g alcohol in 100 ml of blood; this is the diagnostic criterion for intoxication.

Adolescent Medicine

1. Discussing confidentiality with both the teen and his/her parents at the beginning of the visit: the provision of confidential care.
2. A minor is emancipated through enlisting in the **military** or **marriage** or others as stated by local state law.
3. Parental consent is not needed for life or limb-saving treatment under emergency conditions.
4. **HEEADSSS** interview is used to assess psychosocial risks in adolescents: home, education, employment, eating, activities, drugs/alcohol, sexuality, suicide, depression, and safety.

5. **CRAFFT** questionnaire is used for substance use disorder screening in adolescents aged 12–21: CAR, RELAX, ALONE, FORGET, FRIENDS, TROUBLE.
6. **Controversial issues** for which confidential care is generally allowed: contraception, prenatal care, abortion, immunizations, sexually transmitted infections, HIV, substance abuse, and mental health issues; however, confidentiality is not unconditional. Many states allow minors to give informed consent for the aforementioned conditions but will need to check with state law first.
7. **Early adolescent**: preoccupied with self, often demanding increased privacy. **Middle adolescents**: watch for risk-taking behavior, peak peer involvement, and peak parental conflicts. Late adolescents: watch for struggles with their own identity, social interactions, and/or moral issues.

Anxiety

1. **Generalized anxiety disorder (GAD)** refers to excessive and persistent anxiety and uncontrollable worry for at least 6 months not secondary to physiological effects of a substance or medical condition. Its diagnosis requires ≥3/6 symptoms: irritability, sleep disturbance, restlessness, fatigue, difficulty concentrating, and muscle tension. A cut-off score of **≥10** on the **Generalized Anxiety Disorder Assessment (GAD-7)** is an indication for treatment. **Risk factors** for **anxiety**: old age, female gender, and family history of anxiety.
2. **First-line treatments for GAD** include cognitive behavioral therapy, selective serotonin reuptake inhibitor (SSRI), serotonin–norepinephrine reuptake inhibitor (SNRI), or cognitive behavioral therapy in conjunction with either an SSRI or an SNRI. **Pregabalin** and **buspirone** (a partial agonist for 5HT1a receptors) and **quetiapine** are second-line or adjunctive medications for GAD. Other treatments of GAD may include imipramine, trazodone, anxiolytics benzodiazepines (high risks and should only be used in the short-term) like lorazepam → diazepam → clonazepam → alprazolam, and antihistamines such as hydroxyzine.
3. Indications for **referral to psychiatry** include complex or treatment-refractory GAD; **active psychosis; sensitivity, allergy, or intolerance to multiple medical classes; or suicidal ideation**.
4. Reassess **SSRI and SNRI** effects in **4–6 weeks**, can consider **taper off in 6 months** if well-controlled symptoms, and typically treat 3–6 months, or up to 1–2 years or even longer. If a patient carries a depression diagnosis**, anxiety can only be diagnosed once the depression is in remission**. When managing a patient with depression and anxiety, first treat **depression**.
5. After prescribing medications for GAD, we will need to **contact the patient in a week** to guard against suicidal ideation, have a **return visit in 1 month** to ascertain compliance, and monitor for significant adverse events; symptomatic relief usually happens in 4–6 weeks with SSRIs or SNRIs.
6. **Benzodiazepines** (BZDs) are used for acute exacerbation in depression. **Pregabalin, bupropion** (FDA-only approved for depression), and **buspirone** can all be used as augmentative therapy to SSRI or SNRI (duloxetine, venlafaxine) for GAD.

7. Sedatives-hypnotics of benzodiazepines and Ambien (zolpidem), Lunesta (eszopiclone), and Sonata (zaleplon) are usually only for anxiety and/or insomnia as a short-term relief and lack a good safety profile in older adults age 65 and older.
8. **Cognitive behavioral therapy and mindfulness-based stress reduction** are effective for anxiety as well as depression.
9. **Cognitive behavioral therapy** focuses on correcting cognitive distortions (**Thoughts**) and their associated behaviors (**Behaviors**) to improve emotional regulation (**Feelings**), such as activity scheduling and homework challenging and changing cognitive distortions. **Psychodynamic therapy** focuses on conscious and unconscious feelings and past experiences addressing underlying conflicts that are thought to be the source of anxiety. **Cognitive therapy** focuses on working through and correcting false beliefs about him/herself, and working out negative thoughts.
10. **SNRIs** such as **venlafaxine and duloxetine** are also useful in patients with chronic pain and depression.

Depression

1. Diagnosis of depression requires at least **2 weeks' duration with depressed mood or anhedonia (lack of interest or enjoyment)**, plus ≥3 other symptoms of the following: poor concentration, feeling excessive guilt or worthlessness, hopelessness, disrupted sleep, or tiredness or low energy.
2. **Psychomotor agitation** or **retardation** is one of the diagnostic symptoms of depression.
3. Depression interfering with **work** is considered **moderate or severe depression** and should be treated with pharmacotherapy and counseling. Psychotherapy and symptom monitoring are the first-line treatments for mild to moderate depression.
4. Assessment of depression focuses on **identifying potential causes** (like prescribed and/or illicit drug use and psychosocial factors) and **contributing medical comorbidities** (like anemia, hypothyroidism, anemia, chronic infections, and seizures).
5. **First-line medications** in moderate to severe depression include selective serotonin reuptake inhibitors (**SSRI**s), serotonin–norepinephrine reuptake inhibitors (**SNRI**s), **bupropion, and mirtazapine; vilazodone, vortioxetine, and levomilnacipran** may also be used.
6. **Tricyclic antidepressants (TCAs)** amitriptyline, imipramine, and nortriptyline are fatal in overdose; **<10 pills** each time can be prescribed.
7. Citalopram, escitalopram, sertraline, and all **second-generation** antidepressants (venlafaxine, bupropion, mirtazapine, and others) but not TCAs are equally effective for depression.
8. SSRIs can be used for **depression with daytime fatigue and hypersomnolence**. TCAs and SNRIs can be used to treat **chronic pain**.
9. **Dysthymia** diagnosis: symptoms suggestive of depression but failure to meet diagnostic criteria for depression and ≥ **2 years** of duration.

10. Paroxysmal sadness with preserved self-esteem = **bereavement** or **grief**. If symptoms last **≥2 months, antidepressants** are indicated.
11. Depression screening consists of asking if the patient is **depressed** or **has anhedonia**.
12. **Psychosocial stressors** will need **counseling**.
13. **Abrupt discontinuation of SSRI** can cause withdrawal syndrome of **paresthesias**, **tinnitus,** and **vertigo**.
14. Efficient = prasugrel; Effexor = venlafaxine (37.5–225 mg a day).
15. If only partially responsive, may **advance to higher** doses early in the course of anti-depression medication therapy. If no improvement after 6–8 weeks, need to **switch medications** (either the same or a different category of antidepressant).
16. If the risk of recurrence is high, depression medication treatment should be continued for **2 years**.
17. **Remission** definition: no less than **3 consecutive weeks** of absence of both sad mood and reduced interests along with fewer than **3 remaining symptoms** of major depression. **Recovery** definition: at least **4 months** following the onset of remission, during which a relapse has not occurred. Discontinuing therapy for depression can be considered after **6 months of clinical response**.
18. **Augmentation** of **citalopram 20 mg** daily (maximal 40 mg daily) with sustained-release **bupropion, mirtazapine, aripiprazole,** or **buspirone** can be effective for treatment-resistant depression.
19. **Bupropion, mirtazapine, risperidone, and atypical antipsychotics (e.g., aripiprazole, quetiapine, brexpiprazole)** can be used as an add-on treatment to other SSRIs to augment response in depression.
20. **Mild depression treatment**: observation, single modality treatment, or combination therapy. **Moderate or severe depression** treatment: combination therapy.
21. All SSRIs and venlafaxine may increase the risks for suicidality among persons younger than 24 years of age.
22. In suicidal ideation, we will need to **check intent and plan**.

Further Readings and References

1. Alford, D.P., P. Compton, and J.H. Samet. 2006. Acute pain management for patients receiving maintenance methadone or buprenorphine therapy. *Annals of Internal Medicine* 144 (2): 127–134.
2. Nehring, S.M., R.J. Chen, and A.M. Freeman. 2024. Alcohol use disorder. [Updated 8 Aug 2023]. In *StatPearls [Internet]*. Treasure Island: StatPearls Publishing. Available from: https://www.ncbi.nlm.nih.gov/books/NBK436003/.
3. Park, L.T., and C.A. Zarate Jr. 2019. Depression in the primary care setting. *The New England Journal of Medicine* 380 (6): 559–568.

4. Stein, M.B., and J. Sareen. 2015. Clinical practice. Generalized anxiety disorder. *The New England Journal of Medicine* 373 (21): 2059–2068.
5. Winslow, B.T., M. Onysko, and M. Hebert. 2016. Medications for alcohol use disorder. *American Family Physician* 93 (6): 457–465.
6. Zhou, K., P. Jia, S. Bhargava, et al. 2017. Opioid tapering in patients with prescription opioid use disorder: A retrospective study. *Scandinavian Journal of Pain* 17: 167–173.

Chapter 15
Cardiovascular Health

Hyperlipidemia

1. The USPSTF recommends statin for the primary prevention of CVD for adults aged 40–75 years with 1 or more CVD risk factors (i.e., dyslipidemia, diabetes, hypertension, or smoking) and an estimated **10-year CVD risk of ≥ 10%**. The USPSTF recommends that statin is offered for the primary prevention of CVD for selective adults aged 40–75 years who have 1 or more of these CVD risk factors and an estimated 10-year CVD risk of **7.5%–10%**.
2. In clinical ASCVD, prescribe **high-intensity statins or maximally tolerated statins to reduce LDL-C by ≥ 50%** (in very high-risk ASCVD, LDL-C goal is <70 mg/dL), consider adding ezetimibe and/or a PCSK9 inhibitor if necessary to reach the goal.
3. **Major ASCVD events** include recent acute coronary syndrome, history of myocardial infarction, ischemic stroke, and symptomatic peripheral arterial disease (claudication with ABI < 0.85 or previous revascularization or amputation).
4. In patients with LDL-C ≥ 190 mg/dL without ASCVD (regardless of age), prescribe **high-intensity statins or moderate-intensity statins plus ezetimibe to ensure an LDL-C goal of < 100/mg/dL.** Consider adding a PCSK9 inhibitor as appropriate.
5. In patients 40–75 years old **with diabetes** but no ASCVD, if LDL-C ≥ 70 mg/dL, **moderate-intensity statin** should be prescribed and **high-intensity statin (or moderate-intensity statin plus ezetimibe)** should be prescribed for patients **≥50 years** to reduce LDL-C by ≥50%.
6. In patients of 40–75 years old **without diabetes** and LDL-C ≥ 70 mg/dL, need to calculate ASCVD risks: <5% = low risk; 5%–7.5% = borderline risk; ≥7.5%–<20% = intermediate risk; ≥20% = high risk. For intermediate risks, initiating statin to reduce LDL-C by 30%–49%; for high risks, initiating **statin to reduce LDL-C ≥ 50%**. In these patients with **intermediate** risks for ASCVD, **calculate coronary artery calcium (CAC)** score if a decision about statin therapy is

K. Zhou, *Internal Medicine Training Notes and Survival Guide*,
https://doi.org/10.1007/978-1-0716-4039-5_15

uncertain: initiate statin if CAC score ≥ 100 or CAC score 1–99 but age ≥ 55 years.

7. **PCSK9 inhibitor Repatha** (evolocumab) is an alternative or offers an additive benefit option to statin if high-intensity statin therapy is desired.
8. **Diabetes specific risk enhancers:** T1DM > 20 years, T2DM > 10 years, albuminuria >30 μg/g creatinine, eGFR <60 mL/min/1.73 m^2, retinopathy, neuropathy, ABI < 0.9.
9. **Resistance training** lowers LDL and TG.
10. **Risk-enhancing factors for CAD** include a family history of premature ASCVD, CKD, metabolic syndrome, chronic inflammatory conditions, south Asian, LDL-C > 160 mg/dL, hsCRP >2, Lp(a) > 50 mg/dL, apoB >130 mg/dL, and decreased ankle-brachial index (ABI) < 0.9.
11. In persons >75 years without ASCVD, diabetes, or LDL-C ≥ 190 mg/dL, do not initiate statin therapy. **Start or continue statin in all patients ages 75–84 with diabetes or known occlusive vascular disease**. Low- to moderate-intensity statins were associated with a greater reduction in LDL-C levels in people >75 years than in young patients.
12. Statin therapy may be considered in patients **≤30 years old with T1DM and T2DM if end-organ damage or LDL-C > 100 mg/dL**. Initiate moderate or **high-intensity statin for ≥ high-risk patients with diabetes of 20–39 years old targeting LDL-C reduction ≥ 50% and goal < 70 mg/dL**. High risks refer to diabetes without target organ damage but duration of diabetes ≥10 years or another risk factor. Very high risks refer to diabetes with target organ damage, three major risk factors, or early onset T1DM of long duration.

Obesity and Overweight

1. **Exercise alone** is slow in weight loss: **0.1 kg/week**.
2. **Pharmacotherapy** is **indicated** if BMI ≥ 30, or BMI 27–29.9 with at least one obesity-related comorbidities like hypertension, hyperlipidemia, type 2 diabetes (T2DM), or sleep apnea.
3. **Bariatric surgery** is indicated for BMI > 40 or BMI ≥ 35 with T2DM, hypertension or obstructive sleep apnea (OSA).
4. **Risk assessment** in obese patients: existing heart or vascular disease, T2DM, OSA, and high waist circumference with BMI > 40 in males and > 35 in females confer a high risk of mortality and morbidity.
5. **Initial goal** for weight loss: **5%–10%** weight loss over **6 months or at least 10% weight loss at 12 months**. Weight loss of ≥15% is associated with a decreased all-cause mortality rate.
6. **Atkins diet**: low carbs, high fat and protein. **Ornish diet**: low fat. **South Beach Diet**: low carb, high protein, and low fat.
7. **Reduce calories by 500–750 Kcal/day to produce 1–2 lbs/week weight loss**. Moderate-intensity (defined as 50%–70% of maximal heart rate) exercise 75–150 min per week plus resistance training 2–3 times a week is recommended.

8. **Weight loss medications for long-term use**: GLP-1 agonists (semaglutide, liraglutide, tirzepatide), orlistat, phentermine-topiramate, naltrexone-bupropion, and Gelesis100. Short-term use (12 weeks) weight loss medications include phentermine, diethylpropion, benzphetamine, and phendimetrazine. Metformin is commonly used off-label for long-term obesity management.
9. Two FDA-approved **metabolic and bariatric procedures:** Roux-en-Y bypass procedure, and laparoscopic sleeve gastrectomy (LSG). They require screening and supplementing thiamin, vitamin B12, folate, iron, vitamin D, calcium, vitamin A, vitamin E, vitamin K, zinc, and copper.
10. Two FDA-approved **bariatric endoscopic procedures**: intragastric balloons and endoscopic sleeve gastroplasty. Side effects may include nausea/vomiting (20%) and abdominal pain in intragastric balloons while both can cause hiatal hernia and gastric ulcers.

Hypertension

1. **Ambulatory blood pressure monitoring** or home blood pressure monitoring is necessary to confirm a diagnosis of hypertension as white-coat hypertension is common.
2. A **24-hour ambulatory average blood pressure** of ≥130/80 correlates with an office reading of ≥140/90 = diagnosis of hypertension and requires pharmacological treatments in patients <60 years of age.
3. Upon diagnosis of hypertension, **assess cardiovascular risks and target organ damage** including hypertensive retinopathy, vascular bruits, left ventricular hypertrophy, ventricular failure, diminished pedal pulses, kidney functions, and neurologic abnormalities. Routine tests for target organ damage assessments include serum creatinine and eGFR, dipstick urine test with albumin creatinine ratio, and 12-lead EKG.
4. **Resistant hypertension** requires screening for **secondary hypertension** including primary aldosteronism, chronic kidney disease or renal parenchymal disease, renal artery stenosis, obstructive sleep apnea (OSA), and substance/drug-induced hypertension.
5. **Hypertension** (HTN) goals: initiate pharmacological treatments in patients with chronic kidney disease or diabetes mellitus (DM) if blood pressure **≥ 140/90 mmHg**. Patients <65 with blood pressure < 140/90 and 10 years ASCVD risk <10% may be managed with lifestyle modification to reach goal blood pressure < 130/80.
6. **Antidepressants, antipsychotics, NSAIDs, and tyrosine kinase inhibitors** can increase blood pressure.
7. For all patients with diabetes, coronary artery disease, chronic kidney disease, or heart failure, the goal of therapy is the same: **<130/80 mmHg.**
8. In younger patients (<65) with 10 years ASCVD risk <10%, and patients with a history of non-lacunar CVA, lifestyle modification rather than pharmaceuticals may be appropriate if sBP < 140 to get to goal blood pressure < 130/80.
9. In African American patients with hypertension and diabetes, but no proteinuria, a **thiazide diuretic or calcium channel blocker** is preferred as first-line

treatment for hypertension. **ACEi** is the preferred drug for hypertension in chronic kidney disease (CKD), regardless of proteinuria.

10. JNC 8 Guidelines: ≥60 years, treat if blood pressure ≥ 150/90 mmHg. <60 years, treat if blood pressure ≥ 140/90 mmHg. In chronic kidney disease and diabetes, treat if blood pressure ≥ 140/90 mmHg.
11. Thiazide diuretic was more effective than a CCB or ACEI in hypertension control in congestive heart failure
12. Alpha blocker use increases risks for poor cerebrovascular, heart failure, and combined cardiovascular outcomes

Further Readings and References

1. Elmaleh-Sachs, A., J.L. Schwartz, C.T. Bramante, et al. 2023. Obesity management in adults: A review. *Journal of the American Medical Association* 330 (20): 2000–2015.
2. Grundy, S.M., and K.R. Feingold. 2000. Guidelines for the management of high blood cholesterol. [Updated 2022 May 28]. In *Endotext [Internet]*, ed. K.R. Feingold, B. Anawalt, M.R. Blackman, et al. South Dartmouth: MDText.com, Inc.. Available from: https://www.ncbi.nlm.nih.gov/books/NBK305897/.
3. James, P.A., S. Oparil, B.L. Carter, et al. 2014. 2014 evidence-based guideline for the management of high blood pressure in adults: Report from the panel members appointed to the Eighth Joint National Committee (JNC 8). *Journal of the American Medical Association* 311 (5): 507–520.
4. Marshall, B., and N. Bennett. 2020. PURL: How old is too old for statins? *The Journal of Family Practice* 69 (5): 257–259.
5. O'Toole, T., M.D. Kelsey, N.P. Shah, R.W. McGarrah, and N.J. Pagidipati. 2022. Eradicating atherosclerosis: Should we start statins at younger ages and at lower LDL-Cs. *Current Cardiology Reports* 24 (10): 1397–1406.

Chapter 16
Diabetes and Thyroid Dysfunction and Anemia

Diabetes

1. **Screen diabetes** in all adults >45 yo, all patients with BP > 135/80, and overweight or obese starting at age ≥ 35, screen q3y.
2. **Diabetic** patients: limit carbohydrates to 45%–60% of total calories, and saturated fats to less than 7% of total daily calories.
3. **Common diabetes medication categories:** alpha-glucosidase inhibitors (acarbose), biguanides (metformin), bile acid sequestrants (colesevelam), dopamine-2 agonists (bromocriptine), DPP-4 inhibitors (gliptins like alogliptin, linagliptin), meglitinides (glinides like nateglinide and repaglinide), SGLT2 inhibitors (canagliflozin, dapagliflozin, and empagliflozin), sulfonylureas (glipizide, glimepiride, and glyburide). thiazolidinediones (TZDs, like pioglitazone and rosiglitazone), and glucagon-like peptide-1 agonists (GLP-1 agonists, like dulaglutide, liraglutide, semaglutide, exenatide, and lixisenatide).
4. **Thiazolidinediones** (TZDs), sulfonylureas, glinides, and insulin cause weight gain. **HA1c > 9%** should be treated with insulin.
5. The **fasting glucose goal is ≤ 130 in diabetes**, check morning fasting glucose, and increase glargine by 2–4 units every third day if glucose >130 mg/dL.
6. Spot **urine albumin to creatinine** ratio (normal <30) should be checked annually. NPH requires twice daily dosing. Random urine **total protein to creatinine** ratio is normally less than 0.2 mg/mg; if >**3.5** mg/mg, it is nephrotic proteinuria
7. Urine albumin to creatinine ratio 30–300 = **microalbuminuria** while >300 = **macroalbuminuria**.
8. Patients with impaired fasting glucose should have a target **weight loss of 5%–10%** and increase physical activities to **150 min**/week. **Metformin** may be appropriate for impaired fasting glucose in obese patients under 60 years old with at least 1 other risk factor for developing diabetes mellitus (DM), especially, family history, low HDL-C, or others.

K. Zhou, *Internal Medicine Training Notes and Survival Guide*,
https://doi.org/10.1007/978-1-0716-4039-5_16

9. Tight glycemic control lowers **microvascular complications** (eye, kidney, and neuropathy), but is unclear for **macrovascular complications** (heart, peripheral artery disease, cerebrovascular disease).
10. Dual therapy for glucose control is needed if HA1c > 9%. Patients with diabetes and presenting with **symptomatic hyperglycemia** (polyuria, polydipsia, blurry vision, and possibly dehydration and weight loss) should receive insulin.
11. If HA1c is not at goal, may add 1 **rapid-acting insulin injection before the largest meal**, add GLP-1 agonist, or change to premixed insulin 2–3 × /days, 2/3 a.m. + 1/3 p.m. or 1/2 a.m. + 1/2 p.m.
12. When adding **prandial insulin** on basal insulin, if HA1c < 8%, but not at target, consider **decreasing basal** by the same rate.
13. If basal insulin >0.5 u/kg, **prandial insulin** should be added. TZD or SGLT-2 inhibitors to basal insulin may be helpful in those on high doses of basal insulin.
14. Exenatide (GLP-1 inhibitor) and sitagliptin (DPP-4 inhibitor), glimepiride (sulfonylureas), and glinides (nateglinide) are **insulin secretagogues and should not be used together**. This rule likely applies to other medications of the same categories.

Thyroid Abnormalities

1. Indications for treatment of **subclinical hyperthyroidism**: >65 years old with suppressed TSH (<0.1 mU/L to prevent cardiac arrhythmias), <age 65 years with heart disease, osteoporosis, or symptoms. Consideration of treatment in the aforementioned conditions when the TSH is 0.1–0.5 mIU/L.
2. Indications for treatment of **subclinical hypothyroidism**: serum TSH >10 mIU/ml, symptoms of hypothyroidism, positive anti-TPO antibodies, evidence of atherosclerotic cardiovascular disease, heart failure, or risk factors for heart disease.
3. **Thyroid nodule** with increased risk for malignancy: **hypervascularity, punctate calcifications, hyperechogenicity, or irregular borders**.

Anemia

1. **Normocytic anemia** differential diagnoses: mixed micro and macro, anemia of chronic disease, hemolytic anemia with inadequate bone marrow response (check reticulocyte count and haptoglobin), chronic liver disease, renal failure, aplastic anemia, pure red cell aplasia, thyroid disease, myelofibrosis, and multiple myeloma (MM).
2. **Microcystic anemia** with normal red blood cell distribution width (RDW) and high RBC count, do serum hemoglobin electrophoresis for thalassemia.
3. **Mentzer Index** = MCV (fl) /RBC count (millions per microliter); if >13, it is likely iron deficiency anemia (IDA) whereas if <12, it is likely beta cell thalassemia.
4. Thalassemia trait has normal RDW, but normal or high RBC/ferritin.
5. **Macrocytic anemia with hypersegmented neutrophils**: B12 and/or folate deficiency, myelodysplastic syndrome (MDS), hypothyroidism, liver disease, alcohol, drugs (cyclophosphamide, hydroxyurea, and antiretroviral medications)

6. **Spherocytes** may result from **autoimmune hemolytic anemia**. If concerns for autoimmune hemolytic anemia, check LDH, haptoglobin, and direct antiglobulin test (Coomb's test). Coomb's test is done by mixing the patient's red blood cells with anti-human globulin (Ab to IgG and C3).
7. **Iron deficiency anemia**: glossitis, cheilitis, koilonychias (spoon nails). **Burr cell** (acanthocytes) -liver disease. **Dermatitis herpetiformis**: seen in celiac disease (iron deficiency due to malabsorption), also seen in B12 deficiency.
8. **The soluble transferrin receptor** in iron deficiency is elevated, but in anemia of chronic disease (ACD), the soluble transferrin receptor is normal.
9. **Peripheral blood smear** in aplastic anemia: decreased platelet and leukocytes, giant proerythroblast in parvovirus, polychromasia of RBC (HIV, EBV, CMV, non-ABC hepatitis), lack of immature RBC.
10. **Pelger-Huet anomaly** seen in acute myeloid leukemia (AML), chronic myeloid leukemia (CML), and myelodysplastic syndrome.
11. **Target cell** lab: Hgb electrophoresis, liver enzymes; seen in thalassemia, hemoglobinopathy, liver disease (acanthosis).
12. **Intravascular hemolysis** (autoimmune, direct trauma, shear stress, DIC, and toxins) has increased **urine hemosiderin** and urine hemoglobin but decreased **haptoglobin**.
13. **Extravascular hemolysis** (RBCs cleared from the circulation by the spleen and liver) has spherocytes but negative urine hemosiderin and hemoglobin but may have urobilinogen.
14. **Iron deficiency anemia**: microcytic, hypochromic anemia with central pallor of the RBCs.
15. **Hemoglobin electrophoresis** is abnormal when beta-thalassemia is present due to a relative increase in HbF (2 alpha chains and 2 gamma) and A2 but is normal in alpha thalassemia trait. **Thalassemia (trait as well)** will always have low MCV.
16. **Macrocytic anemia** but low normal B12 and folate, **increased homocysteine**, but normal methylmalonic acid = folate deficiency.
17. **Hypoproliferative microcytic anemia**: FLATS- Fe deficiency, lead poisoning, anemia of chronic disease, thalassemia, sideroblastic anemia. **Hypoproliferative normocytic anemia**: renal failure, aplastic anemia, pure red blood cell anemia, thyroid disease, myelofibrosis, myelophthisis, multiple myeloma. **Macrocytic anemia**: B12 and/or folate deficiency, MDS, hypothyroid, liver disease, drugs (chemo meds including cyclophosphamides, hydroxyurea; antiretroviral drugs including zidovudine, stavudine; antimicrobials like valacyclovir, TMP-SMX; anticonvulsants including phenytoin and valproate).
18. **Tear drop cells and dry tap** = myelofibrosis. **Spherocytes**: drug and infection-induced hemolytic anemia or immune hemolytic anemia. **Schistocytes**: TTP-HUS, PNH, DIC.

Further Readings and References

1. Garber JR, Cobin RH, Gharib H, et al. 2012. American association of clinical endocrinologists and american thyroid association taskforce on hypothyroidism in adults. Clinical practice guidelines for hypothyroidism in adults: cosponsored by the American association of clinical endocrinologists and the american thyroid association. Endocr Pract. 18(6):988–1028.
2. Cascio MJ, DeLoughery TG. 2017. Anemia: Evaluation and Diagnostic Tests. Med Clin North Am. 101(2):263–284.

Chapter 17
Respiratory Discomforts

Upper Respiratory Tract Infections

1. **Diphenhydramine** is preferred to second-generation antihistamines, such as fexofenadine or loratadine, for **rhinorrhea**.
2. **Antigenic shift** (only with influenza A) is due to gene reassortment and can cause **severe pandemics**.
3. Differentiation among **influenza, acute HIV seroconversion, and EBV infection**: **severe liver inflammation** and even jaundice often in acute **EBV** infection (infectious mononucleosis); **atypical lymphocytes** in acute **HIV** and **EBV**, but not with influenza; all can have **myalgias** and **arthralgias**, and **thrombocytopenia**.
4. **Bacterial sinusitis characteristics**: symptoms >7 days, tooth pain, unilateral face pain and sinus tenderness, fever, purulent nasal discharge, symptoms worsening after initial improvement. Treatment: Augmentin, amoxicillin, doxycycline, or trimethoprim/sulfamethoxazole.
5. **Centor criteria** for streptococcal throat: If 0–1 of these is present, no testing is indicated and treatment is symptomatic. If 2–3 criteria are present, rapid-strep testing is indicated, with treatment only if positive. If all four criteria are present, treatment with antibiotics is appropriate (as is rapid-strep testing with antibiotics if positive). **Treatment**: Penicillin V 500 mg PO thrice daily for 10 days, cephalexin 500 mg PO twice daily for 10 days.
6. **Lemierre's syndrome** is a rare complication of either viral or **bacterial pharyngitis**: invasive infection by **Fusobacterium necrophorum**, followed by **sepsis** and **internal jugular vein septic thrombophlebitis** (can cause septic pulmonary emboli). **Classic symptoms**: high fevers and rigors after the onset of sore throat. The exam may reveal tenderness over the sternocleidomastoid muscle. Treatment requires stat ENT consult and good anaerobic activity, such as ampicillin-sulbactam or clindamycin.
7. **Acute bronchitis** symptoms can last 1–3 weeks: cough with or without sputum, nasal congestion. **Treatment** for acute bronchitis: non-steroidal anti-

K. Zhou, *Internal Medicine Training Notes and Survival Guide*,
https://doi.org/10.1007/978-1-0716-4039-5_17

inflammatory drugs and first-generation antihistamines (e.g., diphenhydramine) provide general relief; guaifenesin, and tea with honey help with cough symptoms, decongestants [pseudoephedrine (Sudafed) or phenylephrine (Neo-Synephrine and others)] and nasal steroids reduce mucus formation and post-nasal drip.

8. **Influenza** treatment with oseltamivir should be started within the first 48 h of symptom onset (the sooner the better). In hospitalized and sick patients with multiple co-morbidities, oseltamivir started **4 or 5 days after illness onset** still decreases risks for severe outcomes. Prophylaxis with oseltamivir for 5–10 days may be appropriate in high-risk populations.

Pneumonia

1. Diagnostic criteria for **community-acquired pneumonia** (CAP): no hospitalization in the past 2 weeks, **imaging (chest X ray or CT scan) findings** of new infiltrates, and at least two of the following: **fever, cough, chest pain, or dyspnea**.
2. First-line therapy for CAP in an outpatient setting in otherwise healthy adults: **doxycycline or a macrolide** (I do not commonly use either alone in actual clinical practice).
3. In patients with significant comorbidities (diabetes, congestive heart failure, liver disease, immunosuppression, malignancy, asplenia) or recent antibiotics use, **treatment**: **quinolone or a beta-lactam like cefdinir or Augmentin plus a macrolide** (usually azithromycin).
4. **Structural lung disease** vulnerable for: pseudomonas aeruginosa, Burkholderia cepacian, and S. aureus infections.
5. HCAP (healthcare-associated pneumonia, the term is no longer being used): hospitalized for greater than 48 h in the last 90 days, reside in a nursing home or long-term care facility, have received IV antibiotics, chemo, or wound care in the 30 days before infection, or who attend hemodialysis.
6. **Cough** differential diagnoses: (1) **Infectious:** acute bronchitis, upper respiratory tract infections, sinusitis, emphysema, influenza, pertussis, lung abscess, endocarditis with septic pulmonary emboli. (2) **Noninfections**: asthma, PE, COPD, vasculitis, BOOP, malignancy, CHF, GERD.
7. **Common anaerobes** from the mouth and oropharynx include **Peptostreptococcus, Prevotella, Bacteroides, and Fusobacterium**.
8. Procalcitonin <0.1 μg/L is highly suspected of acute bronchitis; >0.3–0.5 μg/L = possible CAP.
9. **CAP treatment**: azithromycin 500 mg × 1 followed by 250 mg × 4 days (a third generation cephalosporin is usually added). Doxy 100 mg bid for 7 days (a third generation cephalosporin is usually added). Moxifloxacin 400 mg, gemifloxacin 320 mg, or levo 750 mg for 5 days. Alternative: Augmentin 2 g bid in combination with a macrolide for 5 days; clarithromycin two 500 mg tablets daily for 5 days.
10. **Barking cough**, like seal sounds, needs moistening, indicates laryngotracheitis (also known as croup), common in ages <6 m to 3 yo; it is from **parainfluenza**

virus infection. **Treatment**: dexamethasone 0.6 mg/kg, max 6 mg, alternative is single dose nebulized budesonide. Additionally, **racemic epinephrine** 0.05 mL/kg per dose, maximum dose of 0.5 mL of 2.25% diluted to 3 mL NS.

11. **Persistent cough** × 2 weeks + vomiting should prompt consideration of **Bordetella pertussis**, also known as whooping cough, it is very contagious. Severe hacking cough with a high-pitched intake of breath that sounds like whoop. If cough duration is <3 weeks → treatment with antibiotics (azithromycin, clarithromycin, or erythromycin). If 3–6 weeks' duration of cough, only give antibiotics to **pregnant women, health care workers, or workers with infants (azithromycin or clarithromycin)**. The same regimen as treatment is used for post-exposure prophylaxis.
12. Sharp right-sided chest pain and nonproductive cough will need to rule out **pulmonary embolism**. Chest x-ray shows **wedge-shaped opacity** next to the periphery = **Hampton's hump** = possible pulmonary embolism. CT angiography is the golden standard in diagnosing pulmonary embolism.

Asthma and Chronic Obstructive Lung Disease

1. **Return of asthma symptoms after bronchodilator** treatment pathophysiology: late phase inflammation of inflammatory cell recruitment.
2. FEV1/FVC ≤ 70% = **obstruction**. TLC or FVC ≤80% = **restrictive lung disease**.
3. **Cough variant asthma** diagnosis requires resolution of symptoms after starting asthma treatment.
4. **Inspiratory flow limitation** indicates an extrathoracic variable obstruction = possible vocal cord dysfunction.
5. **Increased peak expiratory flow** = consider intrinsic restrictive lung disease from increased elastic recoil.
6. COP (**cryptogenic organizing pneumonia**)/BOOP (**bronchiolitis obliterans organizing pneumonia**): patchy bilateral consolidation, nodules, subpleural and peribronchial proliferation of granulation tissue in small bronchioles and inflammation of surrounding alveoli. BOOP is a type of **restrictive lung disease**.
7. **Mild persistent asthma** (symptoms ≥2 days/week, 3–4×/m for night, FEV1 > 80%), **moderate persistent asthma** (symptoms daily, >1×/week during night, 60%–80% FEV1).
8. Flow volume loops. **Well-controlled asthma**: <1× exacerbation per year and symptoms ≤2×/week.
9. **Asthma** not well-controlled: ≥2 exacerbations per year, nighttime wakening 1–3×/week, or daytime symptoms >2×/week. **Asthma treatment**: SABA prn → ICS low dose → ICS low dose + LABA or medium-dose ICS for asthma symptoms → ICS high dose + LABA +/− oral steroids. LTRA can be used as an alternative after SABA prn.
10. A trial of **ICS** improves cough symptoms = consider **asthma** contributing to her chronic cough.

11. Poorly controlled asthma despite being on oral steroids points towards a different diagnosis. Eosinophilia plus ground glass infiltrates will need a lung biopsy to rule out **Churg-Strauss syndrome**.
12. Asthma controller therapies that can prevent asthma exacerbations: ICS, systemic corticosteroids, LABA, LTRA, and **omalizumab** (in severe asthmatics who have **allergies**). Cromolyn and theophylline, SABA, and ipratropium are not controllers.
13. Asthma with known allergies and IgE (**30–700 IU/mL**), **omalizumab** can be used to reduce exacerbations.
14. **Bronchial thermoplasty** is an FDA-approved procedure for patients with **severe asthma uncontrolled** on a combination of ICS and LABA. Dust mites → washing bedding; pollen is usually high in the afternoon.
15. **Exercise-induced asthma** treatments: first line SABA, second line ICS.
16. **Asthma in pregnancy treatment** is the same as regular people. No asthma medication is Category A, Category B medications include inhaled **budesonide and beclomethasone**. Alternatives are LTRA, cromolyn, theophylline, and tiotropium.
17. **Intermittent asthma first line**: SABA. **Mild persistent**: low dose ICS. **Moderate persistent**: median dose ICS or low dose ICS + LABA. **Severe persistent asthma**: medium dose ICS + LABA and referral to an asthma specialist.
18. Maintained control for **3 months minimum** then step-down treatment. Even with well-controlled asthma, a follow-up visit should be in less than **6 months**.
19. Theophylline can be used as an add-on therapy to ICS. Serum concentration of **theophylline** should be checked in the middle of the dosing interval **3–5 days after starting treatment**.
20. **Weight loss** can improve pulmonary mechanics, and quality of life, and decrease exacerbations in asthma.
21. **Diagnostic criteria for allergic bronchopulmonary aspergillosis (ABPA)**: known diagnosis of asthma or cystic fibrosis (CF), **aspergillus skin test positive** or IgE against (A) fumigatus, elevated total serum IgE concentration (>**1000 IU**/mL). Treatment: prednisone 0.5 mg/kg, tapering dose.
22. Treatment for allergic **rhinitis/sinusitis**: intranasal corticosteroids, first/second generation antihistamines, and immunotherapy in refractory cases.
23. Asthma exacerbation typically does not require antibiotic treatment. Antibiotics are used for **pneumonia, purulent sputum** suggesting a bacterial etiology, bacterial sinusitis, or others.
24. **Asthma exacerbation outpatient**: an initial dose of SABA 2–6 puffs × 2 (20 min apart or single dose nebulizer treatment), then assess response peak flow (>80% → continue outpatient SBAA, every 3–4 h for 1–2 days, may use oral steroid with office visit 4–6 days later; 50%–79% → add **oral steroid**, reassess in 2–3 days; <50%, send patient to **ER**).
25. **Asthma and pregnancy**: ICS (Category B), theophylline (Category C), and SABA (Category C) are safe in pregnancy. Oral steroids may cause preterm

delivery. First line Pulmicort. **Zafirlukast and montelukast** are both Category B while zileuton is Category C. Can add LABA in pregnant women.

26. Asthma and surgery: If FEV1 or peak flow **<80%, systemic steroids** may provide lung function optimization before surgery. May need to assess the need for stress dose steroids before surgery.
27. **Montelukast 10 mg daily** (Zafirlukast 20 mg bid) has a flat dose-response curve and a higher dosage or frequency does not provide additional benefits.
28. **Tiotropium bromide** (LAMA) is comparable to LABA but more effective than doubling ICS strength in uncontrolled asthma on single therapy with ICS.
29. **Only BOOP is restcitive interstitial lung disease** while the other three are obstructive interstitial lung diseases: (1) allergic bronchopulmonary aspergillosis (ABPA), (2) obliterative bronchiolitis, (3) cystic Fibrosis, (4) bronchiolitis Obliterans Organizing Pneumonia (BOOP).
30. **Moderate persistent asthma** is treated with either a low-dose inhaled corticosteroid plus a long-acting beta agonist, or a medium-dose inhaled corticosteroid.
31. **For asthma with known allergies and an IgE** level of 30–700 IU/mL, omalizumab should be prescribed.
32. **Mepolizumab is used for severe asthma** with refractory symptoms and an absolute **eosinophil** count greater than 300 cells/μL in the past 12 months or greater than 150 cells/μL at the time of initiation.
33. Severity of obstruction percentages of predicted FEV1 per Global Initiative for Chronic Obstructive Lung Disease (GOLD) criteria for COPD: >80% **mild**, 50%–80% **moderate**, 30%–49% **severe**, <30% **very severe**.
34. COPD staging: **≥2 moderate exacerbations or ≥ 1 leading to hospitalizations** in the previous year = previous stages C and D (now combined as stage E); ≤1 moderate exacerbation and 0 hospitalization = stages A and B. In the 2023 GOLD Guidelines, previous stages C and D were combined into **stage E** for exacerbations and created new guidance based on blood eosinophils.
35. Stage A treatment with LABA or LAMA; stage B treatment with **LABA + LAMA**; stage E treatment with **LABA + LAMA**. In stage E, **if blood eosinophils ≥ 300 cells/μL (≥100 cells/μL in persistent exacerbations despite LABA + LAMA), consider adding ICS**. Persistent exacerbations despite LABA + LAMA + ICS or for patients with <100 eosinophils/μL, **roflumilast** (if FEV1 < 50% and chronic bronchitis) or **azithromycin** (preferentially in former smokers) may be used to prevent exacerbations.
36. COPD exacerbations should be treated with **bronchodilators and prednisone 40 mg** for 5 days. Antibiotics can be used for 5–7 days if increase in sputum volume or purulence or on mechanical ventilation.

Further Reading and Reference

1. Agustí, A., B.R. Celli, G.J. Criner, et al. 2023. Global Initiative for Chronic Obstructive Lung Disease 2023 report: GOLD executive summary. *American Journal of Respiratory and Critical Care Medicine* 207 (7): 819–837.

Chapter 18
Chronic Pain Disorders

Chronic Pain and Palliative Care

1. **Joint swelling** is a major clinical feature of arthritis.
2. **Polyarthritis** refers to five or more joint involvement.
3. **Asymmetric arthritis** (i.e., involving different joints on two sides, e.g., wrist on the right and elbow on the left) is commonly seen in **osteoarthritis**, **psoriatic arthritis,** and **reactive arthritis/spondyloarthritis**.
4. **Inflammatory arthritis** joint aspiration WBC 2000–20,000. Greater than 50,000 is concerning for **infectious** arthritis.
5. **Enthesis** is the connective tissue that attaches a tendon or ligament to the bone. **Plantar fasciitis** is inflammation at the insertion of the plantar fascia at the calcaneus; it is a type of **'enthesitis'**.
6. **The Caprini Score Model** for major surgery predicts venous thromboembolism risks during hospitalization and helps guide decisions of deep venous thrombosis prophylaxis.
7. **Lyme disease** can cause heart blocks; treatment: intravenous ceftriaxone until the heart block resolves followed by a 21-day course of oral therapy.
8. **Patellofemoral pain syndrome**: diffuse knee ache, patella tenderness with crepitus.
9. **Meniscal injury** may cause knee locking.
10. "**1:2:3**" rule: 1 mg IV/SQ morphine = 2 mg po oxycodone = 3 mg po morphine
11. The "**30:20:10:7.5:1.5**" rule refers to equianalgesic dosing of different pain medications: 30 po morphine, 20 po oxycodone, 10 mg IV/SQ morphine, 7.5 po hydromorphone, 1.5 mg IV/SQ hydromorphone. Decrease by 25% during initial conversion to prevent side effects and allow additional pain medication for breakthrough pain.
12. The (microgram-per-hour) dose of transdermal fentanyl patch is about **equal to half of the (milligram-per-day) dose of oral morphine** (i.e., 25 mg oral morphine/24 h = 12.5 μg/h. of transdermal fentanyl).

K. Zhou, *Internal Medicine Training Notes and Survival Guide*,
https://doi.org/10.1007/978-1-0716-4039-5_18

13. **Cholestatic pruritus** treatments: cholestyramine, sertraline, paroxetine, naltrexone, and rifampicin.
14. Opioids are effective for **dyspnea and cough**: codeine, 15–30 mg po q6h prn, given 1/2 h before the desired activity.
15. Opioid-induced nausea treatment: **prochlorperazine** and **haloperidol**.
16. **Methylnaltrexone** (injectable) and **naloxegol** (Movantik, oral) are peripherally-acting μ-opioid antagonists used in **opioid-induced constipation**
17. **Megestrol** acetate (200 mg po q6–8 h) and **dexamethasone (3–4 mg daily)** are used for anorexia.
18. **Gabapentin** can be used for opioid-related **pruritus**.
19. **Testosterone** can be effective for anorexia in patients with AIDS. **Methylphenidate** may help with fatigue.
20. Back pain and risk factors for osteoporosis, plain **X-ray films** of the lumbosacral spine are recommended to rule out **compression fractures**.
21. **Night pain** and **pain worse lying** flat require workup to rule out **malignancy or infection**.
22. **Red flags of low back pain**: age > 50, corticosteroid use, malignancy, fever, endovascular procedure, injection drug use, morning stiffness, symptoms worse at night or when lying flat, saddle anesthesia, bilateral sciatica, bowel/bladder dysfunction.
23. Spinal fusion from ankylosing spondylitis will require workups of **X-ray and even CT scan to rule out a spinal fracture**.

Headache

1. Acute onset of throbbing, one-sided headache that is **disabling** and has known triggers = **migraines**. Common **migraine triggers** include nitrates like hot dogs, xanthene-like dyes, and tyramines like wine.
2. If migraine attacks happen only a few times a year, migraine abortive medications such as "**triptan**" are appropriate treatment; beta-blockers, calcium channel blockers, and tricyclic antidepressants are used for migraine prevention.
3. Migraine daily despite Excedrin (aspirin/acetaminophen/caffeine) daily is likely **medication overuse headache** and should stop Excedrin.
4. **Migraine characteristics**: nausea, unilateral pain, photophobia, debility or throbbing; **PIN** = photophobia, incapacitation, nausea; **POUND** = pulsatile, duration of 4–72 h, unilateral, nausea/vomiting, disabling.
5. **Severe headache with concerns for subarachnoid hemorrhage**: CT head first, and if concerns remain, get a lumbar puncture.
6. If a neurologic deficit from a migraine aura lasts for >24 h = consider **complicated migraine**. Neurologic deficits that do not resolve may have **migrainous infarction** and require brain MRI for diagnosis.
7. Mild to moderate migraine treatment: NSAIDs including aspirin. Moderate to severe migraine treatment: triptans.
8. A combination of **metoclopramide iv and NSAIDs** is the effective abortive option in patients with **migraine** and poorly controlled **hypertension**.

9. A **triptan** is considered effective if the headache is relieved after 2 h, has no recurrence in 24 h, and has tolerable side effects. If the headache lasts and requires a 2nd dose of triptan at the two-hour point, can **increase the initial dosage or add NSAIDs** or other pain meds.
10. Other **abortive** migraine treatments include antiemetics like **Reglan, Compazine, droperidol, ergotamine, calcitonin gene-related peptide (CGRP) antagonists (like erenumab, eptinezumab), NSAIDs, and dihydroergotamines**.
11. Oral formulations of almotriptan, eletriptan, and rizatriptan can relieve migraine headaches quickly. Longer-acting triptans like eletriptan have low headache recurrence rates; frovatriptan and naratriptan are also long-acting triptans.
12. FDA-approved migraine prevention medications include beta blockers like **timolol and propranolol, anticonvulsants like topiramate and valproate, and Botox injections**. Although not approved by the FDA, calcium channel blockers verapamil, flunarizine (not available in the United States), nimodipine, nifedipine, cyclandelate, and nicardipine have been shown effective in migraine prevention.
13. **Pure menstrual migraine** (attacks are purely confined to the peri-menstrual period) versus menstrual-related migraine (attacks that occur in the peri-menstrual period but can occur at other times of the cycle as well) treatments: the triptans (eg. almotriptan, eletriptan, frovatriptan, naratriptan, rizatriptan, sumatriptan, zolmitriptan) as well as an aspirin/acetaminophen/caffeine combination (Excedrin™), NSAIDs, and/or estrogen (once to twice daily for 3–4 days).
14. **Oral contraceptives** in women with migraine with aura have increased risks for **ischemic** stroke.
15. **Cluster headache** (sharp, stabbing, burning, lasting 5 min to 3 h every other day) also known as **suicide headache** pathophysiology: **hyperexcitable posterior hypothalamus. Treatment** of cluster headache: oxygen at 7–10 L or subcutaneous or intranasal triptans.
16. **Trigeminal autonomic cephalalgias**: cluster headache, paroxysmal hemicrania (treatment is indomethacin), and unilateral neuralgiform headache. Gabapentin (800–2700 mg/day), topiramate (50–300 mg/day), and carbamazepine (200–1600 mg/day) may be effective for treatment.
17. **Tension-type headache**: dull, non-throbbing, bilateral band-like, persistent and may last up to a week, and not aggravated by physical activity. **Episodic tension-type headache** is diagnosed if the number of days with headaches is less than 180 per year and less than 15 per month.
18. Treatment for **tension-type headache**: analgesics including Tylenol, aspirin, NSAIDs, but should be limited to 2–3 days a week to avoid medication overuse headache.
19. **Medication overuse headache**: presence of headache more than 15 days a month for $\geq$3 months, Tylenol or NSAIDs use for >15 days a month or ergotamine, triptans, opioids (codeine-based medicines) or combination painkillers for 10 or more days per month.

20. **Idiopathic intracranial hypertension** also known as **pseudotumor cerebri** commonly seen in females aged 20–40 years old, oral contraceptive use, tetracycline, or isotretinoin use. Treatment: lumbar puncture with increased opening pressure, carbonic anhydrase inhibitor.
21. **Cluster headache** comes with **circadian rhythm**.
22. **Red flag symptoms** with a headache that warrants imaging: get an **MRI** brain and possibly LP with CSF studies.
23. Red flag symptoms in headache include **rapid onset of symptoms, a thunderclap headache, concomitant neurological signs and symptoms, neck pain, fever, age > 50, and a new pattern of headache.**

Low Back Pain

1. **Red flags of low back pain**: age > 50, corticosteroid use, malignancy, fever, endovascular procedure, injection drug use, morning stiffness, symptoms worse at night or when lying flat, saddle anesthesia, bilateral sciatica, bowel/bladder dysfunction.
2. **NSAIDs** are proven superior to placebo for pain control in low back pain.
3. Concerns for **soft tissue infection** if uncontrolled back pain or significant impairment in mobility, will need **spinal MRI** to rule out epidural or spinal abscesses and also rarely spinal epidural hemorrhage.
4. **Spondylolysis**: nonunion or fracture of pars interarticularis.
5. **Common causes** of low back pain: lumbar strain, herniated disc, compression fracture, spinal stenosis, spondyloarthritis, neoplasia, infection.
6. **Reactive arthritis** = Reiter syndrome is related to infections caused by Yersinia, Campylobacter, Shigella, Salmonella, or Chlamydia.
7. **Reactive arthritis** has antecedent **gastrointestinal** (GI) or **genitourinary** (GU) infection, check **urine PCR**, and **stool culture** for **campylobacter** or other enteric pathogen; onset of reactive arthritis may lag **3–10** days after an infectious event.
8. **Sacroiliitis and spondylitis** can occur in patients with inflammatory bowel disease.
9. Inflammatory causes of back pain (**spondyloarthritis**): ankylosing spondylitis, psoriatic arthritis, reactive arthritis, and spondyloarthritis with inflammatory bowel disease (**insidious onset of back pain and the presence of enthesitis**).
10. **Straight leg raise** positive refers to the reproduction of symptoms of sciatica at an angle less than 60° with pain radiating below the knee.
11. **Inflammatory arthritis** pain is usually worse in the morning, and better in the day. Osteoarthritis is better in the morning and worse as the day progresses.
12. **Morning stiffness of proximal joints** that improves with activities is suggestive of polymyalgia rheumatica: has high ESR and high CRP but negative CPK, and responds rapidly to low-dose steroids.
13. Patients with **spinal fusion from ankylosing spondylitis are at higher risk for spinal fractures** due to a lack of spinal movements.
14. **Epidural steroid injections** may improve short-term relief in patients with acute low back pain but do not impact the need for surgery.

15. **Concordant nerve root impingement or spinal stenosis 4–6 weeks** after injury requires surgery evaluation.

Gout

1. Synovial fluid **WBC > 50,000** indicates possible infection. The overtly septic range is >100,000 WBC/mm^3.
2. Pathophysiology of gout: **inflammasomes** activate caspase-1 which in turn activates **IL-1 beta**, a proinflammatory cytokine. Treatment of gout can target IL1 using anakinra (IL-1 receptor blocker).
3. 5 days after CABG, a fever of 102 °F together with a painful and swollen right knee, warrants consideration of crystal arthropathy. Aggressive diuresis of congestive heart failure (CHF) causes **intravascular volume contraction and progressive hyperuricemia** → acute gout among adults initially admitted to the hospital free of joint pain.
4. Acute gout attack treatment: **intra-articular or oral steroid, colchicine, or NSAIDs** for a full week; once the attack of gout has subsided, add urate-lowering agent to colchicine. In refractory gout, **anakinra or canakinumab** can be used.
5. Target serum uric acid level is **≤6.0 mg/dL** in gout.
6. Gout is common in menopausal women. A diet high in purine includes **red meat and seafood. Metabolic syndrome and its components** (hypertension, hyperlipidemia, and obesity) increase gout attack risks.
7. **First-line treatment of acute gout attack**: corticosteroids, NSAIDs, and colchicine. A methylprednisolone dose pack 24 mg/day decreases by 4 mg/day, prednisone 20–30 mg/day with a tapering schedule over 1–2 weeks, or intraarticular (triamcinolone 40 mg) can be used in acute gout attack. NSAIDs like indomethacin, ibuprofen, and naproxen can also be used; colchicine-start treatment 1.2 mg → 1 h into treatment, can give colchicine 0.6 mg another dose, followed by colchicine 0.6 mg daily or twice daily until flare resolves.
8. Acute gout most commonly presents as an **acute inflammatory monoarthritis** of the **first metatarsophalangeal joint** (i.e., podagra). Involvement of the **wrist and elbow** occurs late in the disease course of gout. **Alcohol and sugar-sweetened sodas** increase gout attack risks. **Gout**: **needle-shaped** crystal, that appears yellow when the crystal is oriented parallel to the axis of polarized light.
9. **Hypertension** increases gout risk; **diuresis** causes gout flare.
10. Only **≤75%–80%** of patients with acute gout are **hyperuricemic** during **gout attacks**.
11. **Febuxostat** (Uloric) blocks xanthine oxidase, which is metabolized by the **liver**. **Allopurinol** is metabolized by the kidney. **Rasburicase may be used in kidney** failure patients to lower uric acid.
12. **Tophaceous gout** = subcutaneous accumulation of monosodium urate crystals.
13. **Clinical risk factors for gout attacks**: metabolic syndrome, CKD, hemolytic states, increased keratinocyte turnover (psoriasis), and increased neoplastic cell turnover.

14. **Acute gout** treatment: Steroids can be used in chronic kidney disease and when contraindications for colchicine.
15. **Acute gout**: colchicine 1.2 mg at the first sign of flare, followed in 1 h with a single dose of 0.6 mg, then 0.6 mg once or twice daily until flare resolves.
16. **Pericarditis** treatment: colchicine 0.5 mg once (<70 kg) or 0.5 mg twice daily (>70 kg) for 3 mo; can also use high-dose aspirin 750–1000 mg every 8 h. for 1–2 weeks.
17. **Probenecid** (uricosuric) is used for gout prevention: 250 mg bid for 1 week; may increase to 500 mg bid; ineffective in CKD.
18. **Gout**: needle-shaped crystals in gout, negative birefringent under polarized light, yellow when the crystal is parallel to the axis of the polarizer, and blue when oriented perpendicular.
19. **Calcium pyrophosphate deposition disease (pseudogout)**: chondrocalcinosis (cartilage calcification) on X-ray, rhomboid crystals, and weakly positive birefringent under polarized light, blue when parallel to light. Treatment of pseudogout is similar to that of gout.

Further Readings and References

1. Zobdeh F, Ben Kraiem A, Attwood MM, et al. 2021. Pharmacological treatment of migraine: Drug classes, mechanisms of action, clinical trials and new treatments. Br J Pharmacol. 178(23):4588–4607.
2. Hainer BL, Matheson E, Wilkes RT. 2014. Diagnosis, treatment, and prevention of gout. Am Fam Physician. 90(12):831–836.

Chapter 19
Senior Health

Cognitive Decline and Dementia

1. **Dementia** diagnosis is based on progression in **cognitive and functional decline**: progressive decline in both cognitive function and activities of daily living as a result of cognitive decline. Evaluation in dementia includes CBC, LFT, electrolytes, BUN, creatinine, calcium, vitamin B12, and TSH.
2. **Minimal mental status exam (MMSE)** is the best at measuring orientation, attention, and short-term recall; scores **27** or higher are normal, 20–26 is mild dementia, 12–19 is moderate dementia, and <12 is severe dementia. A minimal score of normal can also be 24–27 depending on patients' education level.
3. **Montreal Cognitive Assessment (MoCA)** is another tool used for language assessment in mild **cognitive dysfunction**. It includes naming pictures of three animals, sentence repetitions, and lexical fluency tasks. Scoring: 18–25 = mild cognitive impairment, **10–17** = moderate cognitive impairment, and less than 10 = severe cognitive impairment.
4. **Impaired language, memory, and visual/spatial skills** are commonly seen in Alzheimer's dementia while **social skills like warmth, affability, and social grace and manners** are often retained.
5. Dementia with **Lewy** bodies or diffuse Lewy body disease symptoms: **thinking and behavioral changes** followed by movement dysfunction; **cognitive** changes and **Parkinsonism** at the same time.
6. **Frontotemporal dementia** (FTD also known as **Pick's** disease): early onset of personality disorder, swing between apathy, anger, and disinhibition which typically precedes major cognitive decline and loss of executive functional abilities.
7. **Frontotemporal dementia (Pick's** disease) often starts between age 40 and 65 and has an early onset of **personality disorder**, a combination of emotional blunting, apathy, and periods of behavioral disturbances. Another early manifestation of Pick's disease is **executive dysfunction** while **cognitive testing** can be normal in the early phase. **Amyotrophic lateral sclerosis** symptoms occur

K. Zhou, *Internal Medicine Training Notes and Survival Guide*,
https://doi.org/10.1007/978-1-0716-4039-5_19

in up to **30%** of patients with Pick's disease. Around 30%–50% of people with ALS or FTD will develop both conditions.

8. **Normal pressure hydrocephalus (NPH)** has a triad of gait disorder, urinary incontinence, and cognitive decline. Diagnosis of NPH relies on improvement in gait after **large volume lumbar puncture removing greater than 30 cc CSF**.
9. Patients with dementia typically **lose** their **insight** into memory problems, whereas depressed and anxious patients do not.
10. Deficits in attention and memory can be seen in both **depression and dementia**. Depression can be the early sign of dementia and it requires tests to confirm or rule out memory deficits.
11. Rapidly progressive **dementia**: familial, sporadic, iatrogenic, and infectious etiologies. Additional tests and workups should be performed to correct reversible causes.
12. **Test of attention**: name the months/0–10 in reverse order. **Visual-spatial skills**: drawing a clock or interlocking pentagons.
13. **Treatment for cognitive decline**: cholinesterase inhibitors (donepezil, galantamine, rivastigmine), and NMDA receptor modifier (memantine, used after moderate stage).
14. **Pseudobulbar affect (PBA)**: found in Alzheimer's disease, multiple sclerosis, amyotrophic lateral sclerosis, traumatic brain injury. It is the display of **emotional behaviors without accompanying emotions**, such as crying frequently and randomly/involuntarily. Treatment: **Nuedexta** (dextromethorphan/quinidine)
15. **Nuplazid (pimavanserin)** is used for hallucinations in Parkinson's disease.
16. **Neglect** is the refusal or failure to fulfill a person's obligations or duties.
17. **Adult protection service** (APS) assesses the potential victim's risk, capacity to understand risk and to give informed consent. Doctors and other professionals are **mandated to report abuse or neglect in many states.**

Dizziness

1. Severe acute onset vertigo with a history of low-grade fevers and mild upper respiratory infection symptoms = consider **vestibular neuritis**. **Treatment**: methylprednisolone, anti-emetics, meclizine (use for ≥3 days may prolong dizziness).
2. **Vestibular neuritis**: usually upper respiratory symptoms precede vertigo. **Labyrinthitis** = vestibular neuritis + **tinnitus or even hearing loss**.
3. Pharmacotherapy for **acute vestibular neuritis**: antihistamines (meclizine 25–50 mg q6h), phenothiazine (promethazine 25 mg q12h), anxiolytics like lorazepam dosed at 0.5–1 mg q12h prn, Zofran, **methylprednisolone** taper 100 mg qd for 3 days, tapering by 20 mg q3d, when the last 20 mg for 3 days, do 10 mg for 3 days, then every other day for 4 days.
4. **MRI is better than CT** to visualize the posterior fossa for **acoustic neuroma**.
5. Causes of **peripheral vertigo**: BPPV (cannalith), vestibular neuritis (no hearing loss), labyrinthitis (hearing loss), perilymphatic fistula-barotrauma, chronic unilateral vestibular hypofunction, drugs, Meniere's disease, acoustic neuroma.

6. **Concerning characteristics of vertigo indicating central vertigo**: vascular risk factors, headache, long duration of symptoms, falling to both sides, mild symptoms. Get an MRI head for these situations.
7. Causes of **central vertigo**: thromboembolism, intracranial hemorrhage, brain stem tumors, multiple sclerosis, migraine headache, drugs (anticonvulsants, antidepressants, antihypertensives).
8. **Benign paroxysmal positional vertigo (BPPV) treatment: Epley maneuver** should be performed with the patient looking to **the same side** which proceeds a positive **Dix-Hallpike test**.
9. **Tricyclic antidepressants** (**TCA**) like amitriptyline can prevent **vestibular migraines**. **Hydrochlorothiazide** (HCTZ) is used to prevent **Meniere disease** recurrence. Methylprednisolone is used to improve vestibular neuritis. **Promethazine** can be used for **nausea** from **vertigo**.
10. **Ramsay–Hunt syndrome**: facial paralysis together with painful vesicular skin lesions within the external auditory canal and vestibulocochlear dysfunction. **Treatment**: valacyclovir 1 g tid for 7–10 days + prednisone 1 mg/kg for 5 days. Treatment is essentially the same as Bell's palsy.
11. **Central vertigo** does not cause horizontal vertigo. Nystagmus due to central vertigo is pure **vertical/torsional**.
12. In BPPV, the nystagmus is torsional clockwise for the left side, and counter-clockwise for the right side, with **a vertical up-beating component**. **Torsional nystagmus** = consider posterior semicircular canal BPPV (most common). **Horizontal nystagmus** = consider lateral (horizontal) semicircular canal BPPV. Vertical nystagmus = consider **superior** semicircular canal BPPV (very rare).
13. **Dizziness** differentials: vertigo (central vs. peripheral), presyncope (medication, cardiac, hydration), disequilibrium, nonspecific like psychiatric.
14. **Disequilibrium**: imbalance from sensory deficits like peripheral neuropathy.
15. **Vestibular rehabilitation** is indicated for chronic vertigo. Meclizine is used for acute symptoms and should not be used for more than 3 days.
16. **Saccade**: a rapid movement of the eye; usually indicates vestibular dysfunction.
17. **BPPV** is caused by the loosening of a cannalith in the vestibular system. Diagnosed with positive **Dix-Hallpike maneuver**. Treatment is the **Epley maneuver**.
18. **Peripheral vertigo** nystagmus improves with **gaze fixation** and gets worse with eye closure. Vertical nystagmus is usually specific for central vertigo. **Nystagmus of central vertigo gets worse by fixation of gaze**.
19. **Vertigo from migraine** headaches can be treated with **amitriptyline** for migraine prevention.

Osteoporosis

1. **Screening for osteoporosis** in all women aged 65 and above, men ≥70 yo, ≥50 if weight <125 lbs, current smoker, family history, and fracture if fragility.

Younger women and men **ages 50–69** should consider DEXA scan if **risk factors for serious bone loss**.

2. **Risk of osteoporosis** increases if steroid use ≥5 mg for greater than 3 months, tobacco use, >3 alcoholic beverages per day, and low BMI. **Treatment**: exercise, vitamin D and calcium, tobacco cessation.
3. **Calcium intake for women ≥ 50** is 1200 mg qd, vit D 800 iu. Recheck T score in 2 years after starting bisphosphonates.
4. **After 5 years of bisphosphate, can consider medication interruption** (stop taking the medication) for 1–2 years but not in patients with previous hip, vertebral or multiple non-spine fractures, or increased risk for vertebral fracture, or DEXA scan showing a femoral neck T score of −2.5 or lower. After 10 years on bisphosphonate, if no change in bone density, **stopping bisphosphonate medication is appropriat**e.
5. **Diseases increasing osteoporosis risks**: hemochromatosis, celiac disease, hyperthyroidism, hyperparathyroidism, and hypogonadism.
6. **Medications increasing osteoporosis risks**: corticosteroids, immunosuppressants, proton pump inhibitors (PPIs), and selective serotonin reuptake inhibitors (SSRIs).
7. In addition to hip and spine measurement, DEXA can also measure the density of the **forearm for primary hyperparathyroidism** as it mainly causes loss of the cortical bone.
8. **Z score** is used to evaluate patients under age 50. A **Z score of <2.0** also defines osteoporosis besides a **T score < −2.5**.
9. **Osteoporosis** labs: calcium, phosphorus, PTH, TSH, 24-h urine calcium, ALP, 25-OH vit D, SPEP, UPEP, Cushing disease, hypogonadism, and celiac antibodies.
10. **Celiac disease antibodies**: tissue transglutaminase Abs, IgA endomysial Ab, total serum IgA.
11. **Medications** for **osteoporosis:** calcitonin intranasal 200 iu/day, alendronate 70 mg qwk, risedronate 35 mg qwk or 150 mg qmonth, ibandronate 150 mg qmonth, or zoledronic acid iv 5 mg yearly. If **breast cancer, do raloxifene 60 mg/day**.
12. **Bisphosphonate** causes necrosis of the jaw (dentist clearance before prescription) and atypical femoral shaft fractures.
13. **Calcitonin** is an osteoclast inhibitor that improves bone mineral density (BMD) and reduces vertebral fractures. Denosumab (Prolia) and teriparatide (Forteo) are ok to use in men.
14. **Screening** for osteoporosis in men who have risk factors such as treatment with **corticosteroids, diagnosis of hyperparathyroidism, or X-rays suggesting osteoporosis** is covered by insurance.
15. The National Osteoporosis Foundation recommends that individuals age **50 years and older with a DEXA T-score between −1.0 and −2.5 (osteopenia)** should be treated to improve bone mineral density if the 10-year risk of hip fracture is 3% or greater, or any major osteoporosis-related fracture is 20% or greater.

16. Patients with **vertebral compression fracture or hip fracture** should be treated to prevent further fractures regardless of T-score.
17. **Bisphosphonates are recommended as treatment** for patients with a previous osteoporotic fracture, a T score of < -2.5, and ≥ 50 years who have low bone mass (T score -1.0 to -2.5) and a10-year risk probability of >3% for hip fracture or >20% for major osteoporotic fracture as per the **Fracture Risk Assessment Tool (FRAX)** risk assessment.
18. Patients age 50 and older with a fracture risk of <10% can be treated with **lifestyle modification unless on prednisone ≥ 7.5 mg/d**.
19. **Zoledronic acid and teriparatide** are used in those at highest risk.
20. The risk of **nephrolithiasis** increases with **calcium intake >1500 mg/daily**.

Chronic Kidney Disease (CKD)

1. **Albumin excretion** is moderately increased if the random albumin/Cr ratio is 30–300 mg/L (<30 mg/L is normal). The blood pressure (BP) goal in CKD is 130/80.
2. **ACEis, ARBs, and non-dihydropyridine calcium channel blockers (verapamil and diltiazem)** can reduce proteinuria and progression of CKD. Aspirin is well tolerated by CKD.
3. HIV causes **focal glomerulosclerosis and tubulointerstitial injury**, especially in individuals of African descent.
4. **CKD-EPI** equation is preferred for renal function assessment when GFR >60.
5. Obtain random protein/creatinine ratio (normal < 0.2mg/mg) if **non-albumin proteinuria is suspected** (i.e., Bence Jones proteinuria in multiple myeloma).
6. CKD does not affect lipid recommendations, but **ESRD patients have no cardiovascular benefits from lipid-lowering therapy if no other indications**.
7. Erythropoietin stimulating agents (EPA) increase CVA, stroke, and death, **stop EPA if Hgb >10 or Hgb increases >1 g over 2 weeks**.
8. **$NaHCO_3$ (bicarbonate tablets) should be initiated when serum HCO_3 < 22 mEq/L** to preserve acid-base balance and potentially slow CKD progression.
9. Stage 3a CKD: Na intake <2 g/day, limit K (if hyperkalemia) to 2–4 g/day, restrict phosphorus if P > 4.6 mg/dL, limit Ca intake to <2000 mg/day.
10. Vit D deficiency <10 treatment: ergocalciferol 50,000 iu **weekly for 6–8 weeks**, followed by cholecalciferol **800–1000 u/day**.
11. **Cinacalcet** is used in tertiary hyperparathyroidism; calcitriol is used in very elevated PTH but normal calcium/phosphorus.
12. **Phosphate binders**: aluminum hydroxide, calcium carbonate/acetate, sevelamer, lanthanum. Avoid calcium-based binders in hypercalcemia.
13. A **diuretic** in diabetes can potentiate the antihypertensive and **protein-lowering** effects of ACEis and ARBs.
14. **Mineralocorticoid receptor** blockers and direct **renin inhibitors** (**Aliskiren**) are newer agents that may **improve blood pressure (BP) control** and **decrease proteinuria** in patients with CKD. Both classes increase the risks of hyperkalemia.

15. **24 h urine protein normal is less than 150 mg**. If >3.5 g, it is nephrotic syndrome.

Electrolyte Disturbances

1. **MUDPILES** (high anion gap metabolic acidosis) and **HARDASS** (normal anion gap metabolic acidosis). RTA Type 1 and Type 2 have **low K** while Type 4 has **high K**.
2. In clinical practice: **anion gap (AG) → if high AG → serum osmolarity gap (OG). If normal AG → urine AG = Una + Uk − Ucl.**
3. **Increased AG and increased OG** seen in toxicant ingestion of methanol, ethanol, and ethylene glycol; can also be seen in diabetic ketoacidosis. **Increased AG but normal OG** seen in acetaminophen and salicylate. **Normal or increased AG and increased OG** are seen in isopropyl glycol ingestion. AG vs. HCO_3 determines whether mixed acid-base disorder or not.
4. **Metabolic alkalosis**: loss of H+ from GI/kidney, exogenous alkali, contraction alkalosis, post-hypercapnia. Lab urine Cl, if <20- >saline responsive.
5. **Hypokalemia** is a cause of metabolic alkalosis. **Renal artery stenosis** causes metabolic alkalosis.
6. Causes of **respiratory alkalosis**: pain, fever, trauma, stroke, pregnancy, sepsis, hepatic failure.
7. Normal pH, high AG = high AG metabolic acidosis with compensated alkalosis.
8. Central venous pH + 0.05 = ABG pH.
9. **Low AG metabolic acidosis**: bromism, low albumin, and multiple myeloma. Bromism is the ingestion of excessive bromine-based sedatives (like potassium bromide and lithium bromide) causing CNS impairment like ataxia, confusion, and delusions.
10. For a pure elevated AG metabolic acidosis, the **serum bicarbonate will decrease by the same amount the AG increases**. For example, pH = 7.20, AG 22, Bicarb 8 indicating combined high AGMA and non-AGMA.
11. **Type 1 RTA** defective distal H+ excretion; **Type 2 RTA** decreased proximal HCO_3 absorption; **Type 4 RTA** hypoaldosteronism.
12. Urine AG > 0 = Type 1 and Type 4 RTA; urine AG < 0 = Type 2 RTA. Urine CL is a marker for NH4+; urine AG = urine K+ urine Na − urine Cl
13. **Metabolic alkalosis** = Cushing's disease, Conn disease, or renal artery stenosis.
14. Causes of **metabolic alkalosis**: volume depletion, hyperaldosteronism, hypokalemia.
15. **Bartter syndrome** (low K, hypercalciuria), **Gitelman syndrome** (low K+), **Liddle syndrome** (low K, low aldosterone). All have **metabolic alkalosis**. CO_2 compensation for metabolic alkalosis. $pCO_2 = 0.7\ (HCO_3–24) + 40 + -2$
16. **For metabolic acidosis**, use AG for assessment to decide a plan of care; for **metabolic alkalosis**, use urine chloride for assessment to decide a plan of care. For **respiratory acidosis**, consider three structures: the chest cavity, the central process (CNS), and the lungs and airways.

17. **Normal AG but high OG** metabolic acidosis = consider **isopropyl alcohol** intoxication.
18. **Toluene:** an organic solvent that originally causes an elevated anion gap metabolic acidosis, but later a normal anion gap metabolic acidosis as it results in renal tubular acidosis.

Further Readings and References

1. Post RE, Dickerson LM. 2010. Dizziness: a diagnostic approach. Am Fam Physician. 82(4):361–368, 369.
2. Black DM, Rosen CJ. 2016. Clinical practice. postmenopausal osteoporosis. N Engl J Med. 21;374(3):254–262. https://doi.org/10.1056/NEJMcp1513724. Erratum in: N Engl J Med. 374(18):1797. https://doi.org/10.1056/NEJMx160008.
3. Arceo-Mendoza RM, Camacho PM. 2021. Postmenopausal osteoporosis: latest guidelines. Endocrinol Metab Clin North Am. 50(2):167–178.
4. Berend K, de Vries AP, Gans RO. 2014. Physiological approach to assessment of acid-base disturbances. N Engl J Med. 371(15):1434–1445. https://doi.org/10.1056/NEJMra1003327. Erratum in: N Engl J Med. 2014;371(20):1948.

Chapter 20
GERD, Dermatitis, and Eye Diseases

Gastroesophageal Reflux Syndrome (GERD)

1. Symptomatic acid reflux after 4 weeks of treatment with over-the-counter care with H2 blocker and calcium carbonate, the next step is the addition of a proton pump inhibitor (PPI). EGD is necessary if worrisome symptoms (**bleeding, weight loss, dysphagia, anorexia, odynophagia, vomiting, signs of systemic illness**) or not responding to twice daily PPI after 4 weeks.
2. **PPI** causes hypomagnesemia leading to hypokalemia, hypocalcemia, and **hypoparathyroidism**, increasing the risks for **C. diff** infection, **kidney dysfunction**, **dementia,** and **osteoporosis** as well as **community-acquired pneumonia**.
3. **Medications that increase risks for GERD** include anticholinergic agents, benzodiazepines, beta-blockers, calcium channel blockers, nitrates, prostaglandins, TCAs, and sildenafil.
4. **Differential diagnoses** of GERD: esophageal dysmotility or spasm, scleroderma, achalasia. Tests: endoscopy, esophageal pH testing, barium swallow, and esophageal manometry.
5. **Step-down treatments** for GERD: continue lifestyle modification, and re-endoscopy to confirm the healing of the esophagus, if negative, start H2 receptor blockers.
6. In step-down therapy, maximal doses of H2 receptor blocker treatment should be given initially with **antacids for breakthrough symptoms**.
7. When GERD is treated with PPI, **taking calcium with food** should increase gastric acidity enough to facilitate calcium absorption.
8. **Endoscopy** to screen for dysplasia and early esophageal adenocarcinoma in patients with **Barrett's esophagus**.
9. GERD **complications**: esophageal erosions and ulcers, esophageal stricture formation, Berrett's esophagus, and esophageal adenocarcinomas.
10. If concerns for H. pylori infection, **urea breath test** or **stool Ag test** should be performed 2–4 weeks after the last dose of PPI for GERD.

K. Zhou, *Internal Medicine Training Notes and Survival Guide*, https://doi.org/10.1007/978-1-0716-4039-5_20

11. **H pylori** testing is indicated in **MALT lymphoma, peptic ulcer, certain immigrants, and early gastric cancer**. Additional indications may include: all patients **under age 45 with dyspepsia** (nausea, bloating, and stomach discomfort), **unexplained iron deficiency**, **recurrent idiopathic thrombocytopenia**, **first-degree relative with gastric cancer**.
12. In Canada, the first-line therapy for H. pylori infection is **ClAMet quadruple therapy [clarithromycin (Cl), amoxicillin (A), and metronidazole (Met) plus pantoprazole]** given for 14 days with an efficacy of 80%–85%; the next line of treatment is **bismuth-based quadruple therapy** (PPI, bismuth, metronidazole, and tetracycline) given for 14 days.
13. Patients aged **45 yo and older with dyspepsia** should get EGD.

Dermatitis

1. **Eczema = atopic dermatitis** (pruritic rashes in patients with additional allergic diseases like asthma). **Treatment** can include topical triamcinolone acetonide ointment once to twice daily and antihistamines. Additionally, tacrolimus ointment and pimecrolimus cream can also be used twice daily on the affected areas. **Colloidal oatmeal** is an emollient that can be added to bath water to soften skin and relieve irritation. **Topical steroids** can be used 1–2 times a week during the maintenance phase to prevent flares of eczema.
2. **Treatments for atopic dermatitis**: proper bathing techniques (soak and smear) and avoidance of skin irritants; soak in long baths and smear with mid-high-potency topical steroids.
3. **Treatments for atopic dermatitis**: **mild to moderate potency steroids** include desonide, triamcinolone, fluocinolone; **topical calcineurin inhibitors** like tacrolimus and pimecrolimus; antihistamines oral and topical doxepin.
4. **Super potent topical steroids**: betamethasone augmented. **Potent**: betamethasone, fluocinonide. **Mid strength**: mometasone, triamcinolone, fluocinolone, and hydrocortisone. When systemic steroids are used, **higher doses and at least 2 weeks** duration of treatment are necessary to prevent rebound.
5. **Contact dermatitis**: irritant contact dermatitis vs allergic contact dermatitis.
6. Treatment for **irritant contact dermatitis**: avoidance of the offending agent, application of topical corticosteroids or immunomodulators to relieve dermatitis, and restoration of the normal skin barrier with moisturizers (emollient, bath oils, topical antimicrobials like Silvadene).
7. Calamine lotion and Burrow's solution can have a cooling effect on allergic contact dermatitis.
8. **Bullae** >0.5 cm; **pustules** $\leq$1 cm.
9. **Lichen planus**: shiny, flat-topped, violaceous papules with a lacy white pattern but no vesicles.
10. **Lichen simplex chronicus**: areas of lichenification, history of rubbing the area without exposure to an allergen or irritant as in chronic contact dermatitis.
11. **Dyshidrotic eczema**: pruritic rash that just involves the hands and/or feet.

12. **Pityriasis rosea**: Christmas tree pattern rash; it is a self-limiting papulosquamous disorder. **Pityriasis versicolor**: previously termed tinea versicolor; it is caused by a commensal fungal inhabitant Malassezia, noncontagious.

Common Eye Disorders

1. **Open-angle glaucoma** causes eye pain, haloes, and light sensitivity. **Retinal detachment** causes photopsia (flashes of light) and floaters. **Anterior uveitis** causes eye pain and photophobia.
2. **Central loss of vision** suggests central retinal vein occlusion or vitreous hemorrhage (if sudden) or macular degeneration or cataract if chronic. **Glare** suggests cataracts, corneal edema, or corneal scare.
3. **Floaters** suggest retinal detachment, vitreous detachment, and uveitis. **Flashes** suggest vitreous or retinal detachment or migraine.
4. **Giant cell arteritis** can cause anterior ischemic arteritic neuropathy, and visual field defect is altitudinal (superior or inferior).
5. **Scleritis and iritis** and **keratitis** cause photophobia; **optic neuritis** causes retrobulbar pain and blurry vision. **Scleritis** causes a deep ache in the eye.
6. **Hydroxychloroquine** causes macular degeneration, and should be screened at **baseline and 5 years** after treatment of hydroxychloroquine.
7. **African Americans** should be screened for **glaucoma q2-4 years for age 40–50 and annually if >50 yo**.
8. Crusty, watery eye discharge, preauricular adenopathy is highly suggestive of **viral conjunctivitis**, treatment: cold compression q4h. **Bacterial conjunctivitis rarely causes preauricular adenopathy.**
9. Unilateral redness, discharge, and pain of the eye, no palpable preauricular adenopathy, contact lens wearing too long. Diagnosis: **bacterial keratitis or corneal hypoxia** → urgent ophthalmological evaluation. High risks for Pseudomonas infection. **Patching and topical steroids are contraindicated.**
10. Sectoral hyperemia with no trauma but **subacute pain worse with movements** is **scleritis,** will need ophthalmologist referral for topical steroids. **Episcleritis** is sectoral hyperemia, typically **painless,** and does not need treatment.
11. **Sectoral hyperemia**: erythema involves only a portion, or sector, of the conjunctiva. **Causes** include episcleritis, scleritis, and pterygium. **Episcleritis** is pain-free or mild pain while **scleritis** is deep boring pain.
12. **Macular degeneration**: central vision loss. **Glaucoma** affects peripheral vision and causes near misses with pedestrians.
13. **Causes of peripheral vision loss** include glaucoma, retinitis pigmentosa, eye strokes or occlusions, detached retina, brain damage from stroke, neurological damage like optic neuritis, compressed optic nerve from papilledema like pseudotumor cerebri (increase in intracranial pressure), and concussions.
14. **Topical trifluridine** is used for corneal epithelial herpes simplex infection which is always unilateral.
15. **Diabetic retinopathy treatment**: ranibizumab, bevacizumab, aflibercept (anti-VEGF), or pan-retinal laser photocoagulation. Diagnosis via spectral domain optical coherence tomography.

16. In advanced **dry age-related macular degeneration (AMD)**, **gradual** vision loss occurs because of degeneration changes in the retinal pigment epithelium, Bruch's membrane, and choriocapillaris. Treatment: zinc, copper, zeaxanthin, lutein, vitamin E.
17. In **wet AMD**, abnormal blood vessels grow through Bruch membranes and bleed or leak serous fluid beneath the neurosensory retina → **rapid** distortion, and central vision loss.
18. **Open-angle glaucoma**: dilated examinations to assess the cup: disc ratio of the optic nerve, visual fields, and objective testing of optic nerve status with retinal nerve fiber layer analysis. **Treatment to lower intraocular pressure (IOP)** using beta blockers, alpha-adrenergic, carbonic anhydrase inhibitors (like acetazolamide), and prostaglandins.
19. **Close-angle glaucoma** causes rapid and severe IOP elevation, leading to corneal edema, severe pain, and potential blindness. It is an ocular emergency. **Treatment**: laser argon or YAG to create an iridotomy or surgery to create an iridectomy.
20. **Acetazolamide** causes paresthesia, GI upset, and fatigue.
21. **Entropion** (eyelid turns in) and **ectropion** (eyelid turns out).
22. School-age children should receive regular examinations for **visual acuity and ocular alignment**.
23. **Red eyes** that should prompt urgent ophthalmology referral include **severe pain, visual deficits or loss of acuity, corneal ulceration, hypopyon** (layering of WBC over the inferior iris), and **hyphema** (bleeding).
24. **Pterygium**: irritation, foreign body sensation. **Blepharitis**: morning crusting and discharge, foreign body sensation.
25. **Bacterial conjunctivitis** is often seen in the absence of other allergic symptoms. Topical not oral treatment is the standard of care.
26. **Viral conjunctivitis** is contagious for 1–2 weeks. **Viral keratitis** (herpes simplex or varicella-zoster virus) → po **acyclovir** treatment (+/− topical trifluridine) → **avoid topical steroids except for stromal keratitis**.
27. **Corneal ulceration (bacterial keratitis)** may be secondary to trauma, chronic topical steroid use, other ocular surface diseases (dry eye, ocular cicatricial pemphigoid), or contact lens wearing (G-rod bacterial infection), Staph except for lens contacts (Pseudomonas infection), fungal from trauma or steroid use (candida).
28. **Pseudomonas keratitis** in a contact lens wearer: diffuse corneal edema, purulent corneal abscess, hypopyon.
29. **Acute bacterial conjunctivitis** is usually caused by Pneumococcus and Hemophilus species. Treatment: broad-spectrum antibiotics topically (erythromycin, polymyxin-bacitracin, bacitracin, various fluoroquinolones like ofloxacin, ciprofloxacin) safe. **Topical aminoglycosides** should be avoided because of the high risks of toxic or allergic conjunctivitis.
30. **Neisseria** can cause **hyperacute bacterial conjunctivitis** which is purulent and sight-threatening and requires **urgent ophthalmologist referral.** Chlamydia infection usually leads to chronic conjunctivitis. **Systemic penicil-**

lins or ceftriaxone (1 g im once) for Neisseria infection along with topical **bacitracin** ointment and oral **doxycycline** for presumed chlamydia conjunctivitis are recommended in **Neisseria conjunctivitis**.

31. **Staphylococcal blepharitis** causes chronic eyelid irradiation and redness, loss of eyelashes, and even corneal ulceration. Staphylococcal blepharitis is associated with **conjunctivitis** (staphylococcal marginal keratitis).
32. **Sty also known as hordeolum** = an acute infection (staph) of the hair follicle. **Treatment**: warm compression and topical antibiotics.
33. **Chalazion**: noninfectious blockage of a meibomian gland orifice.
34. Allergic conjunctivitis: bilateral red watery itchy eyes (no pruritus). Nonocular symptoms can include rhinitis and asthma.
35. **Topical steroids** in the eyes can cause glaucoma, cataracts, or infectious keratitis.
36. **Acute recurrent unilateral iritis** is usually seen in HLA-B27-related systemic diseases including seronegative spondyloarthropathies, ankylosing spondylitis, and others. **Bilateral chronic iritis** is usually seen in sarcoidosis and rheumatoid arthritis (RA). **Uvea** = iris, choroid, and ciliary body. **Posterior synechiae** = consider adhesions between the lens and iris.
37. **Acute angle glaucoma** may be precipitated by the use of alpha adrenergics, anticholinergics, and sympathomimetics.
38. **CMV retinitis** should be screened annually in individuals with HIV and $CD4 > 100$ and every 3–6 m for $CD4 < 100$.
39. **Individuals treated with corticosteroids** should be screened q6–12 m for glaucoma and cataracts.
40. Non-infectious **retinal microvasculopathy** (retinal hemorrhages and cotton-wool spots) is the most common ocular manifestation of HIV/AIDS.

Further Readings and References

1. Young A, Kumar MA, Thota PN. 2020. GERD: A practical approach. Cleve Clin J Med. 87(4):223–230.
2. Ständer S. 2021. Atopic Dermatitis. N Engl J Med. 384(12):1136–1143.
3. Bagheri N, Mehta S. 2015. Acute Vision Loss. Prim Care. 42(3):347–361.

Chapter 21
Vaccination, HIV, and Women's Health

Vaccination in Adults

1. **Live attenuated vaccines** include MMR, varicella, zoster, and intranasal influenza; contraindicated in pregnancy and immunocompromised including HIV CD4 < 200 cells/mL.
2. **Relative contraindications to influenza vaccinations**: moderate to severe acute illness with or without fever; history of Guillain-Barré syndrome (GBS) within 6 weeks of previous influenza vaccine.
3. **Amantadine** and rimantadine are only effective against influenza A virus.
4. An adult who received pneumococcal vaccine after age 65 will not need any further revaccination.
5. **Tetanus shot schedule**: 0, 4 weeks, 6–12 months (one should be Tdap). **Tdap** is recommended in all pregnant women during third trimester (27 through 36 weeks of pregnancy) and people with close contact with known exposure to infants.
6. **Meningococcal vaccine types:** (1) meningococcal conjugate or MenACWY vaccines, (2) serogroup B meningococcal or MenB vaccines, (3) pentavalent meningococcal or MenABCWY vaccine.
7. **Conjugate meningococcal vaccine (MenACWY)** is recommended in functional or anatomic asplenia, complement deficiency, complement inhibitor use, and HIV. It requires two doses of primary series, 2 months apart, and should get revaccination every 5 years.
8. Additional indications of **MenACWY** include microbiologist routinely exposed to Neisseria meningitidis, military recruit, college freshmen living in a dormitory, and people traveling or residing in countries in which serogroup A, C, W, or Y meningococcal disease is common.
9. **Bivalent (Serogroup B) meningococcal vaccine**: at-risk patients (complement deficiency, functional or anatomic asplenia, and complement inhibitor use) should get MenB-FHbp (Trumenba) at 0, 1–2 and 6 months, or MenB-4C (Bexasero) at 0, 1 month; if remains high risk, these patients should receive

K. Zhou, *Internal Medicine Training Notes and Survival Guide*,
https://doi.org/10.1007/978-1-0716-4039-5_21

booster dose of MenB vaccine 1 year after series completion and then every 2–3 years thereafter. Healthy adults aged 16–23 may get MenB-FHbp at 0, 6 months or MenB-4C at 0 and 1 month.

10. First-year college students 21 years old or younger who live in a dorm should receive **one dose of MenACWY** if not done at 16+ years old. Additionally, should also **get two doses of the MenB vaccine**, 1 month apart if MenB-4C, at 0 and 6 months if MenB-FHbp.
11. All adults born **after 1957** who have no evidence of immunity should be vaccinated against **MMR**, unless contraindications like pregnancy, cancer, or receiving high doses (>20 mg) of daily corticosteroids. HIV is not a contraindication for MMR.
12. A **second MMR dose (28 days apart from first dose) is indicated** if the patient is: a student in a post-secondary education institution, a healthcare worker, planning to travel internationally, pregnant with no immunity, exposed to measles, previously vaccinated with killed measles vaccine, vaccinated with an unknown type of measles vaccine 1963–1967, household and close contacts of immunocompromised persons.
13. **Live attenuated influenza vaccine (LAIV)** is contraindicated in age <2 or >49, heart disease, lung disease, diabetes, CKD, liver disease, conditions with compromised respiratory function or difficulties handling secretion, aspirin takers.
14. **Respiratory syncytial virus vaccine and monoclonal antibody** indications: (1) a single dose of **RSV vaccine** for adults aged 60 years and older; (2) **Pfizer Abrysvo vaccine** administered September through January in weeks 32 through 36 of pregnancy; (3) one dose of **nirsevimab** for all infants aged 8 months and younger born during or entering their first RSV season; (4) one dose of **nirsevimab** for infants and children aged 8–19 months who are at increased risk for severe RSV disease and entering their second RSV season. Of note, **palivizumab** (once a month during RSV season) for children aged 24 months and younger with high risks for severe RSV disease.
15. Travel in <2 weeks, age < 40 years old and healthy should only get the **HAV vaccine**, but if immunocompromised or liver disease or age > 40 years old, should administer the **HAV vaccine and immunoglobulin**.
16. A vaccinated person but known **nonresponder** after exposure to HBV should get HBV immunoglobulin × 1. Nonresponders with primary hepatitis B vaccine series (i.e., anti-HBs <10 mIU/mL) should complete a second vaccine series or be evaluated to determine if they are HBsAg-positive. If the titer of anti-HBS ≥ **10 mIU/mL**, no treatment is needed. If <10 mIU/mL, give HBV immunoglobulin × 1 and a vaccine booster.
17. The following population needs to **check antibodies 1–2 months after completion of vaccination series for HBV**: immunocompromised, vaccinated in buttocks, infants born to HBsAg positive moms, healthcare workers with contact with blood, sex partners of chronic HBV carriers.
18. Post-exposure of varicella patients should be vaccinated within 3 days of exposure. If contraindications, varicella zoster immunoglobulin should be used.

19. **Vaccination in adults**: influenza, Td/Tdap, MMR, VAR, PCV15, PCV20, HBV, HAV, MenACWY, MPSV4, MenB, Hib.
20. **PCV–naïve adults ≥ 65 years or aged 19–64 years** with certain underlying conditions should be vaccinated with **PCV15 or PCV20**. When PCV15 is used, a dose of PPSV23 should be given typically ≥1 year after. The minimum interval **is 8 weeks after PCV 15 for PPSV 23** and can be considered in an immunocompromising condition for patients aged 19–64 years: chronic lung or heart disease, diabetes, alcoholism, chronic liver or kidney disease, chronic smoker CSF leaks, cochlear implants, sickle cell disease (SCD) or other hemoglobinopathies, asplenia, immunodeficiencies, HIV, leukemia, lymphoma, Hodgkin disease, multiple myeloma (MM), and transplant. If **PCV20** is used, no PPSV23 is necessary.
21. **Varicella vaccine**, a live attenuated virus vaccine, is indicated in adults without known varicella or prior vaccine. If uncertain of immunity, antibody testing should be performed. **Varicella vaccine** should be given at 0, 1–2 months if no known varicella infection history or prior vaccination.
22. **Two doses of HPV vaccination**, at least 6 months apart, are recommended for (routinely for ages 11–12) ages 9 through 14 and catchup vaccination for ages 13–26 who were not adequately vaccinated previously.
23. **HPV vaccination**: two dose regimen for 9–14 yo and three dose regimen for 15–26 yo.
24. The Advisory Committee on Immunization Practices (ACIP) recommends: aged **≥50** years old immunocompetent adults and those aged 19 years or older immunocompromised, **Shingrix (Zoster vaccine recombinant)** should be given two doses, 2–6 months apart unless immunosuppressed or TB diagnosis.

HIV Testing

1. Offer to test everyone for HIV, unless they decline. **Age 13–65** should get an HIV test.
2. **HIV-1,2 Ag differentiation assay** and **rapid HIV Ab test** can be negative in the first few weeks of HIV infection.
3. HIV diagnosis is via **HIV RNA viral load**. HIV incubation period **4–11 days**; antibody positive in **6–12 weeks**.
4. **HIV testing**: HIV RNA, HIV p24 Ag → enzyme immunoassay (EIA): rapid HIV (Ab to HIV-1 and 2) → EIA with western blot.
5. Advice to reduce HIV risks: ask the patient to identify and commit a method to increase condom use.
6. The CDC recommends **pre-exposure prophylaxis (PrEP)** for unprotected sex with people using iv drugs, iv drug abusers, and sex with positive HIV infection.
7. **Pre-exposure prophylaxis PrEP**: Emtricitabine/Tenofovir (Truvada or Descovy). Tenofovir can cause renal insufficiency, additional risks for PrEP include reactivation/worsening of HBV if discontinuation of PrEP, and resistant HIV.
8. **Annual HIV screening** for IVDU, prostitutes, HIV sex partners, and MSM.

9. **Antiretroviral therapy** use reduces HIV transmission to the HIV-negative partner by 96%.
10. **Relative risks for HIV transmission**: insertive fellatio < receptive fellatio < insertive vaginal < receptive vaginal < insertive anal < receptive anal.
11. CSF, pleural, pericardial, peritoneal, synovial, and amniotic fluid are all considered infectious; **saline, sputum, nasal secretions, vomitus, feces, and urine are not considered infectious unless visibly bloody in HIV infection**.
12. **Post-exposure prophylaxis (PEP)** is effective up to **72 h after exposure**; PEP medications: tenofovir, emtricitabine, and an integrase inhibitor (raltegravir or dolutegravir) for **4** weeks. **HIV testing at the time of exposure** and follow-up testing **6** weeks, **12** weeks, and **6** months after exposure.

HIV Treatment

1. **Valganciclovir** can be used to treat CMV retinitis and for second prophylaxis when a patient has a history of CMV retinitis. HIV treatment: three-drug combination of two nucleoside reverse transcriptase (**NRTI**) with one of the following: an integrase inhibitor (**INSTI**), a non-nucleoside reverse transcriptase inhibitor (**NNRTI**), or protease inhibitor (**PI**). **PI should be boosted with ritonavir or cobicistat.**
2. **Tenofovir disoproxil fumarate (DF) and emtricitabine (Truvada)** can decrease GFR and have activity against HBV but not HCV. **Tenofovir and emtricitabine** are active against Hepatitis B.
3. **Tenofovir** DF causes Fanconi's syndrome (hypokalemia, hypophosphatemia, and normal anion gap metabolic acidosis).
4. If **CD4 > 200 and viral load is suppressed**, check CD4 counts every 6–12 months; if viral load >5000, check genotypic resistance, then, if necessary, change the treatment regimen.
5. Patients with **CD4 > 500** are usually asymptomatic and have virtually no risk of developing an AIDs-indicator condition within 18 months, except for TB, cervical cancer, recurrent bacterial pneumonia, or superficial Kaposi sarcoma.
6. **Pneumocystis jiroveci Pneumonia (PJP) treatments/prophylaxis** include TMP-SMX, dapsone, or atovaquone.
7. **CD4 levels and infection in HIV:** If **CD4 < 200**: toxoplasma (prescribe TMP-SMX or pyrimethamine if toxoplasma IgG positive), histoplasma, candida, JC virus, PJP. If **CD4 < 100**, CMV, MAC (azithromycin, clarithromycin, or rifabutin), cryptococcus neoformans, cryptosporidium. If **CD4 < 50**, CMV retinitis (dilated eye exam q6m).
8. After **3** months of HIV treatment, the goal is viral load **undetectable**. If not at goal, will need to check the **genotype** for **resistance**.
9. **Transiently mildly detectable** viral load during treatment may be caused by **false positive HIV RNA test** and thus is generally not a sign of resistance.
10. **Genotype testing** indicated in two situations: newly diagnosed HIV infection to detect transmission of resistant virus; and patients on antiretroviral therapy failing therapies.

11. **Atazanavir** is associated with **unconjugated hyperbilirubinemia** (Gilbert-like). Atazanavir should not be given with an antacid. **Tenofovir** is associated with **nephrotoxicity** and **osteoporosis. Protease inhibitors are** associated with **GI disturbance**.
12. **Hypersensitivity** reactions to abacavir include rash, abdominal pain, nausea, vomiting, and diarrhea → stop the medication and start urgent evaluations.
13. **Genotypic resistance** testing is indicated if viral load increases on the current regimen.
14. The metabolism of **simvastatin** is inhibited by **ritonavir** which can lead to toxicity; whereas pravastatin or atorvastatin can be used together with ritonavir.
15. **Pneumocystis pneumonia (PCP)** prophylaxis: If the patient cannot take TMP/SMX SS due to side effects, **dapsone (100 mg orally twice a week), aerosolized pentamidine, or atovaquone** can be used as alternatives.
16. **Mycobacterium avium complex (MAC)** prophylaxis: effective regimens include **azithromycin** 1200 mg once a week, **clarithromycin** 500 mg twice daily, or **rifabutin** 300 mg daily.
17. **Efavirenz** causes drowsiness, dizziness, abnormal dreams, impaired concentration, and worsens psychiatric disorders.
18. **Non-nucleoside reverse transcriptase inhibitors (NNRTIs), most nucleoside/nucleotide reverse transcriptase inhibitors (NRTIs) and the CCR5 inhibitor maraviroc can cause hepatotoxicity**.

Women's Health

1. **Low-grade squamous intraepithelial lesion (LSIL)**: (1) if age ≥25 years, check HPV. If HPV positive, proceed with **colposcopy** otherwise repeat HPV in a year. (2) If postmenopausal, repeat pap smear in 6 and 12 months, and proceed to colposcopy if **ASCUS** or worse. (3) If 21–24 years old, repeat the cytology in 12 and 24 months. If a serious abnormality (**ASC-H** or **HSIL**) on the 12-month pap smear, or any abnormality (i.e. **ASCUS** or worse) on the 24-month pap smear, proceed to **colposcopy**.
2. ASCUS = Atypical Squamous Cells of Undetermined Significance. HSIL = high-grade squamous intraepithelial lesion. ASC-H = **Atypical Squamous Cells, HSIL cannot be excluded**.
3. Screening for cervical cancer: age 21–65 years with cytology (Pap smear) every 3 years or, for ages 30–65 years with a combination of cytology and HPV cotesting every 5 years.
4. **Cotesting for cervical cancer** screening in a 36-year-old woman: The cytology negative but positive HPV, can be managed in one of two ways: repeat contesting in 12 months, or test immediately for HPV 16 or 16/18 and refer to colposcopy if either HPV test abnormal.
5. **HPV vaccination**: target age 11–12 before sexual activities; "catch-up" vaccinations are approved for both genders ages **9–26**. Two doses, 6 months apart usually; however, for age 15 and older, three (not two) doses at 0, 2, and 6 months are required.

6. **Common menopausal symptoms**: hot flashes, night sweats and vaginal dryness.
7. In menopause, the highest circulating sex hormone is **estrone** via the conversion of androstenedione by peripheral tissues in females. **FSH** may be normal in perimenopausal women.
8. **Estrogen replacement** for menopausal symptoms: initial oral dose 0.625 mg daily, may titrate up if persistent symptoms. Tablets strengths: 0.3, 0.625, 0.9 and 1.25 mg. Dosage quantity should be minimal to its benefits given concerns of side effects. **Estrogen plus progesterone therapy** increases breast cancer mortality after 3–5 years of use; estrogen alone has a more favorable risk-benefit profile even with 7 years' use, but still has lots of side effects **including blood clots, stroke risks, and heart attacks**.
9. **Contraindications** to estrogen use: undiagnosed vaginal bleeding, breast cancer, other estrogen-sensitive cancers, current or previous history of venous or arterial thrombosis, and liver abnormalities.
10. For women on hormone therapy for menopausal symptoms of **≥10 years from menopause onset or ≥60 years old**, hormone therapy is not recommended and likely should be stopped because of the greater absolute risks of coronary heart disease, stroke, venous thromboembolism, and dementia.
11. **Estrogen should be tapered to avoid the return of hot flashes.**
12. Estrogen products: **oral** (conjugated estrogen, esterified estrogen, and estradiol) estrogen, **oral estrogen and progestogen** (progestin or progesterone) combinations, **oral estrogen and selective estrogen receptor modulator**, **transdermal estradiol** patch, transdermal estrogen and progestin combination patch.

Further Readings and References

1. Hunter P, Fryhofer SA, Szilagyi PG. 2020. Vaccination of Adults in General Medical Practice. Mayo Clin Proc. 95(1):169–183.
2. Pneumococcal Vaccine Timing for Adults. CDC. https://www.cdc.gov/pneumococcal/downloads/Vaccine-Timing-Adults-JobAid.pdf (accessed October 20, 2024).
3. Saag MS. 2021. HIV Infection - Screening, Diagnosis, and Treatment. N Engl J Med. 384(22):2131–2143.
4. Pinkerton JV. 2020. Hormone Therapy for Postmenopausal Women. N Engl J Med. 382(5):446–455.

Part III
Specialty Training for a General Internist

As I reflect on my rotations in clinical subspecialties during my internal medicine residency training, I am struck by the depth and breadth of experiences that have shaped my journey as a physician. From cardiology to gastroenterology, nephrology to pulmonology, each rotation has provided me with unique insights, challenges, and opportunities for growth.

Stepping into the world of clinical subspecialties felt like embarking on a journey of exploration and discovery. Each rotation offered a window into a different aspect of internal medicine, with its own set of diseases, diagnostic algorithms, and treatment modalities. From the intricacies of managing complex arrhythmias in cardiology to the nuances of interpreting cancer pathology, I found myself captivated by the depth and complexity of each subspecialty. One of the most rewarding aspects of my subspecialty rotations was the opportunity to expand my knowledge base and deepen my understanding of disease processes, treatment options, and the rapid development of new treatments for disorders. I encountered a diverse array of clinical presentations, from rare and exotic syndromes to common yet challenging conditions, and learned to approach each patient encounter with curiosity, humility, and a commitment to evidence-based practice.

Throughout my rotations, I had the privilege of working alongside expert faculty members, fellows, and co-residents who served as invaluable mentors and role models. They challenged me to think critically, communicate effectively, and perform with precision in the diagnosis and management of complex medical conditions. I embraced each opportunity to expand my knowledge in patient care, refine my clinical skills, and become a more proficient physician. Beyond the clinical aspects of my rotations, I also valued the relationships I forged with my colleagues and mentors. The camaraderie and teamwork within each subspecialty team created a supportive and collaborative learning environment where I felt empowered to ask questions, seek guidance, and grow both personally and professionally. These relationships have enriched my training experience and inspired me to strive for excellence in all aspects of patient care.

As for suggestions for future trainees in internal medicine for subspecialty rotations, emphases remain almost universal on the following aspects: understand the basics via building a strong foundation in pathophysiology; foster a good rapport with patients and their families by demonstrating empathy, compassion, and active listening; stay organized and proactive for workups and treatment plans, and follow-up schedules to ensure comprehensive and timely care; practice clear and empathetic communication when discussing diagnoses, treatment options, prognosis, and supportive care with patients and their families; stay updated and embrace learning opportunities via participation in patient evaluations, treatment planning discussions, and multidisciplinary rounds.

Notes of this section were based on the following resources: the UpToDate and MedScape websites, the Pocket Medicine-The Massachusetts General Hospital Handbook of Internal Medicine, society guidelines, the Medical Knowledge Self-Assessment Program® (MKSAP), and the UWorld®. As I typed, I revised and updated the notes based on the current available guidelines and medical knowledge, and my own clinical experiences. Upon the last moment before submitting the manuscript for publication, I further revised and updated the Chapter of Cardiology based on suggestions of Dr. Dongbo Yu (board-certified cardiologist), and I'm sure, you will appreciate the chapter in its current revised form as I do.

Chapter 22
Hematology and Oncology

1. Acute portal hypertension from **hepatic vein thrombosis = Budd-Chiari syndrome**. Half of Budd-Chiari syndrome is due to acquired **JAK2 mutation**.
2. Paroxysmal nocturnal hemoglobinuria (**PNH**) causes **splanchnic vein thrombosis** and **cerebral vein thrombosis**.
3. **Causes of eosinophilia**: CHINA—connective tissue disease, helminthic infection, idiopathic, neoplasia, allergy. **Hypereosinophilic syndrome** (HES) commonly affects the skin, lungs, gastrointestinal tract, and heart.
4. **Washed erythrocytes** are used in patients with a history of severe **allergic** reactions to transfusions. Washed erythrocytes: most of the plasma, platelets (PLTs), and WBCs are removed and replaced with normal saline (NS).
5. **Leukoreduced and irradiated erythrocytes** are used for **immunocompromised** patients to reduce graft versus host disease (GVHD) in transfusion.
6. **Washed platelet is used for severe allergic transfusion reactions**. In refractory platelet decrease due to alloimmunization, can transfuse HLA-matched platelets.
7. **Nonimmune causes of thrombocytopenia** include sepsis, fever, DIC, splenomegaly, and medications. If due to alloimmunization from previous pregnancies, treatment is HLA-matched PLTs, HLA-compatible PLTs, and PLT crossing match.
8. **Superior vena cava (SVC) syndrome** is usually seen in lung cancer, aggressive lymphoma, thymoma, and primary mediastinal germ cell tumors.
9. **Aromatase inhibitors**: anastrozole, letrozole, exemestane; they cause **debilitating musculoskeletal symptoms**; if this happens, may switch to tamoxifen.
10. Overexpression of **cyclin D1** is associated with **t11:14 chromosome translocation**: diagnostic for **mantle cell lymphoma**.
11. Diagnosis of **chronic lymphocytic leukemia (CLL): peripheral blood smear and flow cytometry** of the peripheral blood with immunophenotypic analyses of circulating lymphocytes; LN and BM biopsy are not needed. **CLL in flow**

K. Zhou, *Internal Medicine Training Notes and Survival Guide*,
https://doi.org/10.1007/978-1-0716-4039-5_22

cytometry: B cell Ags (CD19, CD20, and CD23), co-expression of CD5 (usually a T cell marker), and low levels of monoclonal surface Ig.

12. **Papillary thyroid cancer** follow-up labs: TSH, free T4, and thyroglobulin levels annually, US every 3–5 years.
13. **Sweet's syndrome (acute febrile neutrophilic dermatosis)** is usually seen in hematologic malignancy.
14. **Red blood cell distribution width (RDW) increases in iron deficiency** but is normal in thalassemia. **Metformin** can cause B12 deficiency.
15. **Elevated gamma gap** (>4 g/dL) may indicate plasma cell dyscrasias including Waldenstrom's macroglobulinemia and multiple myeloma. If hyperviscosity occurs, start emergent plasmapheresis.
16. Diagnosis of multiple myeloma (MM): 20% or so patients with multiple myeloma only secretes **a urine light chain with no M spike on SPEP**. As a result, MM diagnosis requires **UPEP with immunofixation or serum-free light chain assay**.
17. Mean corpuscular volume (MCV) is decreased in hemolytic anemia, normal or increased in MDS, and also decreased in hemoglobinopathies.
18. **In megaloblastic anemi**a, first rule out B12/folate deficiency then bone marrow biopsy for myelodysplastic syndromes (MDS).
19. In **antithrombin** deficiency and heparin resistance, **PTT is persistently normal** with heparin drip**.**
20. Thrombophilia evaluation, stop anticoagulation (if appropriate) and **wait at least 2 weeks for thrombophilia tests**.
21. **Active surveillance** (close cancer monitoring and transition to treatment stat if cancer progression) versus **observation** (watchful waiting).
22. **Transformation** of follicular lymphoma to an aggressive non-Hodgkin lymphoma has to be ruled out by **biopsy**.
23. **HER2 expression** occurs in **20%** of gastric cancer and **30%** of gastroesophageal junction tumors.
24. **Iron deficiency anemia diagnosis**: transferrin saturation less than 15%–20% and serum ferritin level <30 ng/mL. Transferrin saturation <20% and ferritin >100 ng/mL indicate anemia of chronic disease.
25. **Prophylactic acyclovir for bortezomib therapy** (increased risk for herpes zoster) after autologous stem cell transplantation.
26. **Hemochromatosis**: atypical presentation of rheumatoid arthritis and osteoarthritis including **hook-like** osteophytes of the second and third metacarpophalangeal joints, increased **transferrin saturation (≥45%), and increased ferritin (≥300 ng/mL in males and above 200 ng/mL in females**).
27. **HbA = $\alpha 2\beta 2$, HbA2 = $\alpha 2\delta 2$, beta thalassemia minor = increased HbA2 (≥3.5%), beta thalassemia major = increased HbF. HbC disease: glutamic acid to lysine mutation in beta globin, causes extravascular hemolysis**.
28. **Paroxysmal nocturnal hemoglobinuria (PNH)** presents with headache, fatigue, and nonspecific abdominal pain, portal vein, or cerebral venous sinus thrombosis. PNH is associated with **5% of MDS and >50% of bone marrow aplasia**.

29. **Alpha thalassemia trait** usually has an Hb of 10ish. **Electrophoresis** in alpha thalassemia trait is normal, with no change in HbA2 and HbF. **Alpha thalassemia** (HbH—3 beta allele deletion; Hb Barts—4 allele deletion)
30. **Sbeta-thalassemia** has HbS of around 60%. Patients with **sickle cell trait** have HbS < 41%. **Sickle cell disease** (SCD) has ≥90% HbS.
31. Pancytopenia + macrocytic erythrocytes + hypersegmented neutrophils = consider **megaloblastic anemia** ⇒ check B12 and folate. Increased LDH and indirect bilirubin = **ineffective erythropoiesis** and **intramedullary hemolysis** is seen in **megaloblastic anemia**. Methylmalonic acid and homocysteine are both elevated in B12 deficiency.
32. Direct Antiglobulin Test (DAT) with Reflex to Anti C3 and Anti IgG: if positive with **C3** (IgG usually absent) on erythrocytes with agglutinated erythrocytes on peripheral smear = consider cold agglutinin autoimmune hemolytic anemia. **Cold agglutinin autoimmune hemolytic anemia** is commonly seen in lymphoproliferative disorders, such as Waldenstrom's macroglobulinemia, other B cell non-Hodgkin lymphomas, and IgM MGUS ⇒ consider treatment with **rituximab**.
33. In **warm antibody autoimmune hemolytic anemia**, DAT almost always has **IgG** with or without C3. For warm Abs, treat with **prednisone and IVIG and other immunosuppressants** like azathioprine, cyclosporine, cyclophosphamide, mycophenolate, and danazol. Direct antiglobulin test vs indirect antiglobulin test = donor RBC vs donor plasma (alloantibody).
34. Approximately **50% of Budd-Chiari syndrome** and **25% of portal vein thrombosis** are from **myeloproliferative neoplasms** ⇒ consider checking JAK2 V617F gene mutation even without erythrocytosis or thrombocytosis.
35. Genetic counseling and BRCA1 and BRCA2 genetic testing. Before that, genetic counseling is recommended in females with **triple-negative breast cancer diagnosed before age 60 or ovarian cancer at any age.**
36. In **hereditary spherocytosis**, acute viral infections like Parvovirus (**B19**) and **Epstein-Barr** virus and **bacterial infections** like Streptococcus pneumoniae, other streptococci, and Salmonella may trigger a **transient aplastic crisis**. Treatment is **observation**.
37. In patients with **severe symptomatic autoimmune hemolytic anemia**, the autoantibodies typically react against all erythrocytes and can transfuse **incompatible crossmatch blood (still ABO and Rh matched)**.
38. Increase in **PTT** (intrinsic coagulation pathway assessment/time to form blood clots; factors VII and XIII do not belong to intrinsic pathway) not fully corrected with mixing study indicates coagulation factor inhibitor(s) and rarely lupus anticoagulants. Acquired hemophilia A can be treated with **activated factor VII**.
39. **Epidural spinal cord compression treatment**: surgical candidates with a life expectancy ≥3 months should receive **IV steroids Decadron and immediate decompressive surgery**. If not a surgical candidate, do **urgent radiation therapy**.

40. After completion of radiation therapy, we should start breast cancer screening at the **age of 25 years old or 8 years after radiation therapy** whichever is later. If chest wall radiation is between 10–30 years old, get an **annual mammogram and MRI breast**.
41. For **unprovoked pulmonary embolism (PE)**, anticoagulation for 6 months to 1 year; for **provoked PE**, anticoagulation only for 3 months.
42. **Immune thrombocytopenic purpura (ITP)** without evidence of bleeding and PLT > 30–40 × 10^9/L has <15% of chance of becoming more severe thrombocytopenia. Treatment: observation, but can include **prednisone, IVIG, and rituximab**.
43. **Coagulopathy in liver failure** is characterized by increased PTT and PT and **increased VIII levels**.
44. **Infection versus anaphylactic transfusion reaction**: the latter has dermatological, pulmonary, and gastrointestinal effects.
45. Warfarin is safe in breastfeeding; essential thrombocythemia → check **JAK2 V617F analysis**.
46. Surveillance imaging in **stage III colon cancer** after treatment: **CT abdomen and chest every 6–12 months for 3–5 years**.
47. Facial swelling, dyspnea but no stridor, laryngeal edema, or altered mentation = consider **superior vena cava syndrome**. Treatment: may include **biopsy** for diagnosis, chemotherapy, **radiation** or **stenting depending on the urgency and emergency**.
48. **Liver lesion unresectable** due to proximity to hepatic vein, treatment: **conversion chemotherapy** to shrink the tumor to a resectable size and then curative intent surgery with neoadjuvant and adjuvant therapy given before and after curative intent surgery.
49. Patients with early-stage head-neck cancer should be treated with only **surgery or radiation** alone.
50. **Sickle cell disease (SCD) crises**: splenic sequestration crisis, aplastic crisis, hyperhemolytic crisis.
51. **Spherocytes** are seen in hereditary spherocytosis and autoimmune hemolysis.
52. **B cell markers**: CD 19, CD 20, CD33.
53. Chronic **GVHD** occurs at any time in **50%** of post-transplant patients, with increased risk with CMV+. Manifestations of chronic GVHD include skin lichen planus-like or scleroderma-like rash, elevated LFTs, dry eyes, cataracts, genitourinary and musculoskeletal abnormalities, and bronchiolitis obliterans.
54. **SCD-CVA risks**: 1/10 before age 20, ¼ by age 45; secondary prophylaxis is chronic simple transfusion therapy q4-6 weeks with a goal **HbS level of <30% and total Hb level of 9–12.5**. Treat iron overload with **deferasirox, deferiprone, or deferoxamine**. Iron chelation therapy starts after 1–2 years of transfusions, serum ferritin >1000 μg/L, or liver iron concentration >3 mg/g dry weight.
55. **Xerostomia** after chemo treatment: cholinergic meds like **pilocarpine**, and **cevimeline**.
56. Decrease or discontinue testosterone if HCT >54%.

57. Peripheral smear shows **immature cells** plus severe **thrombocytopenia and leukocytosis** = consider **acute myeloid leukemia (AML)**. In AML, blast ≥20%. In APL (chromosome 15 and 17 translocations creating an abnormal fusion gene called PML/RARα), blast is low and has hypergranular promyelocytes.
58. Nodular cord may indicate **superficial vein thrombophlebitis**: consider anticoagulation (low dose, like Xarelto 10 mg daily) for 45 days if superficial vein thrombosis >5 cm, anatomic proximity to deep vein (<5 cm), and medical risk factors.
59. **Erythromelalgia**: burning pain and erythema (sometimes pallor and/or cyanosis), treatment with **aspirin**. Primary due to **hyperexcitable dorsal root ganglia**; secondary due to myeloproliferative disease, hypercholesterolemia, autoimmune, mushroom, or medications (ticlopidine, bromocriptine).
60. **Glioblastoma multiforme** usually presents with **seizures** and manifestations of **increased intracranial pressure** (like headache, unstable mood, and personality change) with rapid decline.

Treatment in Hematology and Oncology

1. Prostate cancer with focal extension to capsule (high-risk PSA ≥20, Gleason score 8–10, extraprostatic extension) Treatment: **GnRH agonist + radiation for 2–3 years**. Low risk and limited volume cancer treatment: **brachytherapy**.
2. **Kidney cancer treatment**: Sunitinib → sorafenib → everolimus.
3. **Ibrutinib** (chemokine CXCL12 and 13 inhibitors) is used in CLL, mantle cell lymphoma, and Waldenstrom's macroglobulinemia.
4. **RAS mutation** status should be tested in metastatic colorectal cancer; if wild type, **cetuximab and panitumumab** may be used**.**
5. **Erlotinib** is effective in metastatic non-small cell lung cancer (**NSCLC**) with EGFR mutation as it inhibits the intracellular phosphorylation of tyrosine kinase of EGFR.
6. **Crizotinib** is a tyrosine kinase inhibitor used for metastatic NSCLC with **ALK** translocations or **ROS1** mutations. **Lorlatinib** is also FDA-approved as first-line therapy for ALK-positive metastatic NSCLC; a recent study showed durable longer benefits from lorlatinib than crizotinib.
7. NSCLC treatment primary first line platinum based (**carboplatin or cisplatin + pemetrexed in adenocarcinoma**) ⇒ consider maintenance treatment with pemetrexed or docetaxel.
8. **Laryngeal cancer** early-stage treatment: radiation alone. Locally advanced: consider chemoradiation + total laryngectomy. Chemo regimens include **cisplatin or cetuximab**.
9. **Colorectal cancer stage 1:** consider **surgery**; stage II and III may need chemo and radiation.
10. **Cervical cancer**: early-stage without spread to the pelvic wall or the low 1/3 of the vagina can be treated with surgery alone; more advanced cancer should receive chemoradiation (including cisplatin) instead of surgery
11. **Malignant SVC syndrome**: endovenous recanalization with SVC stent placement, radiation therapy, supportive cancer, and treatment of the cause.

12. **Locally advanced head and neck cancer:** consider **cisplatin + radiation after surgery**. Early-stage head and neck cancer or some locally advanced cancer: radiation alone after surgery.
13. **NSCLC Treatment**: chemo after surgery; no need for radiation if negative margins; add radiation if no surgery.
14. **Hormone-positive breast cancer** who remains premenopausal after chemo ⇒ consider ovarian suppression (like oophorectomy or leuprolide) + aromatase inhibitor exemestane NOT tamoxifen.
15. **High-grade serous carcinoma**: consider debulking surgery followed by IV and IP cisplatin and paclitaxel.
16. **High-grade poorly differentiated NET** requires systemic platinum-based chemo; octreotide is used for low-grade NET.
17. **Melanoma** with solitary or oligometastatic brain lesion: consider surgery of the brain to remove the tumor.
18. **Localized gastroesophageal (GE) junction cancer:** consider neoadjuvant chemo (**carbo + Taxol**) plus radiation and surgery.
19. **Breast cancer** treatment: doxorubicin and cyclophosphamide (AC) or docetaxel-cyclophosphamide (TC). **DCIS with no LN involvement** treatment: lumpectomy → radiation → aromatase inhibitor (AI). **Breast cancer Her 2+ with brain mets treatment**: pertuzumab (Jerjeta) + trastuzumab [human epidermal growth factor receptor 2 (HER2) antibody].
20. **Advanced breast cancer** recurrent after adjuvant aromatase inhibitor therapy ⇒ consider treatment: letrozole (or fulvestrant) + palbociclib (Ibrance); preferably first line letrozole + palbociclib.
21. **Triple-negative breast cancer** treatment: chemoradiation, but no aromatase inhibitor (AI).
22. Prostate cancer metastasized to bone treatment: **abiraterone (Zytiga)** + leuprolide ⇒ consider leuprolide + docetaxel.
23. **Multiple myeloma** (MM) treatment: **RVD** (Velcade, Revlimid, and dexamethasone) → consider stem cell transplants (**SCT**) → **Revlimid maintenance treatment**.
24. **Philadelphia chromosome chronic myeloid leukemia (Ph + CML)** treatment: imatinib.
25. **Lymphoid blast crisis** (like ALL): TKI in the past → switch to second generation TKI; de novo Ph + ALL⇒ consider **hyper CVAD alternate with methotrexate, cytarabine + Nib (imatinib) or dasatinib**.
26. **Myeloid blast crisis (like AML)**: TKI (dasatinib, nilotinib, bosutinib rather than imatinib) → allogeneic hematopoietic stem cell transplantation (HSCT).
27. **CLL** treatment: bendamustine and rituximab. **AML** treatment: cytarabine + idarubicin.
28. **Pancreatic cancer CT1N0M0** treatment: FOLFIRINOX minus 5-FU with leucovorin (LV).
29. **Adenocarcinoma of colon** treatment: FOLFOX + Avastin → FOLFIRI (**oxaliplatin causes neuropathy**) → cetuximab + irinotecan

30. **Stage IV well-differentiated primitive neuroectodermal tumor (PNET)** to lung. **Treatment**: lanreotide 120 mg monthly → G^A68 scan and peptide receptor radionuclide therapy (PRRT) or capecitabine + Temodar (temozolomide)
31. **Perihilar cholangiocarcinoma** treatment: status post concurrent chemoradiation therapy (CRT) with **5-FU and brachytherapy → capecitabine** maintenance.
32. **Tamoxifen** increases risks for venous thromboembolism (VTE). **Discontinue tamoxifen 2–4 weeks before** any surgery associated with moderate or high risk for VTE.
33. **Waldenstrom's macroglobulinemia, also** known as **lymphoplasmacytic lymphoma,** is a slow-growing type of non-Hodgkin lymphoma. Diagnosis requires the presence of **IgM monoclonal gammopathy and bone marrow infiltration** showing an intertrabecular pattern with small lymphocytes. **Waldenstrom's macroglobulinemia hyperviscosity** treatment: **emergent plasmapheresis.**
34. 20% of patients with essential thrombocythemia (**ET**) develop acquired **vWD**.
35. **VIPoma** has no cardiac involvement and cutaneous telangiectasia compared to **serotonin syndrome**.
36. **Advanced seminoma** should be treated with **bleomycin, etoposide, and cisplatin**.
37. Most patients with **small cell lung cancer (SCLC)** relapse in 1–2 years. Limited stage disease of SCLC is limited to one hemithorax, with hilar and mediastinal lymphadenopathy. **A limited-stage disease** of SCLC can be encompassed in **one tolerable radiotherapy portal**. **Treatment**: combined chemoradiation followed by prophylactic cranial irradiation.
38. **Large B cell lymphoma**: R-CHOP → consider R-ICE (rituximab, ifosfamide, carboplatin, and etoposide phosphate) salvage chemo → consider SCT vs. CAR T therapy.
39. **CD20+ Burkitt lymphoma** treatment: **R-hyper-CVAD** = rituximab plus hyperfractionated (rapidly cycled) cyclophosphamide, vincristine, doxorubicin, and dexamethasone.
40. **Recurrent Hodgkin lymphoma** that responds to salvage chemo [like ifosfamide, carboplatin, and etoposide (ICE) or etoposide, methylprednisolone, high-dose cytarabine, and cisplatin (ESHAP) or bendamustine, gemcitabine, and vinorelbine (BeGEV)] should also be treated with **autologous hematopoietic stem cell transplantation** (**HSCT**).
41. The standard treatment for stage I, II, and III **anal squamous cell cancer**: **concurrent radiation with chemotherapy of mitomycin plus 5-FU**.
42. **Resectable pancreatic cancer** should go for definitive curative resection without prior tissue confirmation.
43. **Gastrointestinal stromal tumor (GIST)** with a relatively high risk for recurrence (location outside the stomach, larger size, and high mitotic index) should be treated with **imatinib for 3 years after tumor resection**.
44. Multiagent systemic chemotherapy with 5-FU, leucovorin, irinotecan, and oxaliplatin (**FOLFIRINOX**) is the treatment for the **metastatic recurrence of**

pancreatic cancer if good performance status. **Gemcitabine** as a single agent therapy can be used for pancreatic cancer with **ECOG ≥2.**

45. **HIT**: Type 1- **heparin-induced PLT clumping** → 1–2 days after heparin use, mild thrombocytopenia; treatment: observation. Type II- **positive heparin-PLT factor 4 complexes**, 5–10 days after heparin use; <1 day with prior heparin exposure, treatment: discontinue heparin, start a direct thrombin inhibitor. Type III- **delayed onset HIT, high titer Ab against heparin-PLT factor 4 complexes** in the absence of circulating heparin ⇒ thrombocytopenia with or without life-threatening arterial or venous thrombosis 5–19 days after heparin cessation.
46. **Superior pulmonary sulcus tumor (Pancoast tumor)** symptoms: shoulder pain, Horner syndrome, invasion of C8-T2 nerves, supraclavicular LN, weight loss. CXR shows an enlarged apical cap and/or bone destruction.
47. **Acute chest syndrome** refers to acute life-threatening respiratory symptoms and fever; **treatment**: PRBC transfusion to target hematocrit ≥30% or hemoglobin ≥10 g/dL, antibiotics, pain control, and oxygen. Additionally, exchange transfusion may be necessary if severe hypoxia, multilobar pneumonia, or failure of improvement despite the aforementioned treatments. After acute chest syndrome, give **hydroxyurea** to decrease vasooclusive episodes, transfusion requirements, and hospitalizations.
48. **Acute chest syndrome transfusion treatment**: SO_2 > 90% transfusion 0–2 u PRBC; ≥85%, transfuse 2–3 u PRBC; <85% + 2 lobes ⇒ consider exchange transfusion.
49. **BRCA mutation carrier status**: annual mammogram and breast MRI beginning at age 25.
50. **Transfusion-associated graft-versus-host disease (GVHD)**: typically occurs 4–30 days after transfusions; manifestations include fever, erythematous/maculopapular rash anorexia, RUQ pain, hepatomegaly, elevated LFTs, and profuse diarrhea. **Treatment**: prevention via using irradiated blood products.
51. For bone metastasis, **parenteral bisphosphonates** (i.e., zoledronic acid, denosumab, pamidronate) or **oral ibandronate** is appropriate. **Zoledronic acid** is contraindicated if creatinine clearance is <35 mL/min.
52. **Chemoradiation of the brain** increases the risks for meningioma and gliomas.
53. Lung cancer with solitary brain metastasis treatment: surgery or **stereotactic radiosurgery**.
54. **Anthracycline** can cause leukemia 5–10 years post-treatment with a preceding MDS phase. **Anthracycline** like doxorubicin causes **local tissue injury and necrosis** from **extravasation**, cardiomyopathy, AML, MDS, and myelosuppression.
55. **Cetuximab and panitumumab** inhibit EGFR via binding to extracellular domain III and are only used in **wild-type** N-RAS, K-RAS, with or without EGFR mutations in colorectal cancer. If RAS or RAF mutation, give **Avastin** (anti-VEGF).
56. **Prostate cancer indications for imaging studies**: PSA ≥20, PSA ≥10 with T2 tumor, a Gleason score of ≥8, or T3 or T4 tumor.

57. **Sentinel lymph node biopsy** is recommended for **melanoma**: 1–4 mm thickness, <1 mm with ulceration, lymphovascular invasion, or more than 1 mitosis/mm^2. If node + or ≥4 mm thickness, give interferon (IFN) alpha.
58. **Peritoneal carcinomatosis** is commonly seen in colorectal, gastric, and gynecological malignancies. Major signs and symptoms of abdominal carcinomatosis include ascites, nodular implants, and infiltration of the peritoneal fatty tissue. **Treatment is cytoreduction surgery and intraperitoneal chemotherapy (HIPEC or EPIC procedures).** In peritoneal carcinomatosis due to primary ovarian cancer, treatments include cytoreduction surgery [tumor debulking along with total abdominal hysterectomy bilateral salpingo-oophorectomy (TAH-BSO), omentectomy, selective lymphadenectomy, and appendectomy] and intraperitoneal administration of platinum/taxane chemo.
59. **Tyrosine kinase inhibitors sunitinib and temsirolimus** are used in metastatic renal cancer.
60. Treat **oligometastatic colorectal cancer** by **surgical** resection.
61. **Platinum-based chemotherapy** such as carboplatin plus paclitaxel or cisplatin plus etoposide is for a **poorly differentiated cancer of unknown primary site**, such as germ cell (testicular) tumor, or poorly differentiated NEC.
62. **Cisplatin versus cetuximab** in head and neck cancer with **radiation**. Cisplatin is the preferred treatment but is contraindicated in chronic kidney disease.
63. Pure observation indicates only possible treatment for symptoms rather than cancer itself. **Surveillance indicates monitoring for the need for cancer treatment**.
64. Adenocarcinoma of the colon into serosa treatment: surgery alone, usually no need for chemo.

Chapter 23
Pulmonology and Critical Care

1. **Massive hemoptysis** refers to 100–1000 cc in 24 h; check CT angio and call interventional radiologist (IR) stat for bronchial artery embolization if it happens.
2. Symptoms of **pulmonary embolism** (PE): pleuritic chest pain, shortness of breath, and cough. **Wells criteria**: clinical signs of DVT, tachycardia, immobility.
3. Diagnosis of **allergic bronchopulmonary aspergillosis** (ABPA): skin test + for aspergillus, **IgE** >417 IU/mL, **eosinophilia** >500/uL, and specific IgG and IgE for aspergillus. **Treatment**: steroid (prednisolone 0.5–1 mg/kg daily) and itraconazole (200 mg bid). Newer agents voriconazole (300–600 mg/day) or posaconazole (800 mg/day) could decrease the need for oral steroids.
4. **Tension pneumothorax** should be suspected in hemodynamic instability with iatrogenic risk factors. Treatment is stat **chest tube**.
5. **Severe allergic reaction**: sudden respiratory failure, hypotension, nausea, and vomiting after allergen exposure, even mild symptoms, treatment: **intramuscular epinephrine 0.5 mg, may repeat q5–15 min**.
6. **Paradoxical vocal cord motion** is often triggered by psychosocial stressors. Diagnosis: flow volume loops consistent with variable extrathoracic airway obstruction. Treatment for acute symptoms: **PEEP +/− heliox (helium + oxygen).**
7. Pectus excavaum, scoliosis → compromised chest wall mechanics/compliance; treatment: non-invasive positive pressure ventilation (NPPV) and pulmonary rehab.
8. **Rheumatoid effusion** (white blood cell counts <5000/uL with predominant lymphocytes); **empyema** (high white blood cell counts >50,000/uL with neutrophil predominance).
9. **Bronchial tree colonization of candida** species is common in critically ill patients receiving mechanical ventilation, usually **no treatment** is necessary.
10. **Dyspnea in end-stage COPD treatment 1st opioids, 2nd alprazolam**.

K. Zhou, *Internal Medicine Training Notes and Survival Guide*,
https://doi.org/10.1007/978-1-0716-4039-5_23

11. **Exudative effusion** etiology: empyema, chylothorax (milky white, increased triglyceride), malignancy, tuberculosis (acid-fast stain).
12. **Respiratory acidosis**: **acute** patient labs with **1 mEq/L HCO_3** increase with ten increase of PCO_2; **chronic** (4–5 days) patient labs with **4 mEq/L HCO_3** increase with ten increase PCO_2.
13. **Massive pulmonary embolism** (PE), hemodynamically unstable (in actual practice thrombolysis/thrombectomy is also used in patients with submassive PE and tachycardia) → do bedside transthoracic echocardiogram, if right ventricular (RV) dysfunction (this step may not be necessary in actual clinical practices) → call for thrombolysis or thrombectomy.
14. **Febrile illness in asplenia** should prompt progressive antibiotic therapy and urgent diagnostic evaluation. Asplenia is susceptible to **encapsulated bacterial infections**, including **Streptococcus pneumoniae, Neisseria meningitidis, and Haemophilus influenzae** infections. Additional encapsulated bacteria include Escherichia coli, Pseudomonas aeruginosa, Capnocytophaga canimorsus, group B Streptococcus, Enterococcus spp., Ehrlichia spp., and protozoa such as the Plasmodium spp. (leading to malaria).
15. **Acute eosinophilic pneumonia (AEP)** usually occurs in smokers; **chronic eosinophilic pneumonia (CEP)** is commonly seen in nonsmokers but has asthma history. Symptoms include fever, cough, dyspnea. Chest X-ray (CXR): AEP -diffuse ground glass changes; CEP—bilateral infiltrates sparing central lungs and perihilar regions. Diagnosis: **eosinophilia >6%**, ESR and CRP elevation. Bronchoalveolar lavage **>25% eosinophil** = consider eosinophilic pneumonia. Treatment: improve in 48 h after **steroids**.
16. **Pulmonary alveolar proteinosis**: a diffuse lung disease due to the accumulation of periodic acid-schiff positive **lipoproteinaceous material** in the distal airspace of the lung. Symptoms are similar to CEP, but CXR shows central opacities (**batwing**). Treatments include whole lung lavage and lung transplant.
17. For moderate persistent asthma, **adding LABA is superior to doubling ICS** in asthma control, lung function, and quality of life (QoL).
18. Aspirin exacerbated respiratory disease (**Samter's triad = rhinosinusitis with polyposis, asthma, and nonsteroidal anti-inflammatory drug (NSAID) intolerance**). Treatment: optimal asthma therapy, surgery for chronic rhinosinusitis, and avoidance of NSAIDs, adding **montelukast**.
19. Nocturnal asthma-like symptoms **differential diagnoses**: true **nocturnal asthma** (wheezing), **GERD** (burning), **OSA** (choking), upper airway cough syndrome (**sinusitis**)
20. Normal peak flow **400 cc in female, 500–600 cc in male**. For asthma exacerbation, systemic oral steroids should be started if peak flow is between <70% (moderate) and <40% (severe). **If peak flow is >70%, the patient can be discharged; if peak flow is <40%, the patient should be admitted.**
21. **COPD treatments**: LABA → LABA + LAMA → LABA + LAMA + ICS if they have blood eosinophils ≥100 cells/μL.
22. **Systemic sclerosis** is associated with **pulmonary hypertension** (preserved lung volume and decreased DLCO) and **interstitial lung disease** (restrictive

lung disease with decreased FEV1, FVC, TLC, and DLCO, but normal FEV1/FVC ratio).

23. Flow volume loop, **fixed** upper airway obstruction (goiter) vs. **dynamic or variable** obstruction (tracheomalacia vocal cord dysfunction).
24. **Acute radiation pneumonitis**: CT shows hazy opacities with extensive ground glass changes; **4–12** weeks after neck or thoracic radiation treatment → **6–12** months later with fibrotic radiation pneumonitis. Treatment: **prednisone 1–1.5 mg/kg daily with a taper over weeks**. Example regimen for treatment: prednisone 40–60 mg daily for 2–4 weeks with a gradual taper over 3–12 weeks.
25. Low-grade **fever**, joint pain, cough, dyspnea, **erythema nodosum** (tender red nodule) = consider **sarcoidosis**.
26. **Churg-Strauss syndrome**: prodromal phase (asthma, allergic rhinitis, recurrent sinusitis); eosinophilic infiltration of multiple organs; vasculitis (subcutaneous nodules, congestive heart failure, neuropathy, necrotizing glomerulonephropathy, and migratory oligoarthritis)
27. **Goodpasture Syndrome** presents with **hemoptysis** and **glomerulonephritis**; no marked increase in ESR, no constitutional symptoms.
28. **Fat embolism syndrome** is diagnosed based on clinical symptoms: CT chest shows **bilateral ground glass opacities** and thickening of the interlobular septa 24–72 h after **fracture.** Symptoms of fat embolism syndrome include **hypoxemia, confusion, and petechiae**.
29. Goals of ventilator setting in **acute respiratory distress syndrome** (ARDS): PEEP 5–15, RR <35, plateau pressure $\leq$30 cmH_2O, pH > 7.2.
30. **Peak = plateau + airway resistance** (bronchospasm, mucous plug, biting of ET tube).
31. Diagnostic thoracentesis is recommended for effusion $\geq$10 mm with no high-risk features. If **loculations, $\geq$ 1/2 hemithorax, or thickened pleura** → consider thoracostomy.
32. **Strategies to correct auto-PEEP**: reducing minute ventilation, increasing expiratory time, using bronchodilators and inhaled steroids to relieve airway obstructions. **Obstructive sleep apnea**: screen with home sleep testing → diagnosis with polysomnography (sleep study).
33. **Interstitial lung disease** is characterized by varying degrees of inflammation and scarring of lung tissues. **Idiopathic interstitial pneumonia (IIP)** includes idiopathic pulmonary fibrosis, desquamative interstitial pneumonia, acute interstitial pneumonia, respiratory bronchiolitis-associated interstitial lung disease, cryptogenic organizing pneumonia, and lymphocytic interstitial pneumonia.
34. **Smoking-related interstitial lung disease** includes **desquamative** interstitial pneumonia, **pulmonary Langerhans** cell histiocytosis, and **respiratory bronchiolitis-associated** interstitial lung disease.
35. **Desquamative interstitial pneumonia (DIP)**: diffuse macrophage filling of alveolar spaces, cough, dyspnea, bilateral ground glass opacities.
36. **Pulmonary Langerhans cell histiocytosis**: thin-walled cyst with nodules and pulmonary hypertension, subacute, evolving during weeks to months. It affects

young adult smokers with pathologies in bronchiolar, interstitial, and pulmonary vascular tissues. It is a myeloid neoplasm (BRAF or other MAPK mutations) with inflammatory properties.

37. **Respiratory bronchiolitis-associated interstitial lung disease (RB-ILD)**: submucosal inflammation of the membranous and respiratory bronchioles with tan-brown pigmented macrophages, mucus stasis, and metaplastic cuboidal epithelium.
38. **Hypersensitivity pneumonitis (HP)**: midlung and upper lung zones with association with environmental exposures. Characteristics of HP include bronchiolocentric and interstitial inflammation on CT scan, lymphocytosis with bronchoalveolar lavage, and biopsy showing airway-centered fibrosis with or without peribronchiolar metaplasia, interstitial pneumonia, and poorly formed granulomas. Hypersensitivity pneumonitis may have no eosinophil.
39. **Idiopathic pulmonary fibrosis**: patches of dense scarring alternating with normal lung tissues on CT, and honeycombing zones, without inflammation or granulomas. Also, we can see bilateral peripheral and basal predominant septal line thickening with honeycombing at the lung bases on the CT scan. Idiopathic pulmonary fibrosis treatment: nintedanib (Ofev) and pirfenidone (Esbriet).
40. **Asthma exacerbation with eosinophil** of 150–300/uL. Treatment: mepolizumab q4 weeks subcu or reslizumab.
41. **Omalizumab** is used for asthma symptoms not controlled with ICS; allergies to perennial aeroallergens; IgE 30–700 u/mL.
42. **Bilevel-positive airway pressure** (BiPAP) is appropriate for **ALS**; it improves QoL and prolongs life.
43. **Cor pulmonale treatment**: O2. **Pulmonary hypertension** treatment: Bosentan.
44. **A thoracostomy** tube is indicated for empyema and tension pneumothorax.
45. **Benzodiazepine intoxication**, no need for flumazenil given short half-life.
46. In patients with hypoxic respiratory failure, the use of noninvasive positive pressure ventilation (NIPPV) is controversial. Hypoxic respiratory failure, awake, diaphoretic, and anxious plus use of accessory muscles → consider intubation.
47. **Pneumothorax** is divided into primary and secondary spontaneous pneumothorax (PSP vs. SSP). For SSP, recurrence is common → consider treatment: chemical/mechanical **pleurodesis** (subpleural bullae/cysts). If surgical candidate, do **video-assisted thoracoscopic surgery (VATS)** to locate and staple or resect blebs followed by mechanical pleurodesis. If not a surgical candidate, treat with a **blood patch or chemical pleurodesis**.
48. If the patient is awake and has **excellent bulbar control (swallows and gags)**, no intubation.
49. For **hypertensive emergencies** without compelling conditions like brain bleeding or aortic dissection, sBP should be reduced by **no more than 25% within the first hour**; then if stable, reduce to 160 mmHg in the next 2–6 h; then cautiously to **normal in 24**–48 h.

50. **Cyanide poisoning**: usually coexposure to CO, common in-house fires with vinyl burning. Diagnosis: increased lactic acid, inappropriately **elevated central venous oxyhemoglobin** saturation (bright red venous blood). Treatment: **hydroxocobalamin** which binds cyanide to produce cyanocobalamin. second line—**sodium thiosulfate**.
51. **CO poisoning treatment**: **hyperbaric oxygen** is indicated if >25%–40% carboxyhemoglobin or pregnant.
52. **Methemoglobinemia** treatment: **methylene blue** is indicated if **methemoglobin >20%–30%.**
53. **Methemoglobinemia**: pulse oximetry < or stays at 85% but SO_2 on ABG is good, the **difference (saturation gap) >5%**; causes include **dapsone**, **nitrates**, and local/topical **anesthetics**.
54. **Daily interruptions in sedation and analgesia** decrease delirium, the need for diagnostic testing, and the amount of time spent on mechanical ventilation and in the ICU.
55. **V/Q scan** is the diagnostic screening modality for **chronic thromboembolic pulmonary hypertension** (CTEPH). **Right heart catheterization** with pulmonary artery pressure measurement and pulmonary arteriography should be performed as a confirmatory test if the V/Q scan is positive for CTPH. Pulmonary CT angiogram in chronic pulmonary embolism provides no benefit. CTEPH = mean pulmonary arterial pressure **≥25 mmHg** but normal pulmonary wedge pressure and left ventricular end-diastolic pressure. **Treatment**: pulmonary thromboendarterectomy.
56. **Empyema** status post **thoracostomy tube**, add instillation of **intrapleural tPA-DNase** (deoxyribonuclease), protocol per interventional radiologist or general surgeon, may require decortication.
57. **Silicosis**: foundries, sandblasting, eggshell calcifications of hilar lymph nodes of CXR. BAL—milky effusion.
58. Medical Research Council Muscle Scale is used for ICU-related weakness.
59. For patients with **exudate** pleural effusion for whom malignancy is suspected but negative cytology: proceed with **thoracoscopy with pleural biopsy**.
60. Indwelling pleural catheter (**PleurX**) works better than **talc pleurodesis** for **recurrent pleural** effusion from terminal cancer.
61. **Neuroleptic malignant syndrome** (days to weeks after starting antipsychotics, rigidity, and hyperreflexia, takes days to resolve) vs. **serotonin syndrome** (has rigidity, but more clonus, with hyperreflexia, resolves in 24 h). Both have hyperthermia, altered mental status, and rigidity. Elevations in creatine kinase, liver function tests (lactate dehydrogenase, aspartate transaminase), and white blood cell count, coupled with a low serum iron level can happen in both syndromes.
62. Patients with **isopropyl alcohol** (non-anion gap but osmolar gap and no acidosis) poisoning can be treated effectively with supportive care.
63. Inhaled **antibiotics** (**tobramycin**) can be used for prophylaxis of acute exacerbations of **bronchiectasis**, but not for acute treatment.

64. Patients with **central sleep apnea** usually have normocapnia or slight hypocapnia.
65. **Apnea hypopnea index** (AHI) is the number of apneas or hypopneas recorded during the study per hour of sleep. AHI of 5–15 is indicative of mild OSA; **≥30** is indicative of severe OSA.
66. Obesity hypoventilation syndrome = daytime hypercapnia with **$PaCO_2 \geq 45$ mm H_2O.**
67. Hilar and mediastinal lymphadenopathy with new interstitial thickening and beading at the lung base = consider **lymphangitic carcinomatosis.**
68. **Portopulmonary hypertension (PoPH)**: chronic vasoconstriction and vascular remodeling of pulmonary arteries with elevated mean pulmonary artery pressure secondary to an increased pulmonary vascular resistance as a result of portal hypertension.
69. **Hepatopulmonary syndrome (HPS)**: acute to chronic diffuse pulmonary capillary vasodilation and shunting leading to hypoxemia.
70. **Right heart catheterization** is reserved for pulmonary hypertension of unknown cause, not necessary if known to be COPD.
71. Tumors invade the proximal airways → **endobronchial narrowing and obstruction** → increasing the risks for **post-obstructive pneumonia**.
72. A symptomatic **primary spontaneous pneumothorax (≤3 cm)** may be initially managed with oxygen therapy at 2–3 lpm and daily chest X-rays. Such patients can be discharged after 48–72 h of clinical stability. If hemodynamically unstable or progressive pneumothorax, perform thoracotomy followed by tube placement.
73. Pulmonary hypertension and **left ventricular hypertrophy** treatment: lisinopril (treat the cause) to decrease the remodeling of cardiac muscles.
74. **Cystic fibrosis** should be considered for chronic asthma-like symptoms, chronic sinusitis, nasal polyps, allergic bronchopulmonary aspergillosis, Burkholderia cepacia, or Pseudomonas infections.
75. **Lymphangioleiomyomatosis** is a rare cystic lung disease in childbearing age or tuberculosis women with thin-walled diffuse small cysts on CT.
76. **High altitude pulmonary edema** treatment: oxygen, rest, descent from high altitude, and vasodilation like nifedipine. May also benefit from diuretic use. Acetazolamide alkalizes urine, causes natriuresis, and decreases bicarbonates from serum. It (**acetazolamide 125 mg bid**) reduces the incidence of adverse altitude effects in **acute mountain sickness** and **high-altitude cerebral edema**, both are brain pathophysiologies related to high altitude.
77. Sequelae of obstructive sleep apnea: **excessive daytime sleepiness** is the strongest indication for **positive airway pressure therapy**.
78. **Endobronchial ultrasound (EBUS)-guided transbronchial** needle aspiration for diagnosing and staging mediastinal and hilar lymphadenopathy with suspected malignancy.

Chapter 24
Nephrology

1. **Monoclonal gammopathy** of renal significance = renal impairment with MGUS. Diagnosis: kidney biopsy. Treatment is needed. Pathology reveals amyloidosis, proliferative glomerulonephritis, immunoglobulin deposition disease, C3 glomerulopathy, and proximal tubulopathy. Treatment is similar to that of multiple myeloma.
2. **Potassium citrate** can be used for calcium oxalate kidney stones.
3. Blood pressure (BP) medications, there are **diminishing effects in BP lowering** if the dose is titrated up from 50%–100% of maximum.
4. Newly diagnosed **membranous glomerulonephropathy** should undergo cancer screening. Membranous glomerulonephropathy is commonly associated with **lung, prostate, and gastrointestinal tract tumors**.
5. HBV, HCV, and lupus can all be related to **membranous glomerulonephropathy**. Anti- **anti-phospholipase A2 receptor (PLA2R)** is a marker for idiopathic membranous glomerulonephropathy. Decreased titers of PLA2R indicate improvement/remission. Treatment: ACEi, Lipitor, and edema management for 6–24 months. If no response after 6–12 months, **immunosuppression** can be considered.
6. For new membranous glomerulonephropathy, conservative therapy with **ACEi and statin for 6–12 months** ⇒ glucocorticoids alternate with alkylating agents (like cyclophosphamide) and cyclosporine can be used.
7. **Balkan endemic nephropathy**, a chronic **tubulointerstitial** disease, is strongly associated with the development of upper urinary tract **transitional cell urothelial cancers**, linked to aristolochic acid.
8. CNS sarcoidosis causes central **diabetes insipidus** (DI); treatment: **desmopressin**. Heparin can cause hypoaldosteronism.
9. Stage 2 hypertension (>140/90 mmHg) usually requires two drugs of different classes for blood pressure control.
10. **C-ANCA = antiproteinase 3. P-ANCA = anti-myeloperoxidase**.

K. Zhou, *Internal Medicine Training Notes and Survival Guide*,
https://doi.org/10.1007/978-1-0716-4039-5_24

11. **Pyroglutamic acidosis** (from long-term acetaminophen use) = mental status change (increased AG in CKD, liver disease, critical illness, poor nutrition). Diagnosis via urine level of pyroglutamic acid. Tylenol chronic leads to the depletion of glutathione.
12. **Salicylate toxicity** = may include respiratory alkalosis or both respiratory alkalosis and increased AG metabolic acidosis.
13. **Acute tubular necrosis (ATN)** has a fraction excretion of **Na >2%**. **Acute interstitial nephritis (AIN)**: UA with numerous renal tubular **epithelial cells** and granular casts; fever, rash, and eosinophilia, can happen **7–10 days** after exposure to **vancomycin**. **Contrast-induced nephropathy** happens within **48–72 h** after contrast dye use.
14. Urine sediment for cast, **granular casts with or without renal epithelial cells** = acute tubular necrosis (ATN).
15. Both oral urea and tolvaptan (very specialty-specific medication) are appropriate for chronic hyponatremia.
16. Stones <1 cm, treatment is calcium channel blocker like **nifedipine** and selective alpha 1A-adrenergic receptor antagonist like **tamsulosin**; 1–1.5 cm requires **extracorporeal shock wave lithotripsy**.
17. **Nephrolithiasis**: **ultrasound** is the initial, and **CT without contrast** is the gold standard test.
18. Increased muscle mass can result in increased creatinine level in the absence of kidney dysfunction ⇒ consider checking **Cystatin C**.
19. In patients with **hypercalciuria** and kidney stones. **Thiazides** increase calcium reabsorption from urine and may prevent kidney stone formation but thiazides also cause hyperuricemia.
20. Incidence of **intracranial aneurysm** is 10%–11.5% in autosomal dominant polycystic kidney disease (ADPKD). **Screening for intracranial aneurysm with MR angiography** is only recommended for patients with ADPKD if family history of aneurysm or SAH or a history of aneurysmal rupture, or high-risk occupations such as bus driver.
21. **Alcoholic ketoacidosis** can be treated with D5 in NS after thiamine.
22. **HELLP** is one type of microangiopathic hemolytic anemia (MAHA).
23. **Preeclampsia**: new onset of hypertension and proteinuria **≥300 mg**/24 h after 20 weeks of gestation; >160/110 mmHg is **severe preeclampsia**. Gestational hypertension has no proteinuria and resolves after 12 weeks after delivery.
24. **Fabry disease**: episodic peripheral neuropathy, angiokeratoma, hypohidrosis, and late ESRD. **Tuberous sclerosis**: angiomyolipoma and cysts, hamartoma.
25. **Adynamic bone disease** (seen in patients with CKD or on hemodialysis) refers to low bone turnover without osteoid accumulation in patients with significant vascular calcifications, symptoms of bone fracture, and pain. Diagnosis is via bone biopsy. **Treatment**: increase PTH, avoid calcium binders, avoid the decrease in PTH, use non-calcium- and non-aluminum-containing phosphate binders, and consider **teriparatide** (PTH 1–34). Increased PTH and increased ALP can exclude adynamic bone disease diagnosis.

26. **Osteitis fibrosa cystica** is caused by the overproduction of **PTH** from hyperactive parathyroid glands leading to increased PTH and ALP.
27. **Mixed uremic osteodystrophy** is a combination of osteitis fibrosa and osteomalacia.
28. **Renal osteodystrophy** includes high bone turnover **osteitis fibrosa** from hyperparathyroidism and low bone turnover **adynamic bone disease** or heavy metal-induced osteomalacia.
29. In CKD, target iron saturation >30%, ferritin >500 ng/mL.
30. **Metabolic alkalosis, check urine chloride** to determine whether this is saline responsive (urine chloride <20). Saline-responsive metabolic alkalosis = usually low urine chloride <15–25 mEq/L. The patient is less likely to respond to saline treatment if urine Cl > 40 mEq/L.
31. **IgG 4 related disease**: dense infiltration of IgG4-positive plasma cells in the affected tissue(s) with or without elevated plasma levels of IgG4, commonly affected organs: salivary and lacrimal glands (**submandibular swelling**), pancreas (**pancreatitis**) and biliary tract, and the kidneys (**tubulointerstitial nephritis**) in middle-aged or older men more often than women. Labs: ANA+, decreased C3 and C4, increased IgE, increased IgG, peripheral eosinophilia. Treatment: steroids.
32. Kidney transplants with **calcineurin inhibitor (CI)** induced hypertension and hyperkalemia via sodium chloride co-transporter activation. Treatment: **hydrochlorothiazide** (sodium chloride co-transporter blocker).
33. Symptomatic hyper-magnesemia happens when Mg >**7 mg/dL**. Treatment: normal saline, furosemide, IV calcium.
34. African American (AA) patients, **hydrochlorothiazide** → amlodipine; but if CKD, do ACEi. The target blood pressure for hypertension, regardless of CAD, DM, or CKD, is **130/80**.
35. **Intermittent hemodialysis** is most efficient for correcting increased K in oliguric AKI. **Continuous renal replacement therapy (CRRT)** is used in critically ill patients with **symptoms** or **electrolyte abnormalities** that are refractory to medical treatments.
36. Lupus CKD followup: **kidney biopsy if Cr increases with no explanation**, **proteinuria** >500/24 h or **active urine sediment** (dysmorphic RBC, erythrocyte casts). If the biopsy shows proliferative lupus nephritis (III, IV), treatment with glucocorticoids and mycophenolate or cyclophosphamide is needed.
37. **Medications** (cimetidine, trimethoprim, cobicistat, dolutegravir, bictegravir, and rilpivirine) **reduce proximal tubule secretion of creatinine**, resulting in increased serum creatinine that is **non**-progressive which means creatinine will return to baseline after medication cessation.
38. **Topiramate** is associated with decreased urinary citrate secretion ⇒ calcium phosphate stones, distal renal tubular acidosis, and increased PTH.
39. **Pseudohyperkalemia** in extreme elevations of WBC or PLT ⇒ consider repeat plasma K+; hyperkalemia has **peak T** and shortened QT interval.

40. Urine K <20 is non-renal loss. If **urine K >20 = renal loss of K**; seen in RTA, renal excretion of bicarb, Hippurate, ketones, aminoglycoside, cisplatin, Gitelman/Bartter syndrome, decreased Mg.
41. **Rapid kidney failure** seen in S. aureus, infection-related glomerulonephritis (IRGN), post-streptococcal infectious glomerulonephritis (PSGN), usually happen in **7–10 days** after oropharyngeal infection, **2–4 weeks** after skin infection. Both IRGN and PSGN are immune-complex mediated glomerulonephritis.
42. Goal blood pressure for >60 yo is <150/90. Patients >65 years old, can set BP goals as appropriate if comorbidities.
43. **Chronic lead nephropathy** is frequently associated with **hyperuricemia**, **hypertension**, and **recurrent gout attacks**.
44. Anion gap (AG) → osmolar gap (OG) → urine AG ($U_{Na} + U_K - U_{Cl}$); metabolic alkalosis, check urine chloride.
45. Kidney transplant recipients should **wait 1–2 years with a stable allograft before attempting conception**. **Calcineurin inhibitors** (tacrolimus and cyclosporine) have been used safely in pregnancy. Mycophenolate mofetil, sirolimus, and everolimus must be discontinued 3–6 months before conception and replaced with **azathioprine**.
46. Discrepancy of urine analysis, UA protein low, but urine Pr/Cr ratio = 4100 mg/g equals **light chain cast nephropathy** from multiple myeloma.
47. **Recurrent gross hematuria** usually occurs in **days** after an upper respiratory tract infection = **IgA nephropathy**, also known as synpharyngitic glomerulonephritis or Berger's disease.
48. The expected **metabolic compensation for chronic respiratory alkalosis**: decreased HCO_3 = 0.4× change in PCO_2. Chronic metabolic acidosis: decrease in PCO_2 = 1.5× change in HCO_3 + 8 +/− 2. Chronic metabolic alkalosis: increased $PaCO_2$ = 0.7× change in HCO_3. Respiratory acidosis chronic: increased HCO_3 = 0.35× change in $PaCO_2$.
49. **Renal transplant referral**: if GFR <30, stage G4 CKD, follow up q3m.
50. BUN **100 mg**/dL, increased Na 147 is likely due to **urea osmotic diuresis**. Urine osmolarity is usually 300–600 Osm/kg.
51. **Indications for kidney biopsy** include glomerular hematuria, severely increased albuminuria, acute or chronic kidney disease of unknown cause, and kidney transplant dysfunction or monitoring.
52. **Cisplatin** (produces crosslinking impairing DNA repair thus no viable DNA replication) induced AKI is characterized by polyuria, tubular injury, hypomagnesemia, proximal RTA with Fanconi syndrome, and happens **7–10 days after administration**. **Bevacizumab** (inhibits VEGF binding to its receptors) causes AKI from **TMA** (thrombotic microangiopathy). **Paclitaxel** (targets microtubules and causes mitotic arrest) causes diffuse interstitial lung disease and peripheral neuropathy (subacute).
53. **ESRD prediction**: age, gender, GFR, and albuminuria.
54. For ESRD with **bilateral kidney solid mass**, treatment with bilateral radical nephrectomy.

55. **Oncogenic osteomalacia** is a paraneoplastic syndrome caused by tumor-induced osteomalacia. It is characterized by **bone pain** and **hypophosphatemia** with **kidney phosphate wasting**, low 1,25-dihydroxyvitamin D and normal 25-hydroxyvitamin D. Mechanism: Tumor secretes fibroblast growth factor 23 (**FGF23**), which inhibits renal tubular reabsorption of phosphate and renal conversion of 25-hydroxyvitamin D to 1,25-dihydroxyvitamin D.
56. In diuretics, **FEurea <35%** indicating prerenal.
57. **Tubulointerstitial process**: a slowly progressive course without a clear inciting event, subnephrotic proteinuria, bloody urine sediment, and atrophic kidneys.
58. Hallmark findings of **interstitial nephritis**: UA may show microscopic hematuria and/or **sterile pyuria** (white cells in the urine without bacteria) and leukocyte casts.
59. **Thyrotoxic periodic paralysis** also known as **hypokalemic periodic paralysis** secondary to thyrotoxicosis; it causes symmetrical proximal flaccid muscle weakness from a sudden **intracellular K shift** (increased Na-K ATPase pump activity) precipitated by strenuous exercise or high carbohydrate meal.
60. **Cerebral salt wasting**, similar to SIADH, but has **hypovolemia**, occurs over a longer time in head trauma patients.
61. Initial management of **rhabdomyolysis-induced** acute kidney injury is normal saline at 200–300 cc/h as appropriate, not bicarbonate.
62. **ANCA-associated glomerulonephritis** is characterized by a **vasculitic prodrome** of malaise, arthralgia, myalgia, skin findings, hematuria, proteinuria, and acute kidney injury.
63. **Systolic-diastolic bruit in the abdomen** with hypertension in a young adult ⇒ consider **fibromuscular dysplasia** which is associated with **aneurysm and/or dissection** and **renal artery stenosis** or **renovascular hypertension**.
64. For unilateral and bilateral atherosclerotic or fibromuscular dysplasia renal artery stenosis, ACEi or ARB is appropriate; concomitant **percutaneous angioplasty with stenting or surgical revascularization** is necessary to shorten the duration of hypertension, if failed optimal medical therapy, intolerant to medical therapy, recurrent flash pulmonary edema or congestive heart failure.
65. **Polystyrene sulfonate** is contraindicated in recent bowel surgery. Nowadays, we use sodium zirconium cyclosilicate (**Lokelma**) 10 mg tid for up to six doses (then 10 mg daily if needed) for hyperkalemia. **May need to avoid the use of Lokelma** in severe constipation, bowel obstruction or impaction, and abnormal postoperative bowel motility disorders because of a lack of research in these conditions.
66. Abdominal compartment syndrome **(≥20 mmHg)** ⇒ consider checking urinary bladder pressure. This is a surgical emergency.
67. Patients with **enteric hyperoxaluria** and **calcium oxalate nephrolithiasis** can be treated with **cholestyramine** or **potassium citrate** (only if hypocitraturia).
68. Patients with chronic kidney disease and normal calcium and phosphate should be treated with active Vit D analogs to reduce elevated PTH and prevent renal osteodystrophy (osteitis fibrosa cystica).

Chapter 25
Cardiology

1. **Cardiac transplant patient** home medications (8 years after cardiac transplantation): tacrolimus, prednisone, mycophenolate mofetil, valganciclovir, TMP-SMX. For transplants, the risk for rejection is the highest within the **first 3–6 months** after transplantation and then within **the first year**. **Biopsy** of the transplant in the first year after cardiac transplantation is needed if concerns for rejection. **If >1 year after transplantation**, patients can develop **allograft vasculopathy** and thus will need **coronary angiography** if concerning symptoms.
2. **Cannon a wave**: A-V dissociation (atria contract against closed tricuspid valve), may be seen in complete heart block, ventricular tachycardia, or junctional rhythm.
3. **Mitral valve surgical repair** is preferred to replacement and is strongly recommended for chronic severe primary mitral regurgitation (MR) in (1) symptomatic patients with severe MR (preferably early before LVEF decline); (2) asymptomatic patients with left ventricular dysfunction (LVEF 30%–60% and/or LVED diameter ≥40 mm); (3) patient going for another cardiac surgery; (4) AFib and/or pulmonary HTN ≥50 mmHg. If asymptomatic severe MR and without LV dysfunction, then surveillance echo q6m to q12m if no other indication for surgery.
4. **Severe MR** = A regurgitant jet over 40% of the left atrium area, >60 mL regurgitant volume or >50% regurgitant fraction, and/or presence of diastolic reversal of pulmonary venous flow.
5. Surgical mitral valve repair is the first-line treatment for MR ⇒ transcatheter mitral valve repair. **Transcatheter mitral valve repair** is approved for significant symptomatic degenerative MR for whom mitral valve surgery poses a **prohibitive risk**.
6. **Percutaneous mitral valve balloon valvuloplasty** or valvotomy for rheumatic mitral stenosis (MS) without significant MR or LAA thrombus.

K. Zhou, *Internal Medicine Training Notes and Survival Guide*,
https://doi.org/10.1007/978-1-0716-4039-5_25

7. **Mitral stenosis** usually stems from either rheumatic mitral disease (progressive valve damage from rheumatic fever while young) or degenerative disease (e.g. mitral annular calcification). The mean pressure gradient (PG) of mitral stenosis (MS) is **5–10 mmHg** in severe mitral stenosis, which is heart-rate dependent (tachycardia worsens mean PG). In rheumatic MS, mitral valve <1.5 cm^2 denotes severe stenosis and <1 cm^2 denotes very severe stenosis. **Treatment is percutaneous mitral balloon valvuloplasty** in favorable anatomy without LAA thrombus or significant mitral regurgitation; otherwise, **surgical MV replacement** should be considered.
8. In **Eisenmenger syndrome**, air filters and meticulous care of all IV lines should be instituted to prevent paradoxical air embolization.
9. Discrepancy between **symptoms typical of severe mitral stenosis** (progressive exertional dyspnea) and **echo findings of only moderate mitral stenosis** ⇒ consider exercise echocardiography.
10. Normal mean **pulmonary artery (wedge) pressure**: 12–16 (upper limit 20) mmHg. Mild pulmonary hypertension: 25–40 mmHg. Moderate pulmonary hypertension: **41–55** mmHg. Severe pulmonary hypertension: >55 mmHg.
11. **Cisplatin side effect**s: neuropathy, bone marrow suppression, ototoxicity, nephrotoxicity, extravasation, VTE, SVT, MI, and cardiomyopathy. **Paclitaxel side effects**: decreased blood counts, hair loss, neuropathy, diarrhea.
12. **Aortic coarctation**: suspect if CXR with "figure 3 sign" and rib notching.
13. **Oral anticoagulation without an antiplatelet agent** is sufficient for the prevention of ACS and VTEs in most patients with high-risk AFib and CAD.
14. **Suspected CAD** with baseline ECG abnormalities, like ST segment depression ≥0.05, LBBB, ventricular paced complexes, digitalis effects, and preexcitation, require stress testing with **adjuvant imaging**.
15. **Effusive constrictive pericarditis** etiologies: idiopathic, infectious, or radiation pericarditis. **Restrictive pericarditis** = abnormal elastic properties of the myocardium and/or intercellular matrix; **constrictive pericarditis** = the external pericardial constraint.
16. **Restrictive pericarditis**: BNP often >100, pulmonary HTN, and thickened myocardium (LVH). **Constrictive pericarditis**: pericardial thickening +/− effusion (occasionally pericardial calcification), annulus inversus on echo (often "septal bounce"). If severe and has no reversible cause in constrictive pericarditis, surgical pericardial stripping may be considered.
17. **Constrictive pericarditis** treatment: NSAIDs → hemodynamic steadiness with right cardiac catheterization for diagnosis → surgical pericardiectomy.
18. **Acute pericarditis** treatment: high-dose aspirin (650 TID) or high-dose NSAIDs + colchicine (weight-based); steroid and/or biologic agents reserved for recurrent or refractory cases. Needs echo to rule out tamponade (hemodynamic instability due to extrinsic fluid accumulation; **not always determined by size but rather the rapidity of accumulation**).
19. Echo criteria for **severe aortic stenosis (AS)**: peak aortic jet velocity >4 m/s (directly measured), mean pressure gradient >40 mm Hg (directly measured),

aortic valve area <1 cm^2 (indirectly calculated from continuity equation most of the time). In patients with echo showing calculated aortic valve area (AVA) <1.0 cm^2 but aortic valve velocity and mean pressure gradient not meeting cut-off for severe AS, one should consider the possibility of **low flow, low gradient severe AS if cardiac output is reduced.** In case of suspected low-flow, low-gradient severe AS and coexisting reduced EF, consider **dobutamine stress echo** to differentiate true vs pseudo severe AS.

20. **Cardiogenic shock secondary to progressive heart failure**: inotropic agents including **dopamine**, **dobutamine**, and **milrinone** may be administered inpatient (usually in the ICU setting); they improve symptoms and quality of life but do not improve (in fact worsen) mortality. Inotropic agents are used for bridging to recovery, transplant, LVAD, or palliative purposes.
21. **VSD**: a loud systolic murmur at the left sternal border that may obliterate S2 (palpable thrill)
22. **Cardiac syndrome X** is characterized by chronic angina and stress test abnormality in the absence of angiographically significant CAD. Stress-induced (also known as **Takotsubo cardiomyopathy**) is acute angina with a negative cardiac angiogram. It is characterized by **acute new-onset LV dysfunction**, often with **angina**, and positive troponin but normal angiogram. Tell-tale imaging finding is "**apical ballooning**" reminiscent of Japanese octopus traps; it usually completely resolves after recovering from stress trigger/critical illness.
23. **Abdominal aortic aneurysm (AAA) repair indications**: (1) symptomatic aneurysm of any size (especially if associated with a peripheral arterial aneurysm); (2) asymptomatic AAA diameter ≥ **5.5 cm in males** (**5 cm in females**); (3) rapid expansion of AAA > 0.5 cm over 6 months; or (4) symptomatic. **Open surgical repair vs. endovascular aneurysm repair (EVAR)**: depends on operative risks, expected life span, and ability to adhere to the monitoring requirement of EVAR. Suprarenal and juxtarenal (open surgical) vs. infrarenal (open surgical vs. EVAR).
24. Indications for **repeat echocardiogram** in congestive heart failure (CHF) if: change in clinical status, >3 months after optimization of heart failure medical therapy and/or revascularization to assess recovery and need for ICD.
25. **Mitral valve prolapses**: late systolic crescendo murmur with midsystolic click.
26. **Marfan syndrome** can cause aortic dissection in pregnancy; if ascending aortic dissection **≥4.5 cm** ⇒ surgery before pregnancy. Pregnancy with an aortic diameter <4 cm does not require intervention.
27. **Papillary fibroelastoma** (usually associated with valves) vs. **left atrial myxomas** (usually pedunculated from fossa ovalis of patients 30–60 years old, usually incidental finding). Both can cause symptoms of embolization; myxoma may cause **constitutional symptoms and/or valvular obstruction** if large.
28. Patients with cyanosis (i.e., Eisenmenger syndrome) have **compensated erythrocytosis with stable hemoglobin** levels. Iron deficiency and resultant

microcytosis is common in Eisenmenger syndrome, treatment: iron sucralfate/gluconate.

29. **In infective endocarditis, cardiac valve surgery** is recommended if persistent infection (repeat blood culture positive) lasting longer than 5–7 days while on antibiotics, **symptomatic HF**, left-sided involvement with **staph**, **fungal** infection, or highly resistant **organism**, new **heart block**, annular/aortic **abscess** (EKG showing **conduction** abnormalities), or **prosthetic valve**.
30. New onset first-degree AV block in aortic valve endocarditis suggests a **perivalvular abscess**.
31. **Cardiac resynchronization therapy (CRT) should meet all the requirements**: LVEF ≤35%; NYHA functional class II to IV HF despite maximal medical therapy for 3 months or at **least 40 days** after myocardial infarction; LBBB with QRS ≥150 ms (more nuanced if QRS 120–150 ms or non-LBBB). CRT requires biventricular pacing with pacing leads in the **RA, RV, and coronary sinus (CS) although direct LV pacing** may become the new standard.
32. Patients with **Type B acute aortic dissection** without evidence of cardiogenic shock should be initially treated with medical therapy to control HR and reduce BP using **beta blockers and nitroprusside**. Type A aortic dissection requires urgent/emergent open surgery repair. Type A aortic dissection may quickly evolve into shock with **Beck's triad** (hypotension, JVD, muffled heart sound) suggesting **cardiac tamponade** (obstructive shock). Treatment: TTE → operating room.
33. Pulmonary stenosis: the preferred treatment is pulmonary balloon valvuloplasty vs pulmonary valve replacement depending on etiology. **Balloon valvuloplasty** is indicated for symptomatic pulmonic stenosis with appropriate valve morphology with a peak Doppler gradient of **≥50** mmHg or a mean gradient ≥30 mmHg. **Surgical pulmonary valve replacemen**t should be considered if the dysplastic valve or moderate or worse coexisting pulmonary valve regurgitation, a small annulus, severe subvalvular or supravalvar pulmonary valvostenosis, or other cardiac lesions requires operative intervention. Pulmonic valve regurgitation is common in TOF after surgery.
34. Hypertrophic cardiomyopathy (HCM): the main concerns are symptoms (due to **LVOT obstruction**) and the risk of **sudden cardiac death** (SCD).
35. **Symptomatic hypertrophic cardiomyopathy** (HCM) **treatment**: beta blocker, nondihydropyridine calcium blockers (verapamil and diltiazem), alcohol septal ablation, open **surgical septal myectomy, or mavacamten**. If hemodynamically unstable, consider IV fluids and phenylephrine. HCM typical symptoms: **dyspnea, syncope, chest pain**. Patients with HCM should be considered for ICD if: massive myocardial wall hypertrophy (**wall thickness ≥30 mm**); **previous cardiac arrest/VT; blunted BP response or hypotension during exercise**; unexplained syncope; nonsustained VT; family history of sudden cardiac death.
36. A subset of HCM presents with hypertrophic obstructive cardiomyopathy (**HOCM**) with asymmetrical hypertrophy, systolic anterior motion (SAM) of the mitral valve, and a left ventricular outflow tract obstruction (LVOT).

Symptoms of LVOT: angina, dizziness, and dyspnea. If symptomatic HOCM hypotension, treatment with **phenylephrine** and **volume infusion** may be necessary whereas positive inotropes including epinephrine, dopamine, and Levophed should be avoided.

37. **Ostium primum ASD** shows fixed splitting of S2, MR, and LAD on EKG. Coronary sinus ASD: R heart volume overload but no MR, EKG normal or incomplete RBBB or first-degree AV block. Ostium secundum ASD: R heart volume overload but no MR, EKG normal or incomplete RBBB or first-degree AV block.
38. **AFib with aberrant conduction** results in an irregularly irregular rhythm and a wide complex tachycardia from bundle branch block, such as rSR in lead V1, deep terminal S in lead I, and V6 with RBBB may be confused with VT if very rapid heart rate.
39. Most common lesions in Turner's syndrome (only one X chromosome) include **bicuspid aortic valve, aortic coarctation, and aortic aneurysm**.
40. Marfan syndrome—**MVP, aortic dissection/aneurysm**. Marfan syndrome: **dilation of ascending aorta** ⇒ Ascending aorta surveillance imaging 6 months after diagnosis with annual surveillance if root **<4.5 cm**.
41. **Symptomatic secondary AV block** necessitates pacemaker regardless of Mobitz Type 1 or 2 blocker. Mobitz Type 2 is automatically an indication for a pacemaker if there is no reversible cause.
42. **Bacterial endocarditis prophylaxis** (needs to meet both requirements): (1) prosthetic heart valves, unrepaired cyanotic congenital heart disease, heart transplant with heart valve disease, history of infective endocarditis; and (2) in dental, respiratory (incision and biopsy), cardiac surgery. The prophylactic regimen includes **amoxicillin 2 g or cephalexin 2 g once 30–60 min before the procedure**.
43. One week after **acute pericarditis**, EKG may show T wave inversion. Acute pericarditis typically has diffuse ST elevation, PR depression, and/or T wave inversion in EKG.
44. Prophylaxis for secondary prevention in the history of **rheumatic fever**. Uncomplicated: for the longer of **5** years or till age 21 with carditis but **no valvular disease**; for the longer of **10** years or till age 21 with carditis and **valvular disease**; for the longer of 10 years or till age **40** for **chronic rheumatic** heart **disease**. Regimen: **penicillin G, benzathine** injection q4 weeks.
45. Preferred antiarrhythmic drugs: no CAD or structural heart disease—flecainide and propafenone; LVH—dronedarone and amiodarone; CAD without heart failure—sotalol and dronedarone; heart failure—amiodarone and dofetilide.
46. **Amiodarone** is generally more effective in rhythm control but needs long-term monitoring (LFT, PFT/CXR, TSH, eye exam).
47. **Sotalol** and **dofetilide**: often need inpatient initiation to monitor QT prolongation to avoid torsade de Pointes.
48. **Culture-negative endocarditis** (Coxiella, Bartonella, fungus, Strep if after antibiotics). **Characteristics**: low-grade fever, fatigue, no growth of blood

culture × 3 sets ≥5 days. Workup: Echo, Q fever serology, rheumatic factor, urinalysis (UA).

49. **Major criteria** for infective endocarditis: + blood culture for typical microorganism (Strep viridans, HACEK, S. aureus, S. bovis), imaging studies showing vegetation, or Q fever serology IgG titer >1:800. **Diagnosis of infective endocarditis** is established if (1) 2 Major Criteria or (2) 1 Major Criterion and 3 Minor Criteria or (3) 5 Minor Criteria are met.
50. **Consider dobutamine stress test** rather than adenosine/regadenoson stress test if: unable to exercise while having reactive airway disease flare-up +/− uncontrolled seizure disorder.
51. **Hyperkalemia** with EKG changes: K 6–7 (prolonged PR interval, peak T); 7–8 (loss of P wave, tall peak T); >9 (widened QRS, sinusoidal wave, cardiac arrest).
52. **Wide complex tachycardia** = SVT with aberrancy, antidromic AV reentrant tachycardia, or VT.
53. **Ventricular tachycardia** EKG: evidence of AV dissociation (more Rs than Ps), precordial concordance, capture beats, or fusion beats favors **VT** and should be treated accordingly. Differentiation of **VT** from others: absence of an RS complex → RS > 100 ms → AV dissociation → look at V1 (LBBB vs. RBBB)
54. **Cough with lisinopril, can switch to ARB. Muscle pain with statin: can change to a different statin** (rosuvastatin and pravastatin show less myalgia), ezetimibe, bempedoic acid, or PCSK9 inhibitor (evolocumab/alirocumab are q 2–4 week subcutaneous injections; inclisiran is q 3–6 months IV).
55. **Angioedema with ACEi**: wait 4 weeks before switching to ARBs under close monitoring. If it's a cough then, can switch right away.
56. **Digoxin-specific antibody (Fab)** fragments indications: life-threatening arrhythmia (e.g. bidirectional VT), end-organ dysfunction due to hypotension, or hyperkalemia >5.5 mEq/L.
57. Preoperative evaluation: Revised cardiac risk index ≤1, or ≥4 Met [climb a flight of stairs (10–12 steps) or walk on level ground at 3–4 mph] = low risk for surgery. If emergent surgery and no active MI, can bypass cardiac evaluation and proceed to surgery.
58. Treatments for **congenital long QT syndrome**: beta blocker, e.g., propranolol, nadolol.
59. **Demand ischemia**: happens in coronary artery spasm, anemic, arrhythmic, coronary embolism, or significant hypertension/hypotension; should **not have cardiac enzyme elevation**. **Peri-infarction pericarditis** treatment: aspirin 625–1000 mg tid.
60. **Cardiac tamponade**: hypotension, tachycardia, increased JVD (with rapid X descent), and pulsus paradoxus. Confirm with echo stat.
61. **Cardiac myxoma**: early diastolic sound; causes systemic embolization, and constitutional symptoms (fever, weight loss, or Raynaud's symptoms from overproduction of IL-6). **Treatment**: surgical excision.

62. **Chest pain differential diagnoses**: ACS, PE, aortic dissection, esophagitis or esophageal rupture, pneumonia, MSK.
63. **Mechanical heart valve**, can continue Coumadin if <5 mg/day during pregnancy; for all other indications of anticoagulation (i.e., AFib, VTE, AFib with mitral stenosis) and ≥5 mg Coumadin, should use LMWH in pregnancy.
64. **Medications for gestational HTN** only if **≥160/110 mmHg** or evidence of end-organ damage. Treatment: **labetalol, methyldopa**. Nifedipine and hydralazine are alternatives.
65. 1–15 months after AICD placement, endothelial damage during insertion can cause **SVC syndrome,** diagnosis via upper extremity venography (CT chest with contrast usually done first). **Treatment**: anticoagulation, extensive ones require thrombolysis, stent implantation, bypass surgery, or extraction of leads and reimplantation.
66. **Subclavian steal syndrom**e: usually due to severe atherosclerotic narrowing/occlusion of the proximal subclavian artery which results in flow reverse in the ipsilateral vertebral artery, more often on the left side. **Symptoms**: exercise-induced fatigue, pain, numbness, coolness, fatigue and vertebral-basilar insufficiency.
67. In **high-risk patients taking DAPT** (history of PUD, GIB, active H. pylori, >65 yo), start PPI.
68. Opening snap after S2, loud first sound → consider **mitral stenosis**. Holosystolic murmur increases with inspiration → consider tricuspid regurgitation (TR). Late peaking systolic murmur 3/6, paradoxical splitting S2 (delayed closure of aortic valve) → consider severe AS.
69. **Perivalvular absces**s: the abscess extends from the aortic valve into the adjacent conduction tissue near the AV node leading to various **heart blocks**.
70. **Ebstein anomaly**: apical displacement of tricuspid valve, atrialization of the R ventricle, decreased R ventricular volume. TR—holosystolic murmur best heard at left second or third intercostal area or subxiphoid area.
71. **Thiazide** diuretics increase the risks for developing diabetes. Adenosine single photon emission CT (**SPECT**) is a nuclear medicine stress test.
72. ACEi can reduce amlodipine-induced edema; **mechanical heart** (aortic or mitral) **valves** with low rates of bleeding = treatment with aspirin and warfarin
73. Current guidelines recommend long-term anticoagulation with warfarin goal INR 2.5 in mitral stenosis with AFib, left atrial thrombosis, or prior thrombosis.
74. **Surgical aortic valve replacement** indications in AR (early diastolic decrescendo murmur): severe AR in symptomatic patients (i.e., dyspnea, decreased exercise tolerance), asymptomatic patients with LVEF <50% or dilated L ventricle with either end-diastolic size >50 mm or end-diastolic dimension ≥65 mm or indexed end-systolic dimension of 25 mm/m^2.
75. **Aortic valve replacement** in AS: stage D1 (mean gradient pressure ≥40 mmHg, AVA <1 cm^2, max Jet ≥4 m/s); asymptomatic patients with critical AS (Vmax >4.5 m/s, mean pressure gradient >50 mmHg, AVA <0.75 cm^2); asymptomatic patients with severe AS and LV dysfunction (LVEF <50%); asymptomatic patients with severe AS and hypotension with exercise;

moderate AS with other concomitant heart surgery; low-flow/low-gradient (mean gradient <30 mm Hg) severe AS with drop in blood pressure with exercise; otherwise, surveillance echo q6–12m.

76. **Asymptomatic severe aortic stenosis and bicuspid aortic valve** can be managed with close follow-up with echocardiogram 6–12 months only.
77. All **bicuspid aortic valves** should be evaluated with echo, CT, or cardiac MRI for possible associated aortopathy (30%–50% have aortic enlargement, while 6% have aortic coaptation). Also **consider first degree family member screening** (~10% probability).
78. **Bicuspid aortic valve** is commonly associated with aortic aneurysm, dissection, and coarctation, management: echo every 6–12 months after CT angiography of the aorta.
79. Patients with **bicuspid aortic valve and AAA** should receive annual imaging if aortic diameter <4.5 cm; ≥4.5 cm or enlargement ≥0.5 cm/year should receive imaging q6m.
80. Symptomatic AS: if no TAVR, **life expectancy is 2–3 years**; need cardiac catheterization before TAVR.
81. **Peripartum cardiomyopathy**: onset of heart failure during the last month of pregnancy or within the first 5 months following delivery.
82. **Mechanical aortic valve** to get high bleeding risk procedures like pancreatic cyst biopsy ⇒ hold warfarin till INR <1.5, do it. If the patient has a mechanical mitral valve, it will need bridge with heparin drip, and restart heparin 24 h after the procedure. **INR numbers** vary depending on valve type and clinical risk profile.
83. **Normal cardiac index** 2.8–4.2 L/min/m^2. **Normal systemic vascular resistance** (SVR) 800–1200 dynes s/cm^5.
84. High-intensity statin increases risks for new-onset DM (usually in patients already with borderline A1c; continue use as benefit >risk). **Pickering syndrome** = flash pulmonary edema in bilateral renal artery stenosis.
85. Risk stratification of asymptomatic patients with WPW pattern on an EKG can be performed with non-invasive tests (e.g., exercise testing or procainamide challenge) and/or EPS to identify those at greatest risk of sudden cardiac death. **Low risk with intermittent loss of pre-excitation during faster HR treatment: no need for further evaluation or treatment.**
86. **Low QRS voltage and conduction defects in patients with LVH → consider infiltrative cardiomyopathy** (sarcoidosis and amyloidosis). AL amyloidosis causes proteinuria (73% of cases) and renal insufficiency (50% of cases).
87. **Multivessel coronary artery disease (MVD)** = greater than 70% stenosis in at least two major coronary arteries with a diameter of ≥2.5 mm or in one coronary artery in addition to greater than 50% stenosis of the left main trunk.
88. Patients with **left main disease** have traditionally been treated with CABG. Other **indications for CABG** include triple vessel disease, and left main equivalent disease (**≥70% stenosis of LAD and LCx artery**)—particularly if left ventricular function is impaired.

89. **Noonan syndrome** has pulmonary stenosis, short stature, variable intellectual impairment, unique facial features, neck webbing, hypertelorism, and other cardiac abnormalities, including hypertrophic cardiomyopathy, ASD, and VSD.
90. **Atrial fibrillation** in **hypertrophic cardiomyopathy (HCM)** should receive warfarin even if CHAD2DS2-VASc score of 0.
91. Asymptomatic HCM, screening with physical, echo, and EKG starts at age 12 to adults, then every 5 years.
92. **Hydralazine** 37.5 mg tid **and isosorbide dinitrate** 20 mg tid improve survival in African American patients with HFrEF.
93. Transthoracic echo is indicated for 3/6 grade systolic murmur, late or holosystolic murmur, diastolic or continuous murmur, and murmurs with accompanying symptoms.
94. **LVH with repolarization abnormalities** or LBBB → cannot do EKG-only treadmill stress test, needs alternative stress modality (e.g. pharmacological SPECT/PET/MRI).
95. Midsystolic flow murmur at left sternal border = ASD; loud holosystolic murmur = VSD. Tricuspid regurgitation = holosystolic murmur.
96. **Consider coronary artery calcium score if intermediate-risk** (≥7.5%–<20%) **or elected borderline-risk (5%–7.5%) 10-year ASCVD and age >40** if it changes clinical management (e.g. **aspirin and statin**).
97. Patients with **end-stage heart failure** should be considered for cardiac transplantation (usually 65 or younger, not absolute) or mechanical circulatory support such as LVAD.
98. **Placement of a continuous flow left ventricular assistive device (LVAD)** reduces symptoms and improves survival in end-stage CHF. Major post-LVAD complications include stroke, bleeding/hemolysis, driveline infection, pump thrombosis, and others (e.g. aortic regurgitation, RV failure, outflow conduit kinking).
99. **Four pillars of HFrEF medical therapy** that improve mortality: beta blocker, ACEi/ARB/ARNI, mineralocorticoid antagonist (MRA), and SGLT2 inhibitor.
100. **Indications for cardiac transplantation**: age < 65–70 yo, no medical contraindications (irreversible pulmonary hypertension, end organ damage despite heart transplant, malignancies within 5 years, active substance abuse, ESRD unless combined heart/kidney transplant), good support and adherence.
101. **Tetralogy of Fallot**: VSD, pulmonary stenosis, overriding aorta, right ventricular hypertrophy. Treatment: closure of VSD, relief of right ventricular outflow tract obstruction (diastolic murmur from pulmonary valve regurgitation).
102. **ASD**: increased central venous pressure, fixed splitting of S2, right ventricular heave, soft systolic murmur.
103. **Cardiac amyloidosis** (usually ATTR) should be suspected in black patients ≥50 year who have left ventricular wall thickening that is not explained by

preloading conditions like hypertension, aortic stenosis, and present with congestive heart failure with preserved ejection fraction.

104. **Ranolazine** (CYP3A4) should be cut to 50% and should not exceed **500 mg** bid when used with CYP3A4 inhibitors (ketoconazole, clarithromycin, ritonavir, verapamil, and diltiazem).
105. **Platypnea-orthodeoxia** etiologies: intracardiac shunting, pulmonary shunting, V/Q mismatch, or a combination of these. **Platypnea-orthodeoxia** in sitting/standing can be from PFO with right to left shunt. Three days after myocardial infarction, **orthopnea and platypnea indicate possible ASD or PFO**, not VSD.
106. Indications for **percutaneous ASD device closure**: the ratio of pulmonary blood flow to systemic blood flow Qp/Qs $\geq$ 1.5 with right heart enlargement and/or symptomatic disease and/or paradoxical embolism but in the absence of irreversible severe pulmonary hypertension or Eisenmenger syndrome.
107. **Differential cyanosis**: toe cyanosis and digital clubbing but normal hands, holosystolic murmur = patent ductus arteriosus (**PDA**).
108. First-degree relatives of **hypertrophic obstructive cardiomyopathy (HOCM)**, echo q 12–18 m starting after age 10 or 12 years. If >21 years, echo q5 years. If with aortic root dilation, first in 6 months, then annually.
109. Ascites in congestive heart failure → concerns for constrictive pericarditis who have an indeterminate echo ⇒ consider **cardiac catheterization for hemodynamic assessment**.
110. For acute limb ischemia, CT/invasive angiography should be performed to determine **surgical embolectomy vs catheter-directed thrombolysis**.
111. **Severe aortic stenosis** = aortic valve area < 1 cm^2, the mean gradient >40 mmHg, or the aortic jet velocity > 4 m/s. Low flow, low gradient but aortic valve area = 0.9 cm^2 ⇒ **consider dobutamine echo**.
112. **TEE** has a much higher sensitivity than TTE in diagnosing infective endocarditis or potential complications (like abscesses), although often TTE should be done first and offers quicker information while TEE is arranged.
113. **ST depression of 1 mm with TIMI score of 1** ⇒ consider exercise stress testing.
114. **Ivabradine** prolongs diastolic time and reduces heart rate; it is used in: **LVEF < 35% and HR ≥ 70 bpm after beta blocker is maximally uptitrated**.
115. ASD: mid systolic or mid-diastolic murmur. VSD: pulmonary edema and acute dyspnea on exertion. PAD has decreased SO_2.
116. **STEMI**: give aspirin, heparin bolus, go straight to cardiac catheterization or tPA, and transfer to PCI facility. EKG diagnosis with supporting clinical and biomarker evidence. **Standard treatment includes immediate cath lab activation, loading aspirin (325 mg) and a P2Y12 inhibitor (clopidogrel, ticagrelor or prasugrel), heparin bolus (usually 4000 units), go straight to cardiac catheterization or tPA if no cath lab available (geographic limitation, inclement weather, e.g.).**
117. For ACS with DES or BMS, DAPT should be 1 year (maybe longer if high risk). If need for interruption of DAPT, **wait at least 1 month for BMS and**

3–6 months for DES (unless emergent surgery; may consider **bridging with IV cangrelor** to minimize gap).

118. **Valsartan-sacubitril (Entresto)**: superior to ACEi/ARB, should be used with caution in patients with **soft blood pressure and dizziness**, need **36-h** "wash-out" period if transitioning from ACEi, monitor for renal function and potassium level after initiation and/or dose escalation.
119. **Type II NSTEMI** (significant cardiac muscle damage from demand-supply mismatch rather than true actual coronary artery atherosclerosis) → **ischemia guided approach**: stress test if TIMI <2 or GRACE risk score < 109; early invasive therapy for intermediate and high-risk patients.

Chapter 26
Gastroenterology

1. **Four typical phases of HBV infection**: immune tolerant, immune active, immune control (inactive), reactivation.
2. **Naloxegol** (Movantik) and **methylnaltrexone** are peripherally acting μ-opioid receptor antagonists used in opioid-induced constipation.
3. HBV without cirrhosis but with **HBeAg+, if DNA > 20,000, and ALT >2 times upper limit normal**, observe 3–6 months if compensated; treat if no spontaneous HBeAg loss or decompensated (current treatment is not effective in inducing HBeAg seroconversion). Treatment with entecavir, tenofovir alafenamide, tenofovir disoproxil fumarate, or Peg IFNalpha to reach HBeAg-, suppress HBV DNA, and normalize ALT. **HBV without cirrhosis with HBeAg-, if DNA > 2000**, will need treatment with the above medications for 1 year or longer. **HBV+ with cirrhosis** requires treatment regardless, usually with **entecavir** preferred for decompensated liver failure while entecavir, tenofovir alafenamide, or tenofovir disoproxil fumarate for compensated liver failure.
4. **Lamivudine**, **telbivudine**, or **tenofovir** is used to prevent vertical transmission in pregnant women with **HBV DNA > 200,000 at 24–28 weeks of gestation**. Tenofovir and telbivudine are Category B. A 2019 NEJM article reported **Tenofovir 300 mg daily from 30–32 weeks of gestation until postpartum week 4** decreased mother-to-child transmission of HBV (no breastfeeding after child delivery). Neonates of HBV mom should receive **hepatitis B immune globulin** intramuscularly and **vaccine** (GlaxoSmithKline) **within 12 h** after birth, repeat both immunizations at **week 4,** and repeat vaccination at **week 24**.
5. **Antiviral therapy** of HBV is also recommended for acute liver failure, cirrhosis, and patients undergoing treatment with certain immunosuppressive therapy or chemo.
6. **Tenofovir or entecavir** is a first-line treatment for immune active HBV infection because of its low resistance rate.

K. Zhou, *Internal Medicine Training Notes and Survival Guide*,
https://doi.org/10.1007/978-1-0716-4039-5_26

7. **Hepatocellular carcinoma (HCC)** surveillance **ultrasound** (every 6 months) with or without alpha-FP for Southeast Asian M ≥ 40 years of age, F ≥ 50 years of age, Sub-Saharan African ≥20 years of age.
8. HBV or HCV and/or cirrhosis: ultrasound every 6 months; nodule <1 cm, need to repeat ultrasound in 3 months; **>1 cm**, consider multidetector computed tomography (MDCT) with contrast/MRI.
9. **Primary biliary cholangitis (PBC)**: **cholestatic liver enzyme** profile with **positive anti-mitochondrial Ab** (↑ ↑ *ALP*), Diagnosis via magnetic resonance cholangiopancreatography (**MRCP**). 10% of PBCs have negative anti-mitochondrial Ab. If high suspicion, other PBC-specific Ab (sp100 and gp210) can help establish the diagnosis with cholestatic LFTs. PBC has an increased risk (up to 19 folds) for hepatocellular carcinoma.
10. **Achalasia** (30–60 yo, chronic, insidious onset); **pseudoachalasia** (etiologies: tumor, amyloidosis, postsurgical status, sarcoidosis)
11. Treatment for diarrhea-predominant IBS is low **FODMAP** (fermentable, oligosaccharide, disaccharide, monosaccharide, and polyols). **Linaclotide** for IBS-C, **lubiprostone** (chloride channel activator in the GI tract) for women with IBS-C ≥ 18 yo, **alosetron** (selective antagonist of a serotonin 5-HT3 receptor) for women with IBS-D ≥ 18 yo. **Linaclotide** is also used in chronic idiopathic constipation.
12. Zenker diverticulum diagnosis is **barium esophagography**.
13. **Platypnea** and **orthodeoxia** = consider hepatopulmonary shunting. Diagnosis via $PaO_2 < 80$ mmHg or A-a gradient ≥15 mmHg, along with intrapulmonary shunting per **echo with agitated saline or microaggregated albumin**.
14. **Acalculous cholecystitis** treatment: cholecystostomy tube placement if not a surgical candidate vs cholecystectomy if surgical candidate.
15. Manage large (>10 mm) hyperplastic polyps as if they are sessile serrated polyps: repeat **colonoscopy in 3 years**.
16. Acute cholangitis with biliary obstruction (biliary dilation) or choledocholithiasis treatment: **ERCP** for biliary decompression. If not possible, do **percutaneous cholangiography** with **biliary tube placement**.
17. **Eosinophilic esophagitis**: dysphagia in asthmatics, food allergies, eczema patients. Diagnosis requires **15 eosinophils/hpf** on biopsy with EGD. Treatment: dupilumab (Dupixent) is the only FDA-approved drug; additional options include a proton pump inhibitor for 8 weeks or swallowing aerosolized topical glucocorticoids ⇒ consider **repeat upper endoscopy 8–12 weeks** after initiating treatment.
18. **Eosinophilic esophagitis**: common in atopic conditions with longitudinal furrows, concentric rings, and whitish papules/exudates that represent eosinophilic microabscess.
19. **Toxic megacolon** in inflammatory bowel disease treatment: IV fluid resuscitation, IV high dose steroids (if not responding, infliximab or cyclosporine), antibiotics, and lastly colectomy.
20. **Microscopic colitis**: non-bloody watery diarrhea in older adults (lymphocytic vs collagenous); diagnosis via **biopsy** showing **lymphocytic** infiltrates (lym-

phocytic colitis) or subepithelial **collagen** bands (collagenous colitis), can be associated with **NSAIDs** or **PPIs** or **SSRIs**. Treatment: **budesonide** oral tablets, may add cholestyramine or bismuth subsalicylate 282 mg tid if not effective.

21. **Microscopic colitis subtypes**: lymphocytic (20 lymphocytes/100 epithelial cells) versus collagenous (colonic subepithelial collagen band >10 μm in thickness).
22. **Autoimmune pancreatitis** is caused by plasma cell infiltration and can also present with sialadenitis (especially in IgG4+ autoimmune pancreatitis) and probable retroperitoneal fibrosis. Treatment: **prednisone** with a taper over 2–3 months.
23. **Acute fatty liver of pregnancy and HELLP** are similar in presentation; treatment: acute delivery of baby, both are related to long-chain 3-hydroxyl coenzyme A dehydrogenase deficiency.
24. **Gallbladder polyps** larger than **1 cm** in size should be treated with cholecystectomy even if asymptomatic. Cholecystectomy is also indicated for **asymptomatic polyps 6–9 mm** if age >60, Indian ethnicity, or sessile polyp including focal wall thickness >4 mm. Gallbladder polyp >8 mm in primary sclerosing cholangitis also requires cholecystectomy.
25. **Chronic pancreatitis** treatment: NSAIDs, low-fat diet, and smoking cessation.
26. **HBV-related polyarteritis nodosa** symptoms: fever, arthralgia, and vasculitis.
27. Indications for chronic **spontaneous bacterial peritonitis (SBP) prophylaxis**: (1) history of SBP; (2) ascitic fluid total protein <1.5 plus any of the following: Na $\leq$ 130, Cr $\geq$ 1.2, BUN $\geq$25, total bili $\geq$3, or Child-Turcotte-Pugh class B or C cirrhosis.
28. Variceal or gastrointestinal bleeding (**regardless of ascites presence**) or **ascitic protein level of less than 1 g/dL** in cirrhosis patients requires 7-day antibiotic prophylaxis usually with ceftriaxone while inpatient.
29. **Anticoagulation can be resumed right after endoscopic hemostasis in gastrointestinal (GI) bleeding**.
30. **Anti-tissue transglutaminase IgA ab** is the most specific for diagnosing celiac disease.
31. Colon cancer after resection should receive surveillance colonoscopy in 1, 3, and 5 years.
32. Pancreatic cyst lesions: **cysts, pseudocyst**. Both cysts and pseudocysts are collections of fluid. A true cyst is a closed structure with a **lining of cells** that separates it from the nearby tissue. A pseudocyst isn't closed and has **no lining of epithelial cells** separating it from the nearby tissue.
33. The two most common pancreatic cystic neoplasms are **mucinous cystic neoplasm (MCN) and intraductal papillary mucinous neoplasm (IPMN)**. Main duct IPMN can be diagnosed based on diffuse dilation of the main duct and mucin exudate. Mucinous cystic neoplasms and **main duct IPMN** should

receive **surgical resection** because main duct IPMN has a malignancy risk of 33%–60%, and mucinous cystic neoplasm has a malignancy risk of 10%–15%.

34. **Stool osmotic gap** <50 mOsm/kg suggests secretory while ≥75 mOsm/kg indicates osmotic: 290—2 × (stool Na+K).
35. **Crohn disease**: patchy, spares rectum, skip lesions, affects entire thickness of the intestinal wall.
36. Patients with uncomplicated **diverticulitis** should undergo colonoscopy **1–2 months** after acute episode to exclude colorectal cancer.
37. **Atrophic gastritis for pernicious anemia** → check for H. pylori-associated autoimmune atrophic gastritis → gastrinemia → gastric carcinoid and adenocarcinoma. Treatment: lifelong **B12 and Fe supplementation**.
38. **5%** of patients with inflammatory bowel disease (IBD) will develop primary sclerosing cholangitis (PSC). **80% of patients with PSC have IBD,** usually **ulcerative colitis**. Most PSCs have a string of beads bile duct with MRCP; however, a minority only involve small ducts of PSC and require liver biopsy for diagnosis because of normal MRCP in these patients. **PSC** is associated with **gastrointestinal cancers, cholangiocarcinoma, and gallbladder polyps**.
39. Treatment for cholangitis is immediate broad-spectrum **antimicrobial** therapy; if no rapid improvement, urgent **endoscopic stone** removal via ERCP should be performed.
40. Patients with **cirrhosis** are at increased risk for **osteoporosis**.
41. **Lynch syndrome**, also known as hereditary non-polyposis colorectal cancer syndrome. Diagnostic criteria: 3-2-1-1 = 3 relatives, 2 generations, at least 1 diagnosed at age younger than 50, and 1 is a first-degree relative. Lynch syndrome is caused by a mutation in the mismatch genes of **MLH1, MSH2, MSH6, or PMS2**. Lynch syndrome-related cancers include colorectal, endometrial, small bowel, ureter (upper tract urothelial carcinoma), and renal pelvis cancers.
42. **Lynch syndrome**: colonoscopy at 20–25 yo or 2–5 year before the earliest age of colorectal cancer in the family (whichever is first, repeat q1y to q2y until age 40). Lynch syndrome diagnosis has to rule out familial adenomatous polyposis (FAP). **FAP colonoscopy starts at 10–12 yo**.
43. Persistent cough can be from GERD; other atypical symptoms of GERD include asthma, globus sensation, hoarseness, throat clearing, and chronic laryngitis. Diagnosis: ambulatory pH testing (laryngopharynx more sensitive to acid).
44. In hepatorenal or end-stage cirrhosis, **ACEi, ARB, and NSAIDs** should be stopped as they decrease renal perfusion.
45. Acute liver failure is defined by **hepatic encephalopathy within 26 weeks of liver injury with INR ≥1.5 but no cirrhosis or preexisting liver disease**. Treatment: supportive care and may require liver transplantation.
46. **Combined mesalamine (oral and topical enema)** is the treatment for mild to moderate active ulcerative colitis.

47. Young patients with **age <60** present with dyspepsia should receive **H. pylori testing** first.
48. Treatment for **amebic liver abscess**: metronidazole plus a luminal agent like paromomycin.
49. **Wilson disease** should be considered if the patient's age is ≤40 years old with unexplained liver disease. Children ≤10 yo with Wilson disease tend to present with acute liver failure; older ≥30 yo presents with **chronic liver disease and/or neurological symptoms**.
50. **Achalasia** treatment: endoscopic pneumatic dilation, or botulinum toxin injection if not a surgical candidate.
51. The mainstay therapy for **intrahepatic cholestasis of pregnancy** is **ursodeoxycholic acid**.
52. **Drug-associated enteropathy** (**olmesartan**) can mimic refractory **celiac disease** (**villous atrophy and increased intraepithelial lymphocytes** in the first part of the duodenum).
53. **Barret esophagus**: no dysplasia- endoscopic surveillance <q3-5y; indefinite dysplasia- repeat endoscopy in 1 year; low- and high-grade dysplasia- treatment with **endoscopic ablation**.
54. **Colonoscopy** at age 40 indications: (1) First degree relative with colon cancer; (2) Advanced adenoma diagnosis <60; (3) Two or more relatives with colon cancer or advanced adenoma diagnosed at any age. Colorectal cancer screening with colonoscopy is recommended starting at age 45 through age 75 for average risk people.
55. **Milan criteria for liver transplantation**: up to three hepatocellular cancer tumors ≤3 cm or one tumor <5 cm, no macrovascular invasion, and no metastasis.
56. **Liver cancer diagnosis**: lesion >1 cm with contrast enhancement in arterial phase and portal venous washout. **Portal hypertension** is a contraindication for surgical resection.
57. **Gastrointestinal (GI) bleeding** after aortic graft surgery should raise the possibility of **aortoenteric fistula**. Symptoms of **herald bleed**: a **brisk bleed** associated with hypotension that stops spontaneously and then is followed later by massive GI hemorrhage. Other causes of **aortoenteric fistula** include aneurysm (most common), foreign body, tumor, radiation therapy, and infection.
58. Fresh blood seen in colonoscopy **(≥0.5 mL/min) ⇒ consider CT angiography GI bleeding protocol**, if the source of bleeding is identified, call an interventional radiologist for embolization.
59. **Mesenteric angiogram** detects bleeding **1 mL/min** as compared to tagged RBC scintigraphy at **0.1–0.5 mL/min**. Slow bleed, do RBC tag study. CTA (CT angiogram GI bleeding protocol) detects bleeding as low as **0.3–0.5 mL/min**.
60. **Push enteroscopy** can be used to diagnose small bowel bleeding. Upper and lower scope negative → push enteroscopy → RBC scan.

61. **Loose stool with hematochezia:** consider ischemic colitis if **hypotensive** episodes; **Treatment**: supportive care; this can also be ileus in sick patients if no hematochezia. Out of proportion central abdominal pain in an 80 yo with coronary artery disease: consider **acute mesenteric ischemia from embolism**.
62. **Indications for TNF inhibitors** infliximab (Remicade), adalimumab (Humira), or certolizumab (Cimzia) in Crohn's disease: moderate to severe ileal Crohn's disease after multiple rounds of tapering prednisone for flares of disease despite treatment with the immunomodulator of azathioprine. If no response or intolerance to TNF alpha inhibitors, treatment with a leukocyte trafficking blocker with natalizumab (Tysabri) or vedolizumab (Entyvio) can be considered. Use budesonide for mild Crohn's disease.
63. Treatments with anti-TNF agents like infliximab, adalimumab, and certolizumab are effective for **induction and maintenance of remission** in Crohn's disease.
64. **FAP: upper endoscopy** should begin at the onset of colonic polyps or **age 20–25 (whichever comes first, repeat q1-3y)**; annual colonoscopy starts at **age 10–11**.
65. **Pathogenic germline CDH1 gene** testing indications: ≥two family members with gastric cancer (including one confirmed diffuse gastric cancer), a diffuse gastric cancer diagnosis in the family before age 40, or having both diffuse gastric cancer and lobular breast cancer in a family (with one diagnosed before age 50). **If a CDH1 gene mutation is identified, prophylactic total gastrectomy at the ages of 20–30 is recommended**.
66. **Functional dyspepsia** diagnostic criteria: bothersome postprandial fullness, early satiety, epigastric pain, and/or epigastric burning for at least 3 days per week. Symptoms started 6 months ago with criteria met for 3 months. Treatment: TCA, SSRI, SNRI.
67. **Cryoglobulinemia** has **Meltzer** triad- palpable **purpura**, **arthralgia**, and **weakness**.
68. In **hepatic adenoma** ≥5 cm in size, need to discontinue estrogen-containing oral contraceptive pill (OCP) → followed by liver imaging q6m for ≥2 years.
69. **CT enterography** combines neutral (low-density) oral contrast with "enteric phase" CT to optimize contrast resolution between mucosa and lumen in the small intestines; it is used in patients with a history of **small bowel obstruction where a lesion or mass is suspected**.
70. **Asymptomatic walled-off pancreatic necrosis** does not need treatment.
71. All patients with **cirrhosis** from any cause should undergo **liver ultrasound q6m with or without alpha-FP**.
72. **High-risk ulcers** are characterized by active arterial spurting or a non-bleeding visible vessel and should be treated endoscopically with **hemostatic clips, thermotherapy, or injection of sclerostats**.
73. **Hepatorenal syndrome** treatment: stop diuretics and lactulose, and give albumin at 1 g/kg/day in divided doses for 2 days. If no response, give Levophed + albumin or midodrine, octreotide, and albumin.

74. **Symptomatic acute pancreatic fluid** collection can be medically treated with bowel rest, jejunal feeding, pancreatic enzymes, octreotide, and rarely pancreatic stenting. Rarely, pancreatic fluid collection persists beyond 4 weeks to become pseudocyst. **If persistent pain despite medical therapy, infected pseudocyst, or obstruction of gastric outlet or biliary tract, surgical debridement and drainage** is indicated.
75. **Sporadic gastric fundic gland polyps** (1–5 mm in size, <10 in number) are associated with PPI use, need reassurance, and no need for treatment.
76. **Chronic mesenteric ischemia**, diagnosis: CT angiography, if equivocal, do splanchnic angiography.
77. Patients with IBS-D should undergo screening for **celiac disease** with serum tissue transglutaminase antibody testing.
78. **Non-occlusive mesenteric ischemia** (hypoperfusion, vasopressors) vs. **ischemic colitis** (**rectal bleeding** and left colon inflammatory changes on CT).
79. **Gallstone pancreatitis** requires laparoscopic cholecystectomy before discharge.
80. Large (>2 cm) adenomas or adenomas with invasive cancer and favorable prognostic features treatment: post polypectomy surveillance colonoscopy in **3–6 months**.
81. **MYH-associated polyposis** is an autosomal recessive disorder: >10 adenomatous colon polyps during a lifetime with increased risks for colorectal cancer.
82. Recent history of cholelithiasis, cholecystectomy, and dilated intrahepatic and extrahepatic bile ducts = consider **choledocholithiasis**. Up to 20% of cholelithiasis patients have choledocholithiasis; 50% of them are symptomatic.
83. **N-acetylcysteine** may improve transplant-free survival in non-acetaminophen-related active liver failure in patients with **Grade I or II hepatic encephalopathy**.
84. **Food stuck** in throat ⇒ consider solid food dysphagia requiring endoscopy for removal.
85. **Acute HBV infection without marked liver dysfunction** (but no increase in INR or hepatic encephalopathy) will resolve in 90% of patients; no need to treat it.
86. **Chronic pancreatitis** treatment: Tylenol → ibuprofen → and/or tramadol → pregabalin or TCA → pancreaticoduodenectomy.
87. **Ulcerative colitis** mild to moderate should be treated with 5-aminosalicylate agents (mesalamine, sulfasalazine, and olsalazine). If **left-sided colitis or proctitis**, give topical therapy with 5-ASA or hydrocortisone suppositories or enemas. If the patient requires repeated glucocorticoids, **start thiopurines** (6-mercaptopurine or azathioprine) or **anti-TNF agents** (no methotrexate).
88. If H. pylori is not eradicated with primary therapy, second line salvage therapy should contain an alternative antibiotic to clarithromycin for at least 10 days: Second line therapies (**bismuth + flagyl + tetracycline + PPI**) or **10-day Levaquin + amoxicillin + PPI**.

89. **Repeat colonoscopy in 3 years** is recommended for (1) adenoma ≥1 cm; (2) ≥3–10 adneomas; (3) tubulovillous or villous adenomas; (4) adenoma with high-grade dysplasia.
90. **Gastric NET** → observe even if hypergastrinemia. **Nutcracker esophagitis** is a hypertonic motility disorder: high amplitude peristaltic contractions **≥220 mmHg**. **Diffuse esophageal spasm (DES)** manometry amplitude contractions of **≥30 mmHg**.
91. **Sporadic nonsyndromic juvenile polyp** (reassurance, no treatment needed) vs. **juvenile polyposis syndrome (JPS)**. JPS diagnosis: (1) ≥3 polyps of colon; (2) Juvenile polyp throughout GI tract; (3) One or more juvenile polyps with a family history of JPS. **Surveillance for JPS**: colonoscopy and EGD q2-3y from age 15 or sooner if symptoms.
92. **Dysphagia**: **oropharyngeal dysphagia—**do videofluoroscopy, treatment-dietary adjustment with food consistencies and incorporation of swallowing exercises. **Esophageal dysphagia** diagnosis via barium swallow, EGD, manometry.
93. **Glucocorticoids** are not effective for maintaining remission in ulcerative colitis. Should be tapered and transitioned to **azathioprine (check TPMP level test first)**, **mercaptopurine** (6MP, check TPMP level test first), or infliximab. TPMP = thiopurine methyltransferase.
94. **Endoscopic ultrasound** is sensitive for detecting insulinomas which are small and solitary and may not be detected by CT scan.
95. **Cardiac causes of ascites** have ascitic fluid protein ≥2.5, whereas in cirrhosis and portal hypertension ascitic fluid protein <2.5. SAAG is <1.1 g/dL in nephrotic syndrome and pancreatic ascites. SAAG >1.1 g/L, if total protein >2.5, it is TB, peritoneal carcinomatosis, pancreatitis; if total protein <2.5, it is nephrotic syndrome. SAAG <1.1 g/L, if total protein >2.5, it's right heart failure and hepatic vein thrombosis; if total protein <2.5, it's cirrhosis.
96. **Maximal doses of Lasix and spironolactone in cirrhosis**: 160 and 400 mg.
97. **Alcoholic hepatitis**: AST/ALT ≥2, usually both <300, increased GGT, bilirubin, and/or INR, leukocytosis with neutrophils.
98. **Cholecystitis** can present with fever, RUQ pain, N&V, and anorexia; however, **jaundice only happens in cholangitis.**
99. **Boerhaave syndrome** also known as esophageal rupture: forceful vomiting followed by chest pain and respiratory distress, subcutaneous emphysema, rapid development of left pleural effusion in hours, and retrocardiac air shadow. **Diagnosis** requires a contrast esophagram.
100. **Epigastric** pain radiating to the back and hematemesis after extended nausea and vomiting ⇒ consider EGD, need to rule out **Mallory-Weiss tear**; most Mallory Weiss tear patients have self-limiting symptoms (24–48 h) of bleeding with spontaneous healing of ulcers.
101. **Smooth tight stricture** in the upper esophagus: consider trauma, mechanical, chemical erosion.

102. **Small intestine bacterial overgrowth** is common in gastroparesis, celiac disease, diabetes, and scleroderma on top of gastric bypasses and gastrectomy surgeries.
103. **Further evaluation is needed for hemorrhoids** in: (1) Anal fissure with atypical features; (2) Rectal bleeding (sigmoidoscopy if age <50 and colonoscopy if age ≥50); (3) Failure to respond after 8 weeks of optimal medical treatment including topical vasodilators (i.e., nitroglycerin, nifedipine), stool softeners, and advice to supplement fiber intake.
104. Treatment for **acute colonic pseudo-obstruction (Ogilvie syndrome)**: serial abdomen examination, NPO, NG tube and rectal tube decompression, neostigmine if no improvement within 48 h; **colonoscopic decompression** can be considered and so does erythromycin iv.
105. GI bleed: EGD biopsy negative for H. pylori can be **falsely negative due to PPI or bleeding**, next step is outpatient urea breath testing or stool Ag after **stopping PPI for 1–2 weeks**.
106. **Caustic or corrosive substance ingestion**: serial chest and abdominal x-ray to rule out perforation. If no perforation, perform an early endoscopy within 24 h in stable patients to assess the severity of esophageal involvement. If perforation, mediastinitis, or severe strictures, consider **esophagectomy**. In **alkali ingestion**, the patient should be screened for **esophageal cancer up to 15–20 years after ingestion**.
107. **Abnormal ALT/AST**: (1) Rule out common liver disease (i.e., drug-induced, ETOH, HBV, HCV, fatty liver disease if AST/ALT <1 → RUQ U/S, hemochromatosis); (2) Nonhepatic (i.e., muscle, thyroid, celiac disease, adrenal) causes; (3) Less common etiology (autoimmune, Wilson disease, check alpha-1 antitrypsin deficiency) → biopsy if persistent elevation.
108. **ALP elevation** → rule out physiologic causes (e.g., pregnancy and postprandial) → if GGT is normal, it is the **bone origin**. If GGT is high, it is from likely **biliary origin** → U/S **dilated bile duct** → MRCP and ERCP. If GGT is high, also check RUQ U/S and **AMA** → if any one is abnormal → **biopsy**; if both are normal, ≥50% increase → **liver biopsy**, ERCP and MRCP; <50% increase → follow up and observation.
109. **Chronic pancreatitis** can lead to splenic vein thrombosis. **Gastric varices** localized to the gastric fundus essentially provide the diagnosis of **splenic vein thrombosis**. Bleeding in such cases can be cured by splenectomy or splenic artery embolization.
110. **Constipation**: First line **bulk-forming** agents with methylcellulose and psyllium → MiraLAX (osmotic **laxative**), Senna or bisacodyl (**laxative**) → milk magnesium and bisacodyl suppository.
111. **Budd-Chiari syndrome** is thrombosis of the hepatic/intrahepatic veins or suprahepatic IVC, commonly seen in 30–40 yo, idiopathic or due to hepatocellular carcinoma, myeloproliferative disease, OCP, pregnancy, or hypercoagulable state. Acute symptoms in patients (20%) include severe RUQ pain, hepatosplenomegaly, jaundice, ascites, and variceal bleeding. **Treatment**:

diuretics, anticoagulation, possible angioplasty with stenting, and possible thrombolytics.

112. **Typhlitis** = neutropenic enterocolitis, neutrophil <500, a life-threatening condition in hematologic malignancies (e.g., leukemia). Typically presents 10–14 days after chemo with fever, RLQ pain, nausea, watery or bloody. Uncomplicated typhlitis, no perforation, peritonitis, or severe GI bleed; treatment is with cefepime or ceftazidime plus Flagyl, bowel rest, supportive care, **empiric C. diff coverage unless negative**; **antifungal coverage is added if fever persists longer than 72 h**.
113. **Secondary lactose intolerance** develops after acute infection or inflammation. Hiatal hernias, GERD, and Barrett's esophagus are associated with the development of the Schatzki ring.
114. Pruritus, fatigue, hepatomegaly, cholestatic pattern = consider **primary biliary cholangitis**. Treatment: **ursodeoxycholic acid** (delays progression), liver transplantation for advanced disease.
115. Common deficiencies in **celiac disease**: iron, calcium, Vit D, folic acid, and rarely thiamine. Obtain **DEXA scan at diagnosis and repeat DEXA** if osteopenia presents 1 year later. Give **pneumococcal vaccine**. Treatment with **dapsone** in addition to **gluten-free diet** for **dermatitis herpetiformis**.
116. **Crampy and periumbilical pain with vomiting** = consider proximal small bowel obstruction (SBO). **Obstipation** = complete bowel obstruction happens 24–12 h after obstruction. Diagnosis of SBO is via chest X-ray upright and supine KUB → if inconclusive, CT with oral or IV contrast. If the change from crampy into persistent pain together with fever, lactic acidosis, and worsening leukocytosis, severe obstruction leading to **strangulation with necrosis** should be suspected. **Water-soluble gastrografin** can be used for therapy. The presence of **contrast in the colon 4–24 h after the test** indicates SBO resolution.
117. Common **non-pancreatic causes of lipase elevation** include renal insufficiency, diabetic ketoacidosis, intestinal obstruction, and ileus.
118. Acute versus chronic **mesenteric ischemia**, diagnosis: CT, MRA, duplex ultrasound, or angiography.
119. **Achalasia** is associated with squamous cell carcinoma of the esophagus. **Atrophic gastritis** is associated with intestinal type gastric cancer and type I gastric carcinoid.
120. African American with abdominal pain after traveling, radiating to left shoulder = consider **splenic infarct from HbSc**. 2 months of bloody diarrhea → colonoscopy revealed superficial ulceration from the rectum (diagnosis of **ulcerative colitis**) → prednisone + 5 ASA.
121. Indications for treatment for **autoimmune hepatitis**: if transaminase >10× upper limit normal, greater than 5× upper limit normal with hyperglobulinemia, necrosis on liver biopsy, or incapacitating symptoms.
122. **Indicators for prophylaxis against stress ulcers in ICU**: coagulopathy (platelet <50,000, INR >1.5, or PTT >2 times control), mechanical ventilation

≥48 h, prolonged ICU stay (≥1 week), traumatic brain injury (TBI) or traumatic spinal injury, thermal injury, Hx of GI bleed, or high dose steroid use.

123. **Colonoscopy with biopsy** for inflammatory bowel disease (IBD), **duodenal aspiration** for small intestine bacterial overgrowth (SIBO).
124. **Dyspepsia** without the use of NSAIDs and **<60 yo** without GERD symptoms should get H. pylori testing. H. pylori gastric ulcer needs a **biopsy to rule out malignancy** if high-risk factors.
125. **Ulcers with high-risk features for rebleeding**: e.g., active bleeding, adherent clot, visible vessel. They typically require endoscopic treatment. Most rebleeding happens in **the first 72 h, may need keep a clear liquid diet for 2 days**.
126. **Common complications of Roux-en-Y bypass**: (1) stomal stenosis (anastomotic stricture at the gastrojejunal anastomosis); (2) cholelithiasis; (3) dumping syndrome.
127. **Angiodysplasia** (AV malformation): commonly seen in >60 yo and can occur in one or multiple areas of the GI tract. It's related to **aortic stenosis or ESRD**.
128. **Air-filled sigmoid colon** with the absence of air in the rectum = consider sigmoid (or cecum) **volvulus**. Risk factors for sigmoid volvulus: old age, institutionalized, neurologic or psychiatric conditions like Parkinson's disease and schizophrenia. **Treatment**: sigmoidoscopy. If the diagnosis is uncertain, do **water-soluble contrast**. If perforation, stat surgery.
129. **Diagnostic paracentesis** should be performed even in the absence of signs of infection, as patients with end-stage liver disease (ESLD) may not be able to mount a typical inflammatory response.
130. **Gingival hyperplasia** is seen in phenytoin, cyclosporine, and calcium channel blockers (CCBs).
131. **Active HBV** may be associated with **serum sickness syndrome** (immune-complex-mediated hypersensitivity reaction): fever, symptomatic polyarthritis, urticarial, and skin rash without mucosal involvement.
132. Unconjugated hyperbilirubinemia → **Gilbert** syndrome (reduced glucuronidation of bilirubin) or **Crigler-Najjar** syndrome (marked unconjugated hyperbilirubinemia). no workup is necessary for Gilbert syndrome if mild unconjugated hyperbilirubinemia.
133. **Gastroparesis** workup: first EGD, then schedule scintigraphic gastric emptying study.
134. **NAFLD** is a diagnosis of exclusion and requires the exclusion of hepatitis B and C.
135. **Low low-carb diet** is associated with an increased incidence of GI upset.
136. **Endoscopy** shows multiple stomach ulcers and thickened gastric folds ⇒ consider checking gastrin level → if >1000 → check gastric pH off PPI for 1 week, if >4, no gastrinoma.
137. Ulcerative colitis flare: empiric antibiotics are only indicated if **severe systemic toxicity** (high fevers, marked leukocytosis with left shift, and/or bandemia), toxic megacolon or peritonitis.

138. **Ileal resection due** to Crohn's disease leads to **B12 deficiency**, bile acid malabsorption and secretory diarrhea. Treatment: **cholestyramin**e (binds bile acids) and vitamin supplements.
139. **Small non-bleeding varices** do not need beta blocker but EGD; medium and large varices and small varices with red halo sign or decompensated liver failure or cirrhosis (jaundice, ascites, variceal bleed, hepatic encephalopathy, hepatorenal syndrome) need beta blocker for variceal bleeding prophylaxis.
140. **Beta-blockers should be discontinued** in refractory ascites, hypotension, serum sodium level <120, hepatorenal syndrome, spontaneous bacterial peritonitis, sepsis, or severe alcoholic hepatitis.
141. **Irritable bowel syndrome** diagnosis is based on defecation and stool symptoms in the previous 3 months, and routine CBC, chemistry studies, TSH, and stool studies for ova and parasites are unnecessary.
142. **Red flags** such as rectal bleeding with iron deficiency anemia, abdominal pain, and weight loss should get colonoscopy, regardless of the presence or not of hemorrhoids, to rule out cancer.

Chapter 27
Infectious Disease

1. Patients undergoing cardiothoracic surgery or orthopedic surgery should be screened for **Staph aureus carrier status in nares**. If positive, should have **preparative decolonization** (mupirocin with or without body wash with chlorhexidine gluconate for 5 days). Both mupirocin and chlorhexidine are effective for decolonization of Staph aureus including methicillin-resistant Staphylococcus aureus (MRSA).
2. **Rifabutin is preferred over rifampin** in patients with HIV due to fewer drug-to-drug interactions. **Prednisone** can be added if immune reconstitution inflammatory syndrome (IRIS) is life-threatening (cardiac, lung, central nervous system symptoms) or involves the precordium or CNS.
3. **Immune reconstitution inflammatory syndrome (IRIS)** may happen 1 month after starting antiretroviral therapy by disseminated **Mycobacterium avium complex (MAC)**; symptoms include fever, chills, fatigue, and weight loss.
4. **Strep throat testing** first then antibiotics even if **4/4 Centor criteria are met**.
5. **Aspergillus** invades blood vessels and causes distal infarction; presents with fever, cough, chest pain, hemoptysis, pulmonary infiltrates, cavitary lung lesions, nodules, and wedge-shaped densities. The most efficient way of diagnosis is **bronchoalveolar lavage (BAL) and biopsy**. Serum aspergillus galactomannan test has a **sensitivity of less than 30%**; blood fungal culture has a sensitivity of less than **1% in invasive aspergillosis**; Beta-D-Glucan (Fungitell) test is sensitive but not specific.
6. **Allergic bronchopulmonary aspergillosis (ABPA)** treatment is corticosteroids and itraconazole (newer agents are voriconazole or posaconazole). **Simple aspergilloma** requires surgical resection or embolization. **Chronic cavitary pulmonary aspergilloma** should be treated with **itraconazole** or **voriconazole**. Chronic necrotizing pneumonia and invasive aspergilloma treatment: **voriconazole**.

K. Zhou, *Internal Medicine Training Notes and Survival Guide*,
https://doi.org/10.1007/978-1-0716-4039-5_27

7. **Leptospirosis** presents with **biphasic illness**: phase I—**flu-like illness**; Phase II—**leptospiral meningitis**, usually develops weeks after exposure—uveitis, rash, conjunctival suffusion, sepsis, lymphadenopathy, kidney injury, and hepatosplenomegaly.
8. **Leptospirosis**: conjunctival suffusion and jaundice. Treatment is penicillin and doxycycline.
9. Knee swelling in Lyme ELISA (sensitive screening test) positive patients; **ELISA test should be confirmed with Western blot (specific confirmatory test)**. IgM is only useful within 4 weeks of symptom onset (beyond 4 weeks, it may be false positive) while IgG is usually present 4–6 weeks after exposure.
10. Lyme disease diagnosis: ELISA → western blot. <4 weeks of symptoms, **IgM 2/3 bands** is diagnostic; ≥4 weeks of symptoms, **IgG 5/10 bands** is diagnostic.
11. **Lyme disease arthritis** is excluded if symptoms have been present for longer than 1 month but IgG negative even IgM positive.
12. Early localized Lyme disease treatment: **doxycycline 10–21 days**; post-Lyme disease syndrome is a poorly understood sequela of Lyme disease from a disordered immunologic response. **CNS Lyme disease** and **Lyme carditis** should be treated with **ceftriaxone**.
13. **Facial palsy or central nervous system infection from Lyme disease** may need lumbar puncture to diagnose neuroborreliosis. Treatment is IV ceftriaxone, cefotaxime, or penicillin.
14. **M. kansasii** causes lung infection mimicking tuberculosis, with cough, fever, weight loss, and cavitary lung disease.
15. **Pelvic inflammatory disease (PID)** symptoms: women with sexually transmitted infection risk presenting with otherwise unexplained pelvic pain, cervical motion and adnexal tenderness, and cervical discharge. Etiologies: N. gonorrhoeae, C. trachomatis, or Mycoplasma genitalium infection. Treatment: **im ceftriaxone 250 mg once + doxycycline 100 mg po bid for 14 days**.
16. **Urethritis from N. gonorrhoeae and chlamydia** treatment: 250 mg ceftriaxone im + 1 g azithromycin po once.
17. **Post-exposure prophylaxis (PEP) for HIV**: tenofovir, emtricitabine, and dolutegravir or raltegravir for 4 weeks; PEP must be started as soon as possible and within 72 h after exposure. The exposed patient should be tested for HIV **immediately, at 4–6 weeks, 12 weeks, and 6 months post exposure** using a fourth-generation assay for HIV testing.
18. **Protease inhibitors** such as darunavir are not recommended for PEP due to higher rates of side effects.
19. **HIV diagnosis**: HIV combination immunoassay for HIV1 and HIV2 ⇒ differentiation immunoassay or if negative, it may indicate window period ⇒ HIV RNA.
20. Tenofovir, emtricitabine, efavirenz are ok for use in pregnancy, so do zidovudine, lamivudine and ritonavir-boosted lopinavir.

21. **Zika mainly causes birth defects**, active symptoms include fever, red eyes, joint pain, headache, and maculopapular rash. Condoms should be used for **≥3 months if the husband has Zika.**
22. **Ramsay Hunt syndrome (herpes zoster oticus)** = facial paralysis and hearing loss in the affected ear from varicella-zoster virus (VZV) infection. **HSV-1** causes **Bell's palsy** and herpes encephalitis; **HSV-2** is more commonly associated with **genital ulcers**, recurrent aseptic meningitis (recurrent benign lymphocytic meningitis) and myelitis. **Treatment for Ramsay Hunt syndrome and Bell's palsy**: valacyclovir (1 g 3 times per day for 7–10 days) and prednisone (1 mg/kg for 5 days). **HSV causes meningitis all year long**.
23. **Painful genital lesions** on the penis with myalgia and malaise: check nucleic acid amplification test (NAAT) for HSV-1 (oral herpes) and HSV-2 (genital herpes).
24. **Q fever** (Coxiella burnetii) causes subclinical to severe pneumonia and occurs after inhalation of aerosolized bodily fluids from infected animals. Treatment: **doxycycline**.
25. **Yersinia pestis** causes pneumonic plague mostly in rural areas in the western United States and parts of Africa and Asia: high fever, pleuritic chest pain, productive cough, and hemoptysis. First line treatment for pneumonic plague (from Y. pestis) is either **streptomycin or gentamicin**.
26. A group of young adults from Nevada presented with fever, cough, blood-tinged sputum = consider **pneumonic plague**. Treatment is **streptomycin or gentamycin**.
27. **Pneumonic tularemia** is part of **tick-borne disease** related to farming or landscaping activities: nonproductive cough, dyspnea, and substernal or pleuritic chest pain. Treatment is streptomycin, gentamicin, doxycycline, or ciprofloxacin for 10–21 days.
28. **Coagulase-negative staphylococcus central line-associated bloodstream infections** (CLABSIs) often resolve with the removal of the catheter—blood culture should be repeated after catheter removal to document clearance of the organism. Alternatively, patients with coagulase-negative staph CLABSIs can be treated with **antibiotics for 5–7 days after catheter removal and 10–14 days in combination with antibiotic lock therapy if the catheter is not removed**.
29. Staph aureus requires intravenous antibiotic treatment for **4–6 weeks** after central line removal.
30. **Tick-borne diseases**: Lyme disease, babesiosis, ehrlichiosis, Rocky Mountain Spotted Fever, anaplasmosis, Powassan, Tick-Borne Relapsing Fever, and tularemia.
31. **Human monocytic ehrlichiosis** is characterized by non-focal febrile illness associated with **decreased WBC, decreased PLT, and increased LFTs**. Antibody testing has a low sensitivity in the first week and usually responds to **tetracycline**.

32. **Ehrlichia infection (ehrlichiosis)** can have leukopenia and elevated liver function tests, erythematous skin rash with central clearing. **Treatment**: doxycycline.
33. **RMSF** causes petechial rash. **RMSF** acute phase can have a negative antibody test. **Testing convalescent serum 14 days** after symptom resolution allows for retrospective confirmation of RMSF.
34. **G-, coccobacilli, bipolar staining**: Pasteurella, Yersinia, and Francisella.
35. 86-year-old female with fever, leukocytosis, retroperitoneal and inguinal lymphadenopathy who turned out to be **EBV positive**. Workups include RPR, EBV virus serology, CMV serology, toxoplasma serology, Lyme serology, QuantiFERON, Histoplasma, Blastomyces, and cryptococcus. She also has a positive Fungitell study.
36. **Blastomycosis** (mainly skin, can also affect lung and other organs) treatment: **itraconazole for 6 months**. If severe pulmonary blastomycosis, treatment is **amphotericin B**.
37. **Disseminated histoplasmosis**: oral ulceration, hepatosplenomegaly, pancytopenia. **Diagnosis**: urine Blastomycosis Ag (95% specificity), blood culture, or biopsy of lesions. **Treatment**: liposomal amphotericin B → de-escalate to itraconazole for several months.
38. **Blastomycosis**: cutaneous, bone, sinus tract, genitourinary lesions, and central nervous system lesions (rare). **Histoplasmosis** causes pancytopenia, lymphadenopathy, and hepatosplenomegaly. **Coccidioidomycosis** causes skin, lymphadenopathy, meningitis, and osteoarticular lesions.
39. **Buccal mucosa and tongue ulcer**: if positive for Histoplasmosis, it is disseminated histoplasmosis. The treatment is liposomal amphotericin B.
40. **Behcet syndrome**: Low-dose prednisone or colchicine is used for oral and genital ulcers; high-dose prednisone and immunomodulating agents are used for more severe cases.
41. **P. falciparum** is seen in Africa; **P. knowlesi** is seen in south and southeast Asia.
42. **Malaria prophylaxis**: (1) sub-Saharan Africa, southern and southeastern Asia (atovaquone, proguanil, doxycycline, mefloquine); (2) areas with chloroquine susceptible P. falciparum (**chloroquine**, hydroxychloroquine); (3) areas without P. falciparum like parts of South America, Mexico, and Korea (**primaquine**).
43. **Typhoid fever**: pulse-temperature dissociation with bradycardia, diarrhea followed by constipation, abdominal discomfort, non-productive cough, mild confusion, and rose spots. **Treatment**: ceftriaxone with azithromycin in combination or Cipro as an alternative.
44. **Brucellosis**: recurring or undulating waves of fever.
45. **Enterovirus** is the most common virus causing **viral meningitis**, usually present between May and November.
46. In patients with known exposure to **anthrax**. **Post-exposure prophylaxis (PEP)** for 60 days with Cipro (pregnant safe), levofloxacin, or doxy.

Additionally, **3 subcu injections of anthrax vaccine should be given 2 weeks apart for PEP**.

47. **Postexposure prophylaxis of HAV**: all persons aged ≥12 months and infants aged 6–11 months traveling overseas; **immunoglobulin** may be given to patients **aged >40 years**.
48. **N. meningitidis prophylaxis indications**: close contact 3–6 feet over ≥8 h, or exposed to respiratory or oral secretions. Prophylaxis should be started within 24 h with Cipro 500 mg once or rifampin 4 doses in 2 days.
49. **Contact with chickenpox**: IV **zoster IgG** in immunocompromised patients within 4 days after exposure or **varicella vaccine** within 3–5 days after exposure.
50. **Vaccination** in 72 h or no more than 7 days after variola (smallpox, airborne precautions) exposure, but is **contraindicated** if CD4 ≤ 50 or severe combined immunodeficiency.
51. M sex with M, prophylaxis for HIV: daily tenofovir and emtricitabine for PREP.
52. **Syphilis diagnosis**: **screening** test (RPR and VDRL) and **confirmatory** tests (FTA, TPPA, EIA). Enzyme immunoassay (EIA)+, rapid plasma reagin (RPR), or venereal disease research laboratory test (VDRL) (non-treponemal test, also known as a screening test); if negative, should be followed by a secondary treponemal test like fluorescent treponemal Ab (FTA) test or Treponema pallidum particle agglutination assay (TPPA).
53. The **fluorescent treponemal antibody absorption (FTA-ABS)** test is always positive after infection; while **rapid plasma reagin (RPR)** should decrease with treatment.
54. What if the EIA (enzyme immunoassay) is positive (detects antibody), the RPR (or VDRL) is negative and the TPPA is positive? Explanations: the patient has a history of treated syphilis; the patient has late latent syphilis (should be treated with Benzathine Penicillin G 2.4 mu IM weekly × 3); the patient was recently exposed to syphilis and the RPR has not yet turned positive. If both screening and confirmatory tests are positive, it may indicate **current or past syphilis infection**.
55. Syphilis treatment: unknown duration—**3 weekly doses im benzathine penicillin**, single dose benzathine penicillin for primary and secondary and early latent syphilis.
56. **Cyclospora** is a cause of traveler's (water-borne and food-borne) diarrhea; it has an incubation period of 1 week, symptoms: crampy abdominal pain, anorexia, bloating, decreased appetite, fatigue, flatulence, diarrhea, and weight loss. Treatment: **DS Bactrim** for 7–10 days.
57. **Atovaquone** for PCP, toxoplasmosis, plasmodium, babesia. **Pyrimethamine** for toxoplasma, PCP, Isospora belli (now known as Cystoisospora belli).
58. **Daptomycin** needs weekly **CPK and creatinine** monitoring. **Nafcillin** requires weekly CBC, **Cr, and LFTs** monitoring.
59. **Rifampin** should be used in combination with another anti-staphylococcal agent when managing **staph osteomyelitis** in the setting of **orthopedic hardware** if the hardware cannot be removed.

60. **Fosfomycin** is used to treat UTI by VRE, MRSA, and resistant Klebsiella. **Minocycline** for multidrug-resistant **Actinobacteria** and **Stenotrophomonas** maltophilia infections.
61. **Chronic prostatitis** treatment: **fluoroquinolones** (FQ) or **Bactrim** for 4–6 weeks; Diagnosis: chronic recurrent UTI with repeated isolation of the same bug from urine. **Acute prostatitis**: acutely ill, with spiking fever, chills, malaise, myalgia, dysuria, irritative urinary symptoms (frequency, urgency, urge incontinence), pelvic or perineal pain, and cloudy urine. Treatment for acute prostatitis: **FQ or Bactrim for 4 weeks**.
62. **Febrile UTI in male** treatment: cefepime + kidney ultrasound or CT with contrast (if kidney function appropriate for contrast) to rule out **hydronephrosis** and other **pathologies**.
63. **Urinary tract symptoms** after urological procedure treatment, if concerns for prostatitis, treatment: Bactrim or Cipro for 6 weeks.
64. **Prostatitis** is divided into **acute bacterial prostatitis, chronic bacterial prostatitis, chronic prostatitis/chronic pelvic pain syndrome, and asymptomatic inflammatory prostatitis**. Acute bacterial prostatitis is characterized by fever, chills, and perineal or low back pain. Diagnosis: **prostate massage** is contraindicated in acute bacterial prostatitis with fever, and CT pelvis and transrectal ultrasound may help rule out prostate abscess.
65. If **sepsis with osteomyelitis**, empiric antibiotics like vancomycin and cefepime should be started even without a biopsy.
66. **Haematopoietic stem cell transplantation** prevention and prophylaxis strategy (HSCT ppx): (1) **posaconazole** 200 mg tid (or fluconazole, voriconazole), continue for months even with recovery of neutrophils; (2) **acyclovir** for 30 days to 1 year; (3) **Bactrim** for 6 months; (4) **Cipro** only if neutropenia and continue until recovery of normal white counts. **Valganciclovir can cause leukopenia**, caution its use.
67. Empiric treatment of **tuberculosis meningitis** consists of **RIPE** (rifampicin (also known as Rifampin), isoniazid, pyrazinamide, and ethambutol) **plus dexamethasone**.
68. **CSF** assay is highly sensitive and specific for **cryptococcal meningitis** which has an opening CSF pressure >**200** (normal opening pressure between 18 and 20 cm CSF). **Chronic meningitis** typically includes TB and Cryptococcus.
69. 9 months of INH = once weekly isoniazid + rifapentine for 12 weeks (directly observed therapy)
70. **Polyoma BK virus causes nephropathy** not diarrhea, diagnosis via BK virus DNA in the **urine** preceding **viremia** by a median of 4 weeks after transplantation.
71. **Cytoplasmic morulae** in leukocytes = consider **ehrlichiosis** and **tick-borne diseases**. **Ring-shaped** parasitic inclusion in RBC = consider **malaria** and **babesiosis**. **Banana-shaped** gametocytes = consider P. **falciparum**. **Intraerythrocytic** tetrad forms = consider **babesiosis**.
72. **Bacteroides fragilis** is obligately anaerobic G- rod.

73. **Candidemia**: (1) Remove IV lines; (2) Start antifungal echinocandin (anidulafungin, caspofungin, micafungin). If the candida species is azole susceptible, can de-escalate to fluconazole to complete the **14-day therapy**. C. glabrata, C. auris, and C. krusei are resistant to azoles.
74. Meningococcal **ACWY** vaccine (quadrivalent) does not cover **serogroup B N. meningococcus**.
75. **Proctitis with concerns of sexually transmitted** infection treatment: **ceftriaxone and doxycycline**.
76. **CMV** causes pneumonitis, colitis, esophagitis, and hepatitis.
77. **Cellulitis**: nonpurulent without systemic signs treatment: clindamycin, penicillins, cephalexin, or dicloxacillin after I & D for abscess if any. Bactrim or doxycycline would be appropriate as well. **Inpatient nonpurulent cellulitis** is commonly treated with iv ceftriaxone or cefazolin.
78. **CAP** due to pseudomonas will need **double coverage** like cefepime and levofloxacin and **coverage** for Streptococcus pneumoniae. **Ciprofloxacin** does not cover **Streptococcus pneumoniae**.
79. **M. marinum** treatment: 3–6 months' clarithromycin with ethambutol.
80. **NMDA encephalitis** symptoms: choreoathetosis, psychiatric symptoms, seizures, and autoimmune instability. Diagnosis via **anti-NMDAR IgG antibodies**. **Treatment** includes corticosteroids, immunoglobulin infusion (IVIG), and plasmapheresis (PLEX).
81. Lacerations and puncture wounds, sustained in fresh and brackish water environments can result in necrotizing infection with **Aeromonas hydrophila**. Treatment: surgery, supportive care, antibiotics for G- like **doxy plus Cipro or ceftriaxone**.
82. It requires the attachment of a tick for at least 36 h to develop **Lyme disease**: treatment in 72 h of a tick bite can prevent the development of Lyme disease.
83. **Chickenpox vaccination**: unless the patient is severely immunodeficient (within 4 months of bone marrow transplantation, CD4 <50 HVI, severe combined immunodeficiency), all others should receive chickenpox vaccination, even for patients on infliximab.
84. **Aerococcus urinae** causes **urinary tract infections**, **bacteremia**, and **endocarditis**, usually seen in old patients with cancer, prostate disease, and other underlying urological conditions, treatment is usually **penicillin** as the microorganism can be resistant to cephalosporins.
85. **CMV** causes retinitis (especially in AIDS), pneumonitis, hepatitis, bone marrow suppression, colitis with bloody diarrhea, esophagitis, and adrenalitis. Approximately 60%–90% of adults have **latent CMV infection**.
86. **Esophageal candidiasis** should be treated with fluconazole 400 mg once, then followed by 200 mg daily for 14–21 days.
87. **Group A Streptococcus** may cause necrotizing fasciitis and should be treated with **penicillin** and **clindamycin**. Clindamycin can also be used in difficult-to-treat cellulitis to suppress toxins.

88. **Mediterranean spotted fever** is caused by Rickettsia conorii subspecies conorii (R. conorii) infection in June through September; manifestations: fever, myalgia, and headache shortly followed by maculopapular rash.
89. **Cipro** or **Levaquin** is the preferred antimicrobial for **recurrent cystitis** (>3× in 12 months) when Bactrim resistance is high or a patient has been treated with antibiotics for urinary tract infection in the previous 3 months.
90. **Active TB** must undergo **adequate TB treatment for 2 weeks and have three consecutive negative sputum smears to be considered non-contagious**.
91. **Disseminated coccidioidomycosis** (Valley fever in California and Southwestern USA) most commonly presents with skin lesions, involvements of joints, bones, and meningitis. Diagnosis can be made with **endospore-containing spherules in blood smears**.
92. The etiology of **coccidioidomycosis** is Coccidioides immitis. Coccidioides immitis meningitis diagnosis via **CSF IgG complement fixation** (positive in 90% of patients). Treatment is fluconazole. **Histoplasmosis urine Ag** has 95% specificity.
93. Treatment of first recurrence of C. diff is oral vancomycin in a tapered and pulsed regimen or vancomycin as a standard course or 10 days of fidaxomicin.
94. **Urine culture** is indicated if pyelonephritis, complicated UTI, recurrent UTI, multiple antibiotic allergies or suspected resistant organisms, pregnant, or undergoing urological procedures.
95. **Asymptomatic babesiosis** does not require treatments; can repeat **PCR** testing in **3 months** and if positive or symptomatic, it is treated with **atovaquone** or **azithromycin** for at least 7–10 days.
96. In most cases of **bacterial gastroenteritis**, no antibiotics or treatment is necessary as the infection usually resolves by itself.
97. **Mycobacterium avium complex** (MAC) treatment: clarithromycin and ethambutol and rifabutin. MAC diagnosis requires at least **two sputum culture positive** or bronchoalveolar lavage positive or positive biopsy. Treatment includes **clarithromycin, rifampin, and ethambutol for a year**. MAC can happen after exposure to hot tub water, causing **acute flu-like symptoms and hypersensitivity pneumonitis**.
98. **M. fortuitum** causes soft tissue infection, and grows <7 days. **M. marinum** is related to **granuloma** from fish tank infection and grows >7 days. **Rapidly growing mycobacterium**: M. fortuitum, M. abscessus (lung infection), M. chelonae (wound infection and keratitis).
99. **Droplet precautions** are indicated for large particle droplets >5 μm in size (N. meningitidis, influenza, adenovirus, Mycoplasma pneumoniae, and Bordetella pertussis).
100. **Airborne and contact precautions** are appropriate for disseminated zoster (≥3 dermatomes) or localized zoster in an immunocompromised patient. Other airborne isolation is required for TB, measles, and chickenpox.
101. **Recurrent UTI** ≥ 3 UTIs over 12 months or ≥2 UTIs in 6 months. They should be treated with **antibiotic prophylaxis for 6 months**.

102. **Actinomyces**: chronic, slowly progressive, **nontender indurated mass**. **Treatment** is penicillin or tetracyclines for 2–6 weeks.
103. **Toxoplasmosis** first line treatment: sulfadiazine and pyrimethamine; second line treatment is Bactrim.
104. **Leucovorin** may be used to prevent toxicity from the use of methotrexate, phenytoin, pyrimethamine, and trimethoprim.
105. **Nocardia** causes infections in the lungs, skin, and brain (abscess). Treatment: Bactrim → amikacin → imipenem.
106. Cephalosporin does not cover Listeria, but penicillin G and ampicillin do.
107. Continuous blood culture positive for MSSA requires a **transesophageal echocardiogram** to look for **endocarditis** with possible complications including leaflet perforation (new conduction abnormalities on EKG), aneurysmal formation, and second infection of other valvar structures.
108. **Enterovirus** previously was divided into polioviruses, Coxsackie A viruses (CA), Coxsackie B viruses (CB), and echoviruses cause gastrointestinal symptoms and arthralgia. **Hantavirus** causes cardiopulmonary syndrome or hemorrhagic fever with renal syndrome 2–3 weeks after exposure.
109. **Parvovirus** commonly causes anemia, but not leukopenia and thrombocytopenia.
110. **Chikungunya fever**: central and South America and Asia via Aedes mosquito (also transmits dengue and Zika), symptoms include chronic polyarthralgia, arthritis, and persistent high fevers. Treatment is supportive.
111. **Lemierre's syndrome** is jugular thrombophlebitis and infection of the lateral pharyngeal spaces from bacterial pharyngitis/tonsillitis per neck CT; has recurrent sore throat and difficulties with eating and/or drinking. It is an ENT emergency and typically treated with Unasyn, Decadron 10 mg iv once followed by Decadron 4 mg iv q6h, needs urgent ENT consult.
112. **Mycobacterial infection** can cause cervical lymphadenitis with neck swelling; it is more gradual.
113. **Fever in a returning traveler differential** diagnosis: malaria, yellow fever, dengue, acute HIV, meningococcal disease, typhoid fever, acute schistosomiasis, Katayama fever (acute schistosomiasis).
114. Fever, eosinophilia, urticarial lesion and angioedema, freshwater drinking, and Africa = consider **acute schistosomiasis**.
115. **Influenza**: during flu season, when **≥2 residents** of a facility develop a flu-like symptom in 72 h, screening for flu in the facility is recommended. If confirmed, initiation of prompt **prophylaxis with Tamiflu for 14 days or 10 days** after the onset of illness in the last person infected, whichever is longer.
116. Close contact of **TB**, skin test within a week: + if ≥5 mm, repeat in 8–12 weeks; if interferon-gamma release assay (QuantiFERON-TB Gold), should be repeated 4–6 weeks.
117. **Syphilis**: a patient exposed within 90 days before diagnosis of primary and secondary (latent presumptive syphilis); **latent syphilis in a sex partner should receive presumptive treatment**. If ≥90 days after exposure, the per-

son should get tested (if negative, no treatment needed) or presumptively treated if unable to follow up or serologic test results are not immediately available. Treatment with **penicillin 2.4 million units 1 dose** (or **doxycycline 2 weeks**) for primary syphilis, im weekly × 3 doses for second syphilis, **and 3–4 million iv q6h for 2 weeks for tertiary syphilis** (an alternative is ceftriaxone).

118. Syphilis after appropriate treatment: should see **RPR titer drop by 4-fold within 6–12 months** of treatment and thus requires repeat **RPR in 6 months** to monitor treatment response.
119. **Strongyloidiasis** causes peripheral eosinophilia and gastrointestinal and pulmonary symptoms. Its diagnosis requires ELISA for IgG antibodies, duodenal biopsy, or aspirate.
120. **Babesia microti** has a Maltese cross; Malaria has ring-shaped trophozoites in RBCs.
121. **Leishmania donovani**: insidious onset and progression with fever, malaise, weight loss, and splenomegaly.
122. Low C. diff risk antibiotics include Bactrim, tetracycline, macrolides, and aminoglycosides.
123. **Traveler's diarrhea** includes ETEC, campylobacter, and salmonella. Treatment includes quinolones and azithromycin.
124. **Antibiotics for skin abscess** are indicated in: ≥2 cm, extensive surrounding cellulitis, sepsis, neutropenia, multiple abscess, extremes of ages, or lack of response to incision and drainage.
125. **Norovirus causes vomiting**. **Listeria causes gastrointestinal** symptoms, fever, myalgia, arthralgia, and headache.
126. **Fusarium verticillioides** (infection from maize) can be seen in severely immunocompromised patients with skin breaks exposed to water or soil. Symptoms include refractory fever, skin lesions, and lung disease. Diagnosis requires **skin biopsy (50% sensitivity) or blood culture (40% sensitivity) which grows mold**. Treatment is **amphotericin B +/− voriconazole**.
127. **Ring enhancing lesions in the brain differential diagnoses: abscesses, CNS lymphoma** (single large lesion, related to EBV), **toxoplasmosis** (usually IgG+, IgM−, multiple), **Cryptococcus** (no mass effects, serum and CSF Ag positive in 95% and 99% cases), **histoplasmosis, neurocysticercosis, progressive multifocal leukoencephalopathy** (PML), and others. PML can be seen several weeks after polyomavirus infection at the white matter.
128. **Cryptococcus** in the lung, the next step is lumbar puncture. Treatment for **cryptococcal meningitis**: liposomal amphotericin B + flucytosine for 2 weeks followed by fluconazole for 8 weeks.
129. **Anaplasmosis** (no rash), **Chikungunya** (severe joint pain and stiffness, polyarticular migratory small joint pain), **Dengue** (retro-orbital pain, myalgia, arthralgia, rash appears as fever abates). **Dengue causes retro-orbital pain**.
130. In bacteriuria, when transitioning to oral, oral bioavailability should be good for antibiotic selection. Quinolones, Bactrim, Flagyl, clindamycin, and linezolid have good bioavailability.

131. **Aspergillus** infection is common in the **neutropenic** period after HSCT and lung transplantation. PJP infection is common after transplantation and immunosuppression, especially in the first 6–12 months after transplantation.
132. No antibiotics are needed for simple **furuncle** after incision and drainage in immunocompromised patients.
133. **Ceftazidime** has minimal effects against **Streptococcus pneumonia**.
134. **NAAT** is the most appropriate diagnostic test for genital ulcer disease by herpes simplex virus.

Chapter 28
Rheumatology

1. **Rheumatoid arthritis** treatment: methotrexate, NSAIDs, leflunomide, steroids, hydroxychloroquine/sulfasalazine → consider biological agents including etanercept (Enbrel), infliximab (Remicade), adalimumab (Humira), certolizumab pegol (Cimzia), golimumab (Simponi), abatacept (Orencia), rituximab (Rituxan), tocilizumab (Actemra or Xeljanz), anakinra (Kineret).
2. **Disease-modifying antirheumatic drugs (DMARDs)** include **conventional synthetic DMARDs** (including methotrexate, sulfasalazine, leflunomide, and hydroxychloroquine), **targeted synthetic DMARDs** (JAK inhibitors: tofacitinib and baricitinib), and **biologic DMARDs** (e.g., etanercept, infliximab, adalimumab, rituximab, abatacept, and golimumab)
3. **Treatment algorithm for RA**: use **methotrexate with or without low dose prednisone** (maximum 3 months for steroid) as initial treatment; if failure, **combine MTX with hydroxychloroquine (Plaquenil) and sulfasalazine** or use of biologic DMARD (with or without MTX) or JAK inhibitors (with or without MTX) → switch to other TNF inhibitors.
4. Two-thirds of women with **rheumatoid arthritis** will go into **remission** or achieve low disease activity during **pregnancy** → consider treatment with **etanercept** if flare up.
5. Rheumatoid arthritis treatment: a combination of biologic agents with DMARD to improve functions.
6. **Rheumatoid arthritis** treatment: first line disease-modifying antirheumatic drugs (DMARDs) include methotrexate, hydroxychloroquine, sulfasalazine (causes stomatitis and elevated LFTs), and leflunomide.
7. **Positive CCP** and high titers of antibody with radiographic progression = worse rheumatoid arthritis disease.
8. **Reactive arthritis**, formerly known as **Reiter's syndrome, is characterized** by large joint arthritis, conjunctivitis or uveitis, urethritis, or cervicitis. It is RF-seronegative, HLA-B27-linked arthritis associated with genitourinary and

K. Zhou, *Internal Medicine Training Notes and Survival Guide*,
https://doi.org/10.1007/978-1-0716-4039-5_28

gastrointestinal infections; treatment: NSAIDs → sulfasalazine and methotrexate.

9. **Psoriatic arthritis** treatment: mild use NSAIDs; if skin and/or nail change, use methotrexate.
10. **Milwaukee shoulder** is subacute destructive shoulder arthropathy with large hemorrhagic effusions, calcium phosphate/hydroxyapatite crystal arthropathy; treatment: NSAIDS and repeat arthrocentesis → intra-articular steroids → arthroplasty.
11. **Familial Mediterranean fever** is a hereditary form of recurring fever and serositis including peritonitis, pleuritis, myalgia, and arthritis. Will need to check serum amyloid A (SAA) protein as well as it can cause second amyloidosis. Treatment: colchicine. If colchicine resistant, may benefit from IL-1 inhibitors (canakinumab, anakinra, rilonacept).
12. **Polyarteritis nodosa** is manifested with necrotizing arteritis and typical aneurysms in medium (occasionally small)-sized arteries. Its diagnosis is clinical and usually ANCA -; treatment of polyarteritis nodosa is steroids +/– cyclophosphamide.
13. Gastrointestinal symptoms, HBV+, testicular inflammation, renal involvement, negative ANCA, absence of lung disease = consider **polyarteritis nodosa**.
14. HBV-related **polyarteritis nodosa** symptoms: fever, arthralgia, and vasculitis.
15. **Granulomatosis with polyangiitis (GPA)**, formerly known as Wegner's granulomatosis, is **necrotizing granulomas and pauci-immune vasculitis**) causes systemic signs and symptoms of malaise, fatigue, and myalgia. It affects the upper respiratory tract, lungs, and kidneys (pauci-immune crescentic necrotizing glomerulonephritis). Diagnosis: **cytoplasmic antibody (c-ANCA) against proteinase 3 (PR3)** is specific for GPA, but may also be positive for perinuclear-staining ANCA (p-ANCA) against myeloperoxidase (MPO). **Treatments**: nonsevere—steroids and methotrexate; severe—steroids and cyclophosphamide or rituximab; use steroids and rituximab in relapse; and in remission, use rituximab. **Plasmapheresis** may be indicated if **rapid progressive kidney disease**.
16. **Granulomatosis with polyangiitis** is suspected in patients with ≥2 of the following: nasal or oral inflammation, abnormal chest x-ray, abnormal urinary sediment, and granulomatous inflammation on biopsy of artery or perivasculature. Diagnosis via biopsy.
17. Granulomatosis with polyangiitis is often a mild and limited disease. Treatment includes **methotrexate induction and then treatment with azathioprine**. In severe disease, rituximab can be used.
18. Symptoms and diagnosis of **microscopic polyangiitis (MPA)** are similar to GPA, but **MPO-ANCA (p-ANCA)** is positive in 50%–75% of patients with MPA. Both can cause nongranulomatous **necrotizing pauci-immune necrotizing crescentic glomerulonephropathy**. Treatment is similar to GPA.

19. **ANCA-associated vasculitis includes** granulomatosis with polyangiitis (GPA), microscopic polyangiitis (MPA), and **eosinophilic granulomatosis with polyangiitis** (Churg Strauss syndrome). Testing includes complement 3 and 4, hepatitis B and C viruses and HIV, TB testing, ANA, cryoglobulin, and anti-GBM.
20. **Takayasu arteritis** versus giant cell arteritis: Takayasu has an onset age of 15–25 years while giant cell arteritis happens late in life. In **giant cell arteritis**, jaw claudication (superficial temporal artery), visual changes (ophthalmic arteries), and polymyalgia rheumatica are common but also can affect chest arteritis leading to congestive heart failure (subcranial GCA).
21. **Systemic sclerosis** can have gastric antral vascular ectasia.
22. **Pegloticase** is a uricase, given as IV q12wks. If pegloticase is used, we should start **colchicine**, prednisone, or NSAIDs as prophylaxis for gout attacks.
23. Gouty arthritis with chronic kidney disease can be treated with prednisone 40 mg daily for 5 days. Recurrent **gout attack prevention**: may increase allopurinol from 400 to 800 mg daily.
24. **Gout**: NSAIDs are the first line of treatment, and colchicine is a second line treatment. Intra-articular steroid is a safe and preferred treatment for acute gout flare-ups in chronic kidney disease.
25. **Gout**: colchicine may not be effective if a gout attack of greater than 12–24-h duration. **Gout treatment**: colchicine, NSAIDs, oral steroids, intra-articular steroids, systemic steroids. Low-fat dietary products are good for gout prevention. If severe and refractory gout attacks or contraindications to other treatments, off-label use of **IL-1 inhibitor anakinra or canakinumab** may be effective. Interleukin-1 Trap Rilonacept and IL-1 inhibitor **anakinra** were also effective in **recurrent pericarditis**.
26. In the absence of active disease and once target serum urate is reached, **colchicine should be continued for the longer of the following**: 6 months, 3 months after reaching target urate if no tophi, 6 months after reaching target urate in a patient with baseline tophi that has resolved.
27. Xanthine oxidase inhibitor **Febuxostat** is contraindicated with the use of azathioprine (significantly increased concentration).
28. Angiotensin receptor blockers (**ARBs**) and calcium channel blockers (**CCBs**) but not angiotensin-converting enzyme inhibitors can **lower serum urate** levels.
29. **Shrinking lung syndrome**: chronic insidious dyspnea with low lung volume, possibly due to diaphragm dysfunction.
30. **Soft tissue mass in the abdomen**: IgG4-related disease (retroperitoneal fibrosis) is characterized by IgG4-producing plasma cell infiltration and organ enlargement, fibrosis, and dysfunction. Check serum IgG4. Related diseases included pancreatitis, sclerosing cholangitis, retroperitoneal fibrosis, and mass lesions in intra-abdominal organs.
31. **IgG4-related disease**: lymphoplasmacytic infiltration and enlargement of various structures.

32. Causes of **secondary Raynaud's**: SLE, scleroderma, rheumatoid arthritis, Sjogren syndrome, dermatomyositis, polymyositis.
33. Monojoint **osteoarthritis** treatment: topical diclofenac together with or without joint steroid injections. Chronic monoarticular arthritis in a person with lots of outdoor activities will need to rule out **Lyme disease**.
34. **High-dose steroids** must be initiated prior to biopsy in temporal arteritis to prevent irreversible vision loss.
35. **Inclusion body myositis** happens in males more often than females, usually >50 years old with CPK level <10–12× upper limit normal. Inclusion body myositis is one type of **idiopathic inflammatory myopathies** (polymyositis, dermatomyositis, and autoimmune necrotizing myopathy). **Mitochondrial myopathy has normal CPK**.
36. **Sjogren syndrome** treatment: artificial tears, sugar-free candies → consider topical cyclosporine, or lifitegrast ophthalmic drops.
37. **Rheumatoid arthritis** is associated with **scleritis** and can lead to thinning of the sclera and perforation and vision threatening.
38. **Chikungunya** is an alphavirus endemic to Asia and Africa; it causes **synovitis** and **tenosynovitis** like rheumatoid arthritis.
39. **Libman Sacks endocarditis**: episode(s) of mononuclear blindness in SLE—valvular dysfunction or thickening from the large verrucous lesions near the edge of the valve (mitral valve more common). **Typical lesions** are made of immune complexes, mononuclear cells, fibrin, and platelet thrombi.
40. **Mycophenolate mofetil** has to be stopped 3 months before pregnancy.
41. Side effects of **pregabalin**: weight gain, peripheral edema, lethargy, and dizziness.
42. **Relapsed polymyalgia rheumatica**: increase prednisone to the last pre-relapse dose for 4–8 weeks and then taper.
43. **Primary angiitis of the central nervous system**: gradual progressive neural symptoms including headache, cognitive impairment, and stroke. Normal labs except CSF showed **lymphocytic pleocytosis** and an **increase in total protein**. Diagnosis via cerebral angiogram showing beading, alternating stenosis with dilation. Treatment is **high-dose prednisone** and cyclophosphamide. Steroid to be weaned off over 3–6 months, cyclophosphamide weaning over 3–6 months, and then start maintenance dose of azathioprine or mycophenolate.
44. **Duloxetine** not gabapentin or pregabalin is FDA-approved for chronic musculoskeletal pain including osteoarthritis.
45. **Adalimumab, certolizumab, golimumab, and infliximab** are more effective than other TNF-alpha inhibitors in treating the combination of bowel and joint manifestations in **Crohn's** disease. **Rituximab in combination with methotrexate** is used to treat **rheumatoid arthritis** who have not adequately responded to a TNF-alpha inhibitor.
46. Three drugs approved by the FDA for fibromyalgia: **pregabalin, duloxetine (SNRI), and milnacipran (SNRI)**.

47. **Mycophenolate mofetil** and cyclophosphamide can be used for systemic sclerosis interstitial lung disease.
48. **Undifferentiated connective tissue disease**: has clinical manifestations of other specific connective diseases (Rheumatoid arthritis, scleroderma, GPA, MPA, SLE, Churg-Strauss syndrome, polymyositis, dermatomyositis, MCTD), but not enough positive features to satisfy diagnostic or classification criteria for any specific disease. Treatment is **NSAIDs +/− hydroxychloroquine**.
49. **Mixed connective tissue disease** is an overlap syndrome which includes features of SLE, systemic sclerosis (SSc), and/or polymyositis in the presence of anti-u1-ribonucleoprotein (anti-U1-RNP) antibodies; 50% MCTD has hand edema and synovitis at onset. MCTD workup includes high-resolution CT scan, echocardiogram, and pulmonary function test.
50. **Antisynthetase syndrome** in patients with **dermatomyositis or polymyositis** is characterized by a commonly abrupt onset of interstitial lung disease, myositis, Raynaud phenomenon, nonerosive inflammatory arthritis, low-grade fever, mechanics' hands. **Anti-aminoacyl-tRNA synthetase and anti-Jo-1** are highly suggestive and specific for the diagnosis of antisynthetase syndrome.
51. **Polymyositis** or **dermatomyositis**: progressive proximal muscle weakness and antisynthetase syndrome. For labs, will need to check aminoacyl-tRNA synthetase antibodies (like anti-Jo-1, anti-SRP, anti-M2).
52. Topical **diclofenac** side effects include skin irritation and rash. Topical **capsaicin** side effects include local irritation to the eye mucous membrane. Intra-articular steroids cause skin hypopigmentation, subcutaneous tissue atrophy, and joint infections.
53. **Calcium pyrophosphate deposition disease** (CPPD) also known as calcium pyrophosphate osteoarthritis (also known as **pseudogout**) treatment: low dose glucocorticoids, low dose colchicine, or NSAIDs.
54. **Calcification** = consider chondrocalcinosis = consider pseudogout → check **ferritin** to rule out hemochromatosis arthritis.
55. **Lofgren syndrome** (**systemic sarcoidosis**): the triad of bihilar adenopathy, migratory polyarthritis, and erythema nodosa. They are the common manifestations of sarcoidosis. Additional symptoms of Lofgren syndrome include fever, fatigue, violaceous tender raised lesions, and pedal edema (bilateral ankle arthritis and erythema nodosum). Treatment of Lofgren syndrome even if fever is **NSAIDs, colchicine, or low-dose prednisone**.
56. The classic triad of **Ig A vasculitis (Henoch—Schonlein purpura)** is purpura, abdominal pain, and arthralgia. Diagnosis requires a biopsy of the affected organ like skin.
57. **DRESS** (drug reaction, eosinophilia, and systemic symptoms) syndrome: delayed type IV hypersensitivity drug reaction with extensive skin rash, multiorgan reaction (including kidney failure and death), fever, lymphadenopathy, and lab abnormalities. **Associated with antiepileptic agents** (carbamazepine, lamotrigine, phenytoin, oxcarbazepine), sulfonamides, anti-TB meds (RIPE),

and some antibiotics. Associated drugs should be discontinued at the first sign of a rash. Risk factors may include diuretic use, chronic kidney disease, and the presence of the **HLA-B 5801 allele** in certain Asians.

58. **Palpable purpura—leukocytoclastic vasculitis** (cutaneous small vessel vasculitis) is caused by drug exposure (penicillins, cephalosporins, sulfonamides, phenytoin, NSAIDs, allopurinol), infection, or idiopathic; no visual involvement.
59. **Enthesitis** may indicate **spondyloarthritis** (ankylosing spondylitis, psoriatic arthritis, IBD-associated arthritis, reactive arthritis). When enthesitis is severe, it may extend along tendons and local ligaments, resulting in dactylitis (sausage digits).
60. **Enthesitis** (inflammation of the tendon to the bone) → dactylitis and tendon and enthesis calcification = consider spondyloarthritis (ankylosing spondyloarthritis, psoriatic arthritis, IBD-associated arthritis, and reactive arthritis).
61. **Dactylitis** (destruction of bone), nail pitting, and onycholysis are common in psoriasis (pencil-in-cup appearance).
62. **Chondrocalcinosis** and hook-like osteophytes involving **MCP** = consider **hemochromatosis**.
63. **Pain** at small hand joints especially second and third MCP, subchondral sclerosis, chondrocalcinosis, hook-like osteophytes on the metacarpal heads = consider **hemochromatosis** arthritis.
64. **Hemochromatosis arthritis** occurs gradually while **HBV-associated** arthritis occurs abruptly.
65. **Recalcitrant psoriatic arthritis treatment**s: methotrexate with TNF alpha inhibitor → consider next line of treatment abatacept (Orencia). **Abatacept** is a soluble chimeric CTLA4 protein (extracellular domain of human CTLA-4) that inhibits CD28-mediated T-cell activation.
66. **Psoriatic arthritis** treatment: methotrexate → consider anti-TNF alpha infliximab → consider abatacept (T cell co-stimulation).
67. **Subacute cutaneous lupus erythematosus**: circular or polycyclic scaly erythematous patches and papulosquamous plaques over the forearm, chest, and upper back in a V-shaped configuration. Subacute cutaneous lupus erythematosus is associated with SLE, and Sjogren syndrome, and could also be drug-induced.
68. **Osteonecrosis**: subchondral radiolucency producing the "crescent sign" = consider subchondral collapse.
69. **Leflunomide** causes peripheral neuropathy.
70. Systemic lupus erythematosus (SLE) with acute onset dyspnea, hypoxia, diffuse lung infiltrate, bronchoalveolar lavage showing predominantly lymphocytes = consider **lupus pneumonitis**. Treatment is rapid and aggressive steroids and/or immunosuppressants.
71. **Systemic lupus erythematosus**: cyclophosphamide is reserved for severe active nephritis to induce remission, followed by **mycophenolate** or possibly **azathioprine** for maintenance therapy.

72. **SLE nephritis** treatment: mycophenolate mofetil, cyclophosphamide, azathioprine, rituximab.
73. **Lupus nephritis** 4 months ago, received cyclophosphamide → consider mycophenolate mofetil (MMF), currently on MMF, azathioprine, and prednisone, but continues to have skin and joint disease. Can be treated with belimumab (BLyS protein inhibitor).
74. **Belimumab** is a B-lymphocyte stimulator (BLyS)-specific inhibitor (inhibitors of BlyS) used in addition to SLE standard therapy with mild to moderate disease activity.
75. **Discoid** lupus erythematosus usually affects the **scalp** and face.
76. SLE = **classic rash erythema and scaling** over the cheeks and bridge of the nose sparing the nasolabial groove.
77. **Adalimumab** is used in rheumatoid arthritis and spondyloarthritis. **Secukinumab** (Cosentyx) is an IL-17 inhibitor and is used in psoriatic arthritis and ankylosing spondylitis.
78. **Colchicine toxicity** when used together with fluconazole and clarithromycin (CYP3A4 inhibitor) includes **renal failure**, **rhabdomyolysis**, and **bone marrow suppression**.
79. Patients on urate-lowering therapy should receive prophylactic agents to prevent **mobilization flare-ups** for 6–12 months. Primary prophylactic options include **colchicine**, low-dose **glucocorticoids** or **NSAIDs**.
80. Diagnosis of **rheumatoid arthritis**: chronic, symmetric, polyarticular joint pain, stiffness, synovitis, evidence of inflammation.
81. **Parvovirus B19 arthralg**ia resolves quickly and rarely lasts for 6 months or longer; look for IgM, not IgG. Parvovirus B19 is common in 87% of adults older than 50 years.
82. **Dermatomyositis** can cause weakness of the oropharyngeal and striated muscles in the upper 1/3 of the esophagus → dysphagia and aspiration.
83. **Lupus dermatitis** treatment: topical steroids → consider addition of hydroxychloroquine → consider addition of prednisone 10–15 mg daily → consider immunosuppression and retinoids (methotrexate, isotretinoin, azathioprine, cyclophosphamide, cyclosporine).
84. **Drug-induced lupus**: procainamide (pleurisy as well), hydralazine, INH, TNF inhibitor, minocycline. Symptoms of drug-induced lupus include malaise, myalgia, and arthralgia. Labs are positive for ANA, especially antihistone antibodies with normal complements.
85. No adjustment of allopurinol during acute attack but **3–4** weeks after.
86. **Still disease**: fever, rash, arthritis, and increased ferritin.
87. Long-term **rheumatoid arthritis** with functional limitation not explained by rheumatoid arthritis, likely from mechanical stress of joint deformities and/or destructions. Need orthopedic referrals.
88. **Stress fractur**e: pain with axial loading at metatarsal. **Morton neuroma**: pain when squeezed simultaneously.
89. **Orthopedic referral for stress fractures** at sites like proximal fifth metatarsal with a high risk of nonunion, and delayed healing.

90. Increased **PTT**, **thrombocytopenia**, and ischemic stroke or venous thromboembolism (VTE) = consider **antiphospholipid syndrome**.
91. **Antiphospholipid syndrome** (**APS**) diagnosis requires ≥1 clinical and ≥1 lab test criterion: clinical thrombosis or complication of pregnancy (≥3 abortions <10 weeks or >1 fetal loss after 10 weeks). Lab: positive moderate high titer **anticardiolipin, positive lupus ab, or positive beta2-GP-1 Ab** on ≥2 occasions at least 12 weeks apart.
92. **Behcet disease** = Recurrent **aphthous ulcers** (>3×/year) plus 2 of the following: **eye** lesions (uveitis, recurrent genital lesions, **skin** lesions, or positive **pathergy** (≥2 mm papule 24–48 h after inserting a 20–25-gauge needle 5 mm in the skin).
93. **Complex regional pain syndrome**: pain, sensation (cold/warm), edema, bone demineralization, and inciting event.
94. Men >50 years old or postmenopausal women, expected to receive corticosteroid at **7.5 mg or more for >3 weeks** should get **bisphosphonates**.
95. **Paget's disease** diagnosis is confirmed by radiographic abnormalities (osteolysis and osteosclerosis) and increased **ALP**. After diagnosis, the patient will need a **bone scan** to determine the extent and distribution of bone lesions.
96. Sore throat, shallow ulcer on the buccal mucosa = consider **stomatitis**; replete **folic acid** while on methotrexate (folic acid 5 mg daily).
97. **Symptomatic vertebral fracture treatment** with NSAIDs, Tylenol, occasional opioids → early pain relief, intranasal calcitonin can be given for 2–4 weeks. Severe cases with refractory pain lasting >6 months may require vertebral augmentation with kyphoplasty or vertebroplasty (may also be offered as inpatient for refractory back pain). Its diagnosis may require **CT and even MRI spine**.
98. **Ankylosing spondylitis** treatment: NSAIDs → consider TNF-alpha inhibitors.
99. **Skin ulcers in rheumatoid arthritis**: **Felty syndrome** (triad of seropositive rheumatoid arthritis, neutropenia, and splenomegaly) vs **pyoderma gangrenosum** (no spleen involvement, no leukopenia).
100. **Red flags of low back pain** will need to check ESR and CRP: ≥50 years old, history of cancer, weight loss unexplained, pain ≥1-month, nighttime pain, unresponsive to therapy, neurological symptoms, IV drug abuser, recurrent UTI (transmission to vertebrae via **Batson's venous plexus**).
101. **Polymyalgia rheumatica**: increased ESR but normal CPK. Has pain and stiffness. **Rheumatoid arthritis patients with myelopathy** require MRI neck to rule out cervical spine instability.
102. **Systemic sclerosis**: anti-SCL 70, anti-centromere, anti-RNA polymerase II and III.
103. **Giant cell arteritis** responds well with low dose prednisone → biopsy of the temporal artery on the affected side is negative → biopsy of the contralateral temporal artery (40% sensitivity). After remission with high dose steroids, **steroids should be tapered over several months, even 1–2 years**.
104. Criteria for the diagnosis **of giant cell arteritis**: >50 years of age, localized headache with fever and **visual disturbance**, ESR >50, tenderness at the

temple, temporal artery biopsy showing necrotizing arteritis with mainly mononuclear cells (3/5 criteria positive = 94% sensitivity and 91% specificity).

105. **Giant cell arteritis** should get yearly **chest X-rays for up to 10 years** to identify patients with thoracic (not abdominal) aneurysms.

Chapter 29
Endocrinology

1. The ADA recommends advancing to **dual therapy for HA1c ≥ 9%**.
2. Diagnosis of **primary adrenal insufficiency**: morning cortisol <5 μg/dL raises suspicion for adrenal insufficiency, check ACTH → if ACTH high, check **21-hydroxylase** → if 21-hydroxylase normal, order CT abdomen to identify cause other than enzyme deficiency. Other causes may include lymphoma, sarcoidosis, histoplasmosis, and TB.
3. A value of morning cortisol <4.8 μg/dL is consistent with adrenal insufficiency; morning cortisol level can be falsely low in cirrhosis because of **low corticosteroid-binding globulin**. If inconclusive, do a **salivary cortisol** level check between 11 p.m. and 1 a.m. or a standard high-dose **ACTH stimulation** (**Cosyntropin**) stimulation test. If after Cosyntropin test remains inconclusive, get **dehydroepiandrosterone sulfate (DHEAs)** measurements.
4. Primary adrenal insufficiency (**Addison disease)** treatment: hydrocortisone 15 mg in the morning and 5 mg in the afternoon, fludrocortisone 0.1 mg once daily. Fludrocortisone is **not needed** for **secondary adrenal insufficiency**.
5. **Antipsychotics** only mildly increase prolactin to around >50; if significant prolactin increases to >100, check brain MRI.
6. Causes of **prolactin increase**: pituitary adenoma, malignancy, sarcoidosis, drugs (antipsychotics, Reglan), hypothyroidism, chest wall injury (burns and herpes), chronic kidney disease, following tonic-clonic seizure or focal seizures.
7. **Prolactinomas** can increase in size during pregnancy (prolactin >200 in pregnancy usually) and can lead to vision loss; thus, close monitoring and formal **visual field testing** should be performed each **trimester**.
8. **Subacute thyroiditis** treatment: beta-blockers, NSAIDs, or less commonly steroids in the acute phase.
9. **Vit D deficiency** etiology: obesity, steroid, phenytoin, and phenobarbital use.
10. **Hungry bone syndrome** = low calcium after parathyroidectomy (low calcium, low phosphorus, normal PTH).

K. Zhou, *Internal Medicine Training Notes and Survival Guide*,
https://doi.org/10.1007/978-1-0716-4039-5_29

11. **Female hirsutism**: check serum **testosterone and DHEAs**; if high DHEAs (>8 ug/mL), check CT abdomen to rule out **adrenal tumor**. A pelvic ultrasound is recommended as the first imaging if testosterone levels >100–150 in females to look for testosterone-producing **ovarian cancer or polycystic ovarian syndrome**.
12. Nonthyroidal illness syndrome also known as **euthyroid sick syndrome**: reduced T3 (in 70% of patients with euthyroid sick syndrome), **increased rT3** (also seen in chronic kidney disease), low or low normal T4 and TSH.
13. **Phenoxybenzamine** (alpha blockade) should be prescribed for 10–14 days before surgery for pheochromocytoma and catecholamine-secreting paragangliomas (tumors near the carotid artery along the nerve pathway).
14. Testosterone deficiency: **measure testosterone at 8 a.m.**, also monitor testosterone levels at **3** months and **6** months, and then annually after starting exogenous testosterone treatment. Normal serum testosterone levels: **300–1000** ng/dL in male and 15–70 ng/dL in female
15. **Indications for parathyroidectomy**: serum calcium level ≥1 mg upper limit normal, CrCl <60, 24 h urine calcium >400 mg, nephrolithiasis or nephrocalcinosis, osteoporosis, and age <50. Surgery is indicated if 24 h urine calcium ≥400 mg/day because primary hyperparathyroidism and familial hypocalciuric hypercalcemia share similar lab test results, and 24-h urine calcium together calcium-to-creatinine-clearance ratio can help differentiate the two diagnoses.
16. Total urine calcium **<200 mg/24 h** and calcium creatinine ratio < 0.01 highly suggestive of **familial hypocalciuric hypercalcemia**.
17. After **parathyroidectomy**, measure **24-h urinary calcium excretion**. If >300 mg/24 h (hypercalciuria), calcium and/or Vit D replacement should be decreased. Hyperparathyroidism causes hypercalcemia and hypophosphatemia, and hypercalciuria and hyperphosphaturia
18. **Cushing syndrome** diagnosis requires two positive tests in 24 h urine free cortisol usually >3× upper limit normal, overnight 1 mg dexamethasone suppression test usually ≤5 μg/dL (absolutely <1.8 μg/dL), and 11 p.m. salivary cortisol testing.
19. Screening for **Cushing disease**: one of the three tests (24 h urine-free cortisol level, overnight 1 mg dexamethasone suppression test, or 11 p.m. salivary cortisol level) → check ACTH.
20. The **hypercortisolism related to psychiatric illness** happens via activation of the hypothalamic-pituitary axis: ACTH usually normal or increased.
21. **Transgender treatment**: discuss fertility preservation options → engage in at least 1 year of **satisfactory social role** of change as well as **compliance with hormonal treatment** (estradiol plus androgen blockers in transfemale).
22. **Pheochromocytoma** diagnosis: 24 h urinary fractionated metanephrine, plasma-free metanephrines. If abnormal labs, get adrenal CT. **False elevation of free normetanephrine** is seen in TCA, SSSI, SNRI, levodopa, buspirone, and prochlorperazine use. Need to stop these medications at least **2 weeks** before testing.

23. **Metformin**: eGFR 30–45 can discuss with the patient about its use; if eGFR <30, we should discontinue its use.
24. **Polycystic ovarian syndrome**: **oral contraceptives** are the first line treatment for hirsutism and acne. May add metformin. Workups include testosterone, DHEAs, FSH, LH, TSH, and hCG.
25. **Incidental pituitary adenoma or mass** need to evaluate hormone deficiency: 8 am cortisol, THS, FT4, FSH, LH, testosterone, and hormone in women, prolactin, and IGF-1. If no hormone excess or mass effects, **repeat MRI in 6 months** if macroadenoma ≥1 cm and **repeat MRI in 12 months** if microadenoma (<1 cm) for growth.
26. **Amenorrhea** workup (common in Turner syndrome): FSH, LH, prolactin. If hyperandrogenism, check testosterone and DHEAs.
27. After pituitary surgery, **SIADH** can happen in 3–7 days.
28. Mechanism of **hypercalcemia in granuloma**: macrophages in granuloma convert 25-hydroxy Vit D into 1,25-dihydroxy-Vit D.
29. Women with T1DM or T2DM who are planning pregnancy should be counseled on risks of the development of **progression of diabetic retinopathy**.
30. **Teriparatide (Forteo)** is indicated for **osteoporosis associated with steroid use**, $T \leq -3.5$, or failed bisphosphonates. **Denosumab** is used in osteoporosis with chronic kidney disease.
31. **Honeymoon phase of T1DM**: low need for basal insulin, we discontinue sliding scale insulin to reduce metabolic stress to functioning beta cells; this may occur shortly after the diagnosis and may last months to years.
32. **Denosumab** binds to the receptor activator of nuclear factor-kB ligand (RANKL) inhibiting the activation of the receptor activator of NF kappa B (RANK) and thus inhibits osteoclast maturing and bone resorption. Denosumab is used for bone metastases and osteoporosis.
33. **Adrenal incidentaloma/mass**: dexamethasone suppression test to rule out **Cushing syndrome**; urinary catecholamines and metanephrines to rule out **pheochromocytoma**; aldosterone to renin ratio to rule out **Conn syndrome**. If asymptomatic adrenal mass, screen with 24-h urine total metanephrine.
34. **Adrenal incidentaloma** or of any size, should be screened for subclinical Cushing syndrome with a 1 mg overnight dexamethasone suppression test. If >5 μg/dL, it is positive ⇒ measuring **ACTH, DHEAs, and urine free cortisol, and 8 mg overnight dexamethasone suppression test** is often required to confirm autonomous cortisol secretion.
35. **Adrenal mass adrenalectomy** indications: size **>4 cm**, density > 10 Hounsfield units, absolute contrast washout <50% at 10 min. **Mitotane** (an adrenolytic, suppressing the adrenal gland) may be used as adjuvant therapy after primary resection.
36. **Gynecomastia** is more common with primary (increased LH) than secondary (marijuana use, alcohol, 5 alpha-reductase inhibitor, H2 blocker, or digoxin use) hypogonadism.
37. **Infertility evaluation** indications: no pregnancy with usual sexual activities after **6** months if age >35 years in females, after **12** months if age <35 years

old in females. Tests include **semen analyses and mid-luteal phase progesterone**.

38. **Hypogonadism** in male workup: total testosterone. If total **testosterone** is <150, and **LH** and **FSH** are low → check MRI brain for pituitary tumor (hypogonadotropic hypogonadism needs MRI pituitary). Only check free testosterone if concerns of **low sex hormone-binding globulin** level, such as in obese patients.
39. **The mixed meal test** looks at endogenous insulin secretion; it is used in **postprandial hypoglycemia** 2–3 years after Roux-en-Y.
40. Complete thyroxine replacement should be weight-based at **1.6 ug/kg (lean body weight)** except in patients 65 years of age and older and/or with a history of heart disease.
41. **Inferior petrosal sinus sampling** (after CRH stimulation) is often recommended before exploratory pituitary surgery to diagnose **pituitary tumors**.
42. To diagnose primary aldosteronism, discontinue spironolactone/eplerenone **6 weeks** before checking the renin aldosterone ratio.
43. **Lymphocytic hypophysitis** is an autoimmune disease seen in pregnancy and postpartum.
44. **Hypomagnesemia** (due to medications, EtOH, or malnutrition) activates G-proteins that stimulate calcium-sensing receptors and **decrease PTH secretion → hypocalcemia**.
45. **DPP-4 inhibitors** (saxagliptin and alogliptin) may increase risks for **congestive heart failure**, especially in chronic kidney disease and heart disease history. DPP-4 inhibitors increase active incretin hormones, GLP-1, and glucose-dependent insulinotropic polypeptides.
46. **Thiazolidinediones** cause fluid retention and may worsen congestive heart failure.
47. Monitoring and assessing **secondary or central hypothyroidism**: check FT4, not TSH.
48. Decrease insulin dose if episodes of hypoglycemia and the patient cannot feel it.
49. **Myxedema coma** symptoms: altered mentation, hypoventilation, bradycardia, hypoglycemia, hyponatremia. **Treatment**: stress dose hydrocortisone, IV levothyroxine, +/− liothyronine.
50. **Falsely elevated HA1c** seen in iron deficiency anemia, anemia, asplenism, uremia, chronic alcoholism, and increased bilirubin.
51. **Goal TSH in papillary thyroid cancer** is 0.3–2. Patients with persistent disease should target TSH <0.1, so does in distant metastasis.
52. After **total thyroidectomy** for thyroid cancer, patients with a high risk for disease recurrence should receive **adjuvant radioactive iodine** therapy.
53. **Amiodarone-induced hyperthyroidism** usually happens during or up to 9 months after treatment with amiodarone. **Treatment** is moderate to high dose prednisone with a taper in 1–3 months.
54. Indications for **metabolic surgery**: T2DM with **BMI ≥ 40** (≥37.5 in Asians) regardless of glucose control, **BMI 35–39** with unsatisfactory glucose control.

55. **Osteitis fibrosa cystic**a = high PTH. People **50–69 years old** should go get a **DEXA** scan if there are risk factors.
56. **Glucose Somogyi effects:** hypoglycemia during the night stimulates the secretion of stress hormones causing hyperglycemia in the morning.
57. Before switching from insulin to oral therapy in patients with ketosis-prone diabetes, **fasting C-peptide and glucos**e levels should be checked.
58. **Hypothyroidism and prolactinoma** both suppress gonadotropin secretion and decrease FSH and LH.
59. Most **thyrotoxicosis** has elevation in both T3 and T4, rarely T3 elevation only.
60. XXY has **hyper-gonadotrophic hormone**. **Hemochromatosis** has **low FSH** and **LH**.
61. Training for a **marathon** in T1DM → **decrease meal time short-acting insulin** dose before exercise and continue the same long-acting insulin dosage.
62. In **primary hyperparathyroidism**, serum 21-hydroxyvitamin D should be kept at >30 ng/dL.
63. **ESRD with diabetes affects the accuracy of HA1c**, and needs to measure fasting, pre and post-prandial glucose.
64. **Continuous glucose monitoring** is useful for patients with postprandial hyperglycemia, dawn phenomena (hyperglycemia between 2 a.m. and 8 a.m. without preceding hypoglycemia), or overnight hypoglycemia.
65. **Diabetes** from **chronic pancreatitis** should be treated with insulin only.
66. **Microprolactinoma in asymptomatic** patients does not require treatment but surveillance.
67. **Amenorrhea and cyclic pelvic pain** in a patient with a history of dilation and curettage or abortion history ⇒ consider vaginal ultrasound to rule out **Asherman syndrome**.
68. **Moderate to severe Graves' disease**, first control symptoms with methimazole. Before RAI therapy, pretreatment with **glucocorticoid** to mitigate the rise in antibodies. Mild Graves' disease may go directly to **RAI** without steroids.
69. Hypercalcemia **>16 mg/dL** with **neurologic symptoms** or **AKI**. The treatment is hemodialysis.
70. In patients with **high risks for osteoporosis**, even stable DEXA after 5 years, continue the same alendronate therapy.
71. Plasma aldosterone concentration to plasma renin activity ratio (PAC/PRA) ≥20 and aldosterone concentration high (>20 ng/dL) indicates a positive screening test for **primary hyperaldosteronism**; then **load** 90 mEq **sodium tablet** over 3 days and check urine aldosterone level, if urine aldosterone concentration >12 μg/day, hyperaldosteronism is diagnosed ⇒ check **CT adrenal protocol**. Treatment is **adrenalectomy (preferred for unilateral disease) or spironolactone or eplerenone**.
72. In primary aldosteronism, **adrenal vein sampling** is needed when imaging unrevealing and **older patients** because of the high frequency of non functioning adrenal incidentalomas.

73. For **central hypothyroidism**, neuroimaging and pituitary hormone testing should be performed before levothyroxine treatment (check for adrenal insufficiency); if low cortisol level, check the Cosyntropin test.
74. Effects of **amiodarone**: decreases T4 to T3 conversions, decreases thyroxine synthesis (treatment is levothyroxine). **Amiodarone-induced thyrotoxicosis Type 1** (AIT1) with increased thyroxine synthesis (treatment is antithyroid with methimazole); **amiodarone-induced thyrotoxicosis Type 2** (AIT2) with destructive thyroiditis (treatment is steroid).
75. **Hypercalcemia** etiology: increased PTH, lithium, Vit D, malignancy.
76. **Urinary chloride** is low in patients with vomiting and high in patients with diuretic use or renal issues.
77. Diabetes on basal and premeal insulin: **basal insulin** is reduced for preprandial (**fasting**) and early **morning** hypoglycemia and the dose of **premeal insulin** is reduced for **postprandial** hypoglycemia.
78. **Orlistat** is used for BMI $\geq$ 30 or 27 with diabetes, hypertension, or hyperlipidemia. It inhibits lipase causing side effects of fat malabsorption and **calcium oxalate kidney** stones.
79. **Medullary thyroid cancer**: once diagnosed, check for metastatic disease, identify co-existing tumors, and check for germline RET mutations. Staging CT if **lymph node involvement or calcitonin >400**, bone scan if **suspecting bone metastasis**.
80. **Acromegaly** increases risks for **gastrointestinal cancer, melanoma,** and **cardiovascular diseases** including congestive heart failure.
81. **Subclinical hypothyroidism** usually should not be treated if the age is >70 years.
82. **Bactrim** can potentiate the effects of **sulfonylureas** which can accumulate in chronic kidney disease.
83. **Pituitary incidentaloma**: >1 cm → check hormones and visual fields; <1 cm → targeted hormone checking if symptomatic; if asymptomatic and <1 cm, only check prolactin.
84. **Nodule in thyroid gland**: check TSH and get thyroid ultrasound → thyroid uptake and I131 scan.
85. **Thyroid nodule**: TSH low → do thyroid scintigraphy or radioactive iodine uptake scans, FNA if cold nodule; TSH high/normal → FNA. A high TSH level (cold nodules) correlates with higher risks for malignancy in thyroid nodules.
86. **Radioactive iodine uptake** measures the accumulation of radioactive tracer in the thyroid; whereas **scintigraphy with either 123-radioiodine or 99mTc-pertechnetate** captures emitted radiation from internal radioisotopes in the thyroid using gamma cameras.
87. **HA1c > 10%** or random glucose >300 → start basal and preprandial insulin.
88. **Copper deficiency** has a clinical presentation similar to B12 deficiency; **zinc supplementation** exacerbates copper deficiency.
89. Early onset of severe osteoporosis and recurrent fragility fractures require evaluation of **second causes of osteoporosis**.

90. **Diabetic patients in intensive exercises**: frequent monitoring of glucose, adequate hydration, consumption of rapid carbs before and during exercise, and if necessary, insulin dose adjustment before exercise.
91. **Triglyceride-induced pancreatitis**: all should receive fluid hydration, and pain control. If triglyceride >1000, if glucose >500, start **insulin drip**; if glucose <500 or severe pancreatitis, order **plasmapheresis** (therapeutic plasma exchange).
92. Severe to moderate hypercalcemia (serum calcium ≥13 mg/dL) = consider malignancy. Mild hypercalcemia (serum calcium ≤11 mg/dL) = consider primary hyperparathyroidism and thyrotoxicosis.
93. **Suppressed serum thyroglobulin** differentiates factitious thyrotoxicosis (thyroxine ingestion) from other forms of thyrotoxicosis with low RAIU. Thyrotoxicosis with low RAIU is seen in (1) **ectopic thyrotoxicosis** from factitious thyroid hormone ingestion, struma ovarii, and, rarely, large deposits of functioning thyroid cancer metastases; (2) **subacute painful thyroiditis, silent lymphocytic thyroiditis**.
94. In Graves' disease after radioactive iodine ablation, **hypothyroidism** can happen between **2 and 3 months** after radioiodine therapy and lasts **2–4 weeks**. Therefore, after radioactive iodine therapy, patients will need to check all TSH, T3, and FT4 to assess hypothyroidism (TSH can be either high or low but **T3 and FT4 are usually low**).
95. **Secondary workup for osteopenia** in males starts with morning **testosterone**. **Urine N-telopeptide** is used to monitor the skeletal response in antiresorptive therapy (bisphosphonates and denosumab) in osteoporosis and predict the onset of osteoporosis.
96. In **subclinical hypothyroidism**, we should repeat TSH. Treatment is indicated for subclinical hypothyroidism in the following conditions: + antithyroperoxidase antibody, goiter, pregnancy, overt symptoms, and cardiovascular disease.
97. **Malignant hypercalcemia** with chronic kidney disease, give **calcitonin** in urgent conditions; give **zoledronic acid** if no chronic kidney disease.
98. **Tricyclic antidepressants** should not be used in older adults for neuropathy, rather use **pregabalin**.
99. Osteoporosis diagnosis is based on a history of low trauma (fragility) fracture or bone density measurement by **DEXA scan at the lumbar spine or hip** (total proximal femur or femoral neck) or less commonly other bones.
100. **FRAX risk assessment** tool for ≥50 years old with osteopenia in the spine, femoral neck, or total hip region not previously treated.
101. **Painless thyroiditis** happens >1 year after pregnancy, and should be treated with beta blocker if symptomatic thyrotoxic.
102. Patients with **sarcoidosis and other granulomatous diseases** may have hypercalcemia. Treatment: prednisone. Likely has hypercalciuria as well.
103. Differentiate statin-induced myopathy versus hypothyroid myopathy is the latter has **minimal to no inflammation**.

104. Acute **intra-pituitary hemorrhage**: severe headache, bitemporal hemianopsia, ophthalmoplegia, panhypopituitarism. Management: **neurosurgery team consultation**, and iv **hydrocortisone stress dose**.
105. **Toxic adenoma or multinodular goiter** who has overt symptoms should have definitive treatment with radioactive iodine ablation or surgical thyroidectomy.
106. Endocrine disorders associated with **obstructive sleep apnea** include hypothyroidism, acromegaly, Cushing syndrome, and polycystic ovarian syndrome (PCOS).

Chapter 30
Neurology

1. **Myasthenia gravis crisis** symptoms: increased generalized and oropharyngeal weakness, respiratory insufficiency worse in supine. Treatment: measurement of **vital capacity q2h** in ICU; wean off ventilator if maximal inspiratory pressure (MIP), also known as negative inspiratory force, stronger than **−30 cmH_2O**; **withdrawal of anticholinesterase inhibitors to rule out cholinergic crisis**; **plasmapheresis or IVIG (still takes days to work), plus high dose steroids**.
2. **Myasthenic crisis** treatment: plasmapheresis or IVIG plus high-dose steroid.
3. **Rituximab** is useful for the treatment of refractory myasthenia gravis, especially if muscle-specific kinase (MuSK) antibodies are positive.
4. **Spontaneous subarachnoid hemorrhage** complications: **rebleed** usually happens in 24 h, **vasospasm** (happens in 20%–40% of SAH patients) is more common after 3 days, seizures, increased intracranial pressure, SIADH. Treatment includes **coiling, stenting, nimodipine, and transcranial Doppler monitoring**, and may also benefit from hypertonic saline infusion.
5. **Cerebral vasospasm** (vasoconstriction syndrome) occurs often 5–10 days after subarachnoid hemorrhage. Symptoms include a sudden change of mentation and acute neurological symptoms, diagnosis via **CT angiography of the brain, treatment may require an interventional intra-arterial infusion of vasodilators (verapamil, nicardipine, papaverine, milrinone, and nimodipine)**.
6. **Reversible cerebral vasoconstriction syndrome (RCVS)**, diagnosis via CTA, MRA. **Treatments**: verapamil, nimodipine. **Digital subtraction angiography in RCVS** can cause transient neural deficits and should be avoided.
7. **Central vertigo** presents with less vertigo but more gait disturbance, disequilibrium, **vertical** and or **torsional nystagmus** with neural symptoms like headache, diplopia, and dysarthria. Peripheral vertigo may cause hearing loss, tinnitus, and mostly torsional nystagmus. BPPV nystagmus can be suppressed with visual fixation and has fatigability.
8. **Brain death diagnosis**: The golden standard is absence of cerebral blood flow via angiogram or scintigraphy, but apnea testing is usually for diagnosis. The

K. Zhou, *Internal Medicine Training Notes and Survival Guide*, https://doi.org/10.1007/978-1-0716-4039-5_30

diagnosis of brain death also requires the clinical manifestations of persistent coma, absence of brainstem reflexes, and lack of ability to breathe independently.

9. **Serotonin syndrome** treatment: supportive care with **benzodiazepines** for sedation; may give serotonin antagonist **cyproheptadine** if supportive care fails.
10. **lhermitte's sign**: transient electric shock sensation along the spine and extremities with neck flexion. It suggests a lesion in the lower brainstem or the upper cervical spinal cord.
11. Diagnosis of **multiple sclerosis**: T2 weighted MRI lesions disseminated in time and space. CSF analyses show **oligoclonal IgG bands** (>95%) and **elevated IgG index** (90%).
12. **Cushing's reflex** (response to increased intracranial pressure): hypertension with widened pulse pressure, bradycardia, and Cheyne-stoke breathing.
13. Patients with **suspected viral encephalitis** should be empirically treated with **IV acyclovir** and broad-spectrum antibiotics while waiting for the results of CSF studies.
14. **Bidirectional nystagmus**, like a fast component to the right with a rightward gaze and to the left with a leftward gaze, is concerned for a central process as is vertical or pure torsional nystagmus.
15. **Carotid Doppler** is of limited use for posterior or cerebella circulation signs (i.e., vertigo, nystagmus, and ataxia).
16. For most patients with **post-concussive syndrome, neuropsychological testing** is not necessary unless history of moderate to severe traumatic brain injury or significant cognitive symptoms, especially if not improving within the expected time frame.
17. **Normal pressure hydrocephalus** gait is similar to Parkinson's disease but wider based.
18. **Weber's test**: sensorineural—localized to the unaffected side; conductive—localized to the affected side. **Renne test**: sensorineural—air > bone normal; conductive—bone > air abnormal.
19. The most common **intracranial hemorrhage** (the most common cause is uncontrolled hypertension) happens in the **basal ganglia** (putamen) followed by the thalamus, pons, and cerebellum. Hemorrhagic stroke symptoms: headache and rapid progression of symptoms.
20. **Cerebral amyloid angiopathy** is the second most common cause of intracranial hemorrhage (ICH), usually in **>75-year-olds** with **multi-lobar ICH**. Hemorrhage usually spares ventricles and deep brain structures (i.e., putamen, thalamus, and pons), and has increased risks for recurrence.
21. In normal aging and mild cognitive dysfunction, we should have no impairment in **activities of daily living**.
22. **Paraneoplastic cerebellar degeneration symptoms**: acute nausea, vomiting, and dizziness, followed by cerebellar signs, dysarthria, and diplopia several days later.
23. **Paroxysmal hemicranias**: unilateral trigeminal distribution with ipsilateral autonomic symptoms. Treatment: **indomethacin**.

24. **Medication overuse headache** treatment: discontinuation of offending agents, start 1–2 weeks' oral steroid and add migraine prevention medications.
25. **Relapsing-remitting multiple sclerosis** with abnormal MRI, check JC virus, if negative, start natalizumab (Tysabri); if positive, start fingolimod (Gilenya). Although it is very rare, fingolimod can still increase the risks for developing **progressive multifocal leukoencephalopathy** (PML).
26. **Fingolimod** (a structural analog of sphingosine, used in multiple sclerosis) side effects: macular edema, first dose **bradycardia**. Avoid fingolimod use in heart block, **infections,** or leukopenia.
27. **Dalfampridine** is used for impaired mobility in multiple sclerosis. **Dextromethorphan quinidine combination** is used for pseudobulbar affect (uncontrolled laughing or crying).
28. **Lateral medullary syndrome (Wallenberg syndrome)**: ipsilateral Horner syndrome, loss of ipsilateral facial pain, loss of contralateral pain, and temperature sensation. **Medial medullary syndrome**: ipsilateral tongue weakness, contralateral hemiplegia, decreased contralateral posture sense.
29. A 60-year-old male with a history of alcohol consumption and falls presented with lethargy, confusion, and focal weakness. We will have to rule out **chronic subdural hematoma** which has an insidious onset with more global deficits.
30. The only required lab test before tPA administration is **plasma glucose**.
31. **Carotid endarterectomy** is recommended for symptomatic patients (TIA, ischemic stroke in the past 6 months) with high-grade (70%–99%) stenosis, and asymptomatic patients with 80%–99% stenosis or progression >80% stenosis despite intensive medical therapy.
32. **Guillain-Barré syndrome (GBS)** causes ascending weakness. With progression, GBS can cause ophthalmoplegia, diplopia and bulbar symptoms (like hoarseness, dysarthria, dysphagia, facial drooping, monotone voice), can also develop **dysautonomia** (i.e, tachycardia, diaphoresis, sluggish pupils).
33. **Tylenol** is the preferred medication for **migraine in pregnancy**.
34. Diagnosis of **myasthenia gravis** consists of **serology** (Ach receptor and muscle-specific tyrosine kinase receptor antibodies) and **nerve conduction studies** in a stepwise manner.
35. **Leptomeningeal carcinomatosis** symptoms: subacute onset (days to weeks) headache and a variety of neurologic signs and symptoms including altered mental status, seizure, and/or multifocal neurological deficits. **Diagnosis**: gadolinium MRI spine and brain → CSF studies.
36. **Posterior reversible encephalopathy syndrome (PRES)** seen in hypertensive encephalopathy/crisis, chemotherapy (i.e., cyclosporine), pre-eclampsia/eclampsia, hematopoietic stem-cell transplantation (HSCT), chronic kidney disease, autoimmune disease, shock → increased fluid migration to the brain parenchyma and subsequent vasogenic edema.
37. **Wernicke encephalopathy**, double vision with **lateral gaze palsy** and **lethargy**, D5 before thiamine can worsen or even cause Wernicke encephalopathy.
38. **Convulsive syncope** evaluation includes history taking, orthostatic signs and physical exam, and EKG.

39. **Valproic acid hyperammonemic encephalopathy** treatment: **lactulose** and **l-carnitine**.
40. **Multiple system atrophy**, also known as **Parkinson's plus syndrome**: rapid development of symptoms with symmetric neural findings of Parkinson's disease. Symptoms: a combination of **Parkinsonism**, **cerebellar ataxia** and **dysautonomia**, and early **postural instability** and **falls**. Compared to Parkinson's disease, **early prominent imbalances, recurrent falls, and cerebellar findings** are common in multisystem atrophy.
41. **Dystonia in Parkinson's disease** (very painful foot contraction) treatment: switch to long-acting levodopa/carbidopa at night.
42. **Diabetic amyotrophy**: pain and weakness, usually seen in well-controlled diabetes, from ischemic injury from nonsystemic microvasculitis.
43. **Asymptomatic complete occlusion of carotid artery** = adequate collateral blood flow which requires no treatment.
44. **Toxoplasma encephalitis**: multiple ring-enhancing lesions with mass effects and edema, commonly affects basal ganglia. **Progressive multifocal leukoencephalopathy** (PML): bilateral white matter lesions, no mass effect, no enhancement or edema.
45. **Early idiopathic Parkinson's disease** = non-motor symptoms, i.e., REM sleep behavior disorder, excessive daytime somnolence, mood disturbance, anosmia and constipation.
46. **Nonpupil sparing vs. pupil sparing**: pupillary fibers of CN III run peripherally and motor fibers exist centrally within the nerve. Nonpupil-sparing CN III nerve palsy involves **nerve compression** from an aneurysm, uncal herniation, or tumor; pupil-sparing CN III **nerve palsy involves vasa vasorum microangiopathy** from diabetes and hypertension and other systemic causes.
47. **Seizure medications** usually like carbamazepine and valproic acid usually **require a taper** when discontinuation.
48. **Familial amyloidosis** is characterized by predominant sensory and motor **peripheral neuropathy** and/or **autonomic neuropathy**. It is diagnosed via genetic testing for mutation of the transthyretin gene.
49. **Myelopathy** to both posterior column and the corticospinal tracts ⇒ diagnosis is B12 deficiency (**subacute combined degeneration of the spinal cord**), **copper** deficiency, or possible **neurosyphilis**.
50. Normal lumbar puncture opening pressure between **18** and **20** cmH_2O in a recumbent position.
51. **Idiopathic intracranial hypertension (Pseudotumor cerebri)** symptoms: visual blurring, diplopia, brief obscurations, **papilledema**, and occasionally CNS IV palsy, CSF opening pressure >25 cmH_2O. **Treatment**: **acetazolamide** (500 mg 2 times daily, gradually titrating up to a maximum of 4 g daily in twice-daily doses), weight loss, **topiramate** (25 mg daily, up to 100 mg bid), **Lasix** 20 mg or 40 mg daily, lumbar puncture, lumbar-peritoneal (LP) and ventriculoperitoneal (VP) shunting, and/or venous sinus stenting. I met a patient who got **venous sinus stenting** from which she developed **dural sinus thrombosis**.

52. **Acetazolamide** causes complications of **hepatic encephalopathy and metabolic acidosis**.
53. Repeat **plasmapheresis** only if symptoms get worse after initial stabilization or impairment. It can cause **significant immunodeficiency** as it depletes immunoglobulins and other immune reactants.
54. **Osteoporosis and seizure** treatment: may only use lamotrigine or Keppra.
55. **Phenytoin** causes dizziness, ataxia, tremors, peripheral neuropathy, cerebellar atrophy, and agranulocytosis.
56. Treatment of **glucocorticoid refractory idiopathic transverse myelitis**: plasmapheresis.
57. **Lamictal** for seizure and depression; **topiramate** worsens psychosis and nephrolithiasis. **Topiramate** does not cause low testosterone or high prolactin.
58. **Post-hypoxic myoclonus** is characterized by prominent action-induced myoclonus with a combination of positive (rapid jerky movements) and negative (lapses in muscle tone) myoclonus.
59. **Dementia** or **cognitive** deficits from **multiple sclerosis** can benefit from **cognitive rehabilitation**.
60. **Haloperidol and other traditional antipsychotics are contraindicated** in **Lewy body dementia**. These medications can worsen confusion, cause heavy sedation, and possibly cause irreversible parkinsonism in Lewy body dementia.
61. Eliquis is recommended for use in cancer patients.
62. **Generalized seizures** (absence seizures and tonic-clonic seizures); **focal seizures** (simple focal seizures, complex focal seizures, and secondary generalized seizures).
63. **Partial seizures** treatment: carbamazepine, gabapentin, and phenytoin. Symptoms of partial seizures include déjà vu, rising epigastric sensations, unilateral clonic movements, or shaking before onset.
64. **Temporal seizure** uncontrolled with two medications management: video EEG for temporal lobectomy.
65. **Alzheimer's disease** CSF has decreased **42-amino acid β amyloid (Aβ42) peptide** and increased **tau protein**.
66. **Migraine prophylaxis** is necessary if migraine attacks $\geq$2 days a week or $\geq$2 times a month.
67. **Primary progressive aphasia** (treatment with a speech therapist) versus dementia.
68. Posterior communicating artery (**PCOM**) aneurysm = **ipsilateral CN III palsy** with **mydriasis**. **Horner syndrome** = partial ptosis, anhidrosis, and miosis.
69. **Withholding anticoagulation** for **4 days to 2 weeks** is recommended for moderate to large brain infarctions.
70. **Status migrainosus** treatment: repetitive IV dihydroergotamine. May need to order a **lumbar puncture** to rule out CNS infections.
71. In **metastatic brain tumor seizure**, give antiepileptic drugs that have no or minimal interaction with hepatic enzymes like Keppra (most often used nowadays), or valproic acid. Carbamazepine and phenytoin are enzyme-inducing

antiepileptic drugs which cause transitory or dose-related liver function abnormality without associated hepatocellular injury in most cases.

72. **Baclofen** will need dosage adjustment in kidney disease and should be avoided if CrCL <30. **Dalfampridine** use should be avoided if CrCL <80.

Chapter 31
Dermatology

1. To diagnose an **autoimmune bullous** disease, two biopsies are performed: lesional skin for histology and perilesional normal skin for direct immunofluorescence.
2. **Pityriasis rosea**: Christmas tree pattern, multiple plaques with collarette scale, self-resolving in 6–8 weeks. **Pityriasis versicolor**: also known as tinea versicolor; treatment: topical anti-seborrheic shampoos or lotions like selenium, sulfide, or ketoconazole.
3. **Pityriasis rosea** resembles secondary syphilis (but no lymphadenopathy) and thus will need to check RPR for syphilis. Pityriasis rosea is usually self-limiting; oral and topical corticosteroids or antihistamines may be used for its treatment.
4. **Erythrasma** is a superficial skin infection from **Corynebacterium** in intertriginous areas; diagnosis via coral-red fluorescence with a wood lamp; **treatment** includes topical erythromycin, clindamycin, mupirocin, fusidic acid, or benzoyl peroxide for localized disease and oral therapy with a single dose of clarithromycin 1 g or erythromycin 250 mg 4 times a day for 14 days for extensive disease. **Melasma** is brown-gray patches over the face of a female which can be related to pregnancy and sunshine, treatment is triple combination cream (hydroquinone 4%, tretinoin 0.05%, and fluocinolone acetonide 0.01%) and avoidance of sunshine.
5. **Painful wheels** = urticarial + bruising = consider vasculitis. Needs biopsy to rule out autoimmune diseases like SLE, and nephritis.
6. **Melanonychia** can be from acral melanoma (Hutchinson sign); it requires a biopsy for diagnosis.
7. **Pruritic urticarial papules** and plaques of pregnancy: symptoms typically last 4–6 weeks and usually abate by second postpartum week. Treatment is low to medium-potency topical glucocorticoids and oral antihistamines.
8. Ursodeoxycholic acid is used in **intrahepatic cholestasis of pregnancy**.

K. Zhou, *Internal Medicine Training Notes and Survival Guide*,
https://doi.org/10.1007/978-1-0716-4039-5_31

9. **Miliaria**: occlusion of eccrine sweat glands. Acute generalized exanthematous pustulosis (AGEP) is medication-related.
10. **Polymorphous light eruption** typically manifests before age 30 in fair-skinned women, fast appearing in spring and early summer. The rash will persist for weeks and resolve without scarring.
11. In immunocompromised patients, Cryptococcosis, histoplasmosis, or penicillium marneffei (now known as Talaromyces marneffei) infection may resemble **molluscum contagiosum** lesions and should be differentiated with a skin biopsy.
12. **Pemphigus foliaceus**: painful itchy blisters with acantholysis, most common in middle-aged adults, scaly papules, crusted erosions (corn flakes), no mucous membrane involvement. **Pemphigus vulgaris** (40–60 years old) and pemphigus foliaceus both have positive Nikolsky signs. Pemphigus vulgaris has flaccid blisters with mucosal involvement and positive antibodies against desmoglein 1 and 3. **Bullous pemphigoid** (>60 years old) has negative Nikolsky sign with linear IgG in the basement member with pemphigoid antigens BP230 and BP180.
13. **Subacute cutaneous lupus erythematosus** is frequently diagnosed as a drug-induced photosensitive rash characterized by erythematous annular scaly patches. Medications like adalimumab, hydrochlorothiazide, ACEi, proton pump inhibitor, NSAIDs and terbinafine can all trigger it.
14. **Actinic keratosis** that does not resolve with cryotherapy or other appropriate therapy requires a biopsy to rule out an invasive neoplasm. Areas with multiple lesions can be treated with topical 5-FU or imiquimod.
15. **Keratoacanthoma**: crusted hyperkeratotic core or central crater of crust and scale treatment → surgical excision.
16. **Lupus pernio** (noncaseating granulomas with minimal lymphocytic infiltration) = sarcoidosis of the central face and nose. **Lupus vulgaris**: purple papules on distal digits exacerbated by cold and moisture = cutaneous tuberculosis (central caseating necrosis).
17. **Basal cell carcinoma** treatment: noninfiltrating—electrodesiccation and curettage; 5-FU and imiquimod for superficial, Mohs micrographic surgery for high risk; vismodegib for locally advanced or metastatic.
18. In **tenosynovitis**, we need to rule out gonococcemia and it requires hand surgery debridement ASAP.
19. **Actinic purpura** is age-related capillary fragility and bleeding under atrophic skin.
20. **Epidermal inclusion cyst** treatment is excision. **Cutaneous abscess** usually does not require antibiotics.
21. **Topical minoxidil** can be used for male or female pattern hair loss.
22. **Transient acantholytic dermatosis** (also known as Grover's disease): red pruritic papules on the chest, flank, and back associated with xerosis heat, and sweating.
23. **Morphea** is a localized form of scleroderma with isolated sclerotic circumscribed plaques.

24. **Scleromyxedema**: deposition of mucin with a large number of stellate fibroblasts in the dermis most frequently associated with paraproteinemia and multiple myeloma or AL amyloidosis, causing waxy yellow red papules overlying thickened skin. **Pityriasis alba** is associated with eczema in young patients.
25. A **wood lamp** is an ultraviolet light source that can be used to evaluate hypo- and depigmentation lesions as in vitiligo.
26. **Dysplastic nevi**: dark brown center and a surrounding ring of light brown, "fried egg" appearance; malignant melanoma presents as macules, papules, or plaques, ≥6 mm in diameter.
27. Three types of common **moles (melanocytic nevi):** junctional (flat), compound (slightly elevated), and intradermal (domed) melanocytic nevi. **Junctional melanocytic nevus**; melanoma in situ (**lentigo maligna**—superficial irregular brown macule); **solar lentigo** is a brown smooth macule. Solar lentigo is from ultraviolet (UV) exposure and no treatment is needed.
28. **Types of melanomas**: superficial spreading melanoma, nodular melanoma, lentigo maligna melanoma, acral lentiginous melanoma, and desmoplastic melanoma.
29. **Morbilliform eruptions** begin 4–14 days after initiation of new medications, coalescing fine monomorphic papules on the trunk and spreading distally and symmetrically.
30. **Psoriasis** with 20% extensive body area involvement treatment: narrow-band UVB phototherapy, Psoralen plus UVA, oral retinoid (acitretin) plus UVA.
31. Patients with **cutaneous only polyarteritis nodosa** (PAN) experience tender subcutaneous nodules from vascular inflammation, stellate erosions, or ulceration from ischemia in the watershed of the affected vesicles, may or may not have livedo reticularis or livedoid purpura. Treatment is oral antihistamine, azathioprine, colchicine, and dapsone.
32. **Erythema nodosum** = panniculitis or inflammation of fat, associated with streptococcus, hormone therapy (oral contraceptives, hormone replacement therapy, or pregnancy), inflammatory bowel disease, sarcoidosis, lymphoma, and medications.
33. **Erythema nodosum:** need chest X-ray to look for lymphoma, sarcoidosis, TB, and fungal infection like coccidioidomycosis.
34. **Erythema multiforme**: can be associated with HSV1 and 2 and mycoplasma infections.
35. **Pitted keratolysis** (caused by Kytococcus sedentarius infection) = bacterial skin infection, crater-like pits with malodor; **aquagenic keratoderma** (carrier status of cystic fibrosis gene with unknown pathophysiology) = white papules and plaques with burning pain, pruritus and hyperhidrosis on palms and rarely soles.
36. **Psoriasis vulgaris** can flare to erythroderma following the use of systemic steroids. The presence of lamellar scale that bleeds when peeled away (Auspitz sign) and nail pitting = erythrodermic psoriasis.
37. **Psoriasis skin change types**: psoriasis vulgaris, inverse psoriasis (red, thin plaques with scale in axilla, intergluteal cleft, perineum, and under the breast

and pannus), sebopsoriasis (scalp, elbow, nasolabial folds, chest and pubic area), guttate psoriasis (0.5–2 cm red plaques erupt suddenly).

38. **Dermatitis herpetiformis**: check G6PD deficiency and give dapsone.
39. **Scabies** treatment: permethrin 5% now and repeat 7–10 days, or al oral ivermectin now and repeat 7–10 days. Post scabetic pruritus treatment: antihistamines, topical glucocorticoids, and oral steroids if severe.
40. **Crusted scabies** (thick crusts of skin that contain large numbers of scabies mites and eggs) is seen in immunocompromised patients, treatment: bathe with 5% permethrin and ivermectin simultaneously.
41. **Rosacea**: chronic pink papules, pustules, erythema, and telangiectasia. Rosacea treatment: topical brimonidine, metronidazole, azelaic acid. Ocular rosacea—ophthalmologist referral.
42. **Porphyria cutanea tarda**: check for underlying disease, especially hepatitis C and hemochromatosis.
43. **Pyoderma gangrenosum** treatment: prednisone 1 mg/kg, steroid-sparing agents, immunosuppressants, intralesional steroids, or high potency topical glucocorticoids.
44. **Severe allergic contact dermatitis** from poison ivy may necessitate 2–3 weeks of taper-dose oral steroids.
45. **DRESS**: drug reaction with eosinophilia and systemic symptoms, 2–6 weeks after exposure, is usually an exuberant morbilliform eruption with prominent facial edema, lymphadenopathy, fever, and in severe cases, hypotension.
46. **Pruritus** in the absence of skin findings should be evaluated for systemic causes. Medication allergies like hydrochlorothiazide, calcium channel blockers, opiates, and NSAIDs can all cause this.
47. **Multiple skin tags** are commonly seen in insulin resistance, pregnancy, and Crohn's disease.
48. **Lipodermatosclerosis** (subcutaneous fibrosis and induration of the skin in the leg, seen in venous stasis and venous ulcers) versus pretibial myxedema.
49. Direct fluorescent antibody and PCR testing can help differentiate between **HSV1, HSV2, and varicella** in 24 h.
50. **Topical tacrolimus** can be used in atopic dermatitis or discoid lupus. Calcipotriene can be used in plaque psoriasis.

Chapter 32
General Internal Medicine

1. **Orthopedic surgery like total knee arthroplasty** requires both intermittent pneumatic compression and low molecular weight heparin during hospitalization and low molecular weight heparin after discharge for 35 days. In actual clinical practices, some surgeons prefer aspirin 325 mg or even 81 mg twice a day for 6 weeks upon discharge to rehabilitation facilities.
2. Only **pregabalin**, **duloxetine** (20 → 30 → 60 mg daily), **tapentadol** (an opioid), and topical **capsaicin** have FDA approval for painful **diabetic neuropathy**.
3. **Methylphenidate** can be used as a rapid-acting **psychostimulant for depression** at the end of life.
4. **Bacterial conjunctivitis**: redness of the conjunctival membrane obscuring tarsal vessels, crusty eyes in the morning, and mucopurulent discharge. Treatment is trimethoprim—polymyxin B or erythromycin or moxifloxacin 0.5% drops bid to qid for 7–10 days.
5. **Olopatadine ophthalmic** drops for seasonal allergies.
6. For **infectious epididymitis**, treat with **ceftriaxone 500 mg im single dose** plus **doxycycline** for 10 days (alternative for doxycycline is azithromycin 2 g single dose) if no history of insertive anal sex; **ceftriaxone** im once plus **fluoroquinolone** for 10 days if history of insertive anal sex.
7. **MMR vaccination** in adults, one dose in regular people, and two doses for health care workers.
8. For women with palpable breast abnormality, if ≥30 years old, perform **both mammography and ultrasound**.
9. **Bariatric surgery** indications: BMI ≥ 40, or ≥35 with comorbidities like type 2 diabetes, coronary artery disease, obstructive sleep apnea, or osteoarthritis.
10. Up to 20% of patients on angiotensin enzyme inhibitors develop a dry cough **1–2 weeks after** initiation of treatment. May trial angiotensin receptor blockers if dry cough with angiotensin enzyme inhibitors.
11. MELD score **≥15**, need a referral to liver transplant. MELD score **≥20**, all but urgent and life-saving surgeries should be avoided.

K. Zhou, *Internal Medicine Training Notes and Survival Guide*,
https://doi.org/10.1007/978-1-0716-4039-5_32

12. **Premature ejaculation** treatments: SSRI, TCA, and topical anesthetic agents (like lidocaine).
13. **Postmenopausal vasomotor symptoms** treatment: estrogen, SSRIs, SNRI, and gabapentin.
14. **Preoperative EKG** is reasonable for patients with known CAD, arrhythmia, PAD, CVA, or structural heart disease.
15. EKG is the only diagnostic study that is routinely recommended in patients with **syncope**.
16. As a secondary prevention of atherosclerotic cardiovascular disease, **aspirin should be initiated as soon as possible** before percutaneous intervention (PCI) and then continued indefinitely at a dose of 81–325 mg daily.
17. For the primary prevention of cardiovascular disease, the USPSTF recommends selectively offering low dose aspirin (75–100 mg orally daily) in adults aged 40–59 years with a 10% or greater 10-year CVD risk but not in adults 60 years or older.
18. **Corneal abrasions** can cause sudden onset of pain and foreign body sensations.
19. The validity of cross-sectional studies is compromised by **recall bias and confounding errors**. Cohort study looks at relative risk and case-control looks at odds ratio.
20. **Recurrent unilateral epistaxis** may be a sign of neoplasm and warrants endoscopy of the nose.
21. **Systemic exertion intolerance** disease diagnosis: impaired social function for 6 months, post-exertional malaise and fatigue, unrefreshing sleep not relieved by rest.
22. **Post-Lyme disease syndrome**: fatigue, arthralgia, myalgia, and impaired memory or cognition that can last for years after treatment for acute infection.
23. Urgent surgery may be appropriate **30 days after bare metal stents and 3 months after drug-eluting stents** with P2Y12 inhibitor hold.
24. Audible post-oropharyngeal secretions ("**death rattles**") are common at the end of life and are best managed with family education and reassurance.
25. Age ≥50 years old immunocompetent adults and aged ≥19 years immunocompromised, **Shingrix (Zoster vaccine recombinant)** should be given two doses, 2–6 months apart.
26. **Central vertigo** has nystagmus with an immediate onset (no latency), longer duration (>1 min), no fatigability with visual fixation, and vertical or horizontal directionality without a torsional component. Diagnosis via **MRI/MRA** of the posterior circulation.
27. One-time HIV screening for adolescent and adult patients, and **every 3–6 months repeat testing in sexually active MSM**.
28. **Moderate intensity statin** is indicated for 40–75-year-olds (without known ASCVD or diabetes) if ASCVD risk 5%–7.5% in select patients and >7.5%–20% and accompanied by the presence of ASCVD risk-enhancing factors; goal for LDL-C drop by 30%–49%. **High-intensity statin** is indicated in diabetes with age 50–75 years-old (moderate intensity for age 40–<50), LDL-C ≥190 mg/dL, ASCVD risk ≥20%; goal for LDL-C drop by >50%. **PCSK9 inhibitor** is an

alternative to and adds additive benefits to statin if high-intensity statin therapy is desired.

29. **Low to moderate intensity statin** is recommended in: ≥75 years old, chronic kidney disease, and use of medications with known interaction with statin (diltiazem).
30. Treatment of **somatic symptom disorder**: acknowledging the patient's symptoms, building a therapeutic relationship via frequent scheduled visits, cognitive behavioral therapy, and avoiding further testing.
31. Severe refractory dyspnea, appropriately dosed oral opioids like **morphine** and **hydromorphone** are first line therapy for **symptomatic relief** in hospice care.
32. Patients with **obesity or overweight** exam: weight, height, waist circumference, blood pressure, HA1c, fasting glucose, and lipid profile.
33. **Adult ADHD**: persistent inattention and/or hyperactivity-impulsivity. **Treatment**: methylphenidate and cognitive behavioral therapy (CBT). Methylphenidate should not be prescribed if recurrent substance use or at high risk for serious adverse effects (arrhythmia, resistant hypertension). Atomoxetine (Strattera), bupropion, and tricyclic antidepressants can be used when stimulants are contraindicated in ADHD.
34. Positive likelihood ratios of 2, 5, 10 correspond to an increase in disease probability of 15%, 30%, and 45%, respectively.
35. **Length time bias** is common in chronic cancer like prostate cancer; lead time bias is common in cancer/disease with early detection and diagnosis.
36. Non-orthopedic surgery who are at high risk for postoperative venous thromboembolisms (VTEs) as defined by **Caprini score**, deep VTE prophylaxis with low molecular weight heparin or unfractionated heparin together with intermittent pneumatic pump therapy are recommended.
37. Radiation-induced nausea and vomiting treatment: **prochlorperazine** and **Zofran**. If chemotherapy-induced, **olanzapine** can also be used.
38. **Neurocardiogenic or vasovagal syncope** usually has prodromal symptoms like nausea and diaphoresis, and afterwards fatigue and generalized weakness are typical.
39. **Rheumatoid arthritis** is commonly associated with **scleritis** which can be vision-threatening and lead to thinning of sclera and perforation.
40. **Meniere's disease** is characterized by episodic vertigo lasting 20 min to 24 h with tinnitus.
41. **Hydrocolloid or foam dressings** are superior to standard gauze dressings for pressure ulcers.
42. **Bridging for surgery** if CHA2DS2-VASc Score ≥5 or 6, mechanical heart valve, recurrent ischemic stroke, DVT, or PE in 3 months.
43. **Auditory symptoms** are not present in vestibular neuritis while **labyrinthitis** has auditory symptoms.
44. **Hydromorphone** is the preferred opioid to treat cancer-related pain in patients with chronic kidney disease; **fentanyl** patch only in **opioid-tolerant** patients.
45. **Central retinal vein occlusion**: painless blurry vision or vision loss; **bacterial endophthalmitis**: decreased vision and hypopyon.

46. **Persistent postural perceptual dizziness**: non-vertiginous dizziness or imbalance that worsens with personal motion, upright positing, and movement of objects for at least 3 months. **Treatments**: Vestibular balance rehabilitation therapy (VBRT), SSRI, or SNRI.
47. **Medical cannabis** (dronabinol and nabilone) is licensed for sale in the USA and is used for the treatment of chronic noncancer pain.
48. **Asymptomatic popliteal cyst** does not require treatment.
49. When **constipation** symptoms do not respond to osmotic and stimulant laxative therapy, the chloride channel activator **lubiprostone** can be considered. FDA approved medications for opioid-induced constipation: **naloxegol** (Movantik), **methylnaltrexone** (Relistor), and **lubiprostone** (Amitiza).
50. Autism spectrum disorder diagnosis: repetitive nonpurposeful behaviors and **deficiencies in communication and social interaction**.
51. **Lichen planus** (associated with HCV infection) can affect skin, nails, mucosa; white lines and patches (**Wickham striae**), or painful erythema and erosions. **Lichen sclerosus**: white atrophic patches on the genital and perinanal skin (figure 8 shaped in general apperance).
52. Opioid risk assessment is necessary before naloxone prescription and evaluation.
53. No **intracranial stenting** in the middle cerebral artery even 95% stenosis. Medical management with DAPT initially remains the standard of care for high grade large cerebral artery stenosis with the exception of mechanical thrombectomy and stenting when appropriate in acute stroke patients.
54. Women aged 65 and older and younger postmenopausal women with **FRAX ≥9.3%** should get screened for osteoporosis.
55. Decreased hearing, stuffiness, and discomfort in the ear, but no inflammation = consider **otitis media** with effusion. **Etiology**: either viral or allergy-related factors. **Treatment**: observation and symptomatic management. If persistent symptoms ≥12 weeks → consider **myringotomy with tympanostomy tubes**.
56. **Topical lidocaine** is a first line treatment for postherpetic neuralgia. **Topical capsaicin** is a first line treatment for **localized neuropathic pain**. The second line treatment of gabapentin causes drowsiness and dizziness. Gabapentin is a first line treatment for **systemic neuropathic pain.** Gabapentin is FDA-approved for **postherpetic neuralgia, adjunctive therapy in the treatment of partial seizures, and moderate to severe restless leg syndrome**.
57. **Uveitis**: unilateral eye pain, redness, photophobia ⇒ consider circumferential redness around the border of sclera and cornea (cornea limbus) also known as ciliary flush.
58. **Scleritis** has bilateral redness across the entire sclera, but not ciliary flush.
59. **FABER test result indications**: **sacroiliac** joint pain, **sacroiliitis**, groin pain with external rotation (iliopsoas bursitis, hip osteoarthritis), posterior hip impingement.
60. **Carpal tunnel syndrome** treatment: **nocturnal wrist splint →** consider steroid injection or po steroid → consider surgery if motor weakness or atrophy of the thenar eminence or refractory to conservative treatments.

61. **Bipolar depression** treatment: quetiapine monotherapy or combined olanzapine and fluoxetine.
62. **Suspected obstructive sleep apnea**: keep head of bed at 30°, careful use of sedatives, continuous pulse oximetry. CPAP only if hypoxia or apneic episodes.
63. **Massage therapy** is better than lumbar support for low back pain.
64. For prednisone <10 mg/day, stress-dosing glucocorticoid is not required, even for high-risk surgery.
65. In **terminally ill** patients, feelings of guilt, hopelessness, helplessness, and worthlessness may distinguish depression from anticipatory grief (**periods of joy**).
66. **Propranolol** can reduce situation-specific anxiety symptoms, but not as monotherapy for **panic attacks as it needs SSRIs**.
67. **Non-bacterial upper respiratory tract infection** treatment: chlorpheniramine-pseudoephedrine (Sudafed).
68. **Somatic symptom disorder** (symptoms >6 months); **illness anxiety disorder** has minimal or no somatic symptoms.
69. **Tilt table testing** for suspected reflex syncope triggered by standing, unexplained episodes of syncope in a high-risk setting, recurrent syncope with no organic heart disease.
70. HBV vaccination requires three doses of vaccination then as needed; if necessary, can check titers for re-vaccinations.
71. **Lipid panel every 4–6 years** is recommended in men aged 35 and older regardless of risks and both men and women aged 20 and older with risks for coronary artery disease. **Glucose level check every 3 years** is recommended in asymptomatic adults aged 35–70 years who are overweight or obese.
72. A **repeat fasting lipid** panel should be obtained **1–3 months after statin** to see adherence and its effectiveness.
73. Older patients with visual difficulties should be referred to see an ophthalmologist to rule out **glaucoma and macular degeneration**.
74. Artificial nutrition and drugs (**dronabinol or megestrol**) do not improve mortality or morbidity or quality of life in cancer patients with cachexia.
75. **Bileaflet mechanical aortic valve** in normal sinus rhythm without other risk factors for stroke: no bridging needed. **Mechanical mitral valve or mechanical aortic valve** with additional risks (hypercoagulable state, atrial fibrillation, previous venous thromboembolism, left ventricular ejection fraction <35%) does need bridging.
76. **Insomnia** treatment: sleep hygiene counseling → sleep restriction counseling.
77. **Cerumen impaction** treatment only if symptomatic or the tympanic membrane needs to be visualized.
78. **Cancer surgery like laparotomy for colon cancer resection**: **low molecular weight heparin 40 mg daily for 28 days after surgery**.
79. **Achilles tendinopathy** typically presents with burning heel pain and stiffness that worsen with activity and better with rest.

80. **Bacterial conjunctivitis** (mucopurulent, bilateral, otitis media, no adenopathy). **Viral conjunctivitis** (watery, unilateral, pharyngitis, adenopathy, sandy and itchy). **Allergic conjunctivitis** (bilateral, chemosis, itching).
81. **Presbycusis** is symmetric and age-related affecting high frequencies of hearing.
82. **Visual problems** can be seen in endophthalmitis; **ophthalmoplegia** can be seen in orbital cellulitis; **preseptal cellulitis** only has anterior (in front of the ocular orbit) soft tissue infection.

Chapter 33
Gynecology and Andrology

1. An **absent cremasteric reflex** suggests testicular torsion.
2. No cervical cancer screening in ≥65 years old with adequate screening which is defined **as three consecutive negative cytology** pap smear results or **two consecutive negative cytology plus HPV test results** within the last 10 years.
3. **Trichomonas vaginitis** treatment: 2 g metronidazole once, redo **NAAT within 3 months**.
4. **Cyclic mastalgia** related to menstruation treatment: education, reassurance, and appropriate breast support. **Danazol** is approved for persistent severe cyclic breast pain unrelieved by conservative management.
5. Patients with **noncyclic mastalgia** with focal breast pain but no palpable mass should undergo **breast ultrasound** because approximately 1% of such patients may have breast cancer at the site of pain.
6. **For breast mass/cyst** do **mammogram** for women ≥30 years of age, do **ultrasound** if <30 years of age, do mammogram → ultrasound for age ≥ 40.
7. Women with **dense breasts and other risk factor**s that impart a lifetime risk for breast cancer of 20%–25% or higher should also undergo **breast MRI** in addition to screening mammography.
8. **Chronic pelvic pain syndrome (CPPS)** is characterized by chronic pelvic pain and intermittent voiding symptoms without evidence of infection. **Treatment**: pregabalin, gabapentin, and nortriptyline. Additional treatments include antibiotics, anti-inflammatory agents, alpha-blocking agents, and 5-alpha reductase inhibitors.
9. **Valvovaginal candidiasis**: vulvar edema, fissures, excoriations, thick white curdy vaginal discharge, pH ≤ 4.5–4.0.
10. **Vaginal pH** >4.5, thin and homogenous discharge, positive whiff (10% KOH → fishy odor) = consider the diagnosis of **bacterial vaginosis** which requires ≥20% clue cells; **treatment** is metronidazole or clindamycin.
11. **Trichomoniasis**: copious, malodorous, pale yellow or gray frothy discharge with vulvar itching, burning, and postictal bleeding.

K. Zhou, *Internal Medicine Training Notes and Survival Guide*, https://doi.org/10.1007/978-1-0716-4039-5_33

12. A **female sexual disorder** requires both **significant distress** and the **persistence** of **symptoms** not explained by a nonsexual mental disorder.
13. **Unilateral right-sided varicocele**, needs CT to rule out tumor and thrombosis.
14. MSM tests: annual genital and extra-genital exam, chlamydia, gonorrhea, syphilis, and HIV infection test, HAV, HBV. If HIV +, check HCV.
15. **Anovulatory abnormal uterine bleeding** treatment: oral contraceptives, if contradictory, do progestin-containing IUD → consider endometrial ablation.
16. **DHEAs > 8 ug/mL** indicate a possible androgen-producing tumor in women.
17. Male **hypogonadism** diagnosis requires at least two different occasions of **testosterone** tests at 8 am. If <40 years with a serum total T <250 ng/dL or >60 years with a serum total T <150 ng/dL, will need a brain MRI to look for abnormalities of the pituitary gland.
18. **Mammogram false negative** rate is around 10%–20%. A breast mass needs a **core biopsy even if** the **mammogram** is **negative**.
19. **Erectile dysfunction first line treatment**: weight loss, exercise, smoking cessation, psychotherapy, and phosphodiesterase-5 (PDE5) inhibitors.
20. **Erectile dysfunction in benign prostate hyperplasia (BPH)** treatment: tadalafil, a phosphodiesterase-5 inhibitor, for both conditions.
21. Erectile dysfunction in a patient with **nocturnal penile tumescence** is mood and/or situation related. Treatment is **psychotherapy**. Sildenafil first line and alprostadil second line treatment for erectile dysfunction in general unless contraindications.
22. **Two types of intrauterine devices (IUD)** available: hormone-free (like copper IUD), or with levonorgestrel.
23. In a woman with hysterectomy taking systemic (oral or transdermal) estrogen therapy for menopausal symptoms, **concurrent progestin** is not indicated to prevent endometrial cancer.
24. Statins are teratogenic and should not be used in pregnancy.
25. In women **≥35 years** old with risk factors or anovulatory bleeding ⇒ consider **endometrial biopsy**.
26. Anovulation and contraindications to combination oral contraceptives, give **progestin-containing IUD**, oral progestin like **medroxyprogesterone acetate may be used to promote withdrawal bleeding for women** who wish to get pregnant.
27. Long-acting reversible contraceptives are progesterone-only forms of contraception that include **depot medroxyprogesterone acetate** injections, **subcutaneous** implants, and **progestin-containing intrauterine devices**, return of fertility may take **10 months**; weight gain is a common side effect.
28. **Estrogen contraceptives** are contraindicated in breast cancer, liver disease, migraine with aura, uncontrolled hypertension, and venous thromboembolism, and ≥35 years of age who smoke 15 cigarettes a day.

Part IV
The Universal Admitter in Hospital

My journey to a hematology/oncology fellowship did not work out for a multitude of reasons. After carefully weighing the pros and cons of multiple potential career paths, I decided to be a full-time hospitalist. The transition to a hospitalist allowed me to embrace a new role in patient care, one that would see me at the forefront of managing acutely ill patients during their most vulnerable moments. Although my original plan was to work as an academic hospitalist, I instead have worked as a hospitalist at multiple community hospitals and healthcare systems after graduation from my internal medicine residency training. Working as a hospitalist at community hospitals has continued to foster my independent thinking and practices and build my confidence as a team leader when taking care of acutely ill patients with multiple comorbidities. During this process, I have enjoyed the fulfillment of providing comprehensive and compassionate care to patients across a wide spectrum of medical conditions.

As a hospitalist, I have had the privilege of taking care of patients at their most critical junctures, navigating complex medical scenarios, and coordinating multidisciplinary care to optimize patient outcomes. Whether it's managing acute exacerbations of chronic illnesses, diagnosing and treating life-threatening infections, or providing end-of-life care with dignity and compassion, each day presents a new challenge and an opportunity to make a meaningful difference in the lives of my patients. The dynamic nature of hospital medicine allows me to engage with patients from diverse backgrounds and with a wide range of medical needs, fostering a deep sense of connection and fulfillment in my practice. I am grateful for the opportunity to serve as an advocate for my patients, guiding them through their hospital stays with empathy, expertise, and unwavering commitment to their well-being.

Over the years, my role as a hospitalist has evolved into a universal admitter and acute medicine caregiver at hospitals more and more often. Besides providing care to patients with acute congestive heart failure, pneumonia, and COPD exacerbation, I have been working as the attending physician provider for patients with neurological emergencies (especially acute stroke and intracranial bleeding), abnormal heart rates and rhythms, various cancers on active chemotherapy and/or radiation treatment, and acute severe and complicated infections. I recognized the need for further knowledge and training as an internal medicine hospitalist in the fields of neurology, EKG, hematology/oncology, and infectious diseases. With continuous lifelong learning from specialists' recommendations and suggestions and my experiences over the years as a hospitalist, I reorganized and revised my notes during and after residency training for neurology, advanced EKG, hematology/oncology, and infectious disease. These chapters were all grouped into this section of The Universal Admitter in Hospital.

When I was ready to submit this book for publication, my colleague encouraged me to devote a section about communication in medical practices. As an experienced hospitalist, we both agree that effective communication is of the same if not greater importance as good patient care and it is part of good patient care. The practice of medicine is not only about medical knowledge, but also excellent communication with patients (and patients' family members), other healthcare providers, and associated personnel in the healthcare field. The characteristics of an excellent physician does not only include excellence in medical knowledge, but also communication. While I strive to be a dedicated hospitalist with a passion for high-quality, patient-centered care, I am grateful for the lessons, knowledge, and skills learned, the experiences gained, and the growth opportunities that have shaped me into the physician I am today.

Chapter 34
The Neurology Ward

1 Neurological Assessment, Airway, Ventilation, and Sedation

1. Mental status is made up of **arousal** or consciousness (wakefulness) and **awareness** (ability to understand and follow commands). For coma patients, we need to assess **responsiveness** (Glasgow Coma Scale), **muscle tone** and **reflexes**, and check labs including serum chemistries, CBC, coagulation, EtoH, ABG, urinalysis (UA), urine toxicology, CXR, CT head.
2. **Neurological exam**: level of consciousness, brain stem assessment, evaluation of motor tone and reflexes (asymmetry?), appraisal of breathing patterns, motor and sensory exams, NIHSS.
3. **Brainstem assessment**: **pupillary** pinpoint raises concern for pontine damage (additional causes include stroke, drug overdose, or organophosphate poisoning); large pupil unreactive indicates midbrain damage or **CN III compression** while dilated reactive pupils indicate pretectal lesions and stimulants like cocaine and methamphetamine, and hallucinogens. **Corneal** reflex (CNV and CN VII) can be performed with a normal saline drop. Eye movement-spontaneous, oculocephalic reflex (side rotation checks CN III, VI, and VIII while flexion and extension examine CN III, IV, and VIII; Doll's eyes caution C-spine instability). **Vestibulo-ocular reflex (VOR)**; cold caloric testing is partial VOR and checks for CN III and medial longitudinal fasciculus. **Cough reflex** (checks CNX). **Gag reflex** (checks CN IX and X).
4. **Breathing**: neurogenic hyperventilation—lesion over midbrain and pons. Cluster (Biot) breathing—lesion over pons. Ataxic breathing—lesion over medulla.
5. **Unstable cervical spine**, enlist expert help with additional stabilization at the shoulder. If a difficult airway is anticipated, call for help.

K. Zhou, *Internal Medicine Training Notes and Survival Guide*,
https://doi.org/10.1007/978-1-0716-4039-5_34

6. **Brain ischemia**: avoid hypotension and hyperventilation, bolus fluid before intubation, ketamine or etomidate is preferred for induction, and maintain normocapnia.
7. Elevation of bed to 30°, preoxygenation with high flow nasal cannula oxygen or nonrebreather mask before intubation.
8. **Indications for intubation**: oxygenation, ventilation, or airway protection failure, and anticipated neurological or cardiopulmonary decline. A **GCS score ≤ 8** is also an indication for endotracheal **intubation**. **Induction** with ketamine 2 mg/kg, etomidate, or propofol. **Paralytic** agents: succinylcholine 1.5 mg/kg, rocuronium 1.2 mg/kg, propofol 2 mg/kg each.
9. **Glidoscope intubation**. (1) Induction: give propofol 100–150 mg → give paralytic rocuronium 36–60 mg (induction time 60–90 s) or succinylcholine 80–100 mg (30 s). (2) Feel the lash, ask to see movement or not → tilt head and neck, widely open mouth, bagging to see air in the face. (3) Bagging if CO_2 increases and to maintain SO_2. (4) Put glidoscope (C shape) in the center of the tongue and mouth, pull up → slide the tube along the C-shape glidoscope, see, and put in. Once in, inject 5 cc (half) air to secure → bagging → start low tidal volume ventilation at 6–8 mL/kg predicted body weight (PBW) and set cuff pressure to 20–30 cmH_2O.
10. **Rapid sequence induction**: Pre-oxygenation, pretreatment medications, induction with sedation, muscle relaxation agents, intubation, primary and secondary confirmation, and post-intubation ventilator management. Pretreatment medications are used to mitigate reflex sympathetic responses like an increase in intracranial blood pressure; they may include lidocaine 1.5 mg/kg 60–90 s before intubation and fentanyl 2–3 mg/kg 30–60 s before intubation. Paralytic agent succinylcholine (45 s before intubation) or rocuronium (60 s before intubation) is usually given immediately after or simultaneously with induction agents.
11. **Rapid sequence intubation agents**: etomidate, drug of choice for elevated intracranial pressure (ICP); propofol is a vasodilator; thiopental is a vasodilator, decreases cerebral metabolic rate of O_2 (MRO2); ketamine with concurrent sedation is safe in ICP elevation; succinylcholine is a type of depolarizing neuromuscular blocker via binding postsynaptic cholinergic receptors and it can increase ICP.
12. Ventilation, target $SO_2 > 94\%$, target premorbid pCO_2, pH 7.3–7.4, **hyperventilation only for herniation to prevent lung injury**.
13. **Goals**: no hypoxia $PO_2 > 300$ mmHg, provide FiO_2 at 0.5 to keep SO_2 above 94%. PCO_2 lowest to 20 mmHg if hyperventilation.
14. **Hemodynamic** goals in brain injury patients with ventilation: intracranial pressure (ICP) < 23 mmHg, mean arterial pressure (MAP) 80–110, cranial perfusion pressure (CPP = MAP − ICP) between 60 and 70 mmHg.
15. **Sedation meds**: propofol, and benzodiazepines (BZDs) like midazolam, dexmedetomidine, and barbiturates decrease ICP, whereas **fentanyl or remifentanil may increase ICP**. Analgosedation with fentanyl or remifentanil (if possible, avoid sedatives like propofol dexmedetomidine) should be considered

as a first-line measure in intubated patients for sedation and analgesia. **Daily sedation interruption** should be performed except deep sedation in patients with increased intracranial pressure, refractory seizures, and neuromuscular blockade use.

16. Prolonged infusion of **lorazepam** can cause **metabolic acidosis** and prolong ICU stay.
17. If intubation is unsuccessful, try supraglottic airway with **laryngeal mask airway**; if still unsuccessful, try **emergent cricothyroidotomy**.
18. **Succinylcholine** should be avoided in longstanding neuromuscular **weakness** or disuse **atrophy** as it can cause **hyperkalemia**.
19. **Succinylcholine** causes **malignant hyperthermia** and **hyperkalemia**. **Valproic acid** concentration can be drastically decreased with the use of **meropenem**.
20. When using neuromuscular blocking agents like **cisatracurium**, continuous infusion of **midazolam** and **fentanyl** is needed to achieve adequate sedation and analgesia. The use of cisatracurium requires monitoring the **train of four** with a peripheral nerve stimulator to monitor the degree of **paralysis**.
21. Sedation and analgesic weaning: wean each agent by about **25%** per day; phenobarbital causes cardiorespiratory suppression.
22. **Propofol is the preferred drug** to control ICP over 24–48 h in TBI ventilated patients.

2 Neuromuscular Emergencies

1. **Bulbar** (lower motor neuron disease) and **pseudobulbar** (upper motor neuron disease, also affect cranial nerves V, VII) palsy affect cranial nerves IX, X, and XII. Check the Gag reflex, tongue, speech, and jaw jerk. **Bulbar palsy**: fascicular Gag reflex, unilateral raspy voice, tongue atrophy and fasciculation, bilateral nasal voice, and normal jaw jerk response. **Pseudobulbar palsy**: increased Gag reflex, spastic tongue, increased jaw jerk, spastic dysarthria.
2. **Acute non-traumatic weakness etiology**: glucose, PO4, CPK, and PTH; multiple sclerosis (MS), Guillain-Barré syndrome (GBS), myasthenia gravis, botulism, stroke, seizure, **infection**, **acute transverse myelitis**, acute demyelinating encephalomyelitis.
3. Critical abnormal values for bedside pulmonary function tests: vital capacity <20 cc/kg, **maximal inspiratory pressure > −30 cmH$_2$O**, maximal expiratory pressure < 40 cmH$_2$O.
4. **Central nervous system** infection manifestations: fever, headache, altered mentation, meningismus? **Lumbar puncture** stat is needed.
5. Spinal cord compression or ischemia is a neurological emergency.
6. **Myasthenia gravis crisis** management: ICU care, BiPAP, once intubated, stop anticholinesterase (anticholinesterases increase secretions making extubation difficult); may need plasmapheresis, IVIG, high dose corticosteroids.

7. **Myasthenia gravis crisis**: increased generalized and oropharyngeal weakness, respiratory insufficiency worse in supine. Treatment: measurement of **vital capacity q2h** in ICU, wean off ventilator if maximal inspiratory pressure (MIP) also known as negative inspiratory force stronger than **-30 cmH$_2$O, withdrawal of anticholinesterase inhibitors to rule out cholinergic crisis, plasmapheresis or IVIG (still takes days to work), plus high dose steroids**.
8. A **cholinergic crisis** refers to an over-stimulation at a neuromuscular junction from an excess of acetylcholine (ACh) because of the use of anticholinesterase medications like edrophonium (Tensilon) or organophosphate.
9. **Intubation for airway protection**: oropharyngeal weakness, diaphragmatic weakness. **Assessment of muscle**: atrophy, fasciculation?
10. **GBS** with rapid progressive respiratory failure requires rapid sequence intubation and should avoid the use of succinylcholine (rather using rocuronium); GBS may require pressor support because of autonomic instability.
11. **GBS and MG** on ventilator treatments are **plasmapheresis** or **IVIG**. For MG patients with dyspnea, will need to differentiate cholinergic crisis (intubation necessary) from myasthenic crisis (BiPAP treatment).

3 Acute Ischemic Stroke

1. **Acute ischemic stroke** checklist: vitals, O$_2$ > 94%, determine last known well time, NIHSS, CT without contrast or CT code stroke (includes CT angiography head and neck), labs, **alteplase** (tPA) or **tenecteplase** (TNK). Target blood pressure before starting tPA/TNK is <185/110 mmHg, and after tPA/TNK administration is <180/105 mmHg
2. **Transient ischemic attack (TIA)**, assess ABCD2 score: age > 60, BP > 140/90, clinical features (unilateral = 2), duration (≥60 min = 2), diabetes = 1. **Start aspirin 81–325 mg daily alone if ABCD2 score < 4**; if ≥4, give dual antiplatelet therapy with aspirin and Plavix for 21 days then single agent antiplatelet therapy. If **thrombocytopenia**, only low-dose aspirin may be prescribed. If intracranial **large artery atherosclerosis with stenosis** of 70%–99%, DAPT for 90 days followed by single-agent antiplatelet therapy is recommended.
3. **TIA treatment and workup**: ASA, clopidogrel, or ASA/dipyridamole, in combination with 80 mg Lipitor qd (moderate intensity in age >75), carotid imaging, echo, permissive hypertension, telemetry, consider 30 days ambulatory cardiac monitor, encourage smoking cessation.
4. **IV tPA delivery**: vital q15 min, 0–9 mg/kg (maximal 90 mg), 10% bolus over 1 min, rest given over 1 h infusion. Stop tPA immediately if neurological deterioration (hemorrhagic conversion >60%). **NIH > 20 = 17% intracranial hemorrhage risk after tPA**, needs head CT and interventions to lower intracranial pressure (check with a neurologist) if hemorrhagic transformation.
5. After tPA, TNK, or mechanical thrombectomy, the patient will need **bed rest for 24 h**.

6. If **hemorrhage concerns** (50% mortality rate if it happens) after tPA administration, check PT/PTT, PLT, fibrinogen, type, and screen, and give **cryoprecipitate and platelet** if confirmed hemorrhagic transformation with CT (check with **neurosurgeon**).
7. **Endovascular therapy (intra-arterial thrombectomy)** criteria: give tPA/TNK if eligible, **large vessel occlusion of the internal carotid artery or proximal middle cerebral artery (M1) or possible (benefit unknown) posterior circulation or M2/M3, Alberta Stroke Program Early CT Score (ASPECTS) ≥3, possible also needs NIHSS ≥6**. The therapeutic window for mechanical thrombectomy: ideally **within 6 h** of symptoms onset and may be up to **24 h**.
8. If tPA/TNK is administered, no anticoagulation or antiplatelet for 24 h before **repeating CT head without contrast**; avoid indwelling urinary catheters, nasogastric tube, and intra-arterial catheters for **4 h after tPA/TNK administration**.
9. tPA/TNK requires the last known well time within a 3–4.5 h therapeutic window. Exclusion criteria for tPA/TNK: blood glucose <50, active bleeding, history of intracranial hemorrhage, **NIHSS > 25, major head trauma or prior stroke in the previous 3 months**.
10. Stroke imaging: **DWI** shows the high-intensity signal of stroke within 3–30 min and lasts 6 h–4 weeks; **DWI-FLAIR mismatch** indicates stroke time < 4.5 h and is a candidate for tPA. Development of **hyperintense** signal on FLAIR is a sign of **vasogenic edema** which typically happens after 4.5 h since the onset of stroke. CT perfusion and MRI **DWI with FLAIR** (rapid tests for stroke of unknown duration) for endovascular procedures (mechanical thrombectomy vs tPA or both) 6–24 h after stroke.
11. Hyperdensity of artery (**dense artery sign**) on non-contrast CT = **ischemic stroke**, indicates embolic or atherosclerotic occlusion of an artery, usually middle cerebral artery (MCA), posterior cerebral artery (PCA), vertebral artery, or basilar artery. **CT angiography (CTA) spot sign** is a sign of intracerebral hemorrhage.
12. **ASPECTS score** (total 10) is used for MCA stroke: caudate, lentiform nucleus (pallidum + putamen), internal capsule, M1-3, M4-6, insular cortex. Striatum = caudate + lentiform nucleus. Every region's involvement is counted as **−1**. ASPECTS score of **≤7** indicates poor prognosis in 3 months with high risks for hemorrhage and more likely to benefit from thrombolysis. ASPECTS score ≤4 indicates a high risk for symptomatic hemorrhage and mortality.

4 Acute Hemorrhagic Stroke

1. **Acute hemorrhagic stroke** includes intracranial hemorrhage (ICH) and subarachnoid hemorrhage (SAH).
2. Intracranial hemorrhage (ICH) etiologies: chronic **hypertension** (bleeding usually happens at basal ganglia, pons, thalamus, and cerebellum), cerebral

amyloid angiopathy (bleeding usually happens at the medium sized blood vessels and lobar areas of the brain, common in >70 years old), **coagulopathy**, vascular anomalies, sympathomimetic drugs (cocaine and methamphetamine). **BP control** target 140–180 mmHg for systolic in acute hemorrhagic stroke. **Reverse anticoagulation** if INR > 1.4, **consult neurosurgery**. Use **labetalol** and **nicardipine** but not nitroprusside in blood pressure (BP) control.

3. **ICH complications**: herniation with brain stem compromise, airway compromise, hematoma expansion, increased intracranial pressure, secondary brain injuries of seizures, fever, and hyperglycemia.
4. **Coagulopathy reversal**: antiplatelet—consider DDAVP (0.4 mg/kg) but not platelet (PLT) transfusion unless neurosurgery if the patient is taking antiplatelet agents. Rivaroxaban, apixaban can be reversed with andexanet alfa (Andexxa) or prothrombin complex concentrate **(PCC, Kcentra) 30 iu/kg**. Protamine for the last dose low molecular weight heparin (LMWH) < 8 h or heparin <2 h in ICH. NOAC management in acute hemorrhagic stroke: **idarucizumab** for dabigatran, **andexanet alfa** for Xarelto and Eliquis; Kcentra, and less commonly emergent dialysis, or rVIIa 80 ug/kg or FEIBA (factor VIII inhibiting bypass agent). **Warfarin reversal** with vitamin K and PCC in intracranial hemorrhage. If oral anticoagulant was taken less than **2 h** ago, consider **charcoal** (50 mg).
5. **Neurosurgery indications**: bleeding in cerebellum >3 cm, decline in neuro exam, supratentorial ICH with mass effects or compressing effects, or hydrocephalus. The best time window for neurosurgery was reported to be **7–24 h** after ictus.
6. **ICH** in the basal ganglia including putamen, lobar ICH, or thalamic ICH is considered as **supratentorial**.
7. **Hematoma expansion** occurs in close to 40% of patients with ICH during the first 12 h. Routine seizure prophylaxis at the moment is not recommended in ICH unless active seizures during hospitalization. **ICH with a GCS <8** should be treated with an emergent external ventricular drain (EVD) to keep ICP <22 mmHg. Goal cerebral perfusion pressure is between 50 and 70 mmHg.
8. ABC/2 method for **estimating ICH hematoma volume**. If the hematoma area on the slide is about 25%–75%, this slide is considered half a hemorrhage slice. If <25%, the slice is not considered a hemorrhage slice.
9. Prophylaxis heparin should be started **1–4 days** after hospitalization when hemostasis has been documented (check with a neurosurgeon or neurologist before ordering as it varies in clinical practice) in ICH patients. A **CTA spot sign** is defined as unifocal or multifocal contrast enhancement with contrast CT; a CTA spot sign indicates acute intracerebral hemorrhage.
10. **Lumbar puncture** may be performed if CT head is negative for SAH but history suggests it: **xanthochromia** takes ≥12 h to develop, and does not clear with time.
11. **SAH**: neurosurgical consultation; CT/CT Angiogram head for aneurysm. **Need bed rest**, **nimodipine** 60 mg po q4h (via NG tube), transcranial doppler, seizure prophylaxis (controversial as phenytoin causes poor cognitive outcome in

SAH; Keppra use data are limited) for a **short period until** the **aneurysm** is secured; **reverse coagulopathy** (goal platelet ≥50,000); treat pain and anxiety; target **sBP <160 mmHg** or MAP <110 mmHg, fentanyl use; no nitroprusside which increases intracranial pressure (ICP); has **a rebleed risk of 8%–23% in the first 72 h** after the SAH, with a mortality rate of ≤60%; consider external ventricular drain (EVD) for hydrocephalus → transfer to neural care unit (may benefit from hypertonic saline infusion or mannitol 1 g/kg IV).

12. Causes of **neurological decline** in SAH: **re-bleed** risk 12%–15% in the first 24 h, acute hydrocephalus, seizure, cardiopulmonary complications (neurogenic pulmonary edema/cardiomyopathy; cardiovascular collapse may indicate cerebral herniation).
13. If there is an unavoidable delay in the **obliteration of aneurysm** and the patient is free of recent MI, DVT, pulmonary embolism, or any other hypercoagulable state, administer a **time-limited course (<72 h) of antifibrinolytic agent (TXA)** until the aneurysm is secured.

5 Elevated Intracranial Pressure and Brain Herniation

1. Elevated intracranial pressure (ICP) diagnosis: **ICP >22 mmHg sustained for 5 min**. **Cerebral perfusion pressure** = MAP−ICP. Cushing's triad = increased sBP (widened pulse pressure), bradycardia, irregular respirations.
2. Increased ICP causes herniation: **subfalcine** (cingulate, frontal lobe), **uncal** (temporal lobe), **central** (tentorial), **tonsillar**, upwards **transtentorial** (cerebellar lesion) herniations.
3. **Herniation symptoms**: pupillary dilation, unequal pupils, posturing, **Cushing** response (hypertension, bradycardia, irregular respiration).
4. Clinical signs and symptoms of **increased ICP** or **herniation**: headache (HA) → Glasgow Coma Scale (GCS) scores decrease; irritability, ipsilateral change of eye, vomiting, photophobia, nystagmus, diplopia, lethargy, and seizure. **Contralateral pupillary size** change and ipsilateral hemiparesis (**Kernohan notch phenomenon** from midbrain compression on the opposite side).
5. **ICP waves**: P2 (intracranial compliance wave) >P1 (normal arterial pulsation wave) indicates poor compliance and impending herniation.
6. **Elevated ICP treatments**: consider ABC, avoid hypotension and hypoxia, head of bed >30° with head midline; if brain tumor, add steroids in cerebral edema. Consider **mannitol** (0.5–1 g/kg + serum Osm q4–6h), or hypertonic saline (check Na 4–6 h); may benefit from brief (<2 h) hyperventilation (goal $PaCO_2$ of 30–35 mmHg). Consult neurosurgery stat for possible placement of external ventricular drain (EVD) and surgical decompression. If ineffective and not responding, consider **sedation on continuous EEG**, hyperventilation (goal $PaCO_2$ 25–30 mmHg), hypothermia (32–34°) with brain O_2 monitoring <6 h, and revisiting goals of care.

7. **Osmolarity > 320 or osmolar gap > 20** indicates no benefit from mannitol but rather kidney injury from mannitol.
8. **Serum Na** can be increased to up to **160 mEq/L**; **propofol** is the preferred sedation in intracranial pressure control for sedation as it decreases the cerebral metabolic rate of O_2 consumption.
9. **Prolonged hyperventilation** can cause brain ischemia in intracranial hemorrhage and bleeding.
10. Mannitol dosage **1 g/kg IV piggy bag over 5–15 min** (usually followed by 1 L of normal saline to prevent side effects) with goal for osmolar gap **<20 mOsm/**kg; hypertonic **saline 30 mL with IV push over 10–20 min** with goal serum Na < **160 mEq**/L. Hypertonic saline causes pulmonary edema, coagulopathy, metabolic acidosis, thrombophlebitis (if peripheral iv infusion), and osmolar demyelinating syndrome if corrected rapidly and requires taper once improved.
11. **Traumatic brain injury (TBI) with herniation concerns**: BP 95/43, given 150 ml 3% NS over 10 min or 23.4% NS as 30 cc IV over 2 min; an alternative is to give 20% mannitol at 1 g/kg IV bolus. Brief (<2 h) hyperventilation with goal $PaCO_2$ of 30–35 mmHg may also be appropriate.
12. Glasgow Coma Scale (GCS) <8 is **severe TBI**; GCS 9–12 is **moderate TBI**; GCS 13–15 is **mild TBI**.
13. Moderate traumatic brain injury (TBI) should be admitted to the neuro ICU with trauma and neurosurgery services, and be monitored with hourly neurological examination. Moderate-severe TBI requires hourly neurological checks with emphasis on **GCS and pupillary examination** together with repeat head CT in 6 h.
14. At risk for herniation, **hyperventilation with** a **respiratory rate of 20** is appropriate.
15. **TBI target goals**: O_2 and BP, SO_2 > 90%, sBP > 110 mmHg for 15–49 yo and >70 yo, >100 mmHg for 50–69 yo. PLT >100, $PaCO_2$ 35–40.
16. **Prophylaxis regimen in TBI for seizur**e: phenytoin 20 mg/kg load then daily doses, fosphenytoin, or Keppra, stop after 7 days.
17. **Hemorrhagic cerebral contusions** are usually seen in the frontal or anterior temporal lobes ("salt and pepper" appearance with mixed density of blood on CT head).
18. CT or MRI **angiography/venography** indications: penetrating head injury, venous sinus injury, neurological symptoms not explained by CT head, select C-spine injuries with concerns for vascular damage, petrous bone fracture, Le Fort II and III facial fracture, vascular damage in intracranial hemorrhage.
19. **Neurosurgery indications**: acute subdural hematoma (SDH) >**10 mm** thickness or >5 mm midline shift, acute epidural hemorrhage >**30 cm^3** or >**15 mm** thickness or >**5 mm** midline shift, cerebellar hemorrhage with mass effects, cerebral contusions with intracranial hemorrhage and >**5 mm** midline shift or herniation.

6 Meningitis and Encephalitis

1. Lumbar Puncture (LP) with four tubes of cerebral fluid collection: **tube 1**—RBC and WBC with differential; **tube 2**—protein, glucose, lactate; **tube 3**—gram stain, antigens, cultures, Indian ink if fungal infection suspected, Herpes simplex PCR, IgM for viruses; **tube 4** is a repeat of tube 1. Normal LP opening pressure <20 cmH_2O, WBC <5, Pr <50, glucose/serum glucose >2/3. **Fungal and tuberculous meningitis** have significantly high protein in CSF.
2. **Herpes encephalitis**: temporal lobe edema with hemorrhagic transformation. Herpes encephalitis can have changes in mood, personality, or behavior on top of typical fever, headache, confusion, and possible seizure.
3. **Abscess of the brain management**: metronidazole, ceftriaxone/cefepime, vancomycin, neurosurgery consult.
4. Vancomycin and **TMP-SMX** can be used in patients with severe penicillin allergy (aztreonam can be used for G−).
5. Fever, headache, hallucinations, and altered mental status indicate possible **viral encephalitis**, need to order acyclovir 10 mg/kg **ideal body weight** q8h IV.
6. Treatment for **bacterial meningitis**: ceftriaxone 2 g iv q12h + vancomycin 15–20 mg/kg iv q12h (if alcoholic or >50 yo or immunocompromised, add ampicillin 2 g q4h), steroid **dexamethasone** 10 mg IV q6h × 4 days must be started before or with first dose antibiotics. Add **acyclovir** IV if unsure about herpes meningitis status.
7. 95% of patients with **meningitis** have at least two out of the following four symptoms: **fever, neck stiffness or pain, altered mentation, and headache**.
8. TMP-SMX is used for **PJP infection, toxoplasmosis, listeriosis, and nocardiosis**, especially if penicillin allergies.

7 Targeted Temperature Management

1. **Targeted temperature management** (TTM) indications: comatose patients who achieve a return of spontaneous circulation (ROSC) after cardiac arrest; goal temperature: 32–34 °C, or 36 °C.
2. **Absolute contraindications** for TTM: rapid neurological recovery; illness that precludes meaningful recovery; contraindications for ICU admission; greater than 12 h following arrest.
3. Phases of **therapeutic hypothermia**: (A) initiation-start cooling immediately, analgesia/sedation, recognize and treat shivering; (B) maintenance- close monitoring of blood pressure, O_2, volume, glucose, K, seizures (continuous EEG is recommended in all TTM); (C) rewarming, begin 24 h after induction at a controlled slow rate of 0.2–0.5 °C/h, monitor blood pressure, electrolytes, and glucose.

4. **Common complications or physiological changes of TTM**: bradycardia (use beta agonist), arrhythmia (happens if T < 33 °C), and cold diuresis with electrolyte disturbances, coagulopathy, and insulin resistance. Serum K 3.0–3.5 is acceptable in TTM. **Arterial blood gas in TTM requires temperature corrections**.
5. After the return of spontaneous circulation (ROSC) following cardiac arrest, start cooling as rapidly as possible to **32–34** °C **or 36** °C **for 24 h**.
6. Acceptable sites for **temperature monitoring** in TTM: endovascular via **pulmonary artery** (PA) catheter, **bladder** via Foley, **rectum**, esophagus (continuous)
7. Start TTM, check **cEEG** in patients with seizure or paralyzed; **CT head** (5% post-cardiac arrest patient with intracranial hemorrhage) to rule out intracranial hemorrhage.
8. **Sedation**: stable, use **propofol**; unstable, use **midazolam**. **Analgesia and sedation dual purposes**: fentanyl or remifentanil infusions.
9. **Shivering control**: sedation → analgesia → buspirone, **meperidine**, IV **magnesium** → propofol, midazolam → neuromuscular blockade. Baire Hugger.
10. The target of **36° in TTM is** preferable to 32° in surgical bleeding, ICH, and hemorrhagic diathesis.
11. Antishivering medications for therapeutic temperature management: **Meperidine** is good at controlling shivering. **Buspirone** 30 mg q8h, and **magnesium** target 3–4 can also be used for **anti-shivering**.
12. To counter shivering, schedule an **antipyretic** agent (acetaminophen or NSAID) every 4–6 h around the clock, **buspirone** 30 mg q8h, iv **magnesium** sulfate to maintain a serum magnesium level of 3–4 mg/dL, and **skin counterwarming** using a heated (maximum of 43 °C) forced-air blanket.
13. **Dexmedetomidine** has addictive anti-shiver effects when used together with **meperidine**.

8 Acute Spinal Cord Injuries

1. Etiologies for spinal cord injuries include **cancer, infection, and trauma**.
2. Cancers of the breast (21%), lung (19%), prostate (7.5%), renal (5%), gastrointestinal (4.5%), thyroid (2.5%) and lymphoma commonly **metastasize to the spine**. Around 10% of patients with primary multiple myeloma (MM) and osteosarcoma present with **extramedullary disease**.
3. Cranial and spinal nerve dysfunction can also be due to **leptomeningeal metastases** which require lumbar puncture with fluid analyses and have a poor prognosis.
4. Abnormalities involving **continuous two vertebral bodies** and disc space = consider **infection as the cause**.
5. **Neoplastic epidural spinal cord compression** treatment: give dexamethasone 10 mg iv once now followed by 4–6 mg iv q6h. **Stat neurosurgery and**

radiation oncology consults; if surgical candidates with an expected survival of at **least 3 months**, initial **decompressive surgery followed by radiation** improves the probability of ambulation compared to radiation alone.

6. **Spinal cord injury without radiographic abnormality (SCIWORA)**: Young patients are at high risk for spinal cord injury (SCI), even with negative radiographic abnormalities on CT.
7. SCIWORA treatment: non-surgical but **spinal motion restriction with collars, braces, or orthosis for up to 3 months**. SCIWORA is most commonly seen in children at the cervical spinal cord and may have transient or persistent neurological symptoms.
8. **Quadriplegia**: ensure proper ventilation, airway, motor, sensation, sphincter. Airway-respiratory function.
9. **Acute myelopathy** of numbness and weakness in both of her legs requires urgent lumbar puncture with cerebrospinal fluid analyses.
10. **Nontraumatic hemorrhage in the spinal cord or canal**: myelitis, vascular malformation, spinal tumors, coagulopathy, syringomyelia. Diagnosis via MRI spine with contrast.
11. **Restrict spinal motion in a collar** if ambulation or intoxication, focal midline bony pain/tenderness, focal neurological deficit/symptoms, or distracting non-spine traumatic injury.
12. **Neurogenic shock** with traumatic spinal cord injury above the **T6** level pathophysiology: **sympathectomy** (sympathetic preganglionic neurons in T1 through L2–3) resulting in **unopposed vagal tone** leading to hypotension, warm dry skin, bradycardia; it's a diagnosis of exclusion.
13. **Spinal shock** refers to the loss of the spinal reflexes below the level of injury. It happens hours to days after SCI and lasts 1–3 weeks. It usually has pink and warm skin.
14. During the complete head-to-toe evaluation in trauma patients, look for **step-offs of vertebra, areas of focal tenderness, and priapism**.
15. **Cervical spine clearance** requires a cervical spine CT scan if any of the following: intoxicated? focal neurological deficit? altered level of consciousness? distracting injury? posterior tenderness to palpation? (these five criteria in combination are called the **Nexus criteria**)
16. **Canadian cervical spine rule**s for cervical spine clearance: if age > 65 years old, dangerous mechanism, or paresthesia in extremities, order cervical spine CT scan. Additionally, if **unable to sit in the emergency department or walk at any time, dangerous trauma etiology, or delayed neck pain**, order a cervical spine CT scan. Lastly, if the patient is unable to actively **rotate the neck 45 degrees** to left and right, order a cervical spine CT scan.
17. **Treatments for spinal cord injury**: decompression of the spinal cord; surgical stabilization of unstable ligaments and bony injury; minimizing secondary complications; treatment of neurogenic bowel and bladder; stress ulcer and venous thromboembolism (VTE) prophylaxis; no neuroprotective drugs and no steroids necessary.

18. **Mean arterial pressure (MAP) for spinal cord injury** should be 85–90 mmHg for 7 days after spinal cord injury.

9 Status Epilepticus

1. **Etiologies of seizure**: hypoxia, hypertensive emergency, autoimmune encephalitis, paraneoplastic (brain tumors), electrolyte disturbance, renal failure, CNS infection, stroke, intracranial hemorrhage (ICH), traumatic brain injury (TBI), drugs, or cardiac arrest.
2. Status epilepticus is defined as **5 min of continuous seizing or ≥2 discrete seizures between which there is incomplete recovery of consciousness.**
3. Drugs **that lower seizure threshold** include theophylline, imipenem, high-dose penicillin G, cefepime, quinolones, metronidazole, isoniazid, tricyclic antidepressants (TCAs), bupropion, lithium, clozapine, flumazenil, cyclosporine, lidocaine, bupivacaine, and others.
4. **Classification of status epilepticus**: **generalized convulsive** status epilepticus (GCSE); **focal motor** status epilepticus; **myoclonic** status epilepticus (MSE); **absence** status epilepticus.
5. Urgent treatments for **status epilepticus**: lorazepam **0.1 mg**/kg iv (maximal single dose **4 mg**, usually give the maximal dose in seizure), clonazepam 1 mg IV, can repeat once at 3–5 min; midazolam 10 mg IM, diazepam PR 10–20 mg. **Levetiracetam**: **40–60 mg/kg** as a single with a maximal maintenance dose of 1500 mg bid can also be used.
6. If seizure continues, in addition to the above, **fosphenytoin** 20 mg/kg IV at up to 150 mg/min; **phenytoin** 20 mg PE/kg iv (im), may give additional 5 mg/kg; **phenobarbital** 20 mg/kg IV, may give additional 5–10 mg/kg; and/or **levetiracetam** 1–3 g IV. If **status epilepticus** continues, start **intubation** and **ventilator management** with **midazolam** for refractory patients (order continuous EEG meanwhile). Midazolam load 0.2 mg/kg, maintenance dose 0.05–2 mg/kg/h.
7. For treatment of **nonconvulsive status epilepticus (NCSE)**: lorazepam 0.1 mg/kg (max 4 mg at a time) combined with one of the following: fosphenytoin at 20 mg/kg, valproate 40 mg/kg, Keppra 2500 mg IV over 15 min, or lacosamide 400 mg over 15 min.
8. **Status epilepticus** treatments: midazolam, lorazepam, diazepam ⇒ consider fosphenytoin, phenytoin, or valproic acid ⇒ consider continuous EEG, phenobarbital, propofol, or midazolam. Intubation and ventilation management are necessary if unresponsive.
9. Side effects: **midazolam causes prolonged sedation** especially in liver and kidney disease as well as tachyphylaxis (rapidly diminishing response to continuous doses) within 24–48 h. **Propofol causes hypotension** and **propofol infusion syndrome**. **Pentobarbital** causes severe **hypotension**, gastric stasis, and metabolic acidosis with a long half-life.

10. **Long-acting anti-epileptic drugs** (AED): fosphenytoin, Vimpat (Lacosamide), and Keppra are good options for chronic seizure treatments.
11. **Non-epileptic spells**: conscious patient with purposeful movements but poorly coordinated thrashing (volitional behavioral problems or non-volitional somatization disorders) in seizure patients.
12. **Pyridoxine (vitamin B6)** deficiency is a cause for seizures in children.
13. **Diazepam** and **lorazepam** contain propylene glycol which causes hypotension and metabolic acidosis. **Midazolam** can be given intramuscularly. **Phenobarbital** causes ileus, immunosuppression, cardiotoxicity, and hemodynamic instability.

Further Readings and References

1. Venkatasubramanian, C., Lopez, G.A., O'Phelan, K.H. et al. 2020. Emergency neurological life support: Fourth Edition, Updates in the approach to early management of a neurological emergency. Neurocrit Care 32, 636–640.
2. Lopez G. A., Venkatasubramanian C. 2019. Emergency Neurological Life Support (ENLS) Version 4.0. Manuscript. Neurocritical Care Society.
3. Greenberg SM, Ziai WC, Cordonnier C, et al. 2022. Guideline for the management of patients with spontaneous intracerebral hemorrhage: a guideline from the american heart association/american stroke association. Stroke. 53(7):e282–e361.
4. Further learning course: Emergency Neurological Life Support (ENLS) Version 5.0. https://learn.neurocriticalcare.org/courses.

Chapter 35
Advanced EKG for Hospitalist

1 General Sequence in EKG Readings

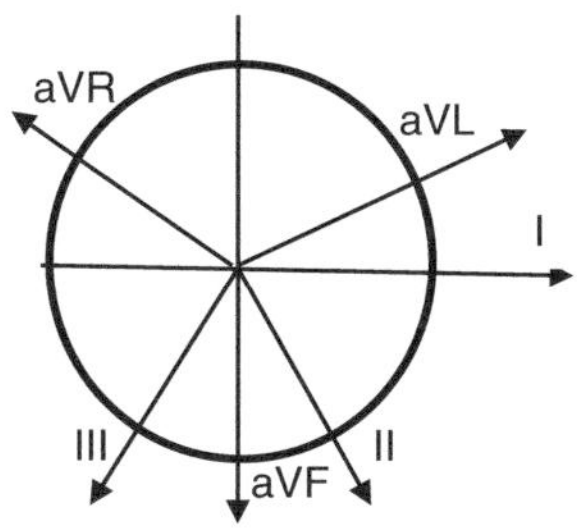

1. **System approach for EKG: rate, rhythm, intervals, axis, chamber enlargement, PQRST waves.**
2. **EKG reading sequence**: Waveforms, duration, amplitude, morphology. Morphology (P, QRS, J, T waves), intervals, QTc < ½ RR intervals, J point (beginning of repolarization), TP segment is the reference point (isoelectric point of recording).
3. 12 Lead EKG: **Standard or bipolar limb leads**: I, II, III. **Augmented or unipolar limb leads** aVR, aVL, aVF. **Precordial leads**: V1-6. **Rhythm leads**: V1, II, V5; V1 and II have prominent P wave
4. Einthoven's Law: lead I + lead III = lead II; aVR + aVL + aVF = 0.
5. First event is left to right depolarization of the interventricular septum → consider simultaneous depolarization of left and right ventricles.
6. **Rate**: heart rate (HR) = 300/# of big boxes between beats, irregular ventricular rhythm uses 10 s rule × 6 is HR. Five boxes is 1 s.
7. **Axis**: normal −30°– +90°. A QRS axis that lies between +180 and +270 is called an "extreme axis" or "superior axis".

K. Zhou, *Internal Medicine Training Notes and Survival Guide*,
https://doi.org/10.1007/978-1-0716-4039-5_35

8. **Determining axis**: *Quadrant approach*: looks at lead I and aVF. If QRS in lead I is + and aVF is −, assess QRS in lead II [predominantly positive = normal axis (−30° to 0°); predominantly negative = LAD (−90° to −30°)]. *Equiphasic approach*: identify the equiphasic lead → determine lead 90° (second lead) away from the most equiphasic lead; if QRS in the second lead is positive, the second lead direction is the QRS axis; if negative, QRS axis is 180° away from the direction of the second lead.
9. **Indeterminate axis**: when all limb leads have equiphasic QRS, low voltage, poor R wave progression, tall P waves, and unusual axis, commonly seen in COPD.
10. Enlargement vs. hypertrophy: atrial enlargement, ventricular hypertrophy.
11. **P wave** axis normal +30° to +75°; >75° = consider RAE; <30° = consider LAE. Lead II is a great place to look for changes in atrial enlargement. Right atrial enlargement (RAE) > **2.5 mm** in inferior leads; left atrial enlargement (LAE) > **110 ms in any lead**. Normally, the P wave in **V1 is biphasic** (one small box for atrial enlargement assessment). P wave is usually **upright in leads I and II, inverted in lead aVR**.
12. Ventricular hypertrophy: bundle of His then depolarization of ventricles, look at the precordial leads; **V1** (tall R plus right axis deviation in right ventricular hypertrophy) **and V6** (tall R plus left axis deviation in left ventricular hypertrophy) **for ventricular hypertrophy**.
13. Right ventricular hypertrophy (RVH) is associated with poor R wave progression; left ventricular hypertrophy (LVH) is associated with delayed intrinsic deflection of ≥50 ms (normal <50 ms).
14. **Criteria for LVH**: dominant S wave in V1 + dominant R wave in V5 or V6 ≥ 35 mm
15. **Criteria for RVH**: dominant R wave (>7 mm) in V1 and dominant S wave (>7 mm) in V5 or V6.

2 Sinoatrial Node Dysfunction

1. Sinus node dysfunction: intrinsic dysfunction (treatment: pacemaker) vs. extrinsic causes. **Causes of sinus node dysfunction**: degenerative fibrosis, cardiomyopathy, increased parasympathetic tone (usually during the day time, not on drugs, minimal to no variation during physical activities).
2. **Sinus node dysfunction categories**: sinus bradycardia, sinus pause or arrest (not a multiply of PP interval), sinoatrial exit block (first, second, and third degree), and alternating bradycardia with atrial tachycardia (tachycardia-bradycardia syndrome). Diagnosis: ambulatory EKG monitoring and pacemaker.
3. **Sinus pause or arrest**: no P waves and associated QRS-T, sometimes followed by junctional rhythm or idioventricular rhythm. If <3 s, no need for investigation or treatment. While many regard sinus pause as the same as sinus arrest, some differentiate between sinus pause (<2 s) and arrest (≥2 s).

4. **Sinoatrial exit block (first, second, and third degree):** First-degree block refers to slow transmission but still 1:1 conduction and thus not detectable on surface EKG. Second-degree Type I (Wenckebach type) refers to progressively decreasing P-P intervals followed by a dropped P wave (not a multiply of PP interval); second-degree Type II refers to intermittently dropped P waves with a constant interval (a multiply of PP interval). Third-degree block refers to a lack of sinus impulse conduction to the right atrium leading to long sinoatrial pauses or arrest.
5. Variants of **SA nodal dysfunction**: (A) sinus arrhythmia (variation of PP interval >.12 s, common with digoxin or morphine); (B) wandering atrial pacemaker.
6. Sinus node arrest and prolonged asystole cause syncope. In significant structural heart disease, if a junctional or idioventricular escape rhythm does not promptly emerge in sinus node arrest and prolonged asystole, syncope happens (sinus pause is not a multiply of PP interval).

3 Repolarization Abnormalities and STEMI

1. **Primary** repolarization abnormalities refer to ST and T wave (ventricular repolarization from epicardium to endocardium) abnormalities in the absence of depolarization (QRS) abnormalities, seen in ischemia, myocarditis, drugs, toxins, and electrolyte abnormalities, particularly abnormalities of serum calcium and potassium, as well as abrupt change in other physiological conditions.
2. **Secondary repolarization abnormalities** refer to changes of EKG especially ST and T waves from abnormal structure or function of the ventricular depolarization (abnormal QRS wave): downsloping ST segment and T wave inversion, most commonly seen over hypertrophied ventricles, BBB and pre-excitation.
3. STEMI: **ST elevation** [0.2 mV in men (0.15 mV in women) in V2 and V3 and 0.1 mV in other leads] due to myocardial ischemia or infarction usually occurs with reciprocal ST depression in opposite leads in the direction from those with ST elevation. Other causes of ST elevation include early repolarization (a normal variant) and pericarditis.
4. Ischemia: **ST depression** refers to depression ≥0.05 mV (0.5 mm) in leads V2 and V3 and 0.1 mV (1 mm) in all other leads after J-point.
5. **Contiguous leads**: chest leads V1–V6; lateral leads aVL, I, aVR (ie, lead aVR with reversed polarity); inferior leads II, aVF, and III.
6. **Acute occlusive myocardial** infarction EKG changes: hyperacute T wave (minutes to hours) → ST elevation (0–12 h) → Q wave (1–12 h) → ST elevation with T wave inversion in 2–5 days → T wave recovery in weeks to months.
7. **STEMI equivalent: Wellens Syndrome** deeply inverted or biphasic T waves in leads V2–V3; **posterior STEMI:** prominent ST depression in V1-V4.
8. A benign variant called "early repolarization" or "J-point elevation" can result in **concave** upward ST elevations, particularly in V2–V3. STEMI has **convex** ST elevations.

9. **Subtle anterior STEMI (four variable) tool** helps the differentiation of normal variant ST segment elevation in V2–V4 (early repolarization) from subtle left anterior descending coronary occlusion: R-wave amplitude in lead V4 (**RAV4**), ST elevation at 60 ms after the J-point in lead V3 (**STE60V3**), the computerized Bazett-corrected QT interval (**QTc-B**), and QRS amplitude in lead V2 (**QRSV2**); a value of ≥18.2 indicates subtle anterior STEMI.
10. **LBBB or paced rhythm dis-concordance in secondary repolarization (not ischemia)**: ST-T wave changes are typically in the opposite direction as the QRS complex (dis-concordance) in LBBB. ST elevations in leads with prominent QRS complexes: V1-3 +/− II, III, and aVF. ST depressions and T wave inversions in leads with broad R waves: I, aVL, V5-6.
11. **ST-T changes in the same direction as the QRS complex in LBBB** are highly suggestive of a **primary repolarization abnormality** (e.g., ischemia/infarction).
12. **Diagnosis of myocardial infarction in the presence of LBBB**: Abridged Sgarbossa's Criteria: ST elevation ≥1 mm in a lead with a positive QRS complex (I, aVL, V5, V6) OR ST depression ≥1 mm in V1, V2, or V3.
13. **Intrinsicoid deflection (R wave peak time)** is the duration of time from the beginning of the QRS complex to the peak of the R wave. It represents depolarization in the ventricles from the endocardium to the epicardium. It is typically measured in the precordial leads (<35 ms in lead V1 and <45 ms in lead V6). Commonly larger and delayed in BBB and LVH. **Intrinsicoid deflection** in lead II can be used to differentiate SVT (<50 ms) from ventricular tachycardia (>50 ms); it is useful for the diagnosis of supraventricular tachycardia with aberrancy.
14. **Early repolarization:** J onset (Jo), J peak (Jp), J termination (Jt), ST segment slope with reference to the ST segment 100 ms after Jt (interval M). **Early repolarization is present if all of the following**: (1) end-QRS notch or slur on the down-slope of a prominent R wave, (2) Jp is 0.1 mV in 2 or more contiguous leads except V1 to V3; (3) QRS < 120 ms. *Upward-sloping ST –segment followed by an upright T wave together with end QRS notch or slur is benign whereas a horizontal or downward-sloping ST segment is potentially associated with ventricular fibrillation.*

4 Conduction System Blocks

1. **Normal resting HR** is 50–90 bpm; maximum sinus rate = 220 − age. A rate of 130–150 bpm suggests the possibility of atrial flutter with 2:1 AV block.
2. Conduction system: SA node → atria and AV node → Bundle of His → LBB and RBB. LBB → septum and left anterior fascicle and left posterior fascicle.
3. **Left anterior fascicular block (LAFB)**: QRS is normal, LAD, qR in leads I and aVL; **rS in leads II, III, aVF**; intinsicoid deflection in aVL > 45 ms. **Left posterior fascicular block (LPFB)**: QRS normal, RAD, small rS in leads I and

aVL, **qR in leads II, III, aVF**; intrinsicoid deflection in aVF > 45 ms; no additional evidence of RVH.

4. **RBBB**: V1 is M shaped and V6 has S wave; prominent S wave in I and aVL. RBBB severely limits the diagnosis of RVH in EKG.
5. **LBBB:** QRS > 120 ms, broad R wave in leads I, aVL, and V6, lack of q wave in leads I and V6. LBBB limits the ability to diagnose LVH and STEMI.
6. RBBB usually has secondary repolarizations in V1-2. LBBB usually has secondary repolarizations in leads I, aVL, and V6. LBBB also has leads V1-3 displacing deep S waves with upsloping ST elevation and upright prominent T waves.
7. **Lev's disease**: **sclerosis and calcification** of the cardiac skeleton, usually of aortic and mitral rings at the beginning of the conduction system. **Lenegre's disease**: primary **degenerative disease** of the conduction system, young patients. Both Lev's and Lenegre's diseases cause **complete heart block**.
8. Morphology consistent with neither LBBB or RBBB: (1) QRS ≥ 120 ms: non-specific intraventricular conduction delay. (2) QRS < 120 ms: LAFB and LPFB.
9. **Bifascicular** = RBBB + LAFB or LPFB
10. **Type 2 second degree AV block**: PR is constant, and P waves are intermittently blocked at unpredictable intervals, the block is usually distal to the actual AV node and His Bundle (infra-Hisian block), usually associated with a wide QRS complex.
11. AV conduction ratio: 2:1 block second degree AV block often not possible to tell where the level of block is. A narrow QRS complex in a 2:1 block favors an intranodal location, but not always.
12. **Etiologies for prolonged QT** (should be corrected for HR): congenital long QT syndrome, medications (e.g., class Ia, Ic and III antiarrhythmics, antipsychotics, antidepressants, antiemetics, quinolones, macrolides), hypocalcemia, hypothyroidism, hypothermia.

5 Tachyarrhythmias

1. **Tachyarrhythmias etiology**: <u>*accelerated automaticity*, *re-entry*, *and triggered activity*</u>. The rate of automaticity depends on the rate of phase 4 depolarization, maximum negative membrane potential, and threshold potential.
2. **Normal intrinsic rates of pacemaker sites**: SA node 50–90 bpm, atria 40–60 bpm, AV node/junction 40–60 bpm, ventricle 20–40 bpm. When the sinoatrial node fails to work appropriately, atrial/junctional/ventricular **escape rhythms** take over.
3. Inverted before, after, or hidden P wave ahead of narrow complex QRS, regular rhythm, together with HR 40–60 is ***junctional escape rhythm*. Junctional bradycardia:** HR <40. **Accelerated junctional rhythm** (***AJR***, has normal QRS): HR 60–100. **Junctional tachycardia**: HR > 100.

4. ***Accelerated/enhanced automaticity***: enhanced normal automaticity (hypoxia, ischemia, hypokalemia); abnormal automaticity (non-pacemaker cells) seen in CHF, acute ischemia, and or reperfusion.
5. **Enhanced automaticity rhythms** include sinus tachycardia, atrial tachyarrhythmias (accelerated atrial rhythm and paroxysmal atrial tachycardia with block), and accelerated junctional and ventricular rhythms.
6. **Accelerated ventricular rhythm (*AVR*):** abnormal QRS with HR 50–110.
7. **Atrial tachyarrhythmias:** accelerated atrial rhythm (***AAR***), paroxysmal atrial tachycardia with block (digitalis effects), multifocal atrial tachycardia (MAT).
8. **MAT**: irregularly irregular, three or more distinctly different P wave morphologies, and no one predominant P wave morphology; seen in COPD, pneumonia, CHF exacerbation, PE, and theophylline.
9. **Sinus tachycardia:** discrete P wave, short PR interval, and normal QRS duration.
10. ***Reentry*:** fast and slow pathway- macroreentry (atrial flutter, AVRT), microreentry (AFib, intraatrial reentrant tachycardia). Anatomic reentry (e.g., VT around a post-infarct scar) and functional reentry (e.g., Afib).
11. **Sinus node reentry** (similar to sinus tachycardia but abrupt onset), **atrial flutter** (reentrant circuit in the right atrium), **atrial fibrillation** (multiple leading circle reentrant impulses in the left atrium and pulmonary veins), **AV nodal reentry (AVNRT), ventricular reentry** (ventricular tachycardia and ventricular fibrillation).
12. **Atrial flutter**: the most common reentrant pathway of Aflutter is a counterclockwise circuit encircling the right atrium, passing through the cavotricuspid isthmus (i.e., isthmus-dependent flutter). F wave rate up to 300 bpm. (regular, regularly irregular, irregularly irregular)
13. **SVT**: regular, HR 150–200 bpm, can be as slow as 120 or as fast as 250. P waves can come before, after QRS, or not visible at all.
14. **Typical AVNRT** is slow to fast pathway activation with P waves usually buried within or fused with the QRS complex.
15. **Typical AVNRT**—PAC travels through the slow pathway to Bundle of His → (1) QRS wave with long PR interval; (2) Retrograde along the fast pathway then back to the Bundle of His causing another quick QRS with shortened P′ or even buried P′ waves; (3). The cycle repeats becoming AVNRT.
16. **Atypical AVNRT** is fast to slow pathways with a P wave after the QRS complex.
17. **Atypical AVNRT**—QRS wave → action potential travels retrogradely through the slow pathway, delayed retrograde atrial activation with long RP interval; soon later, normal fast pathway generates a different QRS; cycle repeats forming uncommon fast-slow variant of AVNRT.
18. **ST depression in AVNRT or AVRT** does not indicate myocardial ischemia in most patients.
19. Symptoms of **AVNRT** included palpitations, dizziness, chest pain, and even syncope. Treatments of AVNRT include vagal maneuver, adenosine, verapamil, diltiazem, metoprolol or esmolol → consider catheter ablation, and rhythm control medications.

20. **AVRT**: (1) PAC travels anterogradely through the normal pathway to Bundle of His → narrow QRS complex (orthodromic AVRT) with no delta wave → reentry via accessory pathway causing inverted P wave, repeat. (2) PAC travel antegradely through the accessory pathway to Bundle of His → wide QRS complex (antidromic AVRT) → action potential travel retrogradely to Bundle of His and AV node causing retrograde inverted P wave, repeat.
21. Symptoms of **AVRT** include palpitations, syncope, dizziness, chest pain, and dizziness. Treatments include adenosine, verapamil, beta-blockers, procainamide, or flecainide.
22. **Retrograde P** wave following the QRS complex in orthodromic AVRT.
23. ***Triggered activity***: oscillations are called afterdepolarizations; early (phase 2 and 3) vs. delayed (phase 4) afterdepolarizations
24. **Early afterdepolarization** is caused by prolonged action potential (risks increase with slowed HR); Early afterdepolarization activates polymorphic ventricular arrhythmias torsades de pointes (TdP) which is maintained by a reentrant mechanism.
25. **Delayed afterdepolarization** happens in excess intracellular Ca++ (risks increase with increased HR). Delayed afterdepolarization is associated with myocardial ischemia, digoxin toxicity, and catecholaminergic polymorphic ventricular tachycardia.
26. Differentiation among **increased automaticity, reentry, and triggered activity**: effect of a premature stimulus on tachyarrhythmias.
27. **Six basic types of tachyarrhythmias**: sinus tach, AFib, Aflutter, multifocal atrial tachycardia, supraventricular tachycardia (AVNRT, AVRT, atrial tachycardia), ventricular tachycardia (monomorphic vs. polymorphic). **AVNRT** is similar to junctional tachycardia and the treatment option is catheter-based slow pathway modification. **AVRT** = Wolff Parkinson White syndrome.
28. **Tachyarrhythmias differentiation** (the six questions): rate, regularity, QRS complex, atrial activity, the relationship between P and QRS waves, gradual or abrupt, or rate changes.
29. Evidence of AV dissociation, fusion beats, or capture beats are not always present but are essentially diagnostic for VT. VT has dissociated P waves.
30. Etiologies of wide **QRS complex tachycardia**: underlying BBB, preexcitation (i.e., WPW), ventricular origin of rhythm, left ventricular hypertrophy, pacemaker, uses of drugs prolonging QRS (class Ia and Ic antiarrhythmics), profound hyperkalemia.
31. The maximum predicted sinus rate = 220 − age; ventricular rate of 150 is suggestive of Aflutter with 2:1 block, most SVTs have HR 150–200 bpm, MAT almost always <160 bpm.
32. **Regularly irregular**: Aflutter with 2:1 alternating with 4:1 AV block. Irregularly irregular: AFib, Aflutter with variable AV block in unfixed pattern, MAT, polymorphic VT, rarely sinus tachycardia with frequent premature beats.
33. What is the atrial activity: the same morphology? Retrograde P wave (i.e., downgoing in II and/or upright in aVR)? Strongly suggests SVT with retrograde P wave. Flutter waves? Is there no discernable atrial activity (AFib, SVT, VT)?

34. A very abrupt onset without rate variation is consistent with atrial flutter, SVT, or VT. A very abrupt onset with rate variation is consistent with AFib, Aflutter with variable block, or MAT. Afib usually has an unstable baseline, especially in V1.
35. **SVT vs. VTach**: SVT with aberrancy (aberrant conduction due to WPW or LBBB/RBBB). RS complex → R to S interval > 100 ms → AV dissociation → morphology criteria for VT presentation in V1-V2 and V6.
36. **Atrial and AV nodal (SV) arrhythmias**: (1) Escape atrial beats; (2) Atrial tachycardia; (3) Atrial tachycardia with AV block; (4) Wandering atrial pacemaker; (5) Multifocal atrial tachycardia; (6) PAC; (7) AVNRT.

6 Wave Morphology

1. **P wave morphology**: same P wave = sinus tachycardia; retrograde P wave = SVT; Flutter waves best seen in II, III, aVF, and lead VI; no discernable P wave seen in AFib.
2. Regular rhythms with rapid heart rates are seen in normal sinus tachycardia, SVT, and VT.
3. **Vagal maneuvers and adenosine** may stop AV conduction long enough to see underlying P or flutter waves, helping to diagnose atrial tachycardia and atrial flutter; may abruptly terminate the arrhythmia, strongly suggesting a reentrant mechanism utilizing the AV node (e.g., AVNRT, AVRT). However, a small percentage of atrial tachycardias are also adenosine-sensitive.
4. Long RR followed by short RR then polymorphic VT = **torsades de pointes**.
5. Rate 130, regular narrow QRS complex, no clear atrial activity, abrupt onset, no rate variability = SVT or Afluter with 2:1 block.
6. **Pathologic Q wave**: ≥30 ms (3/4 of one small box) in duration; presence in V1, V2, or V3;or depth ≥ 1/3–1/4 of the R wave height.
7. **R wave progression**- zone of transition (the point where the R:S ratio = 1) normally occurs between V2 and V3, or V3 and V4.
8. **Delayed or absent R wave progression**: anterior or anteroseptal MI, COPD, LVH, left anterior fascicular block, electrode misplacement.
9. **ST-segment elevation**: ST-segment elevation consistent with acute STEMI requires ST elevation at the J point ≥2 anatomically contiguous leads of ≥2 mm in V1, V2, or V3; and ≥1 mm in other leads.
10. **Etiologies of ST elevation other than STEMI**: usually limited to V1-V3 (STEMI, LBBB, LVH, normal variant also known as early repolarization), pericarditis (early stage), LV aneurysm, vasospasm, severe hyperkalemia, hypothermia, Brugada syndrome, Takotsubo cardiomyopathy.
11. **ST depression types**: horizontal, downsloping, upsloping depressions.
12. **Etiologies of ST depression**: ischemia, tachycardia, digoxin, hypokalemia, RBBB/LBBB/IVCD, RVH/LVH.

13. **T wave inversion** should normally be present in aVR. T wave inversion can be normal in III, aVF (if the patient has a QRS axis close to 0°), and aVL if the patient has a QRS axis close to + 90, V1, and V2. The etiology of T wave inversion is similar to ST depression, additionally, also seen in **intracranial hemorrhage, pericarditis** (late stage), and **hypothyroidism**
14. Flattened or biphasic T waves (nonspecific T waves). **Peaked T** wave seen in hyperkalemia, normal variant (usually only affects mid-precordial leads), acute MI.
15. **Low voltage** is defined as the presence of QRS amplitude in all limb leads <5 mm; QRS amplitude in all precordial leads <10 mm.
16. **Etiologies of low voltage**: obesity, COPD, pleural or pericardial effusion, myocardial infiltration (e.g., amyloidosis, sarcoidosis), hypothyroidism.

7 Blood Supply of the Heart

1. **Cardiac blood supplies**: The left circumflex artery and LAD can both supply high lateral walls. PDA supplies inferior and posterior walls. Right dominant circulation (70%): PDA is supplied by RCA. Left dominant circulation (10%): PDA is supplied by LCx. Co-dominant circulation (20%): PDA is supplied by RCA and LCx.
2. EKG leads and infarctions: I and aVL represent **lateral heart (LCx)**, V1-V2 represent **septal heart (proximal LAD)**, V3-V4 represents **anterior heart (LAD)**, V5-V6 represents **apical heart (distal LAD, LCx or RCA)**, II and III and aVF represents **inferior heart (90% RCA and 10% LCx)**, and V1-V3 depression represents **posterior heart (RCA or LCx)**.
3. **High lateral wall** STEMI only ST elevation in I and aVL. The culprit vessel is the LAD or left circumflex artery.
4. **Posterior STEMI:** RCA supplies PDA in 70%, LCx supplies PDA in 10%, and RCA and LCx both supply PDA in 20% of the general population.
5. **SA node blood supply**: 55% by **RCA**, 45% by **left circumflex**. The AV node is usually supplied by RCA.
6. **Type 2 AV block** usually happens when occlusion in **LAD or RCA**.
7. **Posterior MI** is suggested by horizontal ST depression and prominent upright T waves in V1 and V2; R/S ratio >1 in V1 or V2.
8. **Wellens' sign/syndrome = marked biphasic T waves with deep T wave inversions seen in precordial leads, namely V2 and V3 (may also be in leads V1, V4, V5, and V6)** → high suspicion for a very proximal LAD lesion.

Takeaway Messages

1. J point (beginning of repolarization), TP segment is the reference point (isoelectic point of recording).

2. Secondary repolarization abnormalities refer to changes in EKG especially ST and T waves from abnormal structure or function of the ventricular depolarization (abnormal QRS wave).
3. ST elevation [0.2 mV in men (0.15 mV in women) in V2 and V3 and 0.1 mV in other leads] due to myocardial ischemia or infarction usually occurs with reciprocal ST depression in opposite leads in the direction from those with ST elevation.
4. ST depression refers to depression ≥0.05 mV (0.5 mm) in leads V2 and V3 and 0.1 mV (1 mm) in all other leads after J-point.
5. STEMI equivalent: Wellens Syndrome deeply inverted or biphasic T waves in leads V2-V3; posterior STEMI: prominent ST depression in V1-V4.
6. Tachyarrhythmia etiologies: accelerated automaticity, re-entry, and triggered activity.

Further Readings and References

1. Strong, E. *Strong medicine.* EKG Interpretation. https://www.youtube.com/watch?v=W5cw1cAxXIs&list=PLYojB5NEEakXhL1WoDvNPm1cG57pjE0d7. Accessed November 2023.
2. De Ponti, R., J. Marazzato, G. Bagliani, et al. 2018. Sick sinus syndrome. *Cardiac Electrophysiology Clinics* 10 (2): 183–195.
3. Rautaharju, P.M., B. Surawicz, L.S. Gettes, et al. 2009. AHA/ACCF/HRS recommendations for the standardization and interpretation of the electrocardiogram: part IV: the ST segment, T and U waves, and the QT interval: a scientific statement from the American Heart Association Electrocardiography and Arrhythmias Committee, Council on Clinical Cardiology; the American College of Cardiology Foundation; and the Heart Rhythm Society. Endorsed by the International Society for Computerized Electrocardiology. *Journal of the American College of Cardiology* 53 (11): 982–991.
4. Wagner, G.S., P. Macfarlane, H. Wellens, et al. 2009. AHA/ACCF/HRS recommendations for the standardization and interpretation of the electrocardiogram: part VI: acute ischemia/infarction: a scientific statement from the American Heart Association Electrocardiography and Arrhythmias Committee, Council on Clinical Cardiology; the American College of Cardiology Foundation; and the Heart Rhythm Society. Endorsed by the International Society for Computerized Electrocardiology. *Journal of the American College of Cardiology* 53 (11): 1003–1011.
5. Macfarlane, P.W., C. Antzelevitch, M. Haissaguerre, et al. 2015. The early repolarization pattern: A consensus paper. *Journal of the American College of Cardiology* 66 (4): 470–477.
6. Driver, B.E., A. Khalil, T. Henry, et al. 2017. A new 4-variable formula to differentiate normal variant ST segment elevation in V2-V4 (early repolarization) from subtle left anterior descending coronary occlusion—Adding QRS amplitude of V2 improves the model. *Journal of Electrocardiology* 50 (5): 561–569.
7. Meyers, H.P., A. Bracey, D. Lee, A. Lichtenheld, et al. 2021. Ischemic ST-segment depression maximal in V1-V4 (Versus V5-V6) of any amplitude is specific for occlusion myocardial infarction (versus nonocclusive ischemia). *Journal of the American Heart Association* 10 (23): e022866.
8. Makielski, J.C., and L.L. Eckhardt. *Cardiac excitability, mechanisms of arrhythmia, and action of antiarrhythmic drugs*, ed. S. Levy. Waltham, MA: UpToDate. Accessed November 20, 2023.

Chapter 36
Hematology and Oncology for Hospitalist

1 Basic Theories

1. **Microsatellite instability (MSI) versus stable (MSS)**: as compared with MSI, MSS indicates a poor prognosis in colorectal cancer and thus chemotherapy is needed. MSI is the condition of genetic hypermutability (predisposition to mutation) that results from impaired DNR mismatch repair. MSI colorectal cancer usually responds well to immunotherapy while MSS may not.
2. **MSI-high** colon cancer has a more **positive prognosis** compared to MSI-low and microsatellite-stable colon cancer.
3. **Antiemetics** during chemotherapy: Zofran, Compazine (prochlorperazine), and Ativan. **Emend** (fosaprepitant IV) and **Emend** (aprepitant po) are also used in nausea treatment in cancer patients.
4. **Neulasta** = pegfilgrastim; it is used as a bone marrow stimulant for neutropenia. **Neupogen** = filgrastim; it is a white blood cell stimulator. **Neupogen** 5μg/kg subcu once daily for three doses or until ANC >500 cells/mm^3 in neutropenic fever if the hematologist/oncologist approves.
5. For **unprovoked pulmonary embolism** after anticoagulation for 3–6 months, if the patient does not want to stay on anticoagulation, can give aspirin 81 mg daily and give Lovenox 40 mg subcu before flight (1 h before).
6. **Immune thrombocytopenia (ITP)** treatment: prednisone 20 mg daily (acute inpatient treatments inlcude dexamethasone 40mg daily x 4 plus IVIG), Nplate (romiplostim), or Rituximab four doses; if still not working, will recommend splenectomy; vaccination against **meningococcus, streptococcus, H. influenza** before splenectomy.
7. **Pancytopenia** workup: bone marrow biopsy → flow cytometry → abdominal ultrasound to rule out cirrhosis and splenomegaly.
8. Investigation of **thrombophilia**: loss of function mechanisms (antithrombin deficiency, protein C/S deficiency); gain of function mechanisms (Factor V

K. Zhou, *Internal Medicine Training Notes and Survival Guide*,
https://doi.org/10.1007/978-1-0716-4039-5_36

Leiden, prothrombin G20210A, high levels of FVIII); acquired mechanisms (lupus anticoagulant, anticardiolipin antibody, anti-beta 2 glycoprotein I antibody).

9. **Carbamazepine and valproic acid** can cause lupus-like symptoms, and cause pulmonary embolism and venous thromboembolism (anti-histone antibody positive) in patients with recent travel in the past 3 months.
10. **Brain bleed, how long should we hold anticoagulation?** Most patients with an indication for anticoagulation can be started on therapy **7–14 days** after intracranial hemorrhage. Consulting a neurologist is important as the patient may have **amyloidosis** in which **anticoagulation should be avoided**.
11. **ANA +** is seen in systemic lupus erythematosus (SLE), drug-induced lupus erythematosus (DILE), systemic sclerosis (SCL), rheumatoid arthritis (RA), Sjogren's syndrome, mixed connective tissue disease, Hashimoto's, Graves, autoimmune hepatitis, PBC, EBV, HIV, HCV, parvovirus B19, inflammatory bowel disease, and lymphoproliferative disease.
12. **Injectafer** (ferric carboxymaltose injection) is used in iron deficiency anemia at **750 mg on day 1 and day 8 iv**.
13. **Sorafenib** (Nexavar) 200 mg bid is used for **hepatocellular carcinoma (HCC) and renal cell carcinoma (RCC)**. It's a multi-kinase inhibitor that inhibits tumor growth and angiogenesis by inhibiting intracellular Raf kinase (CRAF, BRAF, and mutant BRAF) and cell surface kinase receptors (VEGFR-1, -2, -3, PDGFR-beta, c-Kit, FLT3, RET, and RET/PTC).
14. **Polycythemia vera** usually has low ferritin level (<50), and can be treated with bloodletting 500 cc q2wk; hydroxyurea may also be used. Labs and studies: erythropoietin, JAK2, CBC, ferritin, PFT, CT chest and abdomen and adrenals, echocardiogram.
15. **Lung cancer biopsy**: if pathology reports atypical pneumocytes, this sample will need redo biopsy.
16. **Autoimmune colitis or pneumonitis** from cancer medication (immunotherapy) may require treatment with **prednisone 1 mg/kg daily**.
17. **Induction or adjuvant chemotherapy**: **induction chemo** is the delivery of chemo before definitive surgery or radiation; **adjuvant chemo** is chemo medication after surgery to prevent recurrence. **Palliative chemo** is used to improve quality of life but not to cure cancer.
18. **Pleural effusion** if malignancy will need a screen for metastasis with CT chest, abdomen, and pelvis, or PET.
19. **Anemia may need to** check ANA and rheumatoid factor, SPEP, UPEP, kappa/lambda light chain, HIV, HBV, HCV, immunofixation.
20. **SBRT** (stereotactic body radiotherapy) can be used for **lung cancer, liver cancer, prostate cancer, pancreatic cancer, and kidney cancer**.
21. **BCL2** (B cell lymphoma-2), **BCL6** (B cell lymphoma-6), and **C-myc** genes are commonly checked in lymphoma; they usually indicate aggressive lymphoma with poor prognosis without treatment.
22. **Gene mutations** (75 genes) include EGFR, ALK, ROS1, BRAF, MET, ERBB, and RET are commonly checked in non-small cell lung cancer.

23. Inferior vena cava filter after 3 months should not be removed. **FDA recommends the removal of IVC filters within 29–54 days of their implantation.**
24. **Avoid antidepressants** with tamoxifen, especially fluoxetine, duloxetine, bupropion, or paroxetine; whereas **sertraline, citalopram, escitalopram, and venlafaxine** are reasonable alternatives because they impart lesser degrees of inhibition in CYP2D6 enzyme function which is required for the conversion of tamoxifen to its active form.
25. Direct oral anticoagulant (DOAC): usually we stop DOAC 2–3 days before surgery, and restart 1 day after surgery.
26. **DVT from long-distance travel management**: Xarelto (or other DOACs) for 3–6 months. After anticoagulation treatment, give Lovenox 40 mg subcu right before long distance travel and prescribe aspirin 81 mg daily.
27. **Lymphocytosis** labs: CBC, LDH, CMP, and **flow cytometry** to rule out CLL.
28. **Acute lymphoblastic lymphoma** versus **acute lymphoblastic leukemia** diagnosis depends on the location of the pathology.
29. **PET/CT** is performed to detect cancer, monitor treatment effectiveness, and detect relapses of cancer.
30. **Cancer staging**: Tx = occult carcinoma; T0 = no evidence of primary tumor; Tis = carcinoma in situ.
31. **History taking in cancer patients**: how is the cancer progressing? How is the patient doing (ambulating, energy, weight loss, function, and pain)?
32. **Ramucirumab** (VEGFR2 inhibitor) indications: (A) advanced gastric or **GE junction adenocarcinoma refractory to previous fluoropyrimidine (capecitabine, fluorouracil, doxifluridine, carmofur) or platinum (Cisplatin, Carboplatin)-containing chemo; (B) metastatic lung cancer** (non-small cell) refractory to platinum-based chemo; (C) metastatic **colorectal cancer** progressed with bevacizumab, oxaliplatin, and a fluoropyridine.
33. **Everolimus** (Afinitor) blocks mTOR protein, and is used to treat **kidney cancers** after other drugs like sorafenib or **sunitinib** have been tried. **Everolimus** is also used in postmenopausal ER-positive but Her 2 negative **breast cancer** failing letrozole or anastrozole, **pancreatic** cancer, **gastrointestinal** cancer, and certain **lung** cancer.
34. **Eastern Cooperative Oncology Group (ECOG)** performance status: zero fully active → four completely disabled → five dead.
35. **Karnofsky performance status**: (A) able to carry on normal activity and work → (B) assistance with ADLs → (C) disabilities, unable to care for self: require equivalent of institutional or hospital care, disease may progress rapidly.
36. The presence of **TP53 mutations** without STK11 or EGFR alterations (TP53-mut/STK11-EGFR wt) independent of KRAS mutations represent tumors with highest CD8 T cell density and PD-L1 expression; they are **more likely to respond to PD-L1 inhibitors**.
37. Expression of PD-L1 is more common in **male smokers with adenocarcinoma** histology and are not carriers of EGFR, ALK, ROS, or KRAS mutations.

38. **Co-mutations of KRAS and KEAP1/NFE2L2** indicate shorter survival and duration of response to initial platinum-based chemotherapy and shorter survival from the start of immunotherapy.
39. DVT treatment with Lovenox: 1.5 mg/kg q24h. If MSI is high and PD-L1 high, may give immunotherapy.
40. **Ki-67** is a marker of proliferation and is associated with ribosomal RNA transcription.
41. Patients with **higher Ki-67 scores** (>50%) correlate with **shorter overall survival in colorectal cancer**.
42. **LDH** is involved in cancer initiation and metabolism. It is a marker for **cancer prognosis**.
43. **Portal vein thrombosis** can cause further end-organ damage like varices, GI bleeding, and splenomegaly.
44. **Predictive markers for anti PD-1/anti PD-L1 therapy**: PD-L1 expression, TMB, MMR/MSI, CD8 T cells, EGFR, LAK, ROS proto-oncogen1 (ROS1) translocation.
45. **Melanoma** treatment with BRAF/MEK inhibitor combination therapy, such as **dabrafenib plus trametinib** or **vemurafenib plus cobimetinib,** is effective for BRAF-mutated melanoma and can target disease in the brain.
46. No thrombophilia testing is necessary in venous thromboembolism with a **major transient risk factor** like surgery, trauma, or prolonged immobility.
47. Side effects of **Keytruda**: rash, dyspnea, diarrhea, and fatigue.
48. **5-FU causes myelosuppression**, resulting in serious life-threatening infections and need for transfusion, fatigue, peripheral neuropathy, magnesium wasting, and alopecia.
49. **Capecitabine** is the oral form of 5-FU, used in colorectal, breast, and gastric cancers.
50. Delayed nausea and vomiting after chemotherapy, add **aprepitant** and **olanzapine** to chemo.

2 Oncologic Urgencies and Emergencies

1. **Superior vena cava (SVC)** syndrome: obstruction of SVC from thrombus formation or cancer burden. **Treatments** may include urgent **anticoagulation and interventional or surgical procedures versus chemotherapy/radiation treatment**. For example, small cell lung cancer, lymphoma, and germ cell cancers are treated with initial chemotherapy, non-small cell lung cancer is treated with initial chemotherapy, radiation therapy, or both; whereas thymoma and mesothelioma require urgent surgery.
2. **Brain metastasis**, usually seen with lung cancer, breast cancer, and melanoma, predicts **3–25 months' overall survival**. **Treatment**: give **dexamethasone** 10 mg iv once now followed by 4–6 mg iv q6h. **Stat neurosurgery and radiation oncology** consults are necessary. Depending on the severity of edema and

risks of brain herniation, the patient may require mannitol, head elevation, hyperventilation, or decompression.

3. **Neoplastic** epidural **spinal cord compression** treatment: give dexamethasone 10 mg iv once now followed by 4–6 mg iv q6h. **Stat neurosurgery and radiation oncology** consults are necessary; if surgical candidates with an expected survival of at **least 3 months**, initial **decompressive surgery followed by radiation** improves the probability of ambulation compared to radiation alone.
4. **Tumor lysis syndrome (TLS)** is characterized by hyperuricemia, hyperkalemia, hyperphosphatemia, hypocalcemia, and elevated LDH. It requires continuous cardiac monitoring and measurement of electrolytes, creatinine, and uric acid level **q4-6h**, and may add **loop diuretics**. Treatment emphasizes **IV fluid hydration and allopurinol, febuxostat, or rasburicase**. TLS is commonly seen in **aggressive lymphoma and leukemia, or with the use of targeted therapy** venetoclax (BCL-2 inhibitor) or ibrutinib (BTK inhibitor).
5. **Oncologic emergencies of non-Hodgkin's lymphoma (NHL)**: spinal cord compression, pericardial tamponade, hypercalcemia (adult T cell leukemia/lymphoma), superior or inferior vena cava obstruction, **hyperleukocytosis** (B or T cell lymphoblastic leukemia/lymphoma), airway obstruction (mediastinal lymphoma), **lymphomatous meningitis** and or CNS mass lesion, hyperuricemia and tumor lysis syndrome, **hyperviscosity syndrome** (seen in lymphoplasmacytic lymphoma also known as Waldenstrom's macroglobulinemia), intestinal obstruction, intussusception, ureteral obstruction with unilateral or bilateral hydronephrosis, severe hepatic dysfunction, venous thromboembolism, severe autoimmune hemolytic anemia and or thrombocytopenia (small lymphocytic lymphoma).
6. Abnormal results in non-Hodgkin's lymphoma: (A) **thrombocytopenia, anemia, and leukopenia** due to bone marrow infiltration, hypersplenism from splenic involvement or immune destruction. (B) **hypercalcemia** for human T-cell lymphotropic virus type 1 (HTLV-1) associated adult T cell leukemia/lymphoma, transformed follicular lymphoma, and diffuse large B cell lymphoma (DLBCL). (C) **hyperuricemia** with gout and nephrolithiasis from Burkitt lymphoma and uncommonly with some aggressive NHLs; hyperuricemia and tumor lysis syndrome are more frequent in patients with underlying renal failure. (D) **elevated serum LDH** due to high tumor burden, infiltration of the liver, hemolytic anemia secondary to immune-mediated RBC destruction or association with rapidly growing forms of NHL like DLBCL, transformed follicular lymphoma, $\geq$2–3× upper limit normal→poor prognosis. (E) **large M spikes** seen in lymphoplasmacytic lymphoma also known as Waldenstrom's macroglobulinemia; small M spikes seen in B cell NHLs, particularly small lymphocytic lymphoma (SLL), CLL, and extranodal marginal zone lymphoma.
7. Definition of **blast crisis**: $\geq$20% blasts in peripheral blood or bone marrow; large foci or clusters of blasts on the bone marrow biopsy; presence of extramedullary blastic infiltrates (e.g., myeloid sarcoma, also known as granulocytic sarcoma or chloroma). **CML blast crisis**: 30% is of lymphoid phenotype (ALL) and 70% is of myeloid phenotype (AML).

8. The clinical and morphologic features seen in patients developing **lymphoid blast crisis** [acute myeloid leukemia t(9,22) (q34;q11), BCR-ABL] after a known period with CML are similar to those presenting de novo with Philadelphia chromosome + acute lymphoblastic leukemia (ALL).
9. Transformation to a blastic crisis is suggested by signs and symptoms more typical of **acute leukemia (night sweats, weight loss, fever, bone pain, symptoms of anemia, and bleeding)**.
10. **Lymphoid blast crisis** (30% of CML blast crisis) in Philadelphia chromosome + ALL (Ph+ ALL) treatment: **hyper-CVAD alternating with methotrexate (MTX), cytarabine, and nib (imatinib, dasatinib, and nilotinib)**. Bcr-Abl tyrosine kinase inhibitor (TKI) therapies (imatinib, dasatinib, nilotinib, bosutinib) have side effects of pleural effusions, interstitial lung disease (ILD) and pulmonary arterial hypertension (PAH).
11. **Myeloid blast crisis** (70% of CML blast crisis) treatment: TKI followed by allogeneic hematopoietic cell transplantation (HCT) for eligible patients.
12. Cancer-associated **venous thromboembolism (VTE) usually coexists with thrombocytopenia**. If platelet >50 K/uL, continue anticoagulation; if platelet 25–50 K/uL, anticoagulation should be individualized; if <25 K/uL, need to avoid anticoagulation.
13. **Intramural leiomyoma** with bleeding in a 45 yo requires endometrial biopsy to rule out malignancy.
14. **Immune thrombocytopenia (ITP)** treatment for a patient scheduled for rotator cuff repair: eltrombopag (Doptelet) 40 mg daily for 5 days, surgery can be done on days 8–13. Treat ITP only if platelet (PLT) < 30 K/uL or surgery. Prednisone takes a long time to work. IVIG weekly increases PLT but drops quickly as well. If **bleeding or PLT < 10 K/uL,** may **give methylprednisone 1 g/kg iv × 3 days (alternative is dexamethasone 40mg daily x 4), IVIG, and PLT transfusion at the same time (consult hematologist first)**.
15. ITP, add **eltrombopag** (**Promacta**) 25 mg, then taper off prednisone.
16. 75 yo M with **severe ITP after septic shock** (PLT < 10 K/uL): not responding to PLT transfusion; hematologist was consulted and started Decadron 20 mg once on day 1 then 40 mg iv daily for another 3 days with good improvement (PLT > 50 K/uL after four doses) and hematologist recommended no steroid upon discharge but close follow up.
17. **Indications for PLT transfusion**: major surgery or invasive procedure but no active bleeding ≤50 K/uL; ocular or neurosurgery and no active bleeding ≤100 K/uL; surgery with active bleeding <50 K/uL (usually), <100 K/uL (rarely); stable nonbleeding <10 K/uL; stable non-bleeding but T > 100.4 or undergoing invasive procedure, <20 K/uL.
18. **TTP** should be suspected in a patient present with **MAHA (flow cytometry), hemoglobin < 10 g/dL, and severe thrombocytopenia with PLT < 30 K/uL, with or without symptoms of organ involvement and without an apparent etiology.** Diagnosis via **ADAMTS13 activity level < 10%.** Treatment for acquired TTP: **steroids (hydrocortisone 100 mg iv q8h or Solu-Medrol 1 g**

daily × 3 days or Prednisone 1 mg/kg daily), FFP (large amounts) and plasmapheresis.

19. **Cytokine release syndrome (CRS)** refers to mild to overwhelming systemic inflammatory response from a large and rapid release of cytokines due to severe infections like COVID-19 or **T-cell engaging therapies** like **bispecific T-cell engaging (BiTE)** single-chain antibody constructs (e.g., blinatumomab for ALL and teclistamab for MM) and **chimeric antigen receptor (CAR) T** cells. Typical presentations of CRS include **fever, hypotension, hypoxia, seizure** (Immune effector Cell Associated Neurotoxicity Syndrome, **ICANS**), and eventually multiorgan (heart, lung, liver, kidney) failure and CNS symptoms if untreated. Labs may show cytopenia, elevated creatinine and liver enzymes, coagulation profile abnormalities, and a high CRP.
20. Severe cases of CRS can cause similar presentations as **hemophagocytic lymphohistiocytosis (HLH) or macrophage activation syndrome (MAS)** like high fevers, highly elevated ferritin levels, and hypertriglyceridemia.
21. **Treatment of CRS** is supportive care with intravenous fluid, antibiotics (until infection ruled out), steroids, and consider **tocilizumab (IL-6 receptor antagonist)** and **anakinra (IL-1 receptor antagonist)** if no improvement with steroids.

3 Treatment for Various Types of Cancers

Multiple Myeloma

1. **Multiple myeloma** diagnosis: **>3 g/dL serum M** component or **≥10% clonal plasma cells on bone marrow biopsy** or a biopsy-proven plasmacytoma plus end-organ damage of hypercalcemia, renal failure, anemia, and bone lesions (CRAB features); or ≥60% clonal plasma cell involvement of the marrow, serum free light chain **ratio of ≥100** with involved free light chain level **≥100** mg/L, and/or greater than one focal lesion on MRI regardless of end-organ damage.
2. The diagnosis of **smoldering myeloma (asymptomatic myeloma)** requires ≥3 g/dL and/or ≥500 mg/24 h of urinary monoclonal free light chains and/or ≥10% clonal plasma cells in bone marrow AND no evidence of myeloma-related signs or symptoms requiring therapy.
3. **All smoldering myeloma** (M protein ≥3 g/dL, K or lambda urine FLC ≥ 500 mg/24 h, clonal plasma with 10%–59% in bone marrow) **should get an MRI bone to look for lytic bone lesions**; if >5 mm lesion = MM, needs treatment. If unequivocal, repeat MRI in 3–6 months.
4. A **plasmacytoma** (similar to MGUS but with no M protein) is a localized tumor of plasma cells; it is considered as the intermediate phase between **MGUS** and **multiple myeloma**.

5. The risk of **progression** is low at 5% over **20 years in MGUS**. **Treatment**: Follow up in 6 months to 1 year with repeat labs.
6. **Treatments for multiple myeloma**: patients eligible for transplant should undergo induction therapy followed by autologous HSCT and close observation or maintenance therapy. Relapsed or refractory disease treatments: proteasome inhibitors (carfilzomib or ixazomib), immunomodulatory drug pomalidomide, histone deacetylase inhibitor (panobinostat), and monoclonal antibodies (daratumumab and elotuzumab).
7. **Induction chemotherapy for multiple myeloma**: combinations of immunomodulatory drugs (lenalidomide or thalidomide), proteasome inhibitors like bortezomib (Velcade), dexamethasone, and alkylating agents (melphalan or cyclosporine).
8. **Multiple myeloma treatment**: Ixazomib (Ninlaro) 4 mg day 1, 8, and 16; dexamethasone days 1, 8, and 16; Revlimid 10 mg daily, lovenox 40 mg daily, and acyclovir. Bisphosphonates Zoledronic acid (Reclast) q3m at 4 mg iv.
9. **Multiple myeloma workup**: PET and bone marrow biopsy at lesion, serum and urine electrophoresis, alpha-fetoprotein, PSA, CA19-9, LDH, serum and urine free light chain, IgA and IgM.
10. **The use of bortezomib** (Velcade) requires concomitant administration of **acyclovir** 500 mg qd for the prophylaxis of herpes.
11. **Multiple myeloma** treatment: 8 cycles of RVD chemo (Revlimid, Velcade, Dexamethasone) →consolidation with stem cell transplant × 1 → Revlimid 5 mg daily → increase to 10 mg daily if blood cell counts normal.
12. 88 yo **multiple myeloma with lytic lesion on** Zometa × 2, then monthly Xgeva (denosumab), had frequent infection, started on IVIG, had mouth pain (was told to hold aspirin). He was started on pomalidomide which is a derivative of thalidomide with antiangiogenic and immunomodulation effects. Workups included CMP WNL, LDH 185, KFLC 673 (normal 3.3–19.3 mg/L), LFLC 444.38 (normal 5.7–26.3 mg/L), K/L ratio 0.02 (normal 0.26–1.65), beta 2 microglobulin 1.8. Serum immunofixation essay: lambda light chain, SPEP -, bone marrow biopsy, and flow cytometry. **Treatment**: **RVD** with Revlimid (Lenalidomide) 15 mg day 1–4, Velcade (bortezomib) 1.3 mg/m^2 IV day 1, 4, 8, 11 and dexamethasone 20 mg on the days of Velcade → discontinued due to intolerance of fatigue and started on carfilzomib (Kyprolis) → discontinued and started on daratumumab with Revlimid 4 mg qod; continue acyclovir while on daratumumab. Currently on daratumumab, pomalidomide, and dexamethasone.
13. 62-year-old M with **kappa light chain multiple myeloma** diagnosis several years ago. Upon diagnosis, treatment with RVD × 6 cycles → 6 months later, autologous stem cell transplant → day 100 started on maintenance Revlimid 15 mg daily for 3 years till when SPEP+KLC showed KLC concentration 2100, bone marrow biopsy noted 10% atypical plasma cells without cytogenetic change, PET/CT negative→treatment then with CyBorD (cyclophosphamide, Bortezomib, and dexamethasone) × 4 cycles → then 5 months later, started on weekly daratumumab × 3 cycles → progression, started on carfilzomib/

Revlimid/dexamethasone × 3 cycles → progression, one additional cycle with pomalidomide vs lenalidomide → then started D-PACE × 2 cycles...→ started on CAR-T cell infusion →complicated by **cytokine release syndrome**, C diff, neurotoxicity and compression fractures at T2-L3 → bone marrow biopsy negative, flow cytometry suspicious for measurable residual disease (MRD), biopsy negative → later, developed soft tissue nodules consistent with plasmacytomas, biopsy revealed anaplastic multiple myeloma, CD138+, **treatment**: elotuzumab, pomalidomide, and dexamethasone with good response.

Lung Cancer

1. **Metastatic non-small cell lung cancer (NSCLC) without EGFR or ALK mutations** treatment (can be first line): carboplatin, pemetrexed, pembrolizumab, q3wk × 6; if shrink in size → surgery.
2. For nonsquamous metastatic NSCLC, screen for EGFR, ALK, and ROS1 genes. If EGFR mutation, give **erlotinib (osimertinib is the stand of care in 2024)**; if ALK translocation and ROS1 mutation, give **crizotinib**.
3. **Erlotinib** is effective in metastatic NSCLC with EGFR mutation as it **inhibits the intracellular phosphorylation** of tyrosine kinase of EGFR. **Lorlatinib** is also FDA approved as first line therapy for ALK-positive metastatic NSCLC; recent study showed durable longer benefits from lorlatinib than crizotinib (3rd generation ALK inhibitor alectinib is now commonly used).
4. If no driver mutations, 4 cycles of **cisplatin**-based chemotherapy improve survival (survival advantages) in patients who have undergone successful resection of stage II or III **NSCLC** regardless of histologic type.
5. The current standard treatment of metastatic **NSCLC** without driver mutations and good performance status is **platinum-based** chemo with or without immunotherapy or immunotherapy (pemborlizumab, nivolumab, or atezolizumab) alone: like 4–6 cycles of carboplatin and pemetrexed→then pemetrexed or docetaxel maintenance.
6. **Platinum-based anticancer drugs**: cisplatin, carboplatin, oxaliplatin, nedaplatin, triplatin.
7. 79 yo male had a radical nephrectomy, hx of liver mass sp. radiofrequency ablation (RFA) at the liver, then stage I right lung cancer → lobectomy, chemotherapy with **carboplatin and pemetrexed**; no gene mutation but PD-L1 positive. Lung primary cancer, received nivolumab for 9 months, not getting better, still has nodule enlarging → RFA, bony lytic lesion at hip → radiation therapy.
8. Cancer metastasized to brain → **radiation therapy**.
9. **Adenocarcinoma of the lung** with a history of SLE, received 6 cycles of chemo with carboplatin, pemetrexed, and bevacizumab (Avastin) for 6 cycles, then maintenance therapy of pembrolizumab. This patient also has metastasis to the pancreas and brain for which the patient is being treated with Decadron 2 mg bid.

10. **VEGF mutation** is uncommon in Asian females, or non-smokers with squamous cell carcinoma of the lung as compared to lung adenocarcinoma. **RAS** testing is necessary for both lung and colon cancers.
11. **Bevacizumab** is a monoclonal antibody against VEGF-A. **Bevacizumab** improves outcomes when added to first-line treatment in advanced or recurrent **nonsquamous NSCLC** without targetable molecular abnormality.
12. NSCLC stage IIb: 15% respond to treatment and can be cured → 85% will progress or relapse into stage IV, then **18 months' life expectancy**. Treatment is chemoradiation at the same time, starting chemo, then radiation therapy 5 days a week for 7–8 weeks.
13. In patients with metastatic non-small cell lung cancer, **palliative care** improves both quality of life and survival. **Palliative care does not preclude aggressive care or treatment**.
14. For patients with **small cell lung cancer (SCLC)** who have largely central tumors that are not amenable to resection, combined **chemoradiation** can result in a cure for about 20%–30% of patients. Chemotherapy of **cisplatin and etoposide** is started at the same time as radiation.
15. Most patients with **small cell lung cancer (SCLC)** relapse in 1–2 years. Limited stage disease of SCLC is limited to one hemithorax, with hilar and mediastinal lymphadenopathy. The limited-stage disease of SCLC can be encompassed in one tolerable radiotherapy portal. Treatment: combined chemoradiation followed by prophylactic cranial irradiation.
16. **Prophylactic cranial irradiation** is a standard treatment for patients with metastatic SCLC after chemo.

Colorectal Cancer

1. **Esophageal cancer**: chemoradiation before surgery. **Pancreas and duodenum** cancer: perioperative chemotherapy. **Colon and gastric cancer**: vary in timing for chemo and surgery.
2. For **colorectal cancer** patients, we should look for **KRAS, BRAF, NRAS, MSI, MMR, MLH-1, MSH2, MSH6, and PMS2 hypermethylation**. Example of colorectal cancer pathology: Negative surgical margins, lymphovascular invasion, and perineural invasion negative, deficient MMR, no MLH-1 or PMS-2 protein identified, BRAF-, MLH-1 hypermethylation.
3. **Extensive promoter methylation** was associated with MLH-1 inactivation, MSI, and BRAF mutation.
4. TIIIN1M0 **colorectal cancer**: concurrent chemoradiation → surgery → chemo with FOLFOX: 5-FU, leucovorin, oxaliplatin, and Neulasta. Colorectal cancer starts **chemo after wound closure**: FOLFOX regimen (fluorouracil, folinic acid, oxaliplatin).
5. **Colorectal cancer staging**: Stage I—mucosa, submucosa, or muscle layer of rectal wall. Stage II—IIa through muscle layer to serosa; IIb through serosa to

visceral peritoneum; IIc to nearby organs. Stage III to lymph nodes. Stage IV to distal organs.

6. **Colorectal cancer treatment**: if stage II or lower, just surgery; if stage III, may benefit from chemotherapy; if stage IV, check MSI, KRAS/NRAS/BRAF, if all wild type, can give FOLFOX or FOLFIRI plus **cetuximab or panitumumab** (EGFR inhibitors); if one or more mutated, do **Avastin** (a VEGFR inhibitor). If all fail, start the **BEACON regimen** including binimetinib, encorafenib, and cetuximab (for BRAF V600E–Mutated colorectal cancer).
7. Colorectal cancer T4N2M1 maintenance therapy: **capecitabine** (Xeloda).
8. Metastasized colorectal cancer with **KRAS mutation**: FOLFOX chemo (5-FU, leucovorin, oxaliplatin) + bevacizumab (Avastin). KRAS mutation in colorectal cancer indicates poor prognosis.
9. KRAS/NRAS/BRAF wild type will respond to anti-EGFR therapy with two major medications: **cetuximab and panitumumab**. If any of them is mutated, use **Avastin** (anti-VEGF).
10. Side effects of binimetinib, encorafenib, and cetuximab: **congestive heart failure, myositis, retinitis**.
11. Additionally, if **right-sided colorectal cancer**, it is very aggressive usually and should give **bevacizumab**. If left-sided cancer, may use **cetuximab** or **panitumumab** (if wild type KRAS/NRAS/BRAF) on top of FOLFOX or FOLFIRI.
12. 55 yo M with **stage IV rectal carcinoma with metastatic retroperitoneal and pelvic lymph nodes**, MSS, KRAS wt, BRAF V600E mutant per FoundationOne Liquid CDx. Treatment: FOLFOX 10 cycles with interval improvements→concurrent chemoradiation with capecitabine for 2 months then plan for close surveillance rather than surgical resection given distal nodal disease. On surveillance until CT 3 years later showed new aortocaval lymphadenopathy, thus was started on capecitabine + Avastin for 3 cycles → disease progression, thus received Stereotactic body radiation therapy (SBRT) to aortocaval lymph node for ten fractions, developed DVT. Then, started on FOLFIRI, added bevacizumab 1 month later → disease progression, started **BEACON regimen** binimetinib, encorafenib, and cetuximab.
13. The combination of encorafenib and cetuximab was approved by the FDA for adult patients with previously treated metastatic colorectal cancer with BRAF V600E alteration.
14. 52 yo F with **metastatic adenocarcinoma of the transverse colon to peritoneum, liver, and lung**, presenting with sigmoid colon cancer with partial obstruction. Treatment: Triplet (FOLFOXIRI) Versus Doublet (FOLFOX or FOLFIRI). Appears right-sided, added bevacizumab regardless of RAS mutation status, awaiting MMR and MSS testing.
15. For deficient MMR colon cancer, add **fluoropyridine plus oxaliplatin (immunotherapy should be considered as well)**. MSI high indicates possible Lynch syndrome.
16. 34 yo M with partially **obstructing rectosigmoid mass and omental caking, hepatic lesion, ascites** → CT biopsy confirmed **Stage IV mucinous adenocarcinoma**. MSS on IHC. Treatment: FOLFOX + Avastin, then changed to FOLFOXIRI + Avastin 1 month later. Oxaliplatin stopped due to

neuropathy→started capecitabine (Xeloda) 1500 mg bid, 1 week on 1 week off, discontinued irinotecan, on Xeloda + Avastin for 5 months, then added Vemurafenib on top of Xeloda + Avastin. Diffuse rash → vemurafenib hold for concerns of allergy→resumed vemurafenib + cetuximab for 3 months, disease progression → started on weekly cetuximab 250 mg/m^2 thereafter, plan to start encorafenib 300 mg bid + binimetinib 45 mg bid in the coming week, loading dose with cetuximab 400 mg/m^2 then maintenance dosing 250 mg/m^2 qwk.

17. 52 yo white female, low back pain → CT revealed **omentum mass** → biopsy-proven adenocarcinoma → mass of transverse colon; pathology reports **invasive adenocarcinoma**, moderately differentiated, ulcerated. Treatment: FOLFOX (alternative regimen cisplatin and 5-FU) after EGD/colonoscopy and PET CT. Mediport and fanny pack chemo for 48 h. IHC: positive for cytokeratin 20, CDX2 and p53 and negative for cytokeratin 7, TTF1, GATA3, PAX8, WT1 and estrogen receptors. Additionally, in preparation of personalized therapy in solid tumor, ordered molecular pathology send-out for Omniseq panel.
18. Radiation therapy is used for **localized top or bottom tumors**. **Keytruda** q3wk cycle.
19. **Stage IV adenocarcinoma** of colon treatment: FOLFOX + Avastin, discontinue oxaliplatin after cycle 10 to avoid neuropathy.
20. **Metastatic sigmoid colon adenocarcinoma with metastasis to liver**→left hemicolectomy, FOLFOX 8 cycles→FOLFIRI for three more cycles, then adjuvant therapies stopped→liver recurrence; treatment with FOLFIRI + Avastin for 6 cycles. Because KRAS wt → FOLFIRI + cetuximab → disease progression, start Cetuximab + irinotecan→capecitabine + bevacizumab to preserve irinotecan for future. Capecitabine (Xeloda) dose decreased due to **hand-foot syndrome and abnormal liver function test**.
21. **Metastatic rectal adenocarcinoma to the liver**, started FOLFOX after colostomy, added Avastin. Oxaliplatin was discontinued after 8 cycles due to peripheral neuropathy. 5-FU + Avastin was discontinued due to disease progression→ FOLFIRI + Avastin→disease progression and thus started **Regorafenib** (Stivargo).
22. **Stage IIIc colon cancer** (pT3N2b), MSS (microsatellite stability), EMR (endoscopic mucosal resection), sigmoidectomy→FOLFOX for 6 months and 12 cycles.
23. **Metastatic adenocarcinoma**, PET-CT to assess the **mediastinal nodes and lung nodules**. No uptake in the lung, stage IV sigmoid adenocarcinoma with metastasis to the liver, MSS, RAS/BRAF wild type treatment: FOLFOX + Avastin, stopped 5-FU due to myocardial infarction → bFOL (bolus FU + low dose leucovorin) + Avastin.
24. **No 5-FU in cocaine abusers because of cardiac ischemia concerns**.
25. **Stage IV ascending colon adenocarcinoma with metastasis to mesenteric lymph nodes** and lungs, MSS, RAS wt, and BRAF mutated, initiated FOLFOX, increased to FOLFOXIRI for C2 and FOLFOXIRI + Avastin for C4, discontinued 5-FU given positive cocaine test.

26. 66 yo **Stage IV colon adenocarcinoma with metastasis to lungs, peritoneum, liver, MSS, KRAS G12V mutant**, treatment: started FOLFOX + Avastin, discontinued oxaliplatin after 10 cycles to avoid neuropathy. The patient remained on 5-FU/LV + Avastin → transition to capecitabine + Avastin for 2 months → FOLFIRI + Avastin→trifluridine and tipiracil (Lonsurf) + Avastin due to failing previous treatments.
27. 56 yo with **resected metastatic poorly differentiated cecal adenocarcinoma to bilateral ovaries**, KRAS mutant, MSI-H with sporadic MLH-1 promoter hypermethylation→TAH-BSO, resection of cecum, appendix, a portion of the terminal ileum with ileoascending enterocolostomy and infracolic omentectomy, pT4bN2bM1b, treatment: adjuvant full dose FOLFOX q2wks, cycle 6 no evidence of disease, oxaliplatin decreased to 65 mg/m^2 on cycle 9 and then discontinued on cycle 11. Completed 12 cycles. However, later during follow-up, developed BRBPR and found left colon mass and left hydronephrosis → left ureteral stent placement→initiated nivolumab 3 mg/kg + ipilimumab 1 mg/kg cycle 1–4 are q3wks, followed by nivolumab 240 mg flat dose q2wks.
28. Nivolumab: monitor treatment-related toxicities including **thyroiditis, hepatitis, pneumonitis, and arthritis**.
29. **Assess cancer response to treatment**: location of cancer, size of tumor with CT, PET standardized uptake value (SUV) change.
30. **Rectovaginal fistula** → diverting colostomy treatment.
31. **Invasive adenocarcinoma at the rectosigmoid area**, moderately differentiated, angiolymphatic invasion with tubulovillous adenoma, use CT chest, abdomen, and pelvis together with MRI for staging→consider chemoradiation vs surgery or all (started on **concurrent chemoradiation** for 6 weeks, followed by chemotherapy for 4.5 months, then surgery). Check MSI status, KRAS, BRAF, and HER2 Neu. MSI correlates with Lynch syndrome and may need genetic counseling.
32. **Metastatic adenocarcinoma to the liver with cholangiocarcinoma with gallbladder involvement, peritoneum, and widespread nodes**. Treatment: 4 cycles of palliative gemcitabine.
33. **Rectal adenocarcinoma** pT1pNXcM0 sp. resection with negative margins → recurrence treatment: FOLFOX → surgery of low anterior resection (LAR) → 12 cycles of FOLFOX, send MSI, NRAS, KRAS, BRAF. Given recurrent rectal cancer, recommended FOLFIRI + Avastin, oxaliplatin discontinued after peripheral neuropathy.
34. **Recurrent refractory colorectal adenocarcinoma**, RAS wild type, BRAF -, MSS, rectovaginal fistula, suspicious pulmonary nodule, nonhypermetabolic after 2 cycles of **FOLFIRI and bevacizumab** q14 days. Surveillance detected stage III T3N1bM0 later, treated with **low anterior resection (LAR), FOLFOX chemoradiation** → hepatooligo recurrence later sp. metastasectomy followed by FOLFIRI plus panitumumab, recurrence again → FOLFIRI + Avastin.
35. **Stage IV recurrent splenic flexure colon adenocarcinoma with metastasis to the liver**, pelvic lymphadenopathy, and omentum, KRAS/BRAF wild type, NRAS mutated, MSS, HER2 negative. Treatment: full dose palliative FOLFOX

q2w, 9 cycles completed. Added Avastin for cycles 3–5 then held for gastrointestinal surgery consultation. This patient declined the recommendation for liver resection and hyperthermic intraperitoneal chemotherapy (HIPEC).

36. If **recurrent colorectal cancer pT3N0Mx** is stable, will recommend maintenance 5-FU with or without bevacizumab.
37. Sp colectomy, CT chest, abdomen, pelvis without evidence of metastatic disease, surveillance **q3m** office visit with blood work and every **6 m CT scan for 2 years**.
38. **Post-treatment surveillance** generally is not necessary for appendiceal tumors <2 cm and rectal tumors <1 cm.

Gastroesophageal Cancer, Hepatobiliary Carcinoma, and Pancreatic Cancer

1. Neoadjuvant chemotherapy with **carboplatin and paclitaxel** with **radiation** for esophageal or gastroesophageal junction cancer.
2. **Distal esophageal** locally advanced moderately differentiated **adenocarcinoma** at 35–40 cm from the gastroesophageal junction. Treatment: neoadjuvant chemoradiation→started on **carbo + Taxol** qwk, daily **radiation** for 6 weeks, wait for 4 weeks then repeat PET scan→consider surgery.
3. **Type 2 (true) GE junction adenocarcinoma**, T3N0, MSS, PD-L1 negative (CPS < 1), HER-2 negative by IHC and FISH. Bronchoscopy with EBUS for hilar node positive for MCL-1 (myeloid leukemia 1, an antiapoptotic factor of BCL-2 family); Hx of stage IV mantle cell lymphoma diagnosis 4 years ago. Started **neoadjuvant chemoradiation with modified FOLFOX to eliminate leucovorin and 5-FU secondary to Mantle cell lymphoma** (PRODIGE5/ACCORD1 trial) with complete response; however, surveillance CT revealed bilateral lung nodule indicating metastatic disease (stage IV cancer). Treatment is **FOLFOX-5FU/LV** bolus → **paclitaxel + ramucirumab**.
4. **Stage IV Siewert Type gastroesophageal junction cancer with metastasis to liver and bone and lymph nodes**, MSS, HER2+, PD-L1 negative. Treatment: FOLFOX minus bolus q2 weeks, later discontinued 5-FU/LV due to neutropenia at cycle 3. Trastuzumab was added at C4; Zometa (zoledronic acid) q3m was initiated 2 months later due to bone metastasis. Oxaliplatin was discontinued because of peripheral neuropathy. Currently on only **5-Fu intravenous infusion and trastuzumab**.
5. **Advanced Omniseq looks for MSS, PD-L1, and hundreds of genes. Herceptin use requires echo q3m.**
6. **Esophageal adenocarcinoma**—distal, cT3N1 with bulky regional lymphadenopathy treatment: neoadjuvant concurrent chemoradiation therapy with **carboplatin** qwk and **paclitaxel** qwk and daily **radiation** for 6 weeks→good response→esophagectomy.

7. 50 yo gallbladder cancer, surgery of gallbladder fossa and nearby lymph, and partial liver resection. Radical cholecystectomy revealed falciform ligament and peritoneum nodule adenocarcinoma, pT2dNxMx. The tumor invaded the muscularis propia and extended to perivascular adipose tissue on the peritoneum. Treatment arm 1: gemcitabine + cisplatin + Nab-paclitaxel; arm 2: gemcitabine + cisplatin (current standard of care: can use durvalumab in combination with gemcitabine and cisplatin).
8. Loose stool, add Creon; poorly differentiated esophageal adenocarcinoma treatment can be FOLFOX.
9. **Stage IV pancreatic head adenocarcinoma with metastasis** to liver treatment: gemcitabine + Abraxane qwk.
10. Hepatocellular carcinoma of alcoholic cirrhosis, Child-Pugh C, score 10, cirrhosis, poor liver function→consider hospice.
11. **Metastatic pancreatic body adenocarcinoma to omentum and peritoneum**, MSS, treatment: gemcitabine and nab-paclitaxel (Abraxane), stopped after NSTEMI.
12. **Metastatic pancreatic head adenocarcinoma**, resectable, high risk due to high CA199. Treatment: **FOLFIRINOX**, later 5-FU/LV bolus discontinued, and irinotecan dose reduced to 150 mg/m^2 for neutropenia and diarrhea.
13. **Pancreatic cancer**: <T1N0M0, pT2N2p, treatment FOLFIRNOX minus 5-Fu with LV at 200 mg/m^2, oxaliplatin 65/m^2. FOFIRINOX = leucovorin calcium (folinic acid), fluorouracil, irinotecan hydrochloride, and oxaliplatin. Oxaliplatin (Eloxatin) is a platinum-based antineoplastic agent inhibiting DNA repair and/or synthesis.
14. **Locally advanced pancreatic head ductal adenocarcinoma encasing SMA** treatment: gemcitabine and Abraxane. Diagnosis with CT abdomen → MRCP → EUS/ERCP, cholecystostomy tube, deconditioning, decrease treatment to gemcitabine only. Cholecystitis with cholecystostomy tube placement needs to be permanent due to obstruction.
15. 67 yo M with **metastatic pancreatic adenocarcinoma to liver and peritoneum** treatment: gemcitabine + Abraxane → FOLFIRI vs FOLFIRI + Veliparib (PARP inhibitor preventing DNA repair in cancer cells).
16. 80 yo F with **pancreatic uncinate adenocarcinoma** with abutment of SMV and gastroduodenal artery (GDA), Ca19-9 26.9 at baseline. Started on **gemcitabine + Abraxane** day 1, 8, and 15, q28d cycling with Abraxane at 100 mg/m2 for advanced age; hospitalized later for **gemcitabine-related rash, edema**, concerns for bilateral lower extremity cellulitis → chemotherapy on hold due to toxicity and patient was referred to radiation medicine for **neoadjuvant conformal radiation therapy**.
17. 70 yo F with **perihilar cholangiocarcinoma**, presumed primary sclerosing cholangitis, on the transplant list, sp. concurrent **chemoradiation therapy with 5-FU and brachytherapy** then on maintenance **capecitabine**, decrease to 1000 mg bid, stopped 1 month before **transplantation**. ERCP for stenting in the biliary duct was done due to obstruction from the tumor.
18. 71 yo F with HCV treated with sustained virologic response (SVR), MRI showed 4 × 4.7 × 4.4 cm lesion LR5 segment VII/VIII, CT CAP showed no

distant metastasis. **Surgical resection versus liver-directed therapy→selected radioembolization** with **y90** with excellent radiographic response and only mild restricted diffusion. Liver MRI then noted increased lesion and increased AFP→transcatheter arterial chemoembolization (TACE) → disease progression again on MRI → started **sorafenib**→increased tumor thrombosis→started **pembrolizumab** q3wks, informed patient 16%–18% probability of reducing tumor burden.

19. **Hepatic metastasis with stage IV adenocarcinoma of pancreatic tail** found to have a complex mass involving the lower pole of the right kidney, sp. **right renal artery embolization** to address bleeding from kidney mass. Current treatment: **gemcitabine with capecitabine** with gemcitabine at 1000 mg/m^2 (started on gemcitabine alone, and capecitabine was added due to disease progression and frailty) at days 1, 8, q21days→clinical improvements.

Neuroendocrine Tumor (NET)

1. **Carcinoid tumor** is a rare type of NET usually within the gastrointestinal (65%) or respiratory (35%) systems. Workups: **24 h urine 5-hydroxyindoleacetic acid** (5-HIAA), serum chromogranin (CGA) [elevated in 90% of gastroenteropancreatic NET (GEP-NET)]. Normal serotonin levels in healthy adults range between 71–310 ng/mL.
2. Diagnosis of NET via urinary **secretion of 5-HIAA** (hydroxyindoleacetic acid): 90% sensitivity and 90% specificity for carcinoid syndrome. **Chromogranin A** is elevated in well-differentiated NETs including carcinoids, associated with large tumor burden, and can be falsely positive in proton pump inhibitor takers. Blood serotonin level also has high false positive rates.
3. For NET, GA68 PET/CT is the most sensitive modality. However, GA68 PET/CT is not available in many facilities, as an alternative, **somatostatin receptor scintigraphy (SSRS) in combination with CT** is the next most sensitive modality.
4. **Treatment for the non-resectable disease of NET** includes somatostatin analogs, biotherapy, targeted radionuclide therapy, locoregional treatments including ablation and chemoembolization, and chemotherapy.
5. **Chemotherapy** may be used for inoperable or metastatic pancreatic NET, poorly differentiated NET, and in selected non-pancreatic NETs of high-grade or aggressive clinical course.
6. **Carcinoid** refers to well-differentiated NETs arising in the lung (typical and atypical); whereas WHO prefers the use of **NET** in the GI tract which is used for high-grade or poorly differentiated NETs.
7. **Carcinoid crisis symptoms**: profound flushing, bronchospasm, tachycardia, and widely and rapidly fluctuating blood pressure which can be precipitated by anesthetic induction, handling of tumor, or invasive therapies. **Carcinoid syn-**

drome is primarily associated with metastatic tumors originally in the **midgut** (distal small intestine through proximal colon).

8. **Atypical carcinoid** only applies to the intermediate **NET of the lung.**
9. For NET, it's important to rule out **MEN1, MEN2, and neurofibromatosis-1 syndromes**.
10. In carcinoid syndrome or to delay disease growth in poor surgical candidates, use **somatostatin analogs** that bind to SSTR subtype 2 (high affinity) and 5 (low affinity): **octreotide** and **lanreotide** (long-acting).
11. **High grade NET**, always treat; malnutrition, do PEG. If tumor at the gastroesophageal junction or stomach, do **J tube**.
12. **Pancreatic head high-grade NET metastatic to the liver**, Ki 67 > 30%, treatment: palliative **carboplatin** AUC 6 on day 1 and **etoposide** 50 mg/m^2, dose reduced due to hyperbilirubinemia. Labs during the visit: CA153 = 66, CA19-9 = 4450, CEA = 99.
13. **Gastroenteropathetic NETs**: (1) Well-differentiated NET including carcinoid tumors (in the tubular GI tract) and pancreatic NET (islet cell tumors); (2) Poorly differentiated neuroendocrine carcinoma (NEC).
14. **Grading of NETs**: The histologic grading scheme only uses a proliferative rate to stratify the grades and requires both a **mitotic count** and the **Ki-67** labeling index measurements. European Neuroendocrine Tumor Society grading for GI tract neuroendocrine neoplasms: (1) **Well-differentiated**: low grade with Ki-67 < 3% and mitotic count < 2 per 10 HPF (G1); (2) **Intermediate grade** with Ki-67 3%–20% and mitotic count 2 - 20 per 10 HPF (G2), and (3) **Poorly differentiated** with Ki-67 > 20% and mitotic count > 20 per 10 HPF (G3). **Poorly differentiated** NET = small cell neuroendocrine carcinoma and large cell neuroendocrine carcinoma.
15. **Non-neuroendocrine components**, including adenocarcinomas, signet ring cell carcinoma, and less likely squamous cell carcinoma, are common in **40% poorly differentiated NECs**. **Mixed neuroendocrine–non–endocrine neoplasm (Mi-NEN)** is defined as NEC consisting of a NE component and a gland-forming component (both >30%).
16. **Functioning (hormone-secreting) pancreatic NETs** are classified into insulinoma, gastrinoma, glucagonoma, VIPoma, and somatostatinoma.
17. **Small bowel NET** has a high risk for metastasis; it requires surveillance CT/MRI q6m for 1 year, then q1y for 10 years.
18. **Severe diarrhea differential diagnosis**: NET causing carcinoid syndrome, gastrinoma, and VIPoma.
19. **Evaluation of NET** includes CT, MRI, GA68 PET/CT for somatostatin receptors (SSTRs), **somatostatin receptor scintigraphy,** and bronchoscopy with transbronchial needle aspiration for mediastinal lymphadenopathy.
20. **Poorly differentiated NET** generally expressed fewer SSTRs and are not associated with G68 PET/CT.
21. For **Type 1 gastric NET ≤ 2 cm** (increased gastrin), EGD q6-12m for 3 years, then annually thereafter.

22. The median overall survival of NET is **9.3 years**. Treatments for NET progressed on **somatostatin analogs** include **everolimus, capecitabine and temozolomide (CAPTEM), and PPRT**.
23. **Sunitinib or everolimus** may be used for progressive advanced inoperable or metastatic well-differentiated NET.
24. For patients with symptoms of hormone hypersecretion from a pancreatic NET, **somatostatin analogs** should be used but with caution because of possible worsening glycemic control in **insulinoma**. Treatment is with **diazoxide or everolimus for insulinoma**. For **gastrinoma**, use high-dose proton pump inhibitors; somatostatin can be used in refractory cases.
25. Progressive disease/symptoms: somatostatin analogs (sandostatin and lanreotide) → **everolimus and sunitinib** improve progression-free survival (PFS).
26. Highly symptomatic from tumor bulk and who have rapidly enlarging metastases treatment in NEC: combined chemo with **capecitabine and temozolomide (CAPTEM)** rather than **temozolomide** alone. If hepatic predominant disease can do **hepatic arterial embolization**.
27. Somatostatin receptor-positive pancreatic NET treatment: **peptide receptor radioligand therapy (PRRT)**, a radiolabeled somatostatin analog such as lutetium 177 dotatate, may be used.
28. **High-grade gastroenteropancreatic (GEP) NEC** with a non-esophageal NEC and early-stage disease treatment: **surgical resection followed by 4–6 cycles of adjuvant etoposide plus a platinum drug**.
29. **Metastatic NEC treatment**: cisplatin or carboplatin combined with etoposide; an acceptable alternative is irinotecan plus cisplatin.
30. **Stage IV well-differentiated intermediate grade primitive neuroendocrine tumor (PNET)** to lungs and retroperitoneal nodes. **Treatment**: lanreotide 120 mg qmonth → later, retroperitoneal nodes are increasing in size → GA68 PET/CT scan → peptide receptor radioligand therapy (PRRT) or capecitabine + temozolomide (Temodar), hold lanreotide until PET scan. Then give lanreotide, capecitabine and temozolomide.
31. **Atypical lung carcinoid with metastasis to brain and lung** sp. surgery and whole brain radiation therapy (WBRT), Ki-67 proliferative index 30%, pT1bN2, can start **everolimus**, then **cabozantinib** if progression on everolimus. She is not a candidate for **PRRT** based on lack of PET avid disease on gallium and FDA approval for PRRT is as a second line gastroenteropancreatic NETs (GEP-NETs) treatment only.
32. **Low-grade NET of terminal ileum** sp. hemicolectomy with node + disease, Ki-67 not identified but increased serotonin and neurogranin A levels, return to the clinic in 4 months with labs, **no need for treatment**.
33. 72 yo African American male with multifocal well-differentiated NET with extranodal extension, low grade with zero mitosis. Baseline OctreoScan negative, CGA mildly elevated; baseline Ga-68 Dotatate PET/CT scan noted somatostatin receptor + tumor involving a right-sided mesenteric node and a loop of small bowel→**small bowel resection→continue surveillance** if asymptomatic.

34. **Malignant metastatic well-differentiated low-grade NET of the small intestine metastasized to the liver, peritoneum, and pleura**. Current treatment: cisplatin, irinotecan with cisplatin at 30 mg/m^2, and irinotecan at 65 mg/m^2 on hold for neutropenia (ANC < 1500). This patient was treated with capecitabine at the beginning and found to have progressive disease involving the peritoneum and omentum 3 months later, thus was offered options of cisplatin/irinotecan.
35. 61 yo Caucasian female with gastrinoma with solitary liver metastasis (Segment V) and periduodenal, retroperitoneal lymph node dissection (RPLND) in the setting of MEN-1 and ZES→**GA68 PET/CT showed increased uptake in a solitary lesion in segment V of the liver** as well as an 8 mm periduodenal RPLN, primary duodenal → esophagogastroduodenoscopy with endoscopic ultrasound (**EGD/EUS**) with a 10 mm sessile polyp in D2 biopsy consistent with a well-differentiated low-grade NET Ki 67 < 1% with mitosis 0/10 HPF. Low-grade NET at duodenal bulb with PE/CT scan confined metastasis→surgical resection with periduodenal lymph node dissection, resection of the duodenal tumor, partial hepatectomy segment V and cholecystectomy, gastrin level checkup. Plan of care: **repeat EGD 1–2 months** revealed a 10 mm duodenal sessile polyp which was low-grade NET per biopsy.
36. ZES requires a **higher dosage of pantoprazole 60 mg bid; annual EGD thereafter**.

Breast Cancer

1. Herceptin = trastuzumab (**HER2** is the target of monoclonal antibodies, Herceptin); pertuzumab (Perjeta) also targets HER2.
2. Receptor tyrosine protein kinase ErbB-2, also known as CD340, proto-oncogene Neu, and ERBB2, is a protein that in humans is encoded by ERBB2 gene. Also called **HER2 or HER2/Neu** which is a member of the human epidermal growth factor receptor (HER/EGFR/ERBB).
3. **Hormone/endocrine therapies** in breast cancer: **ovarian suppression** with oophorectomy, luteinizing hormone-releasing hormone (LHRH) agonists (used alone or with tamoxifen or fulvestrant) like goserelin (Zoladex) and leuprolide (Lupron), **suppressing estrogen production** with aromatase inhibitors (mainly in postmenopausal women), **interfering estrogen functions** with selective estrogen receptor modulators (SERMs) like tamoxifen and toremifene, and selective estrogen receptor degraders (SERDs)- fulvestrant (Faslodex) and elacestrant (Orserdu).
4. **Ovarian suppression** with leuprolide or other gonadotropin-releasing hormone agonists combined with **aromatase inhibitors** decreases the risk for breast cancer recurrence in premenopausal patients with early hormone receptor-positive breast cancer after chemotherapy.
5. **Tamoxifen** is used for premenopausal and postmenopausal women and men with ER-positive breast cancer; while aromatase inhibitors are used for ER-positive breast cancer in postmenopausal women. **Fulvestrant** is for postmeno-

pausal women with HR-positive, HER2-negative locally advanced or metastatic breast cancer without previous hormone therapy treatment. **Palbociclib** (Ibrance) is used for HR-positive, HER2-negative advanced or metastatic breast cancer in postmenopausal women.

6. **Ovarian suppression**: triptorelin, leuprolide, bilateral oophorectomy, or ovarian radiation.
7. **Selective estrogen receptor modulators** (SERMs) tamoxifen and raloxifene block estrogen uptake in breast tissue. **Aromatase inhibitors**: anastrozole (Arimidex), letrozole (Femara), and exemestane (Aromasin). **Fulvestrant and tamoxifen** can be used in postmenopausal women to inhibit estrogen receptor functions.
8. **Staging** of breast cancer: stage 0 = DCIS (negative lymph nodes); stage IA = ≤ 2 cm and 0 lymph node involvement; stage Ib = ≤ 2 cm and 1–3 micrometastatic positive lymph nodes (0.2–2 cm); stage II = > 5 cm and 0 lymph node or 2–5 cm and armpit lymph node involvement; stage IIIA: ≤5 cm and 4–9 lymph node involvement; stage IV = distal metastasis.
9. Imaging is recommended for staging **only in Stage III or worse disease or signs and symptoms suggestive of distant metastasis**.
10. **Breast cancer assessments**: biopsy report + surgery pathology report + ER/PR report + FISH for HER2 oncotype.
11. If **PR is positive, ER has to be positive**; if PR is negative, ER can be positive or negative.
12. The Oncotype DX Breast Recurrence Score Test (21 gene diagnosis): **≤25** no chemo (of note, for scores between 11-25, chemo may also provide benefits in premenopausal women); >25 chemo is needed. Alternatively using **lymph node involvement** to guide chemo.
13. Cancer can hide with **radial scar** tissue from biopsy and will have to be removed.
14. Breast cancer after 5 years, follow up q1y.
15. **LCIS/DCIS treatment**: lumpectomy and lymph node biopsy (sentinel lymph node) → chemotherapy for 4 months (follow up in 2 weeks to see whether lymph node shrinks), one-month rest → surgery → estrogen inhibitor therapy (**tamoxifen in premenopausal and postmenopausal, anastrozole after menopause**).
16. **Lumpectomy** has a risk of 41% relapse; **lumpectomy + radiation therap**y is the standard of care with a risk of 7% relapse. ER +, T2 (or 0.5cm to 5 cm in size), LN−→consider oncocyte diagnosis; if **21 gene recurrence score** >25, do **chemotherapy**. Triple-negative, if >0.6 cm, do chemotherapy. HER2+ with ER+/− , if >0.5 cm, do **chemotherapy + targeted therapy with trastuzumab and pertuzumab**. In general, breast cancer treatments include surgery (lumpectomy vs mastectomy) → chemotherapy → radiation → hormonal therapy. If aggressive disease, chemotherapy → surgery → radiation therapy → hormonal therapy (sensitive tissue, thus no RT on hormonal therapy). Chemo before surgery decreases tumor size and microscopic metastasis.
17. Besides known family history of BRCA mutation, male breast cancer, and family or personal cancer history at the ovary, fallopian tube or primary peritoneal

cancer, and two or more relatives on the same side with breast cancer and/or pancreatic cancer, **additional BRCA 1 and BRCA 2 testing indications include**: (1) Patients with breast cancer history: onset ≤50 years old; triple negative cancer at age ≤ 60; Ashkenazi Jewish origin; first degree relative with breast cancer at ≤50 years old. (2) Patients without cancer: one first or second degree relative with breast cancer diagnosed at ≤45 years old; Ashkenazi Jewish origin with family history of breast cancer.

18. For BRCA1 or BRCA2, **breast MRI starts at 25 yo and mammogram at 30 yo**. If positive for breast cancer, check **gene expression assays, 21 gene recurrence score**. If DCIS→consider lumpectomy + radiation→consider anastrozole or tamoxifen.
19. Breast cancer (ER+, HER2-) treatment: docetaxel (**Taxotere) + cyclophosphamide** for 4 cycles.
20. Node negative ER/PR+, HER2- left breast cancer Stage 1, sp. lumpectomy + RT, started on anastrozole.
21. Most early-stage invasive breast cancers are treated with initial **excision followed by radiation and systemic adjuvant chemotherapy**; lumpectomy with radiation vs mastectomy (equally effective).
22. **Axillary dissection** is necessary for breast cancer if ≥3 sentinel node involvement.
23. **Breast cancer chemo regimen**: preferred regimen for ER+ / HER-2 negative—dose dense AC (Adriamycin and Cyclophosphamide) followed by **paclitaxel**; preferred regimen for HER-2 positive—AC followed by paclitaxel + **trastuzumab +/− pertuzumab**.
24. **DCIS without lymph node involvement** treatment: **lumpectomy** with **sentinel** lymph node biopsy, 4–6 weeks later → **radiation therapy** for 7 weeks → **hormonal therapy** for 7–10 years.
25. **Breast cancer relapse** workups: CT, MRI breast, PET.
26. **Chemotherapy + Herceptin** has a 47% response rate. **Chemotherapy + Herceptin + Perjeta** (can cause nose bleed) has a 67% response rate.
27. Chemo regimen for HER2+ **breast cancer: TCHP** q3w × 6 cycles (Taxotere (docetaxel) + carboplatin + Herceptin + Perjeta).
28. **ER+/triple negative breast cancer** chemo regimen = AC + T [Adriamycin, cyclophosphamide, and paclitaxel (Taxol)], q2w × 6 cycles. **Aromatase inhibitors** increase osteoporosis and decrease bone density, and cause hot flashes, joint and muscle pain.
29. **Triple-negative breast cancers of 0.6 cm or greater** in size treatment: adjuvant therapy typically anthracycline-based chemotherapy; a taxane agent like Paclitaxel (Taxol) or docetaxel (Taxotere) can be added.
30. **Women with a history of chest wall radiation** between the ages of 10 and 30 years are at high risk for developing breast cancer and should be **screened annually with MRI and mammogram**. Increased breast cancer risk starts at **10 years after radiation exposure and** peaks at **25–34 years after exposure**.
31. Patients with a history of early breast cancer with findings suspicious for **metastatic recurrent breast cancer** should undergo a biopsy to confirm the diagno-

sis and to assess hormone receptor and HER2 status as these may **differ from** the **original cancer**.

32. **HER2 positive, hormone receptor-negative stage II infiltrating ductal breast cancer** treatment: neoadjuvant chemo with **docetaxel, trastuzumab, and pertuzumab**.
33. **Chemotherapy** is used to decrease metastasis risks in many invasive breast cancers, but in **DCIS the risk of distant metastasis is only 1%**.
34. Indications of **adjuvant chemo**: high tumor grade, extensive lymphatic invasion, large primary tumor size, skin or chest wall involvement, ≥4 lymph node involvement in postmenopausal women, triple negative, ≥5 cm, or with + lymph nodes (any number) in premenopausal women.
35. **Adjuvant chemo**: 2–3 agents given for four to 8 cycles; anthracyclines (doxorubicin or epirubicin), cyclophosphamide, taxanes (paclitaxel and docetaxel).
36. **Aromatase inhibitor side effects** (1/3 of patients discontinued treatment as a result): symmetric arthralgia, joint stiffness, bone pain. **Trastuzumab side effects**: infusion reactions, fever, chills.
37. **HER2 + treatment**: trastuzumab or combined with pertuzumab if tumor size >5 cm, + lymph node involvement or both. For HER2+ and size <3 cm, **paclitaxel + trastuzumab** is a less toxic option.
38. **Locally advanced breast cancer** should get CT and **bone scan**; should be initially treated with neoadjuvant **chemo**, followed by **surgery** and then **radiation** therapy.
39. If **tamoxifen** is used, avoid CYP2D6 inhibiting agents like **bupropion** or **fluoxetine** which may decrease tamoxifen activation.
40. Small cancer in the breast after age 70, no radiation; **give trastuzumab + pertuzumab adjuvant therapy + chemotherapy if HER2+.**
41. **Letrozole (Femara) for 5 or 7–10 years** after breast cancer diagnosis and cure.
42. **Letrozole plus palbociclib (Ibrance)** is the most appropriate treatment for patients with advanced breast cancer that recurs after completing previous adjuvant **aromatase inhibitor** therapy. **Palbociclib** is an oral CDK4/6 inhibitor that is **synergistic with hormonal therapies** in vitro.
43. **Post-mastectomy radiation is needed** if ≥5 cm in size, + margins or skin involvement, inflammatory breast cancer, and/or many positive lymph nodes.
44. For **premenopausal women** who remain premenopausal after adjuvant chemo for high-risk hormone-sensitive breast cancer, **ovarian suppression achieved by surgical oophorectomy or pelvic irradiation** in addition to tamoxifen or an aromatase inhibitor is superior to tamoxifen alone.
45. Combining targeted agents such as CDK4/6 inhibior **palbociclib** or the mammalian target for rapamycin (mTOR) inhibitor **everolimus** improves hormonal therapy effects for metastatic breast cancer.
46. Metastatic breast cancer during aromatase inhibitor use: treatment is **palbociclib plus fulvestrant** if during, and **palbociclib** plus **aromatase inhibitor** if after completion of aromatase inhibitor therapy.
47. **HER2+ advanced breast cancer treatment**: trastuzumab + chemo or antiestrogen therapy. The first line treatment is THP (trastuzumab + pertuzumab + docetaxel). Ado-trastuzumab emtansine (Kadcyla or

T-DM1) = trastuzumab + microtubule inhibitor emtansine for HER2 + as a 2nd line treatment; later, trastuzumab deruxtecan (Enhertu) was found to be better than T-DM1 as a 2nd line in HER2+ metastatic cancer.

48. CA27-29 breast cancer marker high but CT sable and MRI brain stable → no change in the treatment plan may be appropriate.
49. **Breast cancer metastasized to the brain** treatment: Perjeta and Herceptin at the same time, q3m.
50. General rule for breast cancer treatment: no metastasis, no chemotherapy (not always true). **With antiestrogen therapy, do bone scan q2y**.

Cervical Cancer and Ovarian Cancer

1. **Cervical cancer**: stage I is confined to the cervix; stage II invades beyond the uterus but not to the pelvic wall or lower 1/3 of the vagina; stage III extends to the pelvic wall and/or the lower 1/3 of the vagina and/or hydronephrosis.
2. Patients with stage **IA1 disease with vascular invasion and patients with stage IA2 or IB1** disease treatment: radical trachelectomy, also known as cervicectomy; permanent cerclage.
3. Stage IIA cervical squamous cell cancer treatment: radical hysterectomy with pelvic lymph node dissection and para-aortic lymph node sampling, followed by **pelvic external beam radiation and concomitant weekly cisplatin with cervical brachytherapy** during the first week of therapy.
4. **Stage III cervical cancer** treatment: radiation with concomitant platinum-based chemotherapy. **Stage IVB** treatment: palliative cisplatin-based chemotherapy, with radiation for local symptoms, i.e., bleeding or pain.
5. **BRCA1 and BRCA2 and mismatch repair gene mutations** should be checked in all patients with ovarian cancer.
6. **Initial studies for ovarian cancer**: CA12-5, transvaginal and transabdominal ultrasound. For early ovarian cancer, surgical exploration is recommended.
7. **Ovarian cancer**: stage I disease (favorable)—treatment with surgery alone; stage I (unfavorable)—high grade or clear cell→surgery is often needed; Stage II- spread beyond ovaries but confined to the pelvis→surgery is often needed.
8. **Stage I unfavorable and Stage II ovarian cancer** treatments: surgery followed by 3–6 cycles chemo (usually carboplatin and paclitaxel); optimally debulked.
9. **Stage IIIA (spread to lymph nodes) high-grade serous ovarian cancer** treatment: TAH-BSO → 6 months of chemo with cisplatin and paclitaxel.
10. Newly diagnosed advanced ovarian cancer and a BRCA1 or BRCA 2 mutation, after remission after chemotherapy, give **olaparib maintenance therapy**.
11. Relapse 6 months or more after chemo is considered **platinum-sensitive ovarian cancer**. Adding the angiogenesis inhibitor **bevacizumab** improves disease-free survival, but not overall survival, and increases the risks of serious GI toxicities including **esophageal or gastric perforation**.

12. **Platinum-taxane chemo** is recommended for all stages of ovarian cancer. Stage IIIc and Stage IV ovarian cancer who are at high perioperative risk or who have a low likelihood of optimal tumor debulking treatment: **neoadjuvant chemo followed by reevaluation for cytoreduction surgery**.
13. **Stage IIIa high-grade serous ovarian cancer with deleterious BRCA1 germline mutation** found on genetic testing. She was treated with TAH-BSO, and chemo with iv and intraperitoneal **cisplatin and paclitaxel**, 18 months later, the cancer was cured, and she underwent two additional sequential chemotherapies including **carboplatin** and **paclitaxel**, **cisplatin** and **gemcitabine** with addition of **bevacizumab**.
14. Oral poly adenosine diphosphate (ADP)-ribose polymerase (**PARP**) inhibitor **Olaparib** (Lynparza) is FDA-approved as monotherapy for patients with **germline BRCA-mutated advanced ovarian cancer** previously treated with three or more lines of chemotherapy.

Lynch Syndrome

1. Hereditary non-polyposis colorectal cancer (HNPCC), also known as Lynch syndrome, refers to patients with **a germline mutation in one of the DNA mismatch repair genes** (MLH1, MSH2, MSH6, PMS2) or the epithelial cellular adhesion molecule (**EpCAM**) gene.
2. Diagnosis with Amsterdam II criteria: **≥3 relatives with Lynch syndrome-associated cancer (colorectal, endometrial, small bowel, ureter or pelvis)**; 1 first-degree relative, 1 < 50 years old, 2 successive generations; not familial adenomatous polyposis, biopsy-proven.
3. Muir-Torre syndrome, a variant of Lynch syndrome, is characterized by **sebaceous tumors and cutaneous keratoacanthomas** in addition to cancers related to Lynch syndrome.
4. Lynch syndrome: 80 yo F with locally advanced second portion duodenal adenocarcinoma with focal signet ring features; clinical Lynch syndrome confirmed with EpCAM and MSH2 mutations; history of colon cancer in 2002 sp. resection, bilateral breast cancer sp. mastectomy; squamous cell carcinoma of the esophagus sp. chemoradiation followed by minimally invasive esophagectomy. Omniseq panel: + BRCA2, high MSI, PD-L1 2% TPS (24%), TMB 28/mb, CD28 (31%) ⇒ **start treatment with pembrolizumab**.
5. **BRAF V600F mutation favors the diagnosis of Lynch syndrome whereas MLH1 promoter hypermethylation** argues against the diagnosis of Lynch syndrome with the exception of rare endometrial cancer in Lynch syndrome.
6. In colorectal cancer: pMMR = proficient mismatch repair. Patients with **pMMR and BRAF or KRAS mutations** had shorter overall survival than those without mutations, but no difference between pMMR and deficient MMR if BRAF or KRAS wild type.

7. **MSI result of MMR** (DNR mismatch repair) deficient hypermutator phenotype is common in a significant portion of endometrial, colorectal, and gastric cancers and is found in >90% Lynch syndrome (**MSI-high**). Methylation of MLH1 promoter leads to a loss of MLH1 expression → leads to **MSI-positive colorectal cancers.**
8. MSI testing, IHC testing for lost or truncated MMR protein, germline testing are commonly recommended in Lynch syndrome.
9. In patients with loss of MLH1 staining on IHC, check for acquired BRAF mutations and **MLH1 promoter hypermethylation** to distinguish Lynch syndrome (usually no methylation) and sporadic colorectal cancer (methylation). **BRAF mutations** are common in sporadic MSI-H colorectal cancer (40%–87%) but not in Lynch syndrome.
10. Testing for **Lynch syndrome**: CRC with high MSI and/or loss of one of the MMR on IHC; endometrial cancer at age < 60, first-degree relatives with known MMR/EpCAM gene mutation; ≥5% chance of MMR mutation calculated.
11. Lynch syndrome: CRC screening with colonoscopy.
12. **HNPCC mutation testing indication**: a personal or family history or both of additional HNPCC-related cancers, particularly **colorectal, small bowel, or endometrial cancers or transitional cell cancers of the renal pelvis or ureters**.

Myelodysplastic Syndrome

1. **Myelodysplastic syndrome (MDS)** typically has megaloblastic **anemia, hepatosplenomegaly (HSM), and cytopenia** in senior adults.
2. **MDS** anemia has **macrocytosis** and pancytopenia. **Erythropoietin** deficiency has **normocytosis** and low reticulocytes.
3. **MDS with 5q deletion** is low risk for progression or transformation. Treatment includes first-line **lenalidomide**, second-line includes recombinant erythropoietin, and hypomethylating agents like **azacitidine** and **decitabine** (which may worsen blood counts initially and takes 6 months to show effects).
4. High-risk MDS in young patient treatment is **hematopoietic stem cell transplantation (HSCT) → azacitidine**.
5. In **high-risk young patients**, can give allogeneic HSCT. The goal of treatments is to **decrease transfusion requirements and decrease the risks for acute myeloid leukemia transformation**. Immunosuppressive therapy with antithymocyte globulin (ATG, rabbit, and horse), cyclosporine, tacrolimus, prednisone, and alemtuzumab may also be used in patients with MDS.
6. **Immunosuppression** with **antithymocyte globulin** and **cyclosporine**, similar to that used for aplastic anemia, has been shown to decrease transfusion requirements in young patients <65 years.
7. If **ferritin > 1000, give deferoxamine iv or deferasirox oral**.

Leukemia

1. Leukemia diagnosis: presence of ≥25% lymphoblast on **bone marrow** exam. **Cytochemical stains and flow cytometry** distinguish ALL from AML and B cell from T cell ALL.
2. Prognosis for ALL is poor in older adults, worse for those with Philadelphia chromosome t (9;22). Treatment of ALL with Philadelphia chromosome t (9;22): **dexamethasone + tyrosine kinase inhibitor (TKI) dasatinib**.
3. **Asparaginase** is incorporated for adolescents and young adults with ALL but not in older patients. **Anthracycline** (such as daunorubicin), **vincristine,** and **dexamethasone** are part of traditional chemotherapy for pediatric and adults with ALL, not in elder patients. **Hyper-CVAD** (hyperfractionated) is the treatment for ALL including older patients.
4. Chemotherapy with **idarubicin and cytarabine** is used for CML in blast crises with ≥20% blasts (AML).
5. **CLL flow cytometry** will show B cell Ags (CD19, CD20, and CD23), coexpression of CD5 (usually T cell markers), and low levels of a monoclonal surface Ig.
6. **CLL treatment**: bendamustine and rituximab; if relapse, treatment with obinutuzumab + venetoclax, alternative options include oral Bruton kinase inhibitors acalabrutinib or zanubrutinib.
7. **CLL indications for treatment**: symptoms, cytopenia, and bulky lymph nodes. Treatment includes **R-CVP** (rituximab, cyclophosphamide, vincristine, prednisone), BR (bendamustine plus rituximab), ibrutinib for stage IV and III; Involved-field radiation therapy (IFRT) for stage I and II. Additional treatments for CLL include BCL2 inhibitor venetoclax and monoclonal antibodies like rituximab, ofatumumab, and alemtuzumab (used alone or in combination with chemotherapy).
8. In **CLL**, many patients have a decrease in one or more immunoglobulins, more in IgG, IgA, and IgM.
9. 65 yo with CLL, baseline WBC 75, asymptomatic, stage 0 CLL 13q deletion. Treatment: surveillance q6m with CBC, CMP, LDH, and quantitative immunoglobulins. **No treatment is needed**.
10. **Hairy cell leukemia**: cytopenia, splenomegaly without lymphadenopathy, positivity for CD20, CD11c, CD25 and CD103. **Treatment**: **cladribine**, and **pentostatin** both are purine nucleoside analogs. If fails 2 cycles, give **rituximab** and may perform splenectomy for cytopenia.
11. **Hairy cell leukemia** is strongly CD20+→5–7 days course of cladribine or pentostatin.
12. 70 yo **hairy cell leukemia (HCL)** sp. first treatment with 2-CDA (cladribine) × 1 cycle, completed. However, persistent bone marrow involvement, thus offered rituximab × 4 doses and got cured.
13. HCL is a **low-grade B cell lymphoproliferative disorder** that typically presents with splenomegaly, cytopenias, and diffuse bone marrow infiltration.

14. **CML** typically presents in the chronic phase with increased neutrophils or platelets or both.
15. **Chronic myelogenous leukemia (CML)** phases: chronic phase, accelerated phase, or blast crisis. CML → acute leukemia (blast crisis) at 20% of patients a year (acute lymphocytic leukemia rather than acute myeloid leukemia) if untreated, 1% with treatment. **Treatment of CML**: potential cure with allogeneic hematopoietic cell transplantation (HCT); disease control without cure using tyrosine kinase inhibitors; or palliative therapy with cytotoxic agents.

Lymphoma

1. Blood cell cancer categories: myelodysplastic syndrome, AML, ALL, lymphoma. **ITP + CLL = Evans syndrome**.
2. **Hodgkin's lymphoma classification**: classical, lymphocyte rich (best prognosis because of CD20+), lymphocyte depleted, nodular sclerosing. Hodgkin's lymphoma usually is diagnosed in young patients and has Reed-Sternberg cells.
3. Monitor **PET at 3, 6, 12, and 24 months after Hodgkin lymphoma treatment with ABVD**: Adriamycin (doxorubicin); Bleomycin; Vinblastine; Dacarbazine (DTIC).
4. 25 yo M with **Hodgkin lymphoma**, treatment: **ABVD** (Adriamycin, Bleomycin, Vinblastine, Dacarbazine) × 6 cycles, sperm banking before chemo. PET/CT revealed residual lymph node involvement → lymph node dissection → relapsed, started on 3 cycles of **ICE** (ifosfamide, carboplatin, etoposide). Salvage chemotherapy ICE followed by **autologous stem cell transplan**t with prior **CBV** (Cytoxan/cyclophosphamide, BCNU/carmustine, and VP-16/etoposide) conditioning regimen → lymph node relapse → localized radiation → PET no evidence of residual disease → start **brentuximab vedotin** (BV) maintenance, stopped due to worsening neuropathy.
5. **Anaplastic large cell lymphoma (ALCL)** is one type of **T-cell non-Hodgkin's lymphoma**. ALCL is divided into ALK+ ALCL, ALK- ALCL, primary cutaneous ALCL (pC ALCL), and the provisional entity breast implant-associated ALCL.
6. **Non-Hodgkin lymphoma**: malignant neoplasms derived from B cell progenitors, T cell progenitors, mature B and T cells, or rarely mature NK cells.
7. **Non-Hodgkin lymphoma**: B cell lymphoma accounts for 85%; T cell lymphoma accounts for 15% but is very aggressive. High grade (50% mortality, can be cured); low grade (may not need treatment, no cure, slow); intermediate (like Mantle cell lymphoma).
8. Systemic disease of **non-Hodgkin lymphoma** treatment: R-CHOP (cyclophosphamide, doxorubicin, vincristine, prednisone + rituximab), R-CVP (cyclophosphamide, vincristine, prednisone + rituximab), or rituximab (can replace rituximab with obinutuzumab) plus bendamustine.

9. **B cell lymphoma**: **low grade**—no treatment necessary, does not kill, no cure, includes CLL, marginal zone, lymphoplasmacytic lymphoma (Waldenstrom's macroglobulinemia), follicular lymphoma grade I and II; **Intermediate grade**—mantle cell lymphoma; **high grade**— DLBCL, follicular lymphoma grade III; **very high grade**—ALL, Burkitt's lymphoma t(8;14), always treat, kills, 50% cure rate.
10. **Staging**: CLL Rai staging 0-lymphocytosis; I-lymphocytosis, lymphadenopathy; II-lymphocytosis, lymphadenopathy, organomegaly; III- lymphocytosis, lymphadenopathy, organomegaly, anemia; IV-lymphocytosis, lymphadenopathy, organomegaly, anemia, and thrombocytopenia.
11. Other types of lymphoma staging: **Ann Arbor staging system**; I one lymph node region; II 2 lymph node regions of the same side of the diaphragm; III lymph node on both sides of the diaphragm; IV extensive lymph node and bone marrow involvement. Five categories of lymphoma: E-extranodal; S-splenic involvement; A-lack of B symptoms; B-positive B symptoms.
12. **High-grade lymphoma** treatment: R-CHOP, hyperCVAD (hyperfractionated cyclophosphamide, vincristine, doxorubicin, and dexamethasone) + R or high dose methotrexate + cytarabine. 50% cured after the aforementioned treatment → 50% primary refractory + relapsed → consider **salvaged with chemo**: ESHAS, DHAS, DHAC, RICE→consider collect stem cells → consider condition chemo BEAM (carmustine + etoposide + cytarabine + melphalan) → infuse back with collected stem cells; alternative is CAR-T therapy.
13. **Excisional biopsy** is used for the diagnosis of the subtype of lymphoma and guiding treatments. The biopsy specimen is used for **histopathologic, cytogenetic, and FISH, as well as immunophenotype and gene expression profiling**. CBC with differential, ESR, CMP, serum urate, LDH, beta2-microglobulin, and immunoglobulins are commonly checked in lymphoma.
14. **Screen for infections in lymphoma:** HIV, HCV, EBV, HBV, the human T-lymphotropic virus type 1, HHV8. Bone marrow biopsy is preferably done at the iliac crest.
15. **Radiation therapy** is used after chemotherapy as **consolidation** in lymphoma treatment.
16. Transformation to **DLBCL** occurs in **30%–40% of patients with follicular lymphoma. Idelalisib**, a PI3K inhibitor, has a high rate of partial response to relapsed follicular lymphoma after exclusion of transformation.
17. **Lymphoma** treatment: **R-CVP** (rituximab, cyclophosphamide, vincristine, prednisone), BR (bendamustine plus rituximab), ibrutinib.
18. **Nonbulky asymptomatic follicular lymphoma** even at stage IV does not need treatment.
19. Follicular lymphoma with B symptoms treatment: **R-CVP** (rituximab, cyclophosphamide, vincristine, and prednisone). Patient's story: prostate cancer → B symptoms → CT abdomen/pelvis and chest → biopsy of lymphadenopathy → diagnosed with follicular lymphoma with B symptoms → treatment with R-CVP (no Adriamycin doxorubicin).
20. **Large B cell lymphoma treatmen**t: **R-CHOP** → salvage chemo (**R-ICE**: rituximab, ifosfamide, carboplatin, and etoposide) followed by **stem cell trans-**

plantation (bone marrow transplantation) versus **CAR-T therapy** (Chimeric Antigen Receptor T Cell Therapy).

21. Large B cell lymphoma treatment: R-CHOP, soft tissue → radiation therapy.
22. **Ibrutinib (Imbruvica)** can be used for low-grade B cell lymphoma.
23. **Mantle cell lymphoma** treatment: **R-HyperCVAD** alternating with **rituximab plus high-dose methotrexate/cytarabine**.
24. The diagnosis of lymphoma requires **two pathologist** reports to identify low versus high-grade lymphoma.
25. **High-grade lymphoma treatment**: 6 cycles of R-CHOP or 8 cycles of hyper-CVAD (cyclophosphamide, vincristine, doxorubicin, and dexamethasone) alternating with methotrexate and cytarabine.
26. **Aggressive lymphoma**: acutely or subacutely with rapidly growing mass, systemic B symptoms (i.e., fever, night sweats, and weight loss), and/or increased LDH and uric acid. Examples include **diffuse large B cell lymphoma, Burkitt lymphoma, precursor B and T lymphoblastic leukemia and lymphoma, adult T cell leukemia and lymphoma, and certain other peripheral T cell lymphoma**.
27. **Indolent lymphoma**: insidious, presenting only with slow-growing lymphadenopathy, hepatomegaly, splenomegaly, or cytopenias. 50% with extranodal disease, 10%–35% with primary extranodal lymphoma at diagnosis. Examples include **follicular lymphoma, chronic lymphocytic leukemia (CLL), small lymphocytic leukemia (SLL), and splenic marginal zone lymphoma**.
28. **Primary CNS lymphoma** symptoms: headache, lethargy, focal neurological symptoms, seizure, paralysis, spinal cord compression, or lymphomatous meningitis.
29. Diagnosis of NHL based on excisional tissues: (1) **Histology**- nodular or follicular pattern, diffuse pattern, change from a nodular to a diffuse pattern in adjacent nodes; change from a lower to a higher grade of involvement within a single node. (2) **Immunophenotype** via flow cytometry conducted on fresh unfixed single-cell suspensions or immunohistochemistry on tissue sections (CD19, and 20 = B cells). (3) **Genetic studies**.
30. **Bone marrow biopsy** before treatment except for DLBCL: bone marrow involvement occurs in 30%–50% of all patients with NHL, commonly in indolent histologies.
31. **CNS lymphoma**: 76 yo with headache, neck pain, and sparing out → right parietal mass, surgical removal and diagnosis with DLBCL. **Treatment**: DeAngelis regimen (MVP = methotrexate, vincristine, procarbazine, dexamethasone, and leucovorin) or high dose methotrexate × 5, high dose ARA-C (cytarabine) × 2 with a weaning dose of steroids for 4 months → complete remission. Follow-up visits initially q4m then q6m; keep Keppra treatment until 1 year after surgery. If a patient develops a seizure, the patient should be treated with Keppra forever.
32. **Mediastinal lymphoma**: 69 yo, dyspnea → mediastinal mass → VATS biopsy → DLBCL of the germinal center B cell phenotype, Ki-67 70%. **Treatment**: rituximab and dose-adjusted EPOCH (etoposide, prednisone, vincristine, cyclophosphamide, hydroxydaunorubicin = doxorubicin).

33. Rituximab + dose-adjusted **EPOCH** is the first-line treatment for **highly aggressive DLBCL (advanced DLBCL with high risk FISH features) and a prerequisite for autologous stem cell transplantation** in selected patients. Use Pola-R-CHP (polatuzumab vedotin + rituximab + cyclophosphamide + doxorubicin + prednisone) in advanced stage DLBCL.
34. **DLBCL example:** Cytogenetics-BCL2 extra signals, BCL6 and C-myc low levels. First cycle rituximab + EPOCH was complicated with pneumonia and LBBB → pacemaker; after cycle 2 demonstrated complete remission. Restaging PET after cycle 4 with continued complete remission. After cycle 5, developed fever; finished 6 cycles. Post cycle 6, had a fall with febrile neutropenia. We would recommend an **autologous bone marrow transplant**; however, given the patient's low ECOG status, we do not believe she is a candidate at this time.
35. 69 yo with **right axillary mass** otherwise asymptomatic→CT multiple lymph nodes of the axilla with bulky supraclavicular right lymphadenopathy→bone marrow biopsy and aspiration negative, but molecular diagnosis showed major breakpoint region (MBR)→lymph node biopsy showed **follicular lymphoma** grade 1–2. Follicular lymphoma grade: Grade 1 = 0–5 centroblasts/HPF, Grade 2 = 6–15 centroblasts/HPF, Grade 3→15 centroblasts/HPF. The patient did not fulfill **GELF criteria (signs, symptoms, and lactate dehydrogenase/ β2-microglobulin) for treatment**. Check CBC, CMP, LDH q6m with annual CT.
36. **CAR-T cells**, genetically modified T cells expressing chimeric antigen receptor (CAR), are a form of genetically modified autologous immunotherapy that has shown activity against DLBCL.
37. 57 yo Trisomy 12, CLL thrombocytopenia + thrombocytosis, transformation?! Treatment: **rituximab + bendamustine** × 6 cycles.
38. 85 yo with **retroperitoneal lymphadenopathy**, 6.3 cm × 5.9 cm, diagnosis after biopsy as **DLBCL**. Treatment: rituximab + CHOP × 6 cycles, Nulastin for chemo-related neutropenia. Later, developed progressive lymphadenopathy at the left inguinal and soft tissue mass posterior to paraspinal musculature at L3, repeat PET, biopsy again → DLBCL/FL grade 3b; pathology: germinal center phenotype, C-myc negative, CD20+, pAX5+, BCL 6+. Treatment: radiation and does not qualify for curative intent as she is above the limit for **high dose chemotherapy with autologous stem cell transplantation** (HDC-ASCT).
39. 67 yo with **loss of appetite and early satiety with positive direct Coombs test**, hepatitis panel -, diagnosis: autoimmune hemolytic anemia (**AIHA**); treatment: **prednisone 20 mg** tid→splenomegaly 20 cm; bone marrow biopsy revealed **low-grade B cell marginal zone lymphoma**. Pathology: mature B cells, proliferative neoplasm + high-frequency NK cells with heterogeneous expression of CD3 and CD6. Treatment: surveillance.
40. **Stage IV follicular lymphoma** with low tumor burden treatment: surveillance.
41. **Tumor burden** = the number of cancer cells, the size of a tumor, or the amount of cancer in the body.

Head and Neck Cancer

1. Signs and symptoms of **head and neck cancer**: otalgia, dysphagia, pain, weight loss, dyspnea, and neck mass. **Laryngeal cancer** symptoms: persistent hoarseness, dysphagia, chronic cough, hemoptysis and neck mass, stridor, and otalgia. **Sinus tumor** symptoms: epistaxis and unilateral nasal obstruction. **Leukoplakia and erythroplakia** are indicative of oral cancer.
2. **Management (diagnosis and staging) of head and neck cancer**: **panendoscopy** (laryngoscopy, bronchoscopy, esophagoscopy), FNA, CT, MRI, PET, and PET-CT. For example, CT chest and neck → laryngoscopy with biopsy → PET-CT.
3. **Pharynx** = nasopharynx (nose, parotid gland) + oropharynx (tongue, salivary gland, and epiglottis) + hypopharynx (larynx).
4. Stage I and II disease (with no lymph node involvement) of the **oropharynx** (tends to recur locally) treatment: **radiation therapy and surgical resection**.
5. Lymph node involvement or involvement of deeper structures = **stage III or IV** disease.
6. After surgery, **adjuvant radiation or combined chemoradiation** is necessary if positive surgical margins, lymphovascular or perineural invasion, or more demand (T3 or T4) disease. If positive surgical margins and extranodal extension, **postoperative chemoradiation therapy** is preferred over **postoperative radiation therapy alone**.
7. **Nasopharyngeal cancer treatment**: radiation alone for stage I disease and combined chemoradiation for stage II and higher disease.
8. **Cisplatin or cetuximab** [an epidermal growth factor receptor (EGFR) inhibitor] on top of **radiation** improves survival in locally advanced diseases in head and neck cancer.
9. **Cisplatin** has to be dose-adjusted in **chronic kidney disease**.
10. **Early-stage laryngeal cancer** treatment: radiation alone. **Chemotherapy (cisplatin or cetuximab)** is added for locally advanced laryngeal cancer before **total laryngectomy**.
11. 62 yo squamous cell cancer of the head and neck (**hypopharynx**) with metastasis to liver → chemoradiation with **carboplatin and taxol and cetuximab** for 6 cycles→after 12 weeks, do PET, excellent response in the head and neck, but disease progression in liver→**radiofrequency ablation** for 6 weeks or **radioactive microsphere embolization** at liver → 3 weeks later, do immunotherapy. Carboplatin and Taxol were held during weeks 3 and 6 due to neutropenia. Cetuximab completed 2 cycles.
12. Nontender neck mass → PET CT revealed lung nodule → bronchoscopy with biopsy confirmed **squamous cell carcinoma and HPV+**; head neck surgery biopsy lung nodule/mass revealed **metastatic squamous cell carcinoma of the right tonsil**. Treatment: extreme regimen (**carboplatin/5-FU/cetuximab**) vs. carbo/taxol/cetuximab.

13. If **localized squamous cell carcinoma of head and neck cancer**, do **cisplatin** weekly or **cetuximab** or **carbo/Taxol with radiation**; low dose weekly cisplatin 40 mg/m^2 is less toxic than high dose cisplatin 100 mg/m^2 q3wks. Add Decadron on day 2,3,4 and Compazine.
14. 74 yo male with **squamous cell carcinoma of the supraglottic larynx**, cT4N2cM0, stage IVB, was treated with **cisplatin** right away with **concurrent radiation** therapy.
15. **BMX solution** = Benadryl, Maalox, xylocaine 1:1:1 solution.
16. **Squamous cell carcinoma (SCC)** accounts for 90%–95% of lesions in head and neck cancer: well-differentiated (>75% keratinization), moderately differentiated (25%–75% keratinization), and poorly differentiated (<25% keratinization). Rarely, other types including verrucous carcinoma, adenocarcinoma, adenoid cystic carcinoma, and mucoepidermoid carcinoma are diagnosed.
17. For induction chemotherapy in head and neck cancer, a combination protocol using TPF with **docetaxel (Taxotere), cisplatin (Platinol), and fluorouracil** is better than the PF protocol with cisplatin and 5-FU. **Sequential therapy** (TPF followed by concurrent chemoradiation with cisplatin and radiation) should be reserved for very healthy patients with a high risk of distant and locoregional failure.
18. **Severe neutropenia** is common during TPF induction chemotherapy, thus primary prophylaxis with **fluoroquinolone, G-CSF**, or both are needed.
19. In most concurrent chemotherapy alone or after induction chemotherapy, **platinum-based chemo, Cisplatin** 100 mg/m^2 q3wks or 40 mg/m^2 qwk is used. If contraindications with platinum-based chemo like nephrotoxicity, ototoxicity, or neuropathy, **cetuximab plus radiation therapy** is used. Alternatives include **carboplatin, carboplatin plus fluorouracil, or weekly carboplatin and paclitaxel**.
20. 54-year-old recurrent **adenoid cystic carcinoma** has a propensity to travel along nerve trunks. Treatment: **Gamma Knife Stereotactic Radiosurgery (GKSRS).** Adenoid cystic carcinoma is a malignant tumor of the salivary gland. The patient was also on Bactrim bid for osteomyelitis.

Genitourinary Cancer

Prostate Cancer

1. **Androgen deprivation therapy** (ADT) testosterone level goal should be **<50 ng/dL**. Biopsy is recommended if **PSA ≥ 0.35 ng/mL/year increases when < 4 ng/mL, or ≥ 0.75 ng/mL/year increases if ≥ 4 ng/mL**.
2. Spinal cord compression or those with focal symptomatic bone metastases treatment: **external beam therapy** and steroids.
3. **Treatment for prostate cancer**: active surveillance, external beam radiation, and radical prostatectomy, or observation. A PSA **doubling time of less than 3 years** is considered an indication for treatment. Repeat biopsy is typically done at 1 year.

4. Newly diagnosed prostate cancer needs **pathology assessment from two pathologists for Gleason score**. **Treatment**: **Lupron + chemotherapy** extends overall survival from 8 years with Lupron alone to 9.5 years.
5. For patients with metastatic prostate cancer with a **biochemical recurrence** (increase in PSA and no local disease progression), treatment: androgen deprivation therapy (**ADT**).
6. ADT consists of inhibiting androgen synthesis (**GnRH agonist leuprolide**) or locking its receptor [**flutamide or bicalutamide** (Casodex)] with **bilateral orchiectomy** as an alternative, especially in the elderly. ADT is typically combined with **docetaxel** chemo in extensive metastatic disease. Docetaxel causes immunosuppression with contraindications for **hepatic dysfunction and compromised bone marrow** functions.
7. **Antiandorgens**: flutamide, bicalutamide, nilutamide, enzalutamide, apalutamide, and darolutamide.
8. **Progressive metastatic prostate cancer** after being treated with ADT equals **castrate-resistant prostate cancer**, treatment: **docetaxel** with prednisone, CYP17 inhibitor **abiraterone** (Zytiga) plus prednisone, androgen receptor blockade **enzalutamide** (Xtandi), Radium 233 (**Xofigo**), or secondary hormone therapy (steroids and adrenolytics, such as **ketoconazole** and **aminoglutethimide**).
9. **Radium-223 (Xofigo)** is indicated specifically for **bone-limited or bone-predominant symptomatic metastatic disease**.
10. A postoperative serum **PSA level of ≥0.1 ng/mL (update: any measurable amount)** is diagnostic for **residual** or **recurrent** prostate cancer. A rising PSA immediately following surgery has a high likelihood of harboring **distal metastatic disease**; and will need **ADT**.
11. **Prostate cancer** treatment: Lupron (leuprolide), GnRH analog/agonist inhibits GnRH secretion. Dual androgen blockade failed→consider enzalutamide or flutamide (first-generation nonsteroidal antiandrogen).
12. **Biochemical recurrence ≥2 years** after surgery is more consistent with **local recurrence**→consider treatment with **radiotherapy**.
13. High-risk prostate cancer is defined as **PSA ≥ 20, a Gleason score of 8–10, or evidence of extraprostatic extension of cancer**. For these patients, the addition of **ADT (GnRH agonist like leuprolide) to radiation** results in an improvement in 10-year disease-free and overall survival compared to radiation alone.
14. **Prostate cancer germline mutations**: BRCA2, HOXB13, and Lynch syndrome genes.
15. Prostate biopsy via transrectal ultrasound guidance sampling **12 cores from different regions:** assessment for **atypical small acinar** proliferation and **multifocal high-grade intraepithelial** neoplasia.
16. Radiation causes short-term **enteritis** (approximately 20% of men) and **cystitis** (approximately 50% of men) and **erectile dysfunction** (60%–70% of men) by 2 years.
17. Prostate cancer of intermediate or high-risk localized disease treatment: **radiation therapy, and adding GnRH agonist**. If high-risk and very high-risk local-

ized prostate cancer, treatment includes 6 cycles of adjuvant **docetaxel** and radiation and a GnRH agonist. Castrate-sensitive prostate cancer treatment: **ADT and docetaxel**.

18. PSA recurrence = increase ≥2 ug/L→**salvage radiation or surgery** if no metastatic disease. Biochemical recurrence is defined as PSA 0.2 ng/mL or greater followed by another increased measurement at the same level or higher.
19. Progressive disease after treatment with docetaxel→consider treatment with **cabazitaxel (Jevtana) with prednisone**.
20. Lupron → enzalutamide → ketoconazole (old days). Nowadays, if **enzalutamide** is ineffective (after 11 m progression-free), stop enzalutamide and add **abiraterone** (Zytiga) (3 m progression-free) and prednisone (5 mg bid).
21. On enzalutamide, PSA elevation to 263, check CT and bone scan, and switch to **Zytiga + prednisone**.
22. Prostate cancer with bone metastasis: **Lupron + bicalutamide** for antiandrogen (dual antiandrogen) therapy. Update: nowadays, bicalutamide is only used as temporary androgen blocking agent when starting GnRH agonists; for treatment purposes, enzalutamide, apalutamide, or darolutamide is more commonly used.
23. Metastatic prostate cancer to the bone. After **bicalutamide (see above update) and Lupron** for 4 weeks, PSA decreased, the next step may be **docetaxel** plus **Lupron**.

Testicular Cancer

1. **Alpha fetal protein** is usually normal in pure seminoma; **beta-hCG** is elevated only in around **20%** of **pure seminomas**. **Nonseminomatous germ cell tumors**: yolk sac tumor, choriocarcinoma, and embryonal carcinoma. We should check **beta-hCG, AFP, and LDH** in patients with seminoma and nonseminomatous germ cell tumors.
2. **Stage I pure seminoma** treatment: surgery → consider active surveillance; the alternative is adjuvant **radiation or chemotherapy** with 1–2 cycles of carboplatin.
3. **Stage II seminoma** is defined by retroperitoneal lymph node metastases. Treatment: adjuvant **radiation or cisplatin-based combination chemotherapy**. Stage III seminoma (spread into the spermatic cord or scrotum) treatment: cisplatin-based chemotherapy.
4. **Testicular cancer** treatment: radical inguinal orchiectomy and adjuvant bleomycin, etoposide, and cisplatin. The risks for **secondary solid tumors** are increased for the lung, colon, bladder, pancreas, and stomach.
5. **Early-stage non-seminomatous germ cell tumors** treatment: **active surveillance in selected patients, retroperitoneal lymph node dissection (RPLND), or limited chemotherapy with 1 cycle of the BEP regimen (bleomycin, etoposide, and cisplatin).**
6. Patients with **recurrent testicular cancer** are treated with combination chemo (bleomycin, etoposide and cisplatin) and can also be treated with high-dose chemo plus autologous hematopoietic stem cell transplant.

Renal Cell Carcinoma

1. **Renal cell carcinoma (RCC)** treatment: radical or partial nephrectomy, may add sunitinib thereafter.
2. **Ultrasound- complex cyst or solid mass**→CT, **biopsy is only if CT does not indicate renal cell carcinoma**.
3. **Paraneoplastic syndromes in RCC**: anemia, hepatic dysfunction in the absence of liver metastasis (known as Stauffer syndrome), fever, hypercalcemia, erythrocytosis, AA amyloidosis, thrombocytosis, and polymyalgia rheumatica.
4. Small tumors of RCC in frail patients with a high risk of postoperative complications management: **cryoablation, radiofrequency ablation, or even active surveillance**.
5. **Metastatic RCC treatments**: cytoreductive nephrectomy → traditional treatments: sorafenib, **sunitinib**, pazopanib, axitinib, bevacizumab, cabozantinib, and lenvatinib; newer combinations: ipilimumab/nivolumab, axitinib/pembrolizumab.
6. **Recurrent RCC treatment**: nivolumab, VEGF inhibitor lenvatinib or axitinib.

Bladder Cancer

1. Diagnosis via cystoscopy with urine cytology and biopsy of visible tumor or mucosal abnormality. If cancer → **transurethral resection of bladder tumor (TURBT)** and examination to determine histology and depth of invasion.
2. **Bladder cancer treatment**: TURBT + BCG.
3. **Exophytic lesion (Ta)** treatment: TURBT followed by a single dose of intravesical chemo (BCG or mitomycin). **Tis and T1** lesion treatment: TURBT followed by 6 weekly treatments of intravesical chemo (BCG or mitomycin). Repeat cystoscopy 3 months later.
4. **Muscle invasive bladder cancer** treatment: cystectomy with or without cisplatin-based chemo. If progression, give **atezolizumab** (Tecentriq), a monoclonal antibody directed against the PD-L1 receptor. Enfortumab vedotin is approved for recurrent metastatic bladder/urothelial cancer.
5. **Bladder cancer with muscular invasion**→consider chemoradiation: chemo weekly × 6 + radiation daily for 5 days × 7 weeks.
6. **High-grade or recurrent low-grade bladder cancer** treatment: transurethral resection of bladder tumor (**TURBT**) followed by **intravesical chemotherapy (BCG or mitomycin)** for six treatments → **cystoscopy 3 m** after treatment and subsequently at 3–6 months intervals. If recurrent, need **cystectomy** with or without **cisplatin**-based chemo → atezolizumab, an anti–PD-L1 monoclonal antibody.
7. **Bladder cancer recurrence** in 6–12 months after initial TURBT or after one to two courses of BCG infusion should undergo **cystectomy**.

Thyroid Cancer

1. **Papillary thyroid cancer with metastasis** treatment: lenvatinib or sorafenib for differentiated refractory metastatic differentiated thyroid cancer (DTC).
2. Treatments for **differentiated thyroid cancer (DTC)** in both papillary thyroid cancer and follicular thyroid cancer: surgery, thyroid hormone therapy, and selective use of radioactive iodine. **Radioactive iodine** can cure a minority of patients with metastatic cancers. **TSH thyroid hormone suppression therapy** slows disease progression.
3. **Medullary carcinoma of thyroid metastatic to lung and liver**: total **thyroidectomy** for stage II T2NxcM0 medullary carcinoma of the left lobe and Stage III T3NxcM0 papillary carcinoma of the right lobe, **radioactive iodine** at dose 98.7 mLi for papillary cancer → observation → CT recurrence with high calcitonin, started treatment with **cabozantinib** → unable to tolerate due to dyspnea and pleural effusion → started sunitinib, check EKG q1m, urine, calcitonin, mag, CEA, had **T7 bone metastasis** → started **external beam radiation T6-T8** × 1 week to preserve neurological function.
4. **Goal TSH in papillary thyroid cancer** is 0.3–2. Patients with persistent disease or distant metastasis should target TSH < 0.1.
5. After **total thyroidectomy** for thyroid cancer, patients with a high risk for disease recurrence should receive **adjuvant radioactive iodine** therapy.
6. **Thyroid stimulating hormone (TSH)** goal 0.1–0.5 mU/L for 5–10 years in high-risk patients after thyroidectomy. TSH target is 0.1–0.5 mU/L in low-risk patients (with papillary thyroid cancer) but TSH initially should be suppressed to below 0.1 mU/L in high- and intermediate-risk thyroid cancer.
7. **Medullary thyroid cancer**: once diagnosed, check for metastatic disease, identify co-existing tumors, and check for germline RET mutations. Staging CT if **lymph node involvement or calcitonin > 400**, bone scan if **suspecting bone metastasis**.

Further Readings and References

1. Martínez-Carballeira D, Bernardo Á, Caro A, Soto I, Gutiérrez L. 2024. Treatment of Immune Thrombocytopenia: Contextualization from a Historical Perspective. Hematol Rep. 16(3):390–412.
2. Roskoski R Jr. 2024. Targeted and cytotoxic inhibitors used in the treatment of lung cancers. Pharmacol Res. 107465.
3. Parekh DS, Tiger YKR, Jamouss KT, et al. 2024. Updates on Therapeutic Strategies in the Treatment of Relapsed/Refractory Multiple Myeloma. Cancers (Basel). 16(17):2931.
4. Peltomäki P, Nyström M, Mecklin JP, Seppälä TT. 2023. Lynch Syndrome Genetics and Clinical Implications. Gastroenterology. 164(5):783–799.
5. Garcia-Manero G. Myelodysplastic syndromes: 2023 update on diagnosis, risk-stratification, and management. Am J Hematol. 98(8):1307–1325.
6. Al Sukhun S, Temin S, Barrios CH, et al. 2024. Systemic Treatment of Patients With Metastatic Breast Cancer: ASCO Resource-Stratified Guideline. JCO Glob Oncol. 10:e2300285.
7. Posdzich P, Darr C, Hilser T, et al. 2023. Metastatic Prostate Cancer-A Review of Current Treatment Options and Promising New Approaches. Cancers (Basel). 15(2):461.

Chapter 37
The Infectious Disease Consultation

The following clinical vignettes were drafted and modified to represent various clinical scenarios of severe acute infections. Infectious disease consultants and other relevant specialties including but not limited to general surgery, interventional radiology, gynecology, and neurosurgery were commonly involved in the multidisciplinary care of these severe acute infections. The treatment plans of these clinical vignettes were mainly based on infectious disease consultant recommendations. As the actual clinical situation varies, rather than following the management examples of these clinical vignettes, timely consultation with infectious disease physicians and other specialists remains the probable only right choice (unless otherwise unrealistic) and thus is highly recommended.

Additional common recommendations for severe infections during acute inpatient care include the following: (1) follow up with infectious disease in 2 weeks for close monitoring and to determine if the duration of the antibiotics needs to be extended; (2) counsel the patient regarding the side effects of the antibiotics; (3) schedule routine weekly CBC, CMP, ESR, and CRP while on IV antibiotics; (4) revisit routine vaccination schedules; (5) an ophthalmology exam to rule out endophthalmitis is generally recommended for fungemia before or around antibiotic completion (preferably within 1 week of diagnosis).

1 Central Nervous System Infections

Meningoencephalitis

Clinical Vignette A 70-year-old male presented in September with high-grade fever, double vision, and unsteady gait for about 1 day before admission. He drinks alcohol regularly and lives in the countryside. A physical exam revealed some rashes involving lower extremity and his abdomen. His temperature upon presentation was

K. Zhou, *Internal Medicine Training Notes and Survival Guide*, https://doi.org/10.1007/978-1-0716-4039-5_37

103.8 °F and the WBC count was 7.2. Platelet counts were 143, lactic acid was 1.3; liver function tests were within normal limit, glucose 169, creatinine was 1.10.

Workups blood cultures were negative and urinalysis was unremarkable. Imaging studies of chest X-ray and CT head did not reveal any acute findings. Lumbar puncture (LP) with cerebrospinal fluid (CSF) studies showed nucleated cell 303 (neutrophils 84%, lymphocyte 15%), protein 76, glucose 85. CSF culture showed many polymorphonuclear leukocytes (PMNs), no epithelial cells, and no organisms seen on the gram stain with negative culture. CSF meningitis/encephalitis PCR panel was negative. The serum tick-borne disease panel was negative. CSF viral culture, West Nile antibody and PCR, Lyme antibody, and Borrelia PCR were all negative.

Analyses and Treatments Initial empirical coverage with IV ampicillin, IV ceftriaxone, IV vancomycin, and IV doxycycline. Differential diagnoses in this scenario include HSV, VZV, syphilis, Rocky Mountain spotted fever (RMSF), West Nile, Lyme, Ehrlichia, and rat bite fever (Streptobacillus moniliformis). Ampicillin was then discontinued as the PCR panel was negative for Listeria. The RMSF antibody and the tick-borne panel are negative, hence doxycycline was also stopped. Infectious work-ups including tick borne panel, Lyme serology, CSF West Nile, and CSF Borrelia PCR and serology were ordered. RMSF serology, RPR, and HIV screening serology were also added.

Final Diagnosis West Nile IgM of the CSF returned positive while West Nile IgG was negative. In the acute phase of West Nile infection, PCR can be negative. Treatment for West Nile encephalitis is supportive only; antibiotics were stopped.

Aspergillus cerebritis

Clinical Vignette An 83-year-old male presented for headache, left eye vision loss, facial numbness, and ride-sided facial pain.

Workups magnetic resonance imaging (MRI) and magnetic resonance angiography (MRA) brain and neck were notable for anterior right temporal lobe cerebritis versus abscess, diffuse paranasal sinus thickening, and right mastoid effusion. Magnetic resonance venography (MRV) was notable for invasive right sphenoid sinusitis with right orbital apex and cavernous sinus involvement. Lumbar puncture was notable for RBC > 10,000, 100 total nucleated cells, and with negative CSF culture.

Plan of Care neurology, neurosurgery, ophthalmology, ENT, and infectious disease teams were consulted. The patient received right frontotemporal sphenoidal craniotomy for anterior temporal lobectomy for abscess resection with pathology showing no evidence of significant inflammation, fungal organisms, or neoplasm.

The aphthalmologist believes that once someone's vision progresses to no light perception, the chance for vision recovery is negligible.

Clinical Diagnosis right temporal lobe cerebritis with abscesses with possible invasive infection through the right sinuses.

Microorganism Diagnosis fungal culture later revealed prelim 1+ yeast. Tissue culture later grew 1 colony of Aspergillus species.

Treatment initially treated with Flagyl and amphotericin B and IV ceftriaxone. With final results, the patient was treated with voriconazole (pharmacist to dose) with voriconazole level check in 5–7 days for months.

Lyme Meningitis

Clinical Vignette A 74-year-old male with a history of leptomeningitis and meningoencephalitis treated with acyclovir 1 year ago presented for intermittent memory loss of 6 weeks. He also complains of dizziness, headache, and neck pain for 4 days.

Workups MRI brain showed a left leptomeningeal signal increase; lumbar puncture showed eight white blood cells with polymorphonuclear leukocytes (PMNs) at 42% and lymphocytes at 50%. CSF meningitis/encephalitis PCR panel negative. Tick borne pathogen panel negative; however, CSF and serum Lyme IgM and IgG positive with Western blot pending.

Treatments Rocephin 2 g once daily for a total of 2 weeks from the start of therapy.

Aseptic Meningitis Versus Lyme Meningitis

Clinical Vignette A 43-year-old female with a possible tick bite at the right foot interarch while outdoors barefoot. She developed a quarter-size erythematous circular-like rash soon after. About 7–10 days later, she developed fever, chills, sweats, some diarrhea, photophobia and myalgias. Lyme titer was noted to be positive. The patient was then treated with doxycycline for about 11 days but developed continuous fever and some paresthesia in the arms and fingertips. As such, she was sent to the hospital from the outpatient clinic.

Workups CSF study results were abnormal with lymphocytosis, slightly low glucose, and elevated protein. Positive serum Lyme screening test and Western blot IgM are concerning for early exposure. Epstein-Barr titers were also high for early capsid antibodies. Monotest was negative. CBC revealed a white count high at 14.5

with lymphocytosis at 70%, hemoglobin 10.5, and platelet count of 208. Liver enzymes were elevated. The tick PCR panel was negative. MRI brain was not suggestive of severe meningoencephalitis or multiple sclerosis.

Analyses and Treatments (1) **Fever of unknown origin**: Headache photophobia, mild hepatitis, and lymphocytosis were consistent with viral illness especially mononucleosis (Epstein-Barr virus) like viruses versus early tick borne infection. Further workup was appropriate. (2) **Aseptic meningitis:** viral versus early disseminated Borrelia Lyme meningitis: CSF analysis results were consistent with aseptic viral-like meningitis with additional testing in process. The meningitis/encephalitis PCR panel was negative. Clinically patient did improve on doxycycline as an outpatient and after admission, she was treated with Rocephin. After admission, she remained afebrile with improvement in headache, photophobia, and paresthesia. As a result, the patient was continued on Rocephin 2 g daily 14-day course. (3) **Possible Epstein-Barr viral infection** with lymphocytosis and positive early capsid serology. EBV quantification level is still pending. She did have mononucleosis as a child and Monospot is negative thus diagnosis is not clear at this time. No enlarged lymph nodes but mild splenomegaly noted on recent CAT scan; will need follow-up outpatient for lymphoma rule out.

Bacterial Meningitis

Clinical Vignette A 60-year-old male with melanoma on immunotherapy presented with fever, headache, mild expressive aphasia, and confusion.

Workups Lumbar puncture stat revealed gram-positive cocci, neutrophil predominant leukocytosis with low glucose. CSF meningitis/encephalitis PCR panel was negative. CSF culture had no growth. MRI brain revealed no acute process.

Assessment Gram-positive cocci in the CSF study made the pneumococcal infection the most likely diagnosis, although no specific pathogen was isolated on PCR meningitis panel or cultures. This could be early bacterial as well as other opportunistic pathogens. The neurology consultant did not recommend further work-up for mild expressive aphasia. Additional testing for tickborne pathogen Lyme and fungal etiology were later negative for any abnormalities. Although the concern for progressive multifocal leukoencephalopathy (PML) is low clinically, we did check for JC virus in spinal fluid and blood which were negative. Cat exposures at home deserve additional tests of toxoplasmosis and Bartonella which returned negative.

Treatments He was originally started on IV dexamethasone, ceftriaxone, ampicillin, and vancomycin. Because of the probable pneumococcal meningitis without signs of encephalitis clinically or on MRI, the patient was discharged on IV

Rocephin for 14 days for probable pneumococcal meningitis and oral doxycycline for possible tickborne pathogen until labs were final.

2 Intra-abdominal Infections

Polymicrobial Bacteremia from Intra-abdominal Source

Clinical Vignette A 75-year-old male presented with worsening fever, chills, and rigors with headache and transient abdominal pain.

Workups CT abdomen and pelvis with contrast initially did not reveal any acute pathology. Culture originally showed gram-negative bacteremia, but later revealed Gemella morbillorum (facultative anaerobic, similar to viridans Streptococci, associated with colorectal cancer and causes endocarditis) and Fusobacterium. Repeat blood culture 2 days later grew Pseudomonas aeruginosa and Bacteroides thetaiotaomicron. Transesophageal echo did not reveal any obvious signs of endocarditis.

Assessment Because of polymicrobial bacteremia, infection from a gastrointestinal source is highly suspected. CT with IV and oral contrast of the abdomen and pelvis was repeated days later and revealed inflammation around the sigmoid colon with evidence of superior mesenteric vein septic thrombophlebitis. General surgery was consulted and EGD and colonoscopy were recommended as outpatient given the risk of bowel injury in the present state. There were also concerns about gastrointestinal absorption and oral antibiotic tolerability.

Treatments IV meropenem 1 g q8h for at least 2 weeks from the date of negative blood cultures, but may need to be extended pending his intra-abdominal pathology. Repeat CT of the abdomen and pelvis is planned in 2 weeks to evaluate further and determine the final duration of antibiotics at follow-up.

Tubo-Ovarian Abscess (TOA)

Clinical Vignette A 61-year-old female presented with abdominal pain for 2 days and an inability to eat.

Workups Routine labs revealed prerenal azotemia, leukocytosis, abnormal urinalysis (concerning urinary tract infection), and CT without contrast of the abdomen and pelvis revealed concerns for an intra-abdominal abscess on the left side (6.3 × 4.5 × 5.4 cm abscess with associated adjacent fat stranding) which is either a tubo-ovarian abscess or abscess related to colitis. The interventional radiologist placed a drain for the abscess with drain fluid gram stain showed gram + and – rods and cocci; culture eventually grew Streptococcus constellatus.

Treatments Generally, tubo-ovarian abscesses are treated with cefotetan and doxy. Because the source of infection is likely a bowel vs vaginal source, the patient was originally treated with Zosyn which was later transitioned to penicillin G and Flagyl (stopped due to nausea and vomiting) with the culture result of Streptococcus constellatus. The patient was eventually discharged on moxifloxacin 400 mg daily and IV penicillin 24 million units' continuous infusion for 2–4 weeks**.** Drain removal is recommended once its output remains low for 3 days. Surgery is only indicated if the abscess fails to resolve with drain placement after completion of antibiotic treatment.

Polymicrobial Pelvic Abscess Status Post Peritoneal Dialysis Catheter Removal

Clinical Vignette A 65-year-old male with end-stage kidney disease on peritoneal dialysis presented with worsening confusion together with generalized weakness for a week.

Workups, Assessment, and Management His peritoneal fluid analysis was consistent with spontaneous bacterial peritonitis (158 WBC, 80% neutrophils). The fluid culture was negative for growth. Later, the patient received diagnostic laparoscopy with the removal of the peritoneal dialysis (PD) catheter and washout of the abdomen with the placement of a drain, debridement of the PD catheter tract, and placement of a vacuum dressing. Purulence was noted in the pelvis adjacent to the PD site during surgery with surgical tissue culture growing lactobacillus species initially. He was discharged on oral Augmentin. Days later, the patient was readmitted for confusion and was found to have a large pelvic abscess. The interventional radiologist placed a drain with culture showing polymicrobial infection on Gram stain (many gram-positive cocci and few yeasts) but no obvious fecal material or bile was noted. Culture eventually grew predominantly Pseudomonas and Candida tropicalis but other gastrointestinal flora was also noted. Given the fact of polymicrobial infection, infection from gastrointestinal sources (like colorectal flora) was considered. CT scan of the abdomen and pelvis with IV but no oral contrast was thus performed but did not show an obvious leak. Given the size of the abscess, source control may take time even with the placement of an external drain.

Final Treatment Plan Cefepime dosing after dialysis 2 g every Monday, Wednesday, and Friday for a total of 14 days, IV Vanco sliding scale per pharmacy dose for a total of 14 days combined with oral Flagyl 500 mg twice daily for 10 days, and Diflucan 400 mg every other day for 14 days. The interventional radiologist agreed to follow up for drain management and the surgery team agreed to monitor for the need for serial CT scan of the abdomen and pelvis with consideration of oral contrast studies shortly to rule out bowel source/leak.

MRSA Peritonitis from Peritoneal Dialysis Catheter

Clinical Vignette A 63-year-old female with end-stage renal disease on peritoneal dialysis (PD) and a history of recurrent urinary tract infections (UTIs) with drug-resistant pathogens ESBL E. coli presented with weakness and dizziness.

Workups Her PD fluid analysis revealed WBC ≥ 100 cells/uL with ≥50% polymorphonuclear leukocytes.

Assessment She was diagnosed with peritoneal dialysis catheter infection with MRSA peritonitis. Peritoneal dialysis was placed on hold. The patient is physically improving after the initiation of intraperitoneal vancomycin, and thus the addition of rifampin would not be helpful and it does not appear that she requires peritoneal dialysis catheter removal or debridement of the PD catheter tract.

Treatments Vancomycin 2 g daily or 25 mg/L concentration once daily for an additional 14 days. Decolonization with nasal Bactroban cream 2% applied to both nares twice daily the first week of each month and chlorhexidine 4% soap for use in the showers twice per week were also recommended. Typically, monitoring of vancomycin drug levels is not needed if using the above regimen.

Peritoneal Dialysis (PD)-Associated Peritonitis

Peritoneal dialysis (PD)-associated peritonitis has a prevalence of 30%–40% among patients with PD. Signs and symptoms include abdominal pain and cloudy PD fluid. Its **diagnosis** requires 2 out of the following three criteria: clinical features of peritonitis, PD fluid WBC ≥ 100 cells/uL with ≥50% polymorphonuclear leukocytes after a dwell time of ≥2 h, positive PD fluid culture. **Treatment** is intraperitoneal antibiotics like vancomycin for 14 days.

Fecal Peritonitis

Clinical Vignette A 59-year-old female presented with worsening abdominal pain and was found to have recurrent small bowel obstruction. She underwent robotic laparoscopic surgery for lysis of adhesions, enterotomy repair, and Roux-en-Y revision appendectomy. She was later found to have an anastomotic leak to small bowel sites requiring additional repair with signs of fecal peritonitis.

Assessments The patient has increased risks for hospital-acquired pathogens and drug-resistant pathogens with prolonged hospital stay and multiple antibiotic exposures.

Treatments IV Meropenem to cover resistant gram-negative rods, IV Diflucan for the coverage of Candida, and daptomycin for the coverage of MRSA and VRE. Dose adjustment based on weight is necessary for the antibiotics. Serial liver enzyme and CPK monitoring are recommended while on the above antibiotics. Repeat CT of the abdomen and pelvis is also necessary to rule out any retained collections and for source control issues.

MRSA Seroma Infection

Clinical Vignette A 51-year-old female status post recent excision of the excessive skin and subcutaneous tissue in the anterior abdomen with the repair of the open incisional ventral hernia presented with abdominal wall surgical site pain.

Workups CT abdomen and pelvis without contrast showed postoperative changes from the recent pannus resection and ventral herniorrhaphy. The anterior abdominal wall surgical site seroma aspiration culture grew profuse MRSA.

Assessment The patient has been treated with IV vancomycin with improvement. However, due to the patient's chronic kidney disease, vancomycin was stopped and switched to IV daptomycin. The surgery team confirmed that no mesh was used to repair the ventral hernia.

Treatments IV daptomycin for at least 2 weeks.

Complicated Intraabdominal Infection

Clinical Vignette A 59-year-old female with colorectal adenocarcinoma presented for robotic total abdominal hysterectomy with bilateral salpingo-oophorectomy (TAH-BSO). The patient developed postoperative infection from enterotomy jejunum with bile leak requiring repair a week later and a second look washout another week later. She later developed a small bowel fistula with a small intraabdominal fluid collection status post interventional radiologist drain placement.

Assessments Gastrointestinal pathogens or hospital-acquired pathogens are expected.

Treatments IV ertapenem 1 g daily and IV fluconazole 400 mg daily for 2–4 weeks combined with supportive care TPN and bowel rest. Serial serum white counts, CRP, and repeat CAT scans for drainage are recommended.

Strep Intermedius Intraabdominal Abscess

Clinical Vignette A 73-year-old female with endometrial cancer status post chemotherapy underwent laparoscopic total abdominal hysterectomy with bilateral salpingo-oophorectomy (TAH-BSO) recently presented with worsening abdominal pain.

Workups CT abdomen and pelvis with contrast revealed an intra-abdominal abscess. The interventional radiologist placed a drain for the abscess with a culture positive for Streptococcus intermedius. Blood culture was negative and there was no record of bacteremia in the past.

Treatments She was initially treated with IV Zyvox, Rocephin, and Flagyl. Upon discharge, the antibiotic regimen was changed to oral Levaquin 500 mg daily and Flagyl 500 mg 3 times daily for 2 weeks. She may need prolonged antibiotic treatment of 4–6 weeks given the abscess. Oral Levaquin and Flagyl have very good tissue penetration and similar distribution to IV infusion. The interventional radiology team agreed to continue drain management and serial CT scan monitoring during follow-up.

3 Pancreatic Pseudocyst Infections

Sepsis from Intra-abdominal Source + Infected Pancreatic Pseudocyst

Clinical Vignette A 55-year-old male with a history of recurrent alcohol-induced pancreatitis presented with worsening abdominal pain, nausea, and vomiting. Upon presentation, his temperature was 98.3 °F and his WBC count was 14.3.

Workups Blood culture was negative in growth. CT of the abdomen and pelvis with IV contrast only revealed worsening pancreatitis with large peripancreatic fluid collection, the largest of which measured about 14 × 6 × 11 cm together with small bowel dilated loops reflecting ileus. Repeat CT abdomen and pelvis with IV contrast only 3 days later showed increased peripancreatic fluid and mesenteric stranding, thickening of the transverse colon and duodenum, and mild fluid-filled distended small bowel suggestive of ileus. Since admission, the patient has been having intermittent fevers as high as 101.3 °F and his white count continues to rise up to 20.

Treatments He was started empirically on IV meropenem upon admission. IV vancomycin was later added given persistent fever despite being on meropenem. Later, IV Diflucan (400 mg load, then 200 mg daily) was added to the antibiotic regimen for possible Candida overgrowth. Repeating another CT scan of the abdomen and pelvis with IV contrast is recommended if the patient continues to have abdominal pain and leukocytosis.

Infected Necrotizing Pancreatitis

Clinical Vignette A 57-year-old male with recurrent alcoholic pancreatitis with known pancreatic duct perforation and a history of spontaneous bacterial peritonitis with ascitic cultures grew Cutibacterium acnes (formerly Propionibacterium acnes) presented for worsening abdominal pain. Upon presentation, he had leukocytosis with WBC 26 and later also developed a fever of 101.7 F.

Workups Abdominal CT scan revealed increased complexity of pseudocysts with an increase in gas. Blood cultures were negative. 4 days later, the patient underwent debridement of the infected pancreatic pseudocyst with multiple drain placement. Culture from drain fluid later grew coagulase-negative Staph but other bacteria may be present.

Assessment Given known pancreatic duct perforation together with other signs and symptoms, there is certainly a concern for infected necrosis from complex pancreatitis with infected pancreatic pseudocyst. Complex infections likely will take weeks to resolve. Serial CT scans of the abdomen are necessary to help determine the duration of antibiotics but tentatively may require at least 4–6 weeks.

Treatments He was treated with IV cefepime and metronidazole upon admission. The infectious disease consultant recommended stopping IV cefepime and IV Flagyl, switching to IV meropenem 1 g q8h, and adding IV vancomycin per pharmacy for broader empiric coverage. Fungitell study is still pending; empiric antifungal coverage should be considered if the (1,3)-β-d-glucan (BDG) test is significantly elevated. Later, the patient was discharged on IV daptomycin 6 mg/kg once daily, IV ertapenem 1 g once daily for 4–6 weeks; added Culturelle 1 capsule by mouth twice daily while on antibiotics.

4 Diabetic Infections, Osteomyelitis

Actinomyces Foot Infection and Polymicrobial Bacteremia

Clinical Vignette A 56-year-old male presented with a rapidly worsening right great toe diabetic necrotizing infection.

Workups Blood cultures were positive for oxacillin-sensitive Staph epi and Gemella. X-ray upon presentation showed soft tissue gas at first digit but no obvious osteomyelitis. He underwent right first ray amputation with surgical culture growing Actinomyces odontolyticus and surgical pathology negative for osteomyelitis.

Assessment The patient was found to have great toe necrotizing diabetic foot infection and polymicrobial bacteremia. Although the transthoracic echocardiogram was negative for any obvious endocarditis, Gemella is a high-risk organism for endocarditis. As such, a transesophageal echocardiogram was recommended to rule out endocarditis (which was negative).

Treatments The patient was initially treated with IV vancomycin and Zosyn and clindamycin. The antibiotic regimen was changed to IV penicillin G 24 mil units/24 h continuous infusion for 4–6 weeks and oral Levaquin 750 mg once daily for 2 weeks.

Necrotizing Diabetic Left Foot Infection with Myositis: Polymicrobial Wound Infection

Clinical Vignette A 46-year-old female with an intravenous drug use history, type 2 diabetes with recurrent foot infections, and chronic hepatitis C presented with fevers and necrotizing left foot infection. She had a history of left foot infection with fourth toe osteomyelitis from group G strep status post amputation of the fourth toe.

Workups and Management MRI foot showed osteomyelitis at the left second and third metatarsal bones. The patient underwent large debridement down to the tendon and bone as well as left third partial ray amputation. Wound culture and surgical cultures both grew Strep dysgalactiae, Finegoldia magna, and mixed skin flora. Surgical pathology was consistent with acute on chronic osteomyelitis with soft tissue necrosis and abscess. Blood cultures were negative. MRSA nasal screen was positive but wound or blood cultures were negative for MRSA.

Treatments Because of polymicrobial infection, the patient was discharged on IV ceftriaxone 2 g once daily and PO Flagyl 500 mg tid for 4–6 weeks.

Osteomyelitis with no Tissue Growth

Clinical Vignette A 58-year-old female with diabetes mellitus, diabetic polyneuropathy, and diabetic foot ulcerations presented with right second toe swelling, redness, and pain with purulent drainage from the ulcer at the tip.

Workups and Management X-ray of the right foot 3 views showed possible osteomyelitis of the second distal phalanx with evidence of cellulitis. MRI of the right foot with and without contrast showed distal second-toe osteomyelitis and cellulitis with no abscess. The patient underwent a right second-toe amputation. Surgical tissue cultures had no growth. Of note, this patient did have a history of left foot diabetic foot ulceration with underlying osteomyelitis of the proximal phalanx and adjacent first metatarsal head with group G Streptococcus bacteremia status post great toe partial amputation and successful antibiotic treatment in the past.

Treatments The patient was initially empirically treated with IV daptomycin and Zosyn. The antibiotic regimen was changed to oral Augmentin plus oral doxycycline for another 2–3 weeks upon discharge.

Diabetic Foot Ulcer, Cellulitis, and Osteomyelitis of the Left Leg

Clinical Vignette A 56-year-old male with diabetes presented with a left great toe wound infection concerning osteomyelitis.

Workups and Management He received a left great toe incision and drainage followed by hallux amputation by the podiatrist. Blood culture and tissue culture were negative.

Treatments The patient was initially treated with IV vancomycin and Zosyn. Upon discharge, the antibiotic regimen was switched to p.o. Levaquin and p.o. Keflex 500 mg 4 times daily for at least 2–3 weeks, possibly 4–6 weeks depending on follow-ups.

Toe Osteomyelitis, Cellulitis, and Diabetic Foot Ulcer of the Right Foot

Clinical Vignette A 64-year-old male with type 2 diabetes presented with a chronic second right toe diabetic ulcer with a fat layer exposed as well as right leg redness, swelling, and pain.

Workups and Management The podiatrist performed an amputation of the second right toe. Blood culture and tissue culture were negative.

Treatments The patient was initially treated with daptomycin and Zosyn IV. Non-weight bearing for the right forefoot was recommended. Upon discharge, the antibiotic regimen was changed to oral Augmentin and oral doxycycline for another 2–3 weeks.

Fournier's Gangrene of the Scrotum

Clinical Vignette A 60-year-old male with a body mass index (BMI) of 45 and type 2 diabetes mellitus presented with severe pain and swelling in the perineum and scrotal area.

Workups and Management CT of the pelvis with IV contrast revealed scrotal skin thickening, edema, and a large amount of subcutaneous gas highly suspicious for necrotizing fasciitis. The general surgery team was consulted and performed left scrotal area debridement with Foley catheter placement by the urologist. Surgical tissue culture grew many gram-positive cocci, many gram-negative rods, and many gram-positive rods.

Treatments The patient was empirically on IV Zosyn, vancomycin, and clindamycin originally.

IV Zosyn, clindamycin, and vancomycin for were continued until the cultures were finalized. The patient was later discharged on IV antibiotics for another 2 weeks.

Guidelines for Necrotizing Soft Tissue Infections

Alternative names for necrotizing soft tissue infections include necrotizing cellulitis, streptococcal gangrene, gas gangrene (clostridial myonecrosis), necrotizing fasciitis, or myonecrosis.

Diagnosis requires pain out of proportion to clinical signs, crepitus, hypotension, skin necrosis, and hemorrhagic bullae in addition to cellulitis signs and symptoms. Patients may or may not have radiologic evidence of gas in tissue. A timely surgical consult for extensive debridement or multiple amputations is necessary to ensure survival and decrease the risk of prolonged hospitalization.

Treatments surgical debridement and IV vancomycin + Zosyn or meropenem + clindamycin.

Polymicrobial necrotizing infections: vancomycin or linezolid plus one of the following therapies: piperacillin–tazobactam, a carbapenem, or ceftriaxone–metronidazole.

Streptococcus pyogenes infection or traumatic or spontaneous gas gangrene: penicillin together with clindamycin for 10–14 days.

Aeromonas hydrophila (freshwater) infection treatments: doxycycline plus either ciprofloxacin or ceftriaxone.

Vibrio vulnificus (salt water) infection treatments: doxycycline plus either ceftriaxone or cefotaxime.

Skin and Soft Tissue Infection (SSTI) General Information

(1) Group A Streptococcus has a 30%–40% mortality rate, and 50% of patients develop toxic shock.

Treatments Penicillin G + clindamycin combination is superior to either agent alone. Add clindamycin 900 mg iv q8h for antitoxin or toxin suppression (for 48–72 h up to 7 days) even if the isolate is resistant; may use linezolid 600 mg iv q12h for penicillin-allergic patients for toxin suppression. Additionally, may add IVIG days 1–3.

(2) Staphylococcus aureus: No data regarding the benefits of clindamycin or IVIG use in Staphylococcus aureus infection is available.

(3) Clostridial SSTI: Clostridium perfringens is the most common; Clostridium sordellii is commonly seen with black tar heroin use and OB/GYN procedures.

Treatments Penicillin G + clindamycin (never use clindamycin alone); may add metronidazole—variable activity; IVIG use is not supported in the literature and not recommended.

(4) Necrotizing SSTI: Type I: Polymicrobial with predisposing conditions are common (most common type), Fournier's Gangrene (males > females by 6 times). Type II: Monomicrobial occurs with or without predisposing conditions, toxin mediated. Type III: Waterborne (i.e., Vibrio vulnificus, Aeromonas hydrophila). Type IV: Fungal.

SSTI Differential Diagnoses

Vaccine reactions, deep vein thrombosis, superficial thrombophlebitis, contact dermatitis, acute tophaceous gout, calciphylaxis (slow lesion, exquisitely tender), chronic venous stasis, drug reaction (DRESS), fixed drug reaction, pseudocellulitis, lipodermatosclerosis, dependent rubor, malignancy-associated (squamous cell, carcinoid, Sweet syndrome), pyoderma gangrenosum (in the setting of inflammatory disease—biopsy at the lesion edge reveals neutrophilic infiltrate). Lipodermatosclerosis refers to chronic venous stasis, fibrosing panniculitis (acute and chronic forms) inverted Champagne bottle, often stopping at the ankle.

Procalcitonin is not reliable for skin, bloodstream, or CNS infections. Elevated **procalcitonin** can also be seen in **noninfectious conditions** like surgery, trauma, cardiogenic shock, multiorgan dysfunction, pancreatitis (severe), severe systemic inflammatory response syndrome (SIRS), and prolonged resuscitation. These conditions most often do not require antibiotics if there are no clinical signs or symptoms of infection.

5 Other Skin and Musculoskeletal Infections

Recurrent Cellulitis in an Obese Patient

Clinical Vignette A 68-year-old female with recurrent cellulitis on cephalexin 1 g oral three times daily for suppression, obesity with BMI 46.55, and lymphedema was found to have recurrent cellulitis.

Assessment and Management obesity dosing of cefazolin (3 g q8h iv) and toxin mediation with linezolid or clindamycin. Additionally, a CT scan was ordered and ruled out necrotizing infection. Upon discharge, antibiotic regimen was changed to oral cephalexin 1 g four times a day and clindamycin for another 48 h for toxin mediation.

MRSA Abscess of the Hand

Clinical Vignette Intravenous drug abuser (IVDA) with MRSA abscess of the hand concerning tenosynovitis.

Assessment and Management The hand surgeon was consulted and the patient underwent incision and drainage. The patient was treated with IV vancomycin initially. Given the concerns of IVDA, the patient was discharged on IV oritavancin 1.2 g every week (via a peripheral IV) for 2 weeks for better coverage. Additionally, MRSA decolonization was also recommended using Bactroban cream 2% to nares b.i.d. for 7 days, repeat each month, and use Hibiclens soap in the shower 2 times per week (not on the face).

Methicillin Susceptible Staphylococcus aureus (MSSA) Abscess and Bacteremia

Clinical Vignette A 58-year-old male presented with worsening back pain.

Workups MRI spine with IV contrast revealed multiple deep abscesses over the right psoas muscle, paraspinal muscles (T11 through S1), and epidural space (L2–L5) likely from MSSA (no aspiration or drainage done). The patient also was found to have obstructive left-side hydronephrosis for which he received a nephrostomy tube and ureteral stent. His blood culture was positive for MSSA and his urine culture grew E. coli. Additionally, he was found to have bilateral pneumonia.

Management The patient completed 7 days of Gram-negative coverage for UTI with Rocephin despite denying any current UTI symptoms. With the culture results, he was started on nafcillin 2 g IV every 4 h for MSSA bacteremia. He was discharged on nafcillin 2 g IV every 4 h vs nafcillin 12 g continuous IV every 24 h × 8 weeks. Potential side effects of nafcillin include renal dysfunction, liver enzyme elevations, Clostridium difficile diarrhea, and severe neutropenia. Weekly CBC, CMP, ESR, and CRP are recommended for close monitoring while on IV antibiotics. Repeat imaging is necessary if worsening symptoms or inflammatory markers.

Septic Prepatellar Bursa Right Knee

Clinical Vignette A 75-year-old male presented with left kneecap swelling, redness, and pain. **Workup and management:** He underwent incision and drainage with surgical fluid culture and grew Staph aureus, sensitivity pending. Orthopedic surgery was consulted for postoperative care and does not believe that there are any signs of adjacent total knee joint infection.

Treatments The patient has multiple allergies to penicillin and cephalosporins with a documented history of allergies and rashes; would recommend the use of an alternative agent daptomycin 6 mg/kg daily adjusted weight for dosing for 14 days for adequate therapy. This will cover all strains of Staph.

Pyogenic Arthritis of the Knee

Clinical Vignette A 69-year-old female with a gout history and uncontrolled diabetes presented for worsening left knee pain for a month. She was found to have redness, swelling, and tenderness in the left knee.

Workup and Management The orthopedic surgeon performed a joint washout with Gram stain positive for Gram-positive cocci but aspiration fluid culture negative and crystal positive for monosodium urate. Her MRSA nares were negative.

Treatments She was treated with iv vancomycin inside the hospital. Upon discharge, the antibiotic regimen was changed to empiric IV ceftriaxone for 2–4 weeks.

Right Hand Mid Palmar and Thenar Area Abscess with Right Middle Finger Flexor Tenosynovitis

Clinical Vignette A 78-year-old male presented with right-hand pain, swelling, and redness. He was found to have infectious tenosynovitis.

Workup and Management A hand surgeon was consulted and performed incision and drainage of the right-hand mid-palm area and thenar area abscess with debridement of the flexor tendon of the middle finger and right carpal tunnel release surgery. Surgical tissue/abscess culture grew Streptococcus anginosus while blood culture was negative.

Treatments The patient was originally treated with IV clindamycin and IV Zosyn. Upon discharge, the antibiotic regimen was changed to IV ceftriaxone and p.o. clindamycin for 4 weeks.

Right Foot Osteomyelitis with Surgical Tissue Culture Positive for Streptococcus agalactiae

Clinical Vignette A 56-year-old male with diabetes presented with a worsening chronic non-healing wound of the left-right foot.

Workup and Management He underwent transmetatarsal amputation with tissue culture and grew Streptococcus agalactiae.

Treatments The patient was discharged on penicillin continuous infusion of 24 million units over 24 h for 4–6 weeks, and metronidazole 500 mg oral TID for 10 days. Weekly labs including CBC with differential, ESR, CRP, BMET, and LFTs were recommended; wound vac per surgery and wound care services.

Rhizomucor Infection and Abscess of the Third Digit of the Right Hand

Clinical Vignette A 73-year-old male developed an abscess to the third digit of his right hand after "digging in the dirt".

Workups and Management He underwent incision and drainage with wound culture which grew Rhizomucor species together with many Gram-positive cocci, a few Gram-negative bacilli, and few Gram-positive bacilli. The orthopedic surgery team was consulted and performed repeat debridement 4 days later after the results.

Assessment Rhizomucor infections are very serious and angioinvasive. The infectious disease consultant recommended immediate debridement of the infected tissue, down to clean bleeding wound edges.

Treatments AmBisome was used for the treatment of Rhizomucor, and Keflex was used for the presumed bacterial superinfection. The patient's renal function got worse with AmBisome and thus normal saline bolus 500 cc before each AmBisome dose. The infectious disease consultant later further recommended repeat debridement and nail removal vs distal amputation. After improvement of symptoms, the patient was started on delayed-release posaconazole 300 mg p.o. b.i.d. × 2 doses, followed by 300 mg p.o. daily.

MSSA Bacteremia + Acute Encephalopathy + Right Hip Prosthetic Joint Infection with Surrounding Abscess

Clinical Vignette An 80-year-old male status post recent right hip hemiarthroplasty half a month ago presented with altered mental status.

Workups Blood culture was positive for MSSA. CT left hip revealed a loculated collection at the right lateral and posterior pelvic soft tissue size of 13.6 cm also there is a fluid collection at the lateral thigh soft tissue at the level of the right proximal femur measuring 6.5 × 5.5 cm. Fluid aspiration grew MSSA as well.

Management The patient was treated with IV nafcillin and the orthopedic surgery team was consulted for explantation of the prosthetic joint and transesophageal echocardiogram was recommended to rule out endocarditis.

Streptococcal Bacteremia with Left Wrist Streptococcal Arthritis

Clinical Vignette A 37-year-old male status post-operative debridement and synovectomy of the wrist. The patient had prior fusion with hardware in place, which is now removed. Purulence was found in the joint tendons consistent with likely hematogenous seeded infection.

Treatments Rocephin IV 2 g daily for 6 weeks.

Cellulitis of the Left Lower Extremity + Infected Venous Stasis Ulceration of the Left Leg on the Lateral Aspect

Treatments The patient was started on IV clindamycin, IV cefazolin, and IV Levaquin while inpatient. Upon discharge, the antibiotic regimen was changed to p.o. cephalexin 500 mg 3 times daily plus p.o. Levaquin 50 mg every 48 h to complete a total of 2 weeks of antibiotics.

6 Endocarditis

Enterococcus Endocarditis

Clinical Vignette A 76-year-old male was found to have sepsis from Enterococcus bacteremia after a syncopal fall. Due to the presence of a prosthetic valve and implantable cardioverter-defibrillator (ICD), endocarditis is suspected. The patient was later discharged with IV ampicillin and IV ceftriaxone for 6 weeks.

Enterococcus Endocarditis, Discitis

Clinical Vignette The above 76-year-old male later presented with fever and confusion and was found to have a urinary tract infection and enterococcus bacteremia. The patient was originally discharged on Rocephin and ampicillin for home antibiotics for 6 weeks and this was changed to daptomycin alone for convenience of infusion at home. Later, he was also found to have C diff colitis and completed a 10-day treatment of oral vancomycin.

Assessments His enterococcus bacteremia is likely due to a complicated urinary tract infection.

Treatments Daptomycin was discontinued and switched back to IV ceftriaxone 2 g every 12 h plus IV ampicillin 2 g every 4 h for 6 weeks. The patient would need a repeat transesophageal echocardiogram after completion of the antibiotics. A cardiologist was consulted to determine the appropriate time for the valve replacement. If the patient's symptoms are manageable with medical treatment, then perhaps the valve replacement could be delayed until after completion of the IV antibiotics and resolution of the endocarditis. Continue p.o. vancomycin 125 every 12 h while on broad-spectrum antibiotic given a history of C. diff colitis.

Enterococcus faecalis Bacteremia with Possible Mitral Valve Endocarditis

Assessment and Treatments Since the patient has a transcatheter aortic valve replacement (TAVR) valve, and transesophageal echocardiogram (TEE) shows possible mitral valve vegetation, the patient was treated for endocarditis. Continue with the IV Unasyn at a dose of 3 g every 12 renally dosed, and IV ceftriaxone 1 g every 12 renally dosed for 6 weeks.

MSSA Bacteremia + Native Valve Endocarditis

Assessment and Treatments Transesophageal echocardiogram revealed a small vegetation or mass on the aortic valve. Also, a mass on the anterior mitral valve leaflet was suggestive of vegetation which measured about 2.4 cm and was mobile. There was also severe aortic stenosis. Cefazolin dose was adjusted to 2 g every 12 because of acute kidney injury. Nephrology was consulted and their concern is that the patient may have acute interstitial nephritis secondary to cefazolin and request to change the beta-lactam antibiotic to some other form of antibiotic. Due to the concern of possible cefazolin-related interstitial nephritis with renal failure, cefazolin was stopped and changed to daptomycin 8 mg/kg every 48 h for 6 weeks according to the patient's creatinine clearance (9 mL/min).

Enterococcus faecalis Bacteremia + Native Mitral Valve Endocarditis

Clinical Vignette A 78-year-old male presented with a sudden onset of aphasia.

Workups Initial CT was negative but MRI confirmed a punctate area of restricted diffusion consistent with left middle cerebral artery (MCA) embolic stroke. He has no significant weakness. Later, his blood culture grew Enterococcus faecalis (sensitive to ampicillin) for 3 consecutive days. Because of dysphagia, he underwent EGD with duodenal dilatation over the guidewire, and a day later, he had a transesophageal echocardiogram (TEE) showing small vegetation on the mitral valve.

Treatments The patient was started and discharged on IV ampicillin 2 g every 6 h and IV ceftriaxone 2 g every 12 for 6 weeks with repeat TEE towards the completion of the IV antibiotics.

Prosthetic Valve Endocarditis Due to Enterococcus

Clinical Vignette An 80-year-old male with aortic stenosis status post transcatheter aortic valve replacement (TAVR) presented for a large stroke of the left posterior cerebral artery (PCA) territory.

Workups Besides concerns for embolic stroke, the patient was also found to have high-grade enterococcal bacteremia for 3 consecutive days concerning high-grade bacteremia endovascular source. His EKG revealed normal sinus rhythm but a new first-degree AV block. This is considered bacterial prosthetic valve endocarditis until proven otherwise.

Assessment and Treatments IV ampicillin 2 g every 4 h plus IV gentamicin synergy dosed per pharmacy (watch for renal toxicity). This is the preferred regimen per the IDSA guidelines for suspected prosthetic valve endocarditis due to Enterococcus. TEE later revealed aortic valve vegetation. The finding of normal sinus rhythm and a new first-degree AV block could be concerning for early valve abscess. The cardiologist and cardiothoracic surgery teams were consulted for the need for urgent aortic valve replacement.

7 Complicated Urinary Tract Infections (UTIs)

Extended Spectrum Beta-Lactamase E. coli Bacteremia and Complicated UTI

Clinical Vignette A 57-year-old female presented with fever, tachycardia, and hypotension.

Workups and Assessment She was found to have a complicated UTI with ESBL E. coli and bacteremia of ESBL E. coli with obstructive uropathy due to nephrolithiasis. The urologist was consulted and the patient underwent a cystoscopy with right ureteral stent placement. The urologist recommended definitive stone surgery when the infection is appropriately cleared.

Treatments continue IV meropenem while inpatient and change to IV ertapenem for 14 days and start on oral fosfomycin prevention upon completion of ertapenem.

ESBL Bacteremia and UTI

Clinical Vignette A 78-year-old female presented with fever, chills, and weakness for 1 day.

Workups She was found to have ESBL E coli bacteremia from a urinary tract infection. Abdominal CT with contrast did not reveal any obvious obstructive process.

Treatments continue ertapenem 1 g daily for 10–14 days. Fosfomycin was only indicated for uncomplicated cystitis as treatment. Start probiotic 2 tablets daily.

Recurrent UTI with Concerns for Chronic Prostatitis

Clinical Vignette A 76-year-old male with recurrent UTI presented with systolic blood pressure as low as 60 s.

Workups He was found to have recurrent UTI due to Enterobacter cloacae with 3 previous admissions in the last 3 months (urine culture grew the same bacterium). He has benign prostate hyperplasia (BPH) with urine retention requiring a Foley catheter after recent admission. Foley is now removed; he does appear to be on medications for BPH but has some overflow incontinence.

Assessment and Treatments History is concerning for the possibility of chronic prostatitis as this male patient has recurrent UTI from infection of the same microorganism. He was prescribed Levaquin 500 mg daily for the next 4–6 weeks.

Right Hydronephrosis, Hydroureter, and Nephrolithiasis

Clinical Vignette A 56-year-old male presented with fever, chills, and back pain 2 days after cystourethroscopy with lithotripsy, stent placement, and right nephrostomy tube removal.

Workups His urine culture grew Pseudomonas aeruginosa and Candida. His blood culture has been negative.

Treatments He was diagnosed with acute pyelonephritis of the right side and has been treated with cefepime and Diflucan. The susceptibility of Pseudomonas aeruginosa to Ciprofloxacin is intermediate. The patient was eventually discharged on cefepime 2 g every 12 for 10 days plus and Diflucan 200 mg daily for 7 days.

Enterobacter Cloacae Complex Bacteremia + Acute Pyelonephritis Associated with Bilateral Hydronephrosis/Left Ureteral Stent

Clinical Vignette A 76-year-old male with metastatic prostatic cancer, left-sided hydronephrosis status post cystoscopy with stent placement on the left side presented with fever and chills.

Workups Blood and urine culture grew Enterobacter cloacae complex (sensitive to fluoroquinolones and ceftriaxone). CT of the abdomen and pelvis with no contrast showed interval placement of the left-sided ureteral stent, and calculi in both collecting systems which increased in size. The urologist was consulted and placed bilateral nephrostomy tubes and removed the stent from the left ureter.

Treatments continue IV cefepime for 14 days and start fosfomycin 3 g weekly after the completion of cefepime because the patient still has the ureteral calculi which can harbor the bacteria (chronic suppressive antibiotic therapy).

Recurrent Complicated UTI Due to Providencia rettgeri in the Setting of Bilateral Hydronephrosis Left Staghorn Calculi, and Urostomy

Clinical Vignette A 77-year-old male with ileal conduit urostomy presented with confusion and hallucination.

Workups He was found to have bilateral hydronephrosis, left staghorn calculi, and urinary tract infection. Urologist is planning nephrostomy tube placement after Plavix washout and definitive stone treatment at a higher level of care facility. The chart review did not reveal any history of frequent UTIs.

Assessment and Treatments He was empirically started on IV ceftriaxone for 4 days. The antibiotic regimen was then changed to Levaquin 750 mg q48h (renal dose) to complete 12 more days of treatment. Antibiotic prophylaxis likely is necessary given the increased risk for recurrent UTIs after nephrostomy tube placement but he would be at high risk to develop antimicrobial resistance. Certainly, a definitive stone treatment will reduce his risk for recurrent UTIs.

MSSA Bacteremia and Bacteriuria

Assessment Sepsis with acute renal failure and tubular necrosis without septic shock due to MSSA bacteremia. Sepsis was resolved. MSSA rarely causes UTIs. Additional workup is necessary. Transesophageal echocardiogram revealed vegetation. CT scan chest, abdomen, and pelvis revealed only atypical pneumonia. MRI cervical, thoracic, and lumbar spine did not reveal any discitis or osteomyelitis.

Treatments continue IV Cefazolin 2 g q8h for 4–6 weeks for endocarditis.

MSSA Bacteremia and Bacteriuria

Clinical Vignette A 78-year-old male with history of MSSA bacteremia and bacteriuria (negative TEE at that time) status post 14 IV antibiotic treatment presented with fever and chills weeks later.

Workups He was found to have right-sided pyelonephritis with culture 1 of 2 positive for MSSA (repeat blood culture was negative). He was also found to have bilateral hydronephrosis, secondary to obstructing nephrolithiasis for which he underwent cystoscopy, left ureteroscopy, and placement of bilateral ureteral double-J stents.

Assessments infectious disease consultant suspected that the patient had MSSA colonization of his kidney stones causing his recurrent infection. As such, a definitive management of his kidney stones was highly recommended. Given the patient only had 1 of 2 positive blood cultures for MSSA and no obvious endocarditis sequela, TEE was not recommended. Per the report, MSSA in culture was pansensitive and thus Bactrim and Levaquin could be used given their good urinary and deeper tissue penetration.

Treatments Ancef was discontinued, and the patient was discharged on Bactrim 2 double-strength tablets p.o. b.i.d. for 6 weeks. CBC, BMP, ESR, and CRP weekly were ordered for close monitoring while on antibiotics.

UTI Prophylaxis

Clinical Vignette A 68-year-old female has a history of recurrent UTI on Vantin prophylaxis complicated by multiple allergies and a history of drug-resistant infections. She did have a breakthrough infection in June with E. coli AmpC positive again. She otherwise has been doing well since starting on Vantin in March.

Treatments continue Vantin 200 mg daily the first week of each month for UTI prophylaxis. However, if she continues to have breakthrough infections, we will need a change in her antibiotic prophylactic regimen. Meanwhile, continue probiotics, vitamin C, estrogen cream, and frequent voiding for UTI prevention.

General UTI prevention measures
Drink 6–8 glasses of water a day unless contraindicated such as on hemodialysis or congestive heart failure; avoid beverages with caffeine which can cause bladder irritation; avoid constipation and wipe from front to back at all times; consider the addition of vitamin C 2000 mg po daily and/or methenamine Hippurate 1 g po bid to acidify the urine making it less hospitable to bacteria; consider the addition of fosfomycin 3 g po weekly if drug-resistant urine cultures. Additionally, may recommend renal ultrasound and urologist consultation as appropriate.

8 Pulmonary Infections

Mycobacterium Avium in Sputum

Clinical Vignette A female who was born in the 1950s presented with worsening dyspnea and increased sputum back in the 2000s. Her sputum culture grew Mycobacterium avium complex (MAC) at that time. She was evaluated by an outpatient infectious disease doctor and was advised against treatment unless significant symptoms or progressive destruction of lung parenchyma or diminution in pulmonary function tests. The patient later did have some cavitary lung lesions per CT scan after complaining of poor energy, cough with sputum and decreased exercise tolerance. A sputum acid fast bacilli (AFB) smear and culture for 3 consecutive days was recommended. If sputum culture is negative, bronchoscopy with bronchoalveolar lavage should be considered.

Treatment for pulmonary MAC infection requires **a minimum of 13 months of treatment with the goal of therapy for 12 months of consecutive negative sputum cultures**. Sputum testing starts after treatment for 1 month. Susceptibility testing is necessary if the culture is positive for MAC. As such, she was started on **azithromycin** 250 mg daily, **rifampin** 600 mg daily, and **ethambutol** 15 mg/kg body weight daily for MAC cavitary lung disease. She initially had significant heartburn following this antimicrobial regimen; luckily, her heartburn responded well to pantoprazole. The cough resolved and the energy level improved and so did exercise tolerance after the initiation of treatment for MAC.

Of note, per the IDSA guidelines, patients with **the diagnosis of nontuberculous mycobacterial pulmonary disease should be treated** (conditional recommendation with very low certainty in estimates of effects). If treatments are necessary, the physician should have thorough discussion with the patient regarding the uncertainties in the benefits of antimicrobial therapy and the potential of reinfection especially in patients with nodular/bronchiectatic disease. The diagnosis of nontuberculous mycobacterial pulmonary disease requires both nodular or cavitary opacities on chest X ray or bronchiectasis with small nodules on CT scan AND positive culture results ($\geq$2 separate expectorated sputum or $\geq$1 bronchial wash/lavage or pathology demonstrating mycobacterial histologic features and positive culture).

Mycobacterium Avium Intracellulare (MAI) Infection

Clinical Vignette An 80-year-old male with lung adenocarcinoma and an incidental finding of Mycobacterium avium complex (MAC) in sputum who presented for fever and weakness.

Workups Nine months before this presentation, the patient was found to have a small cavitary lesion in the right lower lung on CT scan. He underwent bronchoscopy thereafter with bronchoalveolar lavage acid-fast stain positive for acid-fast bacilli (AFB) and the AFB was identified as Mycobacterium avium intracellulare (MAI). While inpatient, the blood culture was negative.

Treatments The patient was empirically started on IV vancomycin and cefepime. Upon discharge, IV vancomycin and cefepime were stopped and changed to Augmentin 875 mg twice daily for another 10 days. For MAI treatment, the patient was discharged on azithromycin 500 mg on M-W-F, rifampin 600 mg T-T-S, ethambutol 2000 mg on M-W-F. Requests were made to the microbiology lab to keep the blood and sputum cultures for 10 days and perform sensitivity test if culture grows MAI.

Of note, Mycobacterium avium, Mycobacterium avium intracellulare, and Mycobacterium paraintracellulare are grouped together as the Mycobacterium avium complex.

Streptococcus Bacteremia and Associated with Community-Acquired Pneumonia Secondary to Streptococcus pneumonia

Treatments The patient was empirically started on IV vancomycin and ceftriaxone. The blood culture susceptibility showed that Streptococcus was sensitive to penicillin and ceftriaxone. Transthoracic echocardiogram negative for vegetation. As such vancomycin was stopped and the patient was discharged on IV ceftriaxone for 2 weeks.

Aspergillus Pneumonia (on Methotrexate and High-Dose Steroids)

Clinical Vignette A 69-year-old male with rheumatoid arthritis on methotrexate presented for fever, cough, and dyspnea.

Workups He was found to have influenza A and bacterial pneumonia for which he was started on IV methylprednisolone and IV antibiotics. The patient continued to have an active cough with hemoptysis, and worsening respiratory status; extensive workup was initiated and isolation of Aspergillus fumigatus in a single sputum culture was noticed. CT chest revealed an enlarging lung lesion which later became cavitary.

Assessment Isolation of Aspergillus fumigatus in a single sputum does not necessarily imply invasive Aspergillus pulmonary infection, but given the clinical context of worsening chest X-ray, active hemoptysis, and worsening respiratory status together with a cavitary lung lesion, it does certainly suggest this may be now playing a role. The prognosis here is guarded given his worsening respiratory status on high flow and comorbidities.

Treatments IV voriconazole loading dose 6 mg/kg twice daily for two doses by regular doses 4 mg/kg twice daily were initiated and then IV voriconazole was changed to oral therapy in 3–5 days as the patient was improving and the medication was thought to be absorbed well. Dual therapy of voriconazole with IV micafungin 150 mg per day may provide better outcomes but with limited evidence. Other options, such as IV AmBisome, would be high risk for treatment complications and side effects, and would like to avoid this agent if possible.

Loculated Pleural Effusion

Clinical Vignette A 69-year-old male presented with cough, sputum, and dyspnea.

Workups He was found to have a large pulmonary embolism and underwent thrombolysis. Follow-up chest CT revealed loculated pleural effusion. The patient underwent thoracentesis with fluid analysis borderline consistent with empyema but no subsequent pleural fluid analysis for Gram stain and culture. Pigtail chest tube was placed for loculated pleural effusion.

Assessment and Plan He did not have subsequent pleural fluid analysis. Although a partially treated infectious empyema is a concern, the patient's clinical course did not appear to be necessarily consistent with that. Pleural effusions are also common after large pulmonary infarcts and his lung has been expanding after thrombolytic therapy and thoracentesis. The patient is now status post pigtail tube placement for drainage which requires close monitoring via serial X-rays. If the concern for infectious empyema rises, certainly we will have to repeat pleural fluid analysis with Gram stain and culture. Luckily, the patient has remained afebrile and his white count is normal, and thus the antibiotic regimen could be transitioned to Augmentin 875 mg twice daily for another 2 weeks with close follow-ups.

Empyema

Clinical Vignette A 55-year-old male presented with progressively worsening shortness of breath, productive cough with greenish phlegm, and hypoxia with oxygen saturation of 65% while on room air. At admission, the patient's vitals included: temperature 97.3 °F, blood pressure 116/81 mmHg, pulse 118, and respiration 24.

Workups and Management Labs revealed WBC count 13.1. Blood cultures later grew Staphylococcus epidermidis in 1 out of 2 sets. CT chest with IV contrast showed a new large multiloculated left pleural effusion with air present in the left pleural space, extensive consolidation and compressive atelectasis of the left lung. The patient thus underwent left thoracoscopy with partial pulmonary decortication, incision, and drainage. Surgical left-sided pleural fluid culture showed moderate growth of Streptococcus intermedius while surgical left-sided pleural fluid anaerobic culture showed no growth.

Antibiotic Treatments The patient was empirically treated with IV ceftriaxone and metronidazole. He was later discharged on IV ceftriaxone and oral metronidazole for 4 weeks.

Right-Sided Necrotizing Pneumonia

Clinical Vignette A 43-year-old female with alcohol abuse history presented with worsening cough and dyspnea. She was found to have right lower lobe necrotizing pneumonia on CT scan.

Assessment and Plan with the patient's severe alcohol abuse disorder, the origin of this pneumonia is very likely aspiration. With clinical improvement, she was transitioned to IV ceftriaxone and po Flagyl. She was later discharged on 4 weeks of IV ceftriaxone plus 2 weeks of oral Flagyl 500 mg tid.

Bilateral Interstitial Infiltrate Possible Pneumonia + Idiopathic Thrombocytopenic Purpura + Hepatitis B Core Antibody Positive

Clinical Vignette A 71-year-old female was told to come to the hospital because of thrombocytopenia with a platelet count of 8 and a CPK level of 8158. At admission, the patient's vitals included: temperature recorded 98.2 °F, blood pressure 123/68 mmHg, respiratory rate 18, and heart rate 90.

Workups Labs revealed WBC count 10.9. LDH was elevated at 947, and haptoglobin was 77. Serum ferritin was 1489, reticulocyte count was 5.8%. CT chest abdomen and pelvis with IV contrast showed bilateral interstitial infiltrates consistent with edema versus pneumonia as well as a very large adnexal cyst in the pelvis, but no free fluid. Blood culture was negative. The peripheral smear showed no schistocytes. Because of the suspicion for immune thrombocytopenic purpura (ITP), she was started on IV dexamethasone 40 mg daily for 4 days followed by IVIG 1 g/kg for 2 days and Rituxan. Incidentally, the patient was found to have HBsAg −ve, HBcAb total reactive, while HBcAb IgM non reactive. Fungitell study result was noticeably >500.

Assessment and Plan The patient was initially empirically treated with Levaquin and metronidazole for pneumonia. While on Rituxan, entecavir 0.5 mg daily was added. Hepatitis B quantitative PCR by NAAT, Hepatitis B surface antibody, Hepatitis Be antigen and antibody, Hepatitis C serology, and HIV serology were all ordered. In the presence of elevated Fungitell study and bilateral interstitial infiltrates in a person who is immunocompromised, a sputum PJP by PCR was also ordered. Given low platelet, the differential diagnosis of hemophagocytic lymphohistiocytosis (HLH) may be considered which can be associated with EBV and Histoplasma infections. Aspergillus antigen, Blastococcus antigen, Histoplasma antigen, EBV by PCR in the blood, and as well as EBV serology were ordered. Lyme serology and tickborne disease PCR panel were negative. Empirically the patient was continued on Levaquin and metronidazole for possible pneumonia; doxycycline was then added.

Followup Visit Days Later thrombocytopenia etiology remains unclear and did not respond to prednisone, IVIG, N plate, or rituximab. Her platelet continues to be <10 k. The patient was later transferred to a higher level of care.

Right Middle Lobe Lung Abscess

Clinical Vignette A 46-year-old male with Down syndrome presented for cough and dyspnea for a week.

Workups The patient was found to have right middle lobe pneumonia and abscess (large 5 cm rounded air-fluid collection on CT scan). Extensive lab workup was negative but sputum culture showed profuse growth of Candida albicans and serum Fungitell study was indeterminate.

Treatments The patient was treated with IV meropenem in the hospital and later discharged on IV ertapenem 1 g daily and p.o. Diflucan 200 mg daily for 4 weeks. Repeat chest CT was recommended in 2–3 weeks.

Extensive Ground Glass Changes in CT Scan

Clinical Vignette A 76-year-old male with pulmonary fibrosis on methotrexate and tapering dose prednisone for rheumatoid arthritis presented with fever, cough, and worsening dyspnea for a week.

Workups and Initial Treatments CT chest showed extensive ground glass changes. He was diagnosed with bilateral community-acquired pneumonia complicated by immune suppression from taking methotrexate and prednisone. The patient was started on cefepime and azithromycin; later on, prednisone and IV furosemide together with Bactrim were added with improvement in symptoms.

Assessment and Plan The patient presented with high fever and hypoxemia, clinically improving on stress doses of steroids with broad-spectrum antibiotics over the past week since admission. Differential includes common respiratory pathogens Pneumococcus, Haemophilus, and Moraxella, opportunistic pathogens such as pneumocystis, fungal pathogens, Nocardia, and atypical pathogens such as Legionella, mycoplasma, or chlamydia. Animal-associated infections such as Q fever is possible but less likely despite farming history with contact with animals (most commonly infected sheep, goats and cattle in Q fever). The timing of the infection occurring during the latter part of steroid taper is very consistent with Pneumocystis jirovecii pneumonia (PJP) infection. Fungitell assay is also a good screening test for this fungal infection. Sputum for pneumocystis PCR, sputum for fungal stain and culture, and sputum for Nocardia culture were thus all ordered.

Treatments Bactrim double strength 2 tablets 3 times a day for 21 days, continue prednisone slow taper for 21 days pneumocystis protocol. Upon discharge, IV cefepime was switched to Levaquin 500 mg daily for 10 days for empiric antimicrobial and atypical coverage. Hold methotrexate while on antibiotics.

Cavitary Lung Lesion Labs aspergillus galactomannan ag, serum cryptococcal ag, QuantiFERON gold, urine Histoplasma ag, urine Blastomyces ag, Pneumocystis jiroveci pneumonia (PJP), legionella and streptococcus ag, acid-fast stain, and beta-d-glucan.

9 Bacteremia and Back Pain

Streptococcus dysgalactiae Bacteremia

Clinical Vignette A 63-year-old female presented for shaking chills, rigors, and generalized weakness.

Workups Blood culture positive for Streptococcus dysgalactiae in 1/4 bottles, contaminant versus real infection remains to be determined.

Assessment Given the high fever and history of shaking chills and rigors, infection was thought to be more likely. The source of infection was not clear, and thus further workup was needed with a transesophageal echocardiogram to rule out endocarditis which was negative. Meanwhile, CT scan of the chest, abdomen, and pelvis with IV contrast was also performed to look for other sources of infection which were unremarkable. Group C Streptococcus (Streptococcus dysgalactiae) can be part of oral flora; thus Panorex X-ray was ordered and turned out to be non revealing.

Treatments IV Rocephin 2 g daily for 2–4 weeks.

MSSA Bacteremia with Low Back Pain

Clinical Vignette A 69-year-old male with a history of diabetic neuropathy and end-stage renal disease on hemodialysis presented with low-grade fever and chills for the past 3 weeks associated with worsening low back pain.

Assessment and Plan His blood culture returned positive for MSSA for 3 days consecutively; therefore the patient was diagnosed with high-grade Staph aureus bacteremia which raises concerns for secondary sites of infection such as endocarditis and osteomyelitis. Ancef 1 g daily was started as the drug of choice with duration to be determined. The source of infection remained not obvious but could be fistula versus minor scrapes or abrasions from falling on his knees. Transesophageal echocardiogram (TEE) is the best screening method for endocarditis screening. If negative for endocarditis, a short course of 2-week IV antibiotic treatment could be considered for MSSA bacteremia. The patient's lumbar spine pain was somewhat chronic but had exacerbated over the previous 3 weeks upon presentation. Lumbar discitis and/or osteomyelitis were in the differential with MSSA bacteremia. CT lumbar scan findings were somewhat equivocal and would necessitate further imaging with MRI or a gallium scan if possible. If results are suggestive of infectious discitis, prolonged therapy with Ancef likely 6–8 weeks therapy is needed.

MSSA Bacteremia and Low Back Pain

Clinical Vignette An 80-year-old male presented with generalized weakness with a fall after syncope. The physical exam revealed superficial excoriation and abrasion on his left from an IV infiltration about a week ago, and a review of the system was positive for severe low back pain.

Assessment and Plan Blood culture was positive for MSSA. MSSA may be from his superficial excoriation in the left arm from IV infiltration 10 days ago. However, an MRI of the lumbar spine was ordered to rule out any possible osteomyelitis or discitis and a transesophageal echocardiogram was performed to rule out endocarditis. IV cefazolin 2 g tid for a total of 2 weeks to 6 weeks depending on further workup results.

L1–S1 Large Epidural Abscess + L4–L5 Discitis/ Osteomyelitis + Streptococcus Intermedius Bacteremia

Workups Blood cultures grew Streptococcus intermedius (penicillin MIC of ≤ 0.06, ceftriaxone MIC of ≤ 0.12). MRI of the cervical and thoracic spine with and without contrast showed a subtle leptomeningeal enhancement with multilevel degenerative changes. MRI of the lumbar spine with contrast revealed: peripherally enhancing lobulated epidural fluid collection along the dorsal aspect of the spinal canal; extensive clumping, thickening, and enhancement of the cauda equina nerve roots; and multiloculated abscess in the left paraspinal soft tissue at the level of L4–L5. X-ray Panorex showed periapical lucency surrounding the left maxillary first tooth and right maxillary first and second molar teeth; could not completely rule out an abscess. A transesophageal echocardiogram was also ordered with results pending.

Management neurosurgery was consulted stat and performed open L1–S1 laminectomies with bilateral foraminotomies with evacuation of the lumbar epidural abscess and hematoma. Surgical tissue/abscess culture also grew Streptococcus intermedius.

Antibiotic Treatments The patient was initially started on IV cefepime and IV vancomycin. This wasa switched to IV ceftriaxone 2 g daily with culture results. Due to the presence of poor dental hygiene and Panorex findings, the likely source of the bacteremia was from dental origin. The patient was discharged on IV ceftriaxone 2 g daily for at least 6–8 weeks. The patient agreed to follow up with an outpatient dentist as soon as he is discharged from the hospital.

Epidural Abscess

Workups MRI showed extensive epidural abscess extending from thoracic sixth through ninth vertebrae with cord compression resulting in significant neurologic deficits and weakness in both lower extremities. Neurosurgery was consulted stat and the neurosurgeon performed decompression laminectomy right away. Preliminary blood cultures were consistent with Staph aureus MSSA infection. The source of infection may have been secondarily infected hematoma with a history of falls. A transthoracic echocardiogram was performed which was negative for endocarditis. However, additional transesophageal echocardiogram may still be necessary if blood cultures do not sterilize in the next 72 h as well.

Management Per the IDSA, Nafcillin sodium or oxacillin 1.5–2 g IV q4–6 h or continuous infusion or Cefazolin 1–2 g IV q8 h or Ceftriaxone 2 g IV q24 h is the first choice for patients with.

native vertebral osteomyelitis and epidural abscess. In this patient, the antibiotic regimen was changed to nafcillin 12 g continuous drip. Side effects of nafcillin which include rash, diarrhea, C. difficile colitis, liver and kidney impairments were discussed in detail with the patient. Follow serial blood cultures and trend white count and CRP as well. May start probiotics. Defer to the neurosurgery team for regular assessments of her status and repeat MRI postoperatively as needed.

10 Fungemia

Hospital-Acquired Candidemia (Candida albicans)

Clinical Vignette An 85-year-old frail male presented with generalized weakness after a recent hospital stay for a urinary tract infection. While waiting for skilled nursing facility placement, the patient developed a fever. Thus, blood culture was ordered which eventually grew Candida albicans.

Assessment and Plan Hospital-acquired candidemia has a risk of azole resistance. The patient was started on micafungin 100 mg IV daily until final culture sensitivities were available. If no resistance, can switch to Diflucan 400 mg daily. Obtain baseline Fungitell assay, and check fungal MIC panel before switching to oral Diflucan. The duration of the treatment likely is 14 days. Follow serial cultures, trend white counts and CRP, and monitor liver enzymes while on antifungal treatments. An ophthalmology exam to rule out endophthalmitis is generally recommended for fungemia.

High-Grade Candida glabrata Bacteremia + Right-Sided Pyelonephritis Secondary to Candida glabrata + Hydronephrosis Due to Right Ureteral Calculi

Clinical Vignette An 80-year-old male presented with fever, chills, fatigue, generalized weakness, and myalgia for a few days.

Workups CT of the chest abdomen and pelvis with IV contrast showed obstructive 7 mm calculi in the right mid-ureter with moderate right-sided hydronephrosis, prostatomegaly, and cholelithiasis. Blood and urine culture grew Candida glabrata. Fungitell was >500. Urology service was consulted and the urologist performed a cystoscopy with a right-sided retrograde pyelogram with placement of the right ureteral stent and fulguration of the bleeding prostate.

Treatments The patient was initially started on IV cefepime and later was switched to IV micafungin. IV micafungin was continued for 14 days from the first day of negative blood culture.

MSSA Bacteremia and Fungemia (Candidemia albicans)

Clinical Vignette A 54-year-old female was initially admitted to the intensive care unit (ICU) for alcohol withdrawal and septic shock from a urinary tract infection (UTI). While in the ICU, a Foley catheter and midline PICC lines were placed but the patient pulled out all of them due to confusion and encephalopathy. She completed antibiotic treatment with Rocephin for UTI from E. coli. While on the general medicine floor, the patient continued to have persistent confusion and sinus tachycardia with a heart rate of 120–150 s. As such, blood culture was collected and later turned out to be positive for MSSA and Candida albicans but cleared quickly after starting the appropriate antibiotics.

Assessments The source of infection is unknown, but possibly related to a recent central line, Foley catheter, or soft tissue wound infection. Candida albicans was confirmed with good MIC to Diflucan. This is also likely the reason for transient fungemia and bacteremia in this patient. Physical exam did not suggest endocarditis and the patient had no cardiac murmur or other embolic lesions. Transesophageal echocardiogram however does suggest possible pulmonic valve infection. No prosthetic or cardiac devices were noted. Ancef is the preferred drug by the IDSA for the treatment of MSSA. Right-sided endocarditis is generally less complicated and appears to be responding and resolving well to antibiotics.

Treatments Continue 2 g every 8 for 2 weeks per the IDSA guidelines for transient MSSA infection, micafungin for 2 weeks total then likely should continue on oral fluconazole 600 mg a day for additional 4 weeks for concerns of fungal endocarditis. Repeat 2D echo in 4–6 weeks is also recommended. An ophthalmology exam to rule out endophthalmitis is generally necessary in patients with fungemia. Monitor liver enzymes while on antibiotic therapy.

Candidemia

Clinical Vignette A 68-year-old male with a history of left hydronephrosis from left ureteral stone status post cystoscopy with left ureteral stent placement presented with fever and chills 3 weeks later.

Workups CT of the abdomen and pelvis with IV contrast revealed the development of pyelonephritis on the left side with a small locule of gas in the left upper pole of the renal collecting system but no hydronephrosis. Blood culture collected on presentation later grew Candida tropicalis. The urologist was consulted and a stent was later removed.

Treatments continue micafungin iv for 14 days; if MIC is good to Diflucan, may change to oral Diflucan. An outpatient eye exam before or around antibiotic completion is recommended.

11 Other Infections

Pregnant Acalculous Cholecystitis

Clinical Vignette A 28 yo 11-week pregnant woman presented for nausea and right upper quadrant pain for 4–5 days; she was found to have acalculous cholecystitis.

Hospital course: Infectious disease and general surgery teams were both consulted. MRCP was completed without identifiable gallstones. The surgery team recommended outpatient follow-up and outpatient cholecystectomy likely during the second trimester or after childbirth pending her clinical course.

Treatments The patient was treated with Zosyn since presentation which was switched to Augmentin for another 14 days upon discharge.

Nocardiosis

Clinical Vignette A 63-year-old female with metastatic leiomyosarcoma on chemotherapy presented with left leg pain, fevers, and confusion.

Workups She was found to have a fluid collection (deep muscle infection) in the left medial thigh which was drained by an orthopedic surgeon. Cultures showed gram-positive branching rods, implying Nocardia infection. She did work out in the garden.

Treatments Given a history of sulfa allergy but she's shown no allergic reaction, the patient was agreeable to the Bactrim allergy desensitization plan. Three days of Bactrim desensitization went well. The patient was discharged on ertapenem 1 g iv daily for 2 weeks with follow-up with a plan to transition to oral Bactrim; may extend IV therapy longer if a multidrug resistant organism is identified.

Of note, **trimethoprim-sulfamethoxazole (TMP-SMX) IV** is the first line treatment during the acute phase while **meropenem/imipenem** is preferred over ertapenem as an alternative for the treatment of Nocardiosis. Induction **therapy with IV antibiotics for 3–6 weeks** is necessary for severe Nocardia infection until clinical improvement and then switch to oral to complete 3–6 months of antimicrobial therapy in immunocompetent patients with non-central nervous system (CNS) nocardiosis and a minimum of 12 months of antimicrobial therapy in immunocompromised patients or those with CNS disease.

Ring-Enhancing Brain Lesion, Vasogenic Edema

Clinical Vignette A 78-year-old male presented with confusion and agitation.

Workups CT and then MRI head revealed ring-enhancing lesions with vasogenic edema.

Assessments and Plan wide differentials and radiologist readings in combination with various lesions in multiple organs point toward malignancy; however, infection could not be ruled out initially. Blood culture together with cysticercosis and toxoplasmosis serum markers were ordered; additionally, CEA, CA19-9, and hCG and AFP markers were checked. The oncologist was consulted for the new MRI brain findings and recommended Decadron 4 mg iv qid and stat radiation oncology consult.

Rim-Enhancing Cystic Lesion from Neurocysticercosis

Clinical Vignette A 35-year-old male immigrant presented after falling off a ladder with witnessed seizure-like activities at the scene.

Workups MRI brain with and without contrast revealed two brain lesions: approximately 1.8 cm rim-enhancing cystic lesion in the right parietal lobe and an additional small 1.2 cm rounded extra-axial lesion at the vertex adjacent to the posterior right frontal lobe. Infectious disease consultant believes that the brain lesions are either infectious or malignant. Labs include *HIV, Cysticercosis (antibody is negative for this patient), Toxoplasma, Brucella, fungal—coccidioidomycosis, Cryptococcus, Blastomyces, Histoplasma, syphilis, parasite smear, Lyme and tick-borne* were ordered (All of these labs later returned negative). Additionally, a *Panorex X ray* was ordered to rule out hematogenous spread from dental decay. No empiric treatment was started given his clinical stability originally. The patient underwent a right parietal mass and brain biopsy the next day by the neurosurgeon who believed parasite infection was highly likely right after surgery. Pathology eventually revealed granulomatous inflammation with necrosis with parasite features consistent with cysticercosis.

Treatments Albendazole 600 mg oral BID for 10 days, and dexamethasone 6 mg oral daily for 10 days to reduce the risk of seizures with cysts potentially rupturing with antiparasitic treatment. The neurologist recommended levetiracetam 500 mg bid indefinitely.

Mastoiditis

Clinical Vignette A 43-year-old female was initially seen by an outpatient otolaryngologist for persistent left ear pain and bloody drainage from the left ear. She was started on oral levofloxacin and ofloxacin ear drops. She later presented to the hospital with persistent and worsening left ear pain and drainage. Upon presentation, the patient's temperature recorded was 98.6 °F, pulse was 82, blood pressure was 146/100 mmHg, and WBC count was 9.3. A physical exam revealed significant tenderness in the left mastoid area.

Workups A CT scan of the temporal bone with contrast revealed mastoiditis but no evidence of any subperiosteal abscess. The patient was admitted to the hospital and was evaluated by an otolaryngologist who performed myringotomy ventilation tube placement with lavage of the middle ear and tissue collection for culture. The surgical tissue culture later grew group A beta-hemolytic Streptococcus.

Treatments The patient was originally treated with IV ceftriaxone 2 g daily while inpatient. The infectious disease consultant recommended an increase of IV ceftriaxone to every 12 h for a total of 4 weeks. May reduce to 2 g daily after 2 weeks.

C. Diff Colitis

Clinical Vignette A 73-year-old male presented with uncontrolled diarrhea. He was found to have recurrent C. diff colitis and fidaxomicin was started. With minimal improvement, infectious disease service was consulted: cholestyramine 4 g daily for 3–4 days was added and a one-time IVIG was also prescribed. This patient tolerated IVIG and Questran well with improved bowel functions and subjective wellness feeling.

Assessment and Plan Continue fidaxomicin for 14 days and supportive care and nutrition supplements. Can consider adding alternative treatment with IVIG or Questran which may be helpful, but we do not have sufficient evidence for their use in C. diff colitis. Would discontinue probiotics as probiotics confer an increased risk for translocation in C. diff infection without clear benefits per the IDSA guidelines. Continue hand hygiene and isolation while understanding the risk of relapse remains despite every effort to minimize such a risk.

Gram Negative Bacteremia

Clinical Vignette A 46-year-old male with a port for recurrent hypomagnesemia presented with fever, chills, and abdominal distension and not feeling well.

Workups Blood cultures from both the peripheral and the port were collected and all grew gram-negative rods (later turned out to be Ochrobactrum anthropi).

Assessment and Plan The mediport is most likely infected and timely removed and a Port-A-Cath tip was sent for culture. Once the repeat blood culture was negative, a new port was placed on the opposite side. As for discharge, Rocephin 2 g IV daily was continued for 10 days after port removal and then changed to Bactrim DS 2 tablets twice a day for another 10 days based on sensitivity results. Obtain weekly CBC, CMP, ESR, and CRP while on IV antibiotics.

Sepsis with Pasteurella bacteremia

Assessment and Plan The source of infection is unclear but likely due to close contact with a pet cat at home. The patient does have a history of Pasteurella UTI in the past. It remains unclear if this is a central line-related infection but likely would be best to remove the PICC line in the setting of bacteremia and place a new midline in 2–3 days once cultures have been sterilized. There is a higher incidence of endocarditis with this organism so at least a transesophageal echo should be done to look for any signs of valvular heart disease or infection. Meanwhile, plan to continue Rocephin 2 g daily for at least 2 weeks.

Herpes Zoster's Ophthalmicus of the Right Eye

Clinical Vignette An 86-year-old male presented with a sudden onset of right periorbital area redness, pain, and blisters. The affected areas include the upper eyelid and extend to the left forehead and adjacent scalp. With treatments since the presentation, lesions began crusting well with resolving erythema around the crusting, and pain decreased rapidly.

Assessment and Plan IV Unasyn and IV acyclovir were started right away. Additionally, the patient was prescribed moxifloxacin-dexamethasone eye drop 0.5% 1 drop every 8 h. Upon discharge, the treatment was changed to oral acyclovir 800 mg 5 times daily and Augmentin 875 twice daily for 7 days. The patient was told to follow up with an ophthalmologist as an outpatient.

Further Readings and References

1. Bruun T, Rath E, Madsen MB, et al. 2021. Risk Factors and Predictors of Mortality in Streptococcal Necrotizing Softtissue Infections: A Multicenter Prospective Study. Clin Infect Dis. 72(2):293–300.
2. Stevens DL, Bryant AE, Goldstein EJ. 2021. Necrotizing Soft Tissue Infections. Infect Dis Clin North Am. 35(1):135–155.
3. Duane TM, Huston JM, Collom M, et al. 2021. Surgical Infection Society 2020 Updated Guidelines on the Management of Complicated Skin and Soft Tissue Infections. Surg Infect (Larchmt). 22(4):383–399.
4. Edwards G, Freeman K, Llewelyn MJ, Hayward G. 2020. What diagnostic strategies can help differentiate cellulitis from other causes of red legs in primary care? BMJ. 368:m54.
5. Garcia BM, Cruz-Diaz C, Agnihothri R, Shinkai K. 2021. Distinguishing Cellulitis from Its Noninfectious Mimics: Approach to the Red Leg. Infect Dis Clin North Am. 35(1):61–79.
6. Falagas ME, Vergidis PI. 2005. Narrative review: diseases that masquerade as infectious cellulitis. Ann Intern Med. 142(1):47–55.
7. Johnson TM, Byrd TF, Drummond WK, et al. 2023. Contemporary Pharmacotherapies for Nontuberculosis Mycobacterial Infections: A Narrative Review. Infect Dis Ther. 12(2):343–365.
8. Perl J, Harel Z, Nessim SJ. 2022. Peritoneal Fluid Analysis in Peritoneal Dialysis-Associated Peritonitis. JAMA. 328(21):2157–58.
9. Pappas PG, Kauffman CA, Andes DR, et al. 2016. Clinical Practice Guideline for the Management of Candidiasis: 2016 Update by the Infectious Diseases Society of America. Clin Infect Dis. 62(4):e1-50.

Index

K. Zhou, *Internal Medicine Training Notes and Survival Guide*,
https://doi.org/10.1007/978-1-0716-4039-5

B

D

F

G

I

J

K

L

MIX
Papier aus verantwortungsvollen Quellen
Paper from responsible sources
FSC® C105338

If you have any concerns about our products,
you can contact us on
ProductSafety@springernature.com

In case Publisher is established outside the EU,
the EU authorized representative is:
Springer Nature Customer Service Center GmbH
Europaplatz 3, 69115 Heidelberg, Germany

Printed by Libri Plureos GmbH
in Hamburg, Germany